BUILDING RESISTANCE

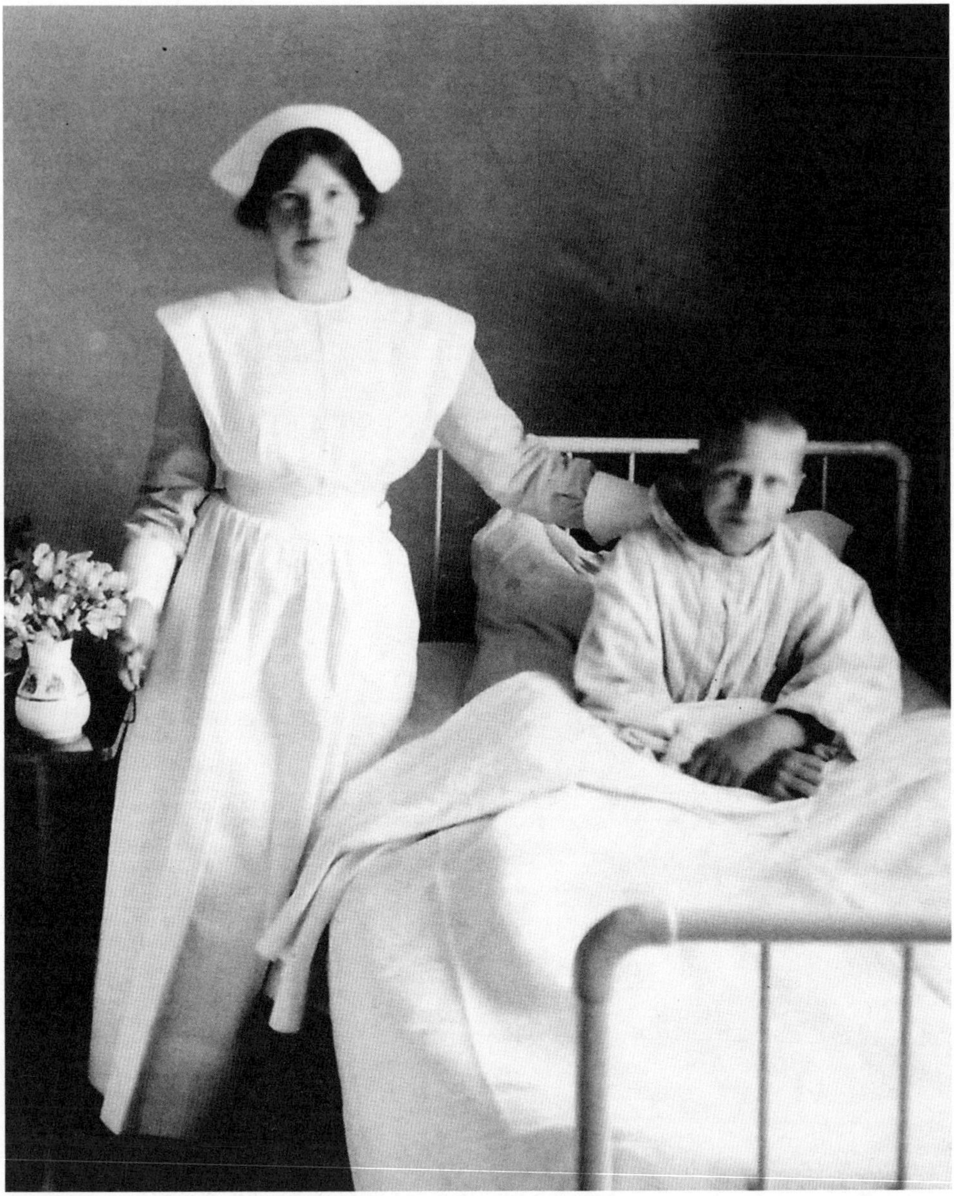

BUILDING RESISTANCE

Children, Tuberculosis, and the Toronto Sanatorium

Stacie Burke

McGill-Queen's University Press
Montreal & Kingston • London • Chicago

ISBN 978-0-7735-5330-9 (cloth)
ISBN 978-0-7735-5331-6 (paper)
ISBN 978-0-7735-5381-1 (ePDF)
ISBN 978-0-7735-5382-8 (ePUB)

Legal deposit second quarter 2018
Bibliothèque nationale du Québec

Printed in Canada on acid-free paper that is 100% ancient forest free (100% post-consumer recycled), processed chlorine free

This book has been published with the help of a grant from the Canadian Federation for the Humanities and Social Sciences, through the Awards to Scholarly Publications Program, using funds provided by the Social Sciences and Humanities Research Council of Canada.

Funded by the Government of Canada | Financé par le gouvernement du Canada | Canada

Conseil des arts du Canada | Canada Council for the Arts

We acknowledge the support of the Canada Council for the Arts, which last year invested $153 million to bring the arts to Canadians throughout the country.

Nous remercions le Conseil des arts du Canada de son soutien. L'an dernier, le Conseil a investi 153 millions de dollars pour mettre de l'art dans la vie des Canadiennes et des Canadiens de tout le pays.

Library and Archives Canada Cataloguing in Publication

Burke, Stacie, 1970–, author
Building resistance : children, tuberculosis, and the Toronto sanatorium / Stacie Burke.

Includes bibliographical references and index.
Issued in print and electronic formats.
ISBN 978-0-7735-5330-9 (cloth).–ISBN 978-0-7735-5331-6 (paper).
–ISBN 978-0-7735-5381-1 (ePDF).–ISBN 978-0-7735-5382-8 (ePUB)

1. Tuberculosis in children – Ontario – Toronto – History – 20th century.
2. Tuberculosis – Treatment – Ontario – Toronto – History – 20th century.
3. Sanatoriums – Ontario – Toronto – History – 20th century. I. Title.

RC309.5.C3B87 2018 362.19699'5009713541 C2017-908068-7
C2017-908069-5

This book was designed and typeset by studio oneonone in Sabon 10.5/14.

To my mom and dad, Dianne and Dennis, with love

Contents

Figures and Tables

Figures

Tables

Acknowledgments

You never know where inspiration will strike. In the late 1990s, nearing the completion of my PhD, I enjoyed my regular Wednesday afternoon distraction at a local country auction in Ontario. One particular Wednesday, I came home with an old photo album, filled with photographs of an anonymous family's memories, probably dating to the 1930s or 1940s. All of the expected photos were there – kids, pets, family portraits, holidays – but there were also unusual photographs of women and men in pyjamas and housecoats, sometimes posed for pictures on a balcony, others in beds. Without doubt, the photos were taken in some sort of institution, and my curiosity was piqued. The people looked happy, smiling for the camera, and seemingly not ill, at least not in any noticeable way. But they were in their pyjamas, and that seemed odd. As someone interested in health, disease, and history, I strongly suspected that these were photos capturing moments at a tuberculosis sanatorium, possibly the old sanatorium that had existed in nearby Gravenhurst. To make a long story short, I traced the provenance of the photos to a tuberculosis sanatorium in southern Ontario. In the process of figuring this out, my inquiries took me to the Archives of Ontario and, from there, I was directed to West Park Healthcare Centre, the health-care institution that had evolved out of the Toronto tuberculosis sanatorium. West Park had made great efforts to curate its long history, establishing a remarkable institutional archive. Putting together a research proposal, undertaking ethics reviews, and applying for funding, with the support of West Park, a new project was born. I would like to extend my sincere gratitude to West Park Healthcare Centre for supporting this research, and to acknowledge West Park's amazing staff for their kind and expert assistance, particularly as the years rolled by.

There are a number of people that I wish to recognize for their support and assistance with this project, particularly Larry Sawchuk and Ann Herring, who have always been such a tremendous source of inspiration and encouragement. For reading selected chapters and providing valuable feedback, I would like to thank Ann Herring, Brenda Chow, and Clay Hammett. For the maps, I am grateful to Richard Maaranen for his expertise. This research was greatly enriched by the skilled assistance of staff at the City of Toronto Archives, the Archives of Ontario, the University of Toronto Archives, and the Fisher Rare Book Library, University of Toronto.

This research would not have been possible without funding provided by the Social Science and Humanities Research Council of Canada. I am also grateful for the support of the Awards to Scholarly Publications Program (Federation for the Humanities and Social Sciences), which provided critical funding for the publishing of this book.

At McGill-Queen's University Press, I will be forever grateful to Mark Abley, the acquisitions editor who offered such a positive and encouraging response to the book proposal that I submitted to the press. Through the years that this manuscript was in preparation, peer review, and revisions, Mark always had kind, thoughtful, and encouraging words, and the very best advice to guide me through the complexities. There would likely not be a book, were it not for Mark. To the three anonymous peer reviewers, I owe a debt of gratitude for their detailed and constructive feedback, helping me to see the manuscript from different perspectives and to think more deeply about disciplinary, theoretical, and methodological issues. The reviewers played a critical role in improving the manuscript and for that, I am truly grateful. As the manuscript moved towards publication, I engaged with more of the McGill-Queen's University Press team, and it was a true pleasure to have the opportunity to work with them. For his fantastic skills and diligence in copy-editing, I owe a debt of gratitude to Ian MacKenzie.

Finally, and more personally, I am grateful to my family, friends, and colleagues for their support and understanding as tuberculosis and the writing of this book occupied my days. For his constant love and support, I thank my wonderful husband, Bill Imperial.

BUILDING RESISTANCE

CHAPTER 1

Building Bodies of Resistance

Going to a hospital resembles a journey to a foreign, exotic land, an often too common pilgrimage in which patients cross into a world of strange rites, miraculous interventions, and frequent death.[1]
~ Guenter B. Risse

Positioning Tuberculosis: The Family Dynamic

Sarah Brown was born in Ontario in 1891 and, at twenty-two years of age, she married twenty-five-year-old Jack Hobbs in the summer of 1913. They made their home in a bustling northern Ontario community and, fourteen months after their marriage, the couple welcomed the birth of their first child, a son they named Bert. Two years later, another son, Sidney, joined the family. Jack Hobbs was industrious, a cabinetmaker by trade, yet he seized an opportunity to start a cartage business, purchasing two trucks and hiring two men to work for him. For the Hobbs family, it seemed, good fortune was in the air. But in 1921, when Sarah was an active homemaker raising her four- and six-year-old sons, tragedy struck. According to Sidney's memoirs, "Mother became very ill to the point where she could not look after her family. The diagnosis, tuberculosis in the blood stream, galloping TB, the dreaded White Plague."[2] With Sarah quickly becoming gravely ill, Jack decided to relocate the family to his parents' farm in rural northern Ontario. They travelled by train, and, after settling Sarah and the boys at the farm, Jack returned home to sell the family's possessions, pay his debts, and rent out their home. Clearly, the spectre of tuberculosis meant that this was no short-term relocation.

At the farm, Bert and Sidney were separated from their mother, the boys living with their grandparents and uncles in the farmhouse, while Sarah and Jack shared a tent on the farm's acreage. Sidney remembered that "everything that was used by them was washed separately and stored separately, including the cutlery." He also recalled that seventy-six days after they had arrived at the farm, and only twenty-four days after his fifth birthday, his mother died in July 1921. While still reeling from the loss of his wife, Jack's attention turned to the nagging stomach pains that he had neglected on account of her illness. Following Sarah's funeral, Jack went to the doctor. The doctor's examination revealed tuberculosis, and Jack was quickly admitted to the sanatorium[3] at Gravenhurst, where he would spend four years apart from his sons trying to build his resistance to the disease before being discharged as "hopeless." Jack returned to the farm for nine months in 1926, before being sent, as a last resort, to the Toronto sanatorium. At that time, Sidney remembered, his father was expected to live only a few more months. In reality, however, "he lingered for three years" before succumbing to pulmonary tuberculosis at the sanatorium.

Because of their parents' tuberculosis, attentions naturally turned to Bert and Sidney, both now TB suspects. It was arranged that the boys would receive yearly chest X-rays, typically in late November or early December, travelling with their uncle "in a 1926 Model T Ford with no heater and hand operated windshield wiper and along the backroads" to the closest city where the travelling clinic made its annual stop. "We looked forward to our jaunts for the X-rays," Sidney recalled, because their uncle enjoyed indulging them "with store candies, cookies, and a silent movie," which "for that era … was a real treat." Bert and Sidney received chest X-rays in 1927, 1928, 1929, and 1930. Their happy excursions to the city ended with the last trip in 1930 when the chest X-rays for both boys in that year returned results that confirmed tuberculosis disease. Elder brother Bert's pulmonary tuberculosis was determined to be in an advanced state, while Sidney's X-ray revealed a suspicious shadow on his lung. According to Sidney, he and Bert were removed from school and advised to "cease all work and physical play." Arrangements were made to have the boys admitted to the Toronto sanatorium, the same distant institution to which their father had been sent and died. Since they faced a six-month waiting list for admission, Sidney remembered that he and his brother "had lots of time to think about our illness." Sidney entered the sanatorium in 1931, when he was fifteen years of age. Unlike his mother and father, however, Sidney would overcome his tuberculosis, successfully building his resistance to the disease, and living a long life well into his eighties.[4]

Children, Tuberculosis, and the Sanatorium: A Case Study

Sidney's vivid recall of the events leading up to his admission to the sanatorium in Toronto is remarkable in its detail, but the sad reality is that his family story was far from unique. Across Canada, in the years when tuberculosis was endemic (continually present and circulating) and before the rise of antibiotic treatments in the 1940s, countless families would be forever changed by tuberculosis. This book considers Sidney's story, along with the stories of hundreds of other children, in a case study of tuberculosis in childhood. The study is focused on the experiences of children who, like Sidney, were diagnosed and hospitalized at the Toronto sanatorium, an Ontario hospital that specialized in tuberculosis care and treatment. Broad in perspective, the study focuses on tuberculous children and their connections with tuberculosis bacteria and the tuberculosis sanatorium (and its staff of doctors and nurses). By focusing on these key areas together, a broad, biosocial[5] perspective on childhood tuberculosis is gained where children, bacteria, and medicine became entangled within the hard architecture of the sanatorium, a concrete place that defined treatment, perseverance, and hope.

This study explores many of the "how" and "why" questions relating to tuberculosis, hospitalization, and treatment among children, the kinds of questions that typically define case studies.[6] In the era before streptomycin, how did children experience tuberculosis infection, disease, hospitalization, and treatment? How did infection and disease affect their bodies, their families, and their lives? Why were they admitted to the sanatorium and how did they experience separation from family and home? How did modern medicine respond as the awareness and understanding of tuberculosis changed? Before antibiotics and cures, what treatments did the sanatorium have to offer and why were those treatments favoured? Aiming for a "rich and holistic account,"[7] this case study pursues detail and description to better understand the lived experience of tuberculosis among child sanatorium patients. In so doing, it follows Lee Peter Ruddin's characterization of the case study as a "study of the particular."[8] In this qualitative case study, in particular, my intentions are not to test or prove specific hypotheses, but, through "rich, 'thick' description" to "illuminate the ... understanding" and perhaps explore "new meaning" in the phenomenon of childhood tuberculosis before antibiotics.[9] This study aims "to enter the world of illness as lived by patients."[10] The qualitative approach expects that the children in this study will "have had unique experiences" and "special stories to tell," that there will be richness and diversity.[11]

Siting and Seating the Case Study

The children represent the focus of this study, but the sanatorium, its staff of physicians and nurses, and the modern medicine that they practised are also critical to consider because, collectively, they play a role in shaping the site or "context" in which the children's experiences took place. Case studies are typically bounded,[12] and what unites or binds these children, despite their potentially unique experiences with infection, signs and symptoms, prognosis, and outcome, is their shared experience of medicine and hospitalization at the sanatorium. Within the sanatorium, the manner in which physicians and nurses chose to treat tuberculosis had a major impact not only on how patients experienced the disease, but also their perception of and response to the hospital itself. As a result, this study explores how and why certain treatments were chosen and the impact of those treatments on body, disease, and experience. Understanding the site of the case study is itself important. Robert Stake advises providing "vicarious experiences for the reader, to give them a sense of 'being there,'" and exploring the aspects of "uniqueness" and "ordinariness" that illuminate the site and its significance.[13]

While local site descriptions and context are important for developing the case study, there are bigger, overarching challenges involved in examining large nineteenth- and twentieth-century medical facilities such as tuberculosis sanatoria. Critical opinion has weighed heavily on interpretations of the medical and social functioning of these institutions. Negative characterizations of such institutions and medicine more generally gained traction with the writings of French philosopher Michel Foucault and American sociologist Erving Goffman,[14] and were powerfully dramatized in popular films such as *One Flew Over the Cuckoo's Nest* (1975) (which is fictitious and based in a psychiatric facility, not a sanatorium, but nonetheless depicts a regimented, oppressive, and downright terrifying institutional life for patients). In the background to her research on Waipiata Sanatorium in New Zealand, Susan Haugh acknowledges Goffman and his writing on the phenomenon of the "total institution," which emphasized "the coercive and regulated aspects of life in which inmates were dehumanised, restricted by a monotonous routine, and rigidly segregated from staff and the outside world."[15] Together, scholars such as Foucault and Goffman, critical of these medical institutions and their organization and treatments, taught us to question these constructed landscapes of medicine, as noted quite powerfully by Haugh: "This context of dissatisfaction with the institutional process has coloured the way that sanatorium narratives have been told. While none of the historians writing since Goffman adhere strictly to his extremely rigid portrayal of institutional life, they do echo Goffman in their description of these institutions by focussing on the elements of routine, discipline, and isolation and the boredom, frustration, and 'institutionalization' that these caused."[16]

In building her argument, Haugh draws on classic studies, including Sheila Rothman's (1994) *Living in the Shadow of Death*, where sanatorium patients became "inmates" suffering through an "infantilizing" hospitalization replete with "humiliation and denigration" and "unrelenting hostility" at an institution that was ultimately viewed as a "waiting room for death."[17] Seeking a more balanced perspective, Haugh notes that Greta Jones's study of an Irish tuberculosis sanatorium and Lynda Bryder's study of British sanatoria are more optimistic, going much further in emphasizing the close sense of community that was shared in hospitalization and illness, the rise of the patient subculture, the romance and friendships, and the dedicated medical and nursing staff that actually really did care for their patients.[18] In the United States, Barbara Bates has similarly described the many benefits offered by the sanatorium, from "the care and support of nurses," the "trusting relationship with a physician," "the comradeship of other patients," and the opportunity to "escape from deleterious conditions at home or at work."[19]

It is precisely this more positive perspective on the role, function, and experience of tuberculosis sanatoria that Haugh emphasizes in her study of New Zealand's Waipiata tuberculosis sanatorium, tempering the perspective on sanatorium hospitalization and helping to dispel some of the common stereotypes. Haugh finds a balance – the sanatorium was neither a perfect place, nor a perfect experience, "but for many of those whose lives had been interrupted by tuberculosis it was the best of all possible worlds"[20] and "offered hope of recovery far more than it created fear of death."[21] Hope, in particular, also surfaced in my own research. Haugh chalks some of the negative characterizations of tuberculosis sanatoria up to individual institutions, because they could vary in fundamental ways, including accessibility for visitors, the ability of patients to take leaves of absence, isolation of the sanatorium, and the status of its funding. Thus, "maltreated and exploited" patients were more often associated with "understaffed and poorly equipped" sanatoria.[22] Such cases were likely fuel to Goffman's fire, and these more dismal sanatoria joined prisons and asylums as "coercive and dehumanising institutions."[23] Yet, as Haugh argues, for most patients, and particularly poor and working-class patients, the sanatorium was a likely source of comfort in tuberculosis:

> Both the staff and the committee that administered the sanatorium placed much emphasis on alleviating those aspects of institutional life that Goffman and others have decried. The sanatorium regime undeniably included elements of discipline and loss of freedoms, and could certainly create a sense of frustration. Yet the willingness of the staff and committee to create a delicate balance between the regime and the happiness of their patients did much to overcome these aspects ... Those who were treated outside a sanatorium community avoided the isolation that institutional care entailed, but suffered the indignity of health inspections, and often lived and died in uncomfortable and undesirable conditions placing at risk the family members who cared for them.[24]

The important point here is the balanced perspective. For those who suffered from tuberculosis, the home was not necessarily better than the sanatorium. And the sanatorium was not necessarily better than the home. But Haugh rejects the notion that the sanatorium was uniformly cruel and tormenting, advising that "while the negative aspects of sanatorium life cannot and should not be denied, nor should its benefits be forgotten";[25] from start to finish the perspective that I gained on the Toronto sanatorium triangulated well with Haugh's perspective and was decidedly less Goffmanesque.

Understanding the historical context of this institutional criticism helps to build that more balanced perspective, and, according to Elizabeth Klaver, this is a critical starting point from which to fairly assess what treatments physicians and nurses pursued and why. "Exactly why did the medical profession find it necessary to quarantine TB patients and to insist on the particular dietary and emotional regime that the patients found so oppressive?," she asks.[26] Without context or explanation, Klaver argues that "medicine comes off as inexplicably mean-spirited,"[27] contributing to the criticism that historic tuberculosis sanatoria offered only punishing regimes of treatment, such as seemingly endless hours of monotonous bedrest. If not directly or indirectly harmful, then, at best, sanatorium treatment might be simply disregarded as ultimately ineffective. Susan Haugh has noted, "The sanatorium experience is often remembered as a misguided, ineffective treatment, the forerunner to the 'chemotherapy revolution' that 'cured' tuberculosis."[28] It is critically important to examine this aspect since it sets the whole tone and context of the sanatorium experience. If medical staff were using treatments that were simply "mean-spirited," then that aspect alone would have seriously compromised patients' beliefs in medicine; but if we understand why the medical and nursing staff were doing what they were doing, why they believed in what they were doing, and how they explained their approach to patients (or patients' families), then we can better understand how such treatments framed hopes for survival and why parents were willing to have their children admitted, often for what would prove to be long-term hospitalization. Since treatments and surgeries ultimately affected the children's experiences, and particularly their bodily experiences with tuberculosis, chapters 5 and 6 explore the medical aspects of the sanatorium.

Methodologically, according to Robert Stake, qualitative case studies may be "naturalistic, holistic, ethnographic, phenomenological, and biographic."[29] Case studies are typically defined by the use of "a full variety of evidence," which, according to Robert Yin, often includes "documents, artifacts, interviews, and observations."[30] This case study of children hospitalized for tuberculosis relies upon a remarkable institutional archive and multiple sources of information to understand their experiences, from their medical and social narratives as captured in patient charts, to archived oral history interviews with those who crossed paths with the Toronto sanatorium, to extensive archival documentation (from the minutiae of the physician-in-chief's memoranda to staff, to his comprehensive memoir of the early history of the sanatorium, to the annual reports of the National Sanitarium Association, and the unparalleled photographic collection of the Toronto sanatorium) and artifacts (such as the pneumothorax apparatus that was used extensively at the sanatorium) that have been curated at West Park Healthcare Centre (the medical institution that developed out of the original Toronto sanatorium). The emphasis on data collection from the institutional archive kept the case study bound and focused on the local, but additional research on medical journal publications (mostly pre-1950) helped to flesh out the changing medical perspective on tuberculosis.

Qualitative case studies typically centre data collection on a small number of persons and, while the number may be small, the study is intense. The patient charts that I worked with as my primary data source offered insights into patients, but unequally, for some patients had thick documentation, others quite thin. Typically, I was privy to only snippets of a patient's life story, perhaps even considerable documentation over a single issue in a patient's life. As a result, while most qualitative researchers would likely balk at my sampling of 822 patient charts (a number that would be perfectly satisfactory to a quantitative researcher), it is important to emphasize the variable nature of the volume of data per case and that only purposefully selected examples have been used to illustrate the themes and interpretations that emerged in this research. Qualitative data were abstracted from the patient charts and, in an ongoing process, themed for content (e.g., "delayed admission," "misdiagnosis," or "deportation"). Comparative and complementary examples of phenomena emerged in the data and were grouped. Unlike quantitative analyses, which involve statistics and tests of significance, "qualitative data are generally content analysed and evaluated subjectively, often in terms of themes, categories or new concepts."[31] The descriptive tendency of this case study will become abundantly evident, for example, when exploring and detailing the medical procedures, an aspect of each patient's story that directly intersects with medicine and its practitioners, physicians and nurses. It would be easy enough to say that some patients had part of their lung collapsed with artificial pneumothorax, but what did that mean in practice and in experience? Physically, how was the body approached and the lung accessed to induce the collapse? What instruments would be needed? Why could a single "smooth" and "glistening" adhesion foil even the best planned artificial pneumothorax surgery? All of these details would contribute to patients' sensory and physical experiences, so "thick" descriptions of the medical procedures were pursued. If the treatments had not been explored – what physicians and nurses were doing and why they were doing it – then one could be left with deep misunderstandings about what was happening at the sanatorium. Returning to Elizabeth Klaver's perspective, tuberculosis treatment might simply appear "mean-spirited."[32]

Underlying paradigms play an important role in seating the case study because such philosophical positionings can influence the type of story told and what aspects of the story are emphasized. According to William Firestone, qualitative research itself is often "rooted in a phenomenological paradigm which holds that reality is socially constructed through individual or collective *definitions of the situation*."[33] This aspect he compares to quantitative research, rooted in a positivist paradigm, "which assumes that there are social *facts* with an objective reality apart from the beliefs of individuals."[34] The goals to uncover "facts" versus "construct" realities shape not only the research process, but also the product. It is precisely because conceptions of reality vary with individual experience that this research explores the diversity of experience – with tuberculosis, hospitalization, family life, and modern medicine. And yet there were also the similarities. The phenomenological paradigm encourages detailed attention to those experiences and, in the instance of this case study, to attempts to understand the "lived experiences" of children hospitalized for tuberculosis. As John Creswell has argued, "We conduct qualitative research because a problem or issue needs to be explored ... We also conduct qualitative research because we need a *complex*, detailed understanding of the issue."[35] While narrative studies typically focus on a single individual and are therefore more biographical, phenomenological studies are often based on multiple persons and their lived experiences.[36] According to Starks and Trinidad, "phenomenological analyses produce rich thematic descriptions that provide insight into the meaning of the lived experience."[37] This qualitative approach expects that the children in this study, for example, will "have had unique experiences" and "special stories to tell," that there will be richness and diversity.[38] Richard Baron argues that, by adopting a "phenomenologic perspective," it may be possible "to enter the world of illness as lived by patients rather than confining ourselves to the world of disease as described by physicians."[39]

As a biological anthropologist, my interest in tuberculosis and childhood is holistic, humanistic, and biosocial, meaning that I am interested in exploring the complex and intersecting effects of both biological and social factors in shaping the children's lived experiences with tuberculosis.[40] Biology, and the relationships struck between *Mycobacterium tuberculosis* (a bacterium) and the body in tuberculosis infection and disease, must be considered in a comprehensive case study because of the role it plays in shaping the whole experience. Some children's bodies managed tuberculosis infection more successfully than others and, as a result, the nature of disease and treatment experiences would also differ. Illness and disease are neither wholly biological nor completely social, both aspects commingling to define experience. A broad, comprehensive underpinning to the biosocial perspective is captured in Singer and Clair's "syndemic" construct where diseases do not occur in isolation, but often overlap and interact in complex ways: "A syndemic is a set of intertwined and mutually enhancing epidemics involving disease interactions at the biological level that develop and are sustained in a community/population *because of harmful social conditions and injurious social connections*."[41] Such "harmful" and "injurious" social features can be captured in Paul Farmer's conceptions of "structural violence," societal inequalities often systematized and ingrained in racism, sexism, and poverty.[42] These types of inequalities typically result in stressors such as "noxious living, working or environmental conditions, or oppressive social relationships," and place the body in a vulnerable position with decreased resistance to a large number of diseases, including infectious diseases such as tuberculosis.[43]

Because this study is biosocially grounded, attention will be paid to both biology (of the body and of the bacterium) and social features, and the terrain that connects them. From the work of the body and the immune system's macrophages, the significant relationship between tuberculosis and measles, the realities of overcrowding and poor homes, and the beliefs in the healing powers of blood and bedrest – all had the potential to shape children's lived experiences with tuberculosis. As a result, part of this story becomes quite biological, delving into the history of treatment and the evolving physiological understandings of the tuberculous body. But it is equally as important to consider the social dimensions, such as the poor living conditions, the destruction of whole families, often through the slow, wasting effects of tuberculosis, and the family and community supports made available to those attempting to cope with the disease.

Sidney's story foreshadows many themes that run through this book, including the struggle with infection and disease in families. This is not coincidental, since tuberculosis has been described as "the quintessential family disease," an infection passed easily between generations, often from parent to child, the children then carrying the legacy of infection on to future generations.[44] Sidney's mother was a likely source of his and Bert's infections, as she was probably infectious for a period of time before her diagnosis, rapid decline, and death in 1921 at thirty years of age; it is equally possible that it was Sidney's father. Tuberculosis is a bacterial disease, most commonly transmitted by either contact (droplet) or airborne (aerosol) routes. Through coughs and sneezes, sufferers with active pulmonary (lung) disease liberated sputum (mucus and saliva) and tuberculosis bacteria from their lungs and respiratory passages. Spending time in confined spaces, such as in a family home, in close contact with a tuberculosis sufferer with cavitary disease (tuberculous cavities in the lungs are typically rife with bacteria) is a risk for transmission because simple proximity increases the chances that droplets will come into contact with vulnerable "portals of entry," such as the eyes, nose, or mouth. Alternatively, tuberculosis bacteria may also become airborne, carried on much tinier droplet nuclei.[45] The aerosol of droplet nuclei can remain suspended in air, moving with air currents and becoming concentrated in the air of poorly ventilated spaces. The very need of our bodies to take in oxygen by breathing defines our vulnerability to tuberculosis infection, since inhaled air containing tuberculosis bacteria may result in their deposition deep in our respiratory tracts and lungs. From that point, an effective immune response to mediate the infection and prevent disease is most critical.

The transmission and bodily experience of tuberculosis is characterized by complexity. Not only, for example, can the human body develop tuberculosis as a result of classical *Mycobacterium tuberculosis* infection, but a related bacterial species, *Mycobacterium bovis*, can also cause tuberculosis in humans. *Mycobacterium bovis* typically circulates zoonotically in animal populations. Infected animals, particularly cattle that live in close association with humans, may pass the infection along when humans consume their milk or meat. For children, consumption of cow's milk was a common risk for tuberculosis infection prior to routine milk pasteurization. While *Mycobacterium tuberculosis* was often associated with lung infection, consumption of *Mycobacterium bovis* in infected milk or meat typically resulted in infection of the gastrointestinal tract (not the lungs). This latter point alludes to yet another complexity of tuberculosis, in the sense that any organ or tissue in the human body may become infected, though lung infections tended to be more common in the history of the disease. Before the rise of antibiotics, tuberculosis was a chronic infection, so once tuberculosis bacteria were in the body, they were typically in the body for life. This did not mean, however, a life of perpetual tuberculosis disease, since the bacteria can express variable levels of activity, depending on the infecting strain of bacteria (some strains are more aggressive than others) and the status of the human immune response (some bodies are more vulnerable or resistant than others) that the bacteria encounter. Based on these conditions, tuberculosis infection may progress in a chronic active state, or fluctuate between periods of activity and latency, or remain chronically latent altogether (never causing active tuberculosis disease). Individuals with latent infection are not infectious, but their infection might become active and their disease infectious if their immune function weakens.

Returning to Sidney's story, a number of other common narratives emerge, including the incapacitation of his mother and her inability to continue to function as homemaker. Her decline had profound effects on the family's stability. As her condition quickly worsened, Jack made the difficult decision to abandon the family home and move in with Sidney's grandparents on the farm.[46] Other families examined in this study were similarly disrupted or fragmented, some without the extended family support that the Hobbs family benefitted from and reliant instead upon orphanages, foster homes, friends of the family, and even sympathetic strangers to care for children when their parents became incapacitated or died because of tuberculosis (or other diseases). Eventually, Sidney's family would be permanently fragmented by tuberculosis, claiming the lives of both of his parents, even as the infection persistently lingered on in the bodies of their children, Bert and Sidney.

Sidney's narrative also touches on aspects of both home and institutional care, as his mother spent her last days in a tent on the farm, firmly separated from her young sons, while his father would later enter a sanatorium. For all of the patients reviewed in this study who were admitted to the sanatorium in Toronto, there were countless others who suffered tuberculosis in their family homes and communities. Some, like Sidney's mother, may have been accommodated in tents, others in shacks, sleeping porches, or well-ventilated screened rooms. At best, separate accommodations were encouraged, though this was seldom possible in homes that were already cramped and overcrowded. Sidney's story also captures the public health efforts to monitor suspected cases of infection and disease through routine testing of known tuberculosis contacts, as well as the role of the sanatorium in the years before antibiotics. Concerns over "responsibility" can be found threaded throughout this book, ranging from responsibility for infection and disease, to accurate diagnoses and advice, the care of the tuberculous, and the support of households experiencing prolonged disability and death. As Poutanen and colleagues note, even the very individual action of "seeking prompt treatment at the earliest sign of disease" to limit the possibility of transmission was conceived as a "social responsibility."[47]

Resistance is another theme in Sidney's family story, and it frames this book as well. Even within Sidney's family, we see many different degrees of tuberculosis resistance and vulnerability. While Sidney's mother succumbed to aggressive disease quickly, his father lingered for many years in a liminal, tuberculous, unwell state, evading all the predictions of his looming demise, at least for a time. Falling under modern medical care at the Toronto sanatorium, Bert and Sidney would both survive tuberculosis, but not without their own struggles and challenges. Sidney, for example, would experience body-altering thoracoplasty surgery. In the early tuberculosis sanatorium era in Canada, before the rise of antibiotics in the 1940s, surviving tuberculosis hinged on resistance, and since resistance is such an important grounding point for this book, it merits introduction.

The Context of Resistance

Resistance is a key, overarching concept that defined how children would experience tuberculosis and influenced the nature of the medical treatments that sanatorium staff would apply. But resistance is also a concept that can be extended to tuberculosis bacteria, and the dynamic struck between bodies and bacteria. At its most basic level, resistance in tuberculosis can be conceived as a biological construct, influenced by the ability to contain a chronic bacterial infection in the body in a latent, inactive state. The reality is somewhat more complex, however, since biological resistance can, in turn, be influenced by prevailing social conditions, situating the health and resilience of bodies in the realities of economics, living and working conditions, diet and nutrition, and social support, all features of life that can increase or decrease vulnerability to many diseases, including tuberculosis. For children who experienced tuberculosis infection, resistance was a key factor linked with health and well-being. The case for resistance is strong. Among those who are latently infected (i.e., those who have contained tuberculosis bacteria in a latent state), there is a lifetime 10 per cent risk (or a one in ten likelihood) that active disease will emerge.[48] Though this risk is significant, it also highlights the much greater probability that disease will not reactivate because, among the majority of individuals, the body is able to continue to maintain the infection in a latent state – testament to the underlying power of the body and its immune defences.[49] At the same time, however, tuberculosis bacteria have also developed their own forms of resistance, including their ability to withstand eradication from the human body, instead sequestered in a persistently long-term latent state. All of this is significant, given that today an astonishing one-third of the global population is infected with tuberculosis bacteria.[50] Should antibiotics become ineffective, and they are waning in that direction, John Grange and colleagues warn "we will very soon be at a very real risk of massive epidemics of tuberculosis that will be exceedingly difficult to control."[51]

The tuberculosis bacterium is one of the most successfully adapted pathogens to infect and affect human populations around the world, but the relationship is far from new. It was long believed that *Mycobacterium tuberculosis* entered human populations via evolution from a related zoonotic species (*Mycobacterium bovis*) around the time that humans began to domesticate animals, cattle in particular, in the Neolithic revolution that began about ten thousand years ago. More recent genetic analyses of the bacterium, however, have pushed the relationship back much earlier. According to a review by Anne Stone and colleagues, mounting evidence, particularly from palaeomicrobiology and studies of ancient DNA (aDNA), suggests that *Mycobacterium tuberculosis* is actually the older of the two pathogens and was present in human populations well before the rise of animal domestication, conservatively estimated at thirty-five thousand years ago, but potentially even earlier in co-evolutionary pathways established between progenitor species and human ancestors in Africa.[52] This book joins the story far more recently, in the sanatorium era, roughly between 1900 and 1950, a time when tuberculosis had long been an established and common disease in Canada.

While humans have generally adapted a biological resistance to tuberculosis bacteria, if their immune systems falter and active tuberculosis disease emerges in vulnerable bodies, then attention shifts to medicine and "resistance building." In the early sanatorium era in which this book is situated there were no antibiotic cures for tuberculosis, so efforts instead focused on building up bodily resistance, playing upon the body's natural abilities to contain and survive tuberculosis infection. Given the high percentage of people who are naturally able to "resist" active tuberculosis, this was a realistic approach. Because of the chronic nature of tuberculosis infection, however, the commitment to maintain resistance had to endure over the long haul of life. Though most people were able to maintain tuberculosis infection in a latent state, the possibility of infection awakening always lingered. There was an ongoing, dynamic relationship between people's immune systems and resident tuberculosis bacteria that could shift over time. Resistance building was not a cure but a survival tactic, which aimed to shift favour to the body to control the chronic bacterial infection.

The medical principles of resistance building were evident in tuberculosis sanatoria, but also extended outside of the sanatorium into homes and communities. With the work of public health, attention was directed at building individual and community resistance to tuberculosis through attempts to improve quality of life, or at least by making the best of challenging circumstances. The capacity for resistance and resistance building was sensitive to the kind of stressors that people faced in daily life. Poor nutrition, bodily struggles with other diseases, a lack of rest, and overwork, in particular, were believed to weaken the body's resisting power and became focal points for public health work. Resistance building focused on those affected by tuberculosis, but also extended the concept more generally by encouraging improvements in living and working conditions, better nutrition, isolating the infectious within homes and institutions, and assisting those who seemed particularly vulnerable by providing, for example, extra milk to children of tuberculous parents. Improving communities became a social concern to build collective resistance in the face of the unrelenting presence of tuberculosis. This approach to resistance building would change significantly with the introduction of antibiotics in the 1940s and 1950s, as the focus shifted to treating the underlying bacterial infection directly, instead of improving and building up individuals and communities to resist infection and disease more generally.[53]

In Canada and elsewhere, resistance building was essential precisely because tuberculosis was so common. Children such as Bert and Sidney were often infected within their family homes, many by mid-adolescence. The movement of tuberculosis infection across generations, from parents to children, is not coincidental, as most adults were vulnerable to reactivations of latent infection at precisely the time in their lives when they were making and raising children. Within the closeness of the family and home, a new, uninfected generation of children would come to be introduced to tuberculosis. Research has suggested that the tendency towards disease reactivation in adolescence and young adulthood is a by-product of the tuberculosis bacterium's evolution, seemingly timing its surge out of latency to ensure its transmission to a whole new generation of vulnerable bodies.[54] Such an evolutionary adaptation helps to explain the persistence of tuberculosis through generational time and the bacterium's tenacious grip once established in human populations.

In this way, the theme of resistance can be read further from the perspective of the tuberculosis bacterium. Within the human body, *Mycobacterium tuberculosis* can become established, almost strategically, within macrophages – phagocytic cells of the human immune system that are intended to engulf and ultimately destroy bacteria. Just as active TB bacteria "consume" the body, macrophages consume TB bacteria. Rather than being destroyed, however, tuberculosis bacteria linger and are lulled into a dormant or latent state within the macrophages. Should the immune system that holds them captive falter, those bacteria may be liberated. The bacterium's persistence is marked by its very livelihood within the macrophage – dormant, but not destroyed. As the sanatorium era transitioned into the antibiotic era of the 1940s and 1950s (and beyond), other themes of bacterial resistance became evident. Early trials with streptomycin revealed that tuberculosis bacteria could quickly gain resistance to this drug; while streptomycin killed the vulnerable bacteria, those with natural (genetic) resistance to streptomycin survived, and their numbers grew until the drug could no longer effectively treat the infection. Recognizing these resistance capabilities, medicine responded with multi-drug treatments, combining streptomycin with other drugs. Even if tuberculosis bacteria could survive streptomycin, it was unlikely that they would also survive all the other drugs used in treatment. Confidence eroded, however, as the strength of resistance revealed itself, first with the rise of multi-drug-resistant strains of tuberculosis bacteria (MDR-TB), then extensively drug-resistant tuberculosis bacteria (XDR-TB), and, most recently and alarmingly, totally drug-resistant tuberculosis bacteria (TDR-TB) that are staunchly resistant to all known drug treatments.[55] Evolving resistance to antibiotic treatments is most worrisome, since it sets limits on the potential to control tuberculosis via one of modern medicine's most ingrained strategies.

Improving Child Health and Well-Being in Ontario

Since this book is focused on children and tuberculosis, it is important to situate the problem of "childhood tuberculosis" in the broader history of concern for child health and welfare that surfaced in places like Ontario in the nineteenth century. Tuberculosis was but one symptom of an overall poor state of infant and child health, as vulnerable youth regularly fell victim to a number of acute infectious diseases, from measles, diphtheria, scarlet fever, whooping cough, typhoid, and diarrheal diseases, to pneumonia, influenza, and smallpox. From the late nineteenth century and into the twentieth century, there were important developments in the area of child health spurred on initially by the work of philanthropists and charitable organizations. From there, the impact of science and professionalization in medicine, public health, and social work further intensified the attentions to, and investments in, improving child health and survival. As a result, this study of childhood tuberculosis and the sanatorium is linked to much broader themes in Canadian family history, such as social welfare, child welfare, and public policy, the sanatorium but one institution among many seeking to improve the lives and well-being of children in Ontario.

Late nineteenth-century Toronto was positioned in the midst of rapid population growth, urbanization, and industrialization, which created hardship and disadvantage, particularly among struggling working-class and destitute families.[56] The loss of parents by desertion or death (including deaths due to tuberculosis), homelessness, mistreatment, neglect, and grinding poverty all weighed heavily on the lives of children, both in urban centres such as Toronto and throughout the province and country more generally. In response, the 1880s saw the rise of a growing reform movement.[57] Working past fatalistic attitudes concerning infant and child survival, middle-class charitable groups, often headed by women and influenced by the example of church-related philanthropic work, attempted to improve the lives of vulnerable children (and also unmarried mothers and widows).[58] Middle-class women who participated in the intensifying social reform movement of the late nineteenth century "sought to right wrongs," particularly the acute social and economic inequalities, that came associated with the industrial revolution in cities such as Toronto.[59]

Alongside the work of charitable groups, the provincial government also formalized a number of Acts intended to improve the well-being of children. Charlotte Neff has examined aspects of Ontario's compulsory education act of 1871, the Industrial Schools Act of 1874, and the Children's Protection Act of 1893. The Acts of 1871 and 1874 were meant to ensure that children received at least a rudimentary education, and both, according to Neff, marked the first intrusions of government into the private lives of families in Ontario. The 1874 Act acknowledged the problem of "parental neglect," and society's collective responsibility for neglected children.[60] Though the Industrial Schools Act would undergo subsequent revisions, the 1874 iteration was notable because it recognized, for the first time in Ontario's history, that children and their behaviour and well-being could be influenced by the actions of their parents. As a result, according to Neff, "the 1874 Act helped pave the way for the 1893 Children's Protection Act, including the concept of the neglected child ... and the acceptance of public responsibility to provide for the care of neglected children."[61] This emphasis on "public responsibility" and its extensions into private family lives marked an important change in ethos and mindset.

In nineteenth-century Ontario, various charities organized by reform-minded citizens sought to improve child well-being through the creation of houses of industry, children's homes, orphanages, and even hospitals.[62] Neff estimates that six private children's homes were receiving provincial support through grants in 1865, increasing to ten in 1871, and eighteen in 1880.[63] According to Neff, Roman Catholic homes were run by nuns, whereas Protestant children's homes "were generally founded and operated by middle-class and upper-middle-class women whose husbands tended to be professionals and members of the local elite."[64] Neff has contended that, first and foremost, Ontario's children's homes functioned to support families, providing a temporary refuge for those families experiencing hardship but not intending to relinquish custody of their children.[65] In her analysis of admissions to one Toronto home, Neff found that, once crises had resolved, between one-third and one-half of the children returned home to their families, most within a year of their admission.[66] In many instances, crises emerged because of the sickness or death of one or both parents, sometimes due to chronic diseases such as tuberculosis,[67] but also acute, epidemic diseases such as influenza.[68]

Such was the circumstance of families without their own extended family supports and few other alternatives in times of illness and death.

In Canada, women were perceived as "the guardians of children's health," and, as such, they were linked to the early rise of children's hospitals.[69] Late nineteenth-century Victorian sensibilities viewed women's philanthropic work with "sick, needy children" as "an acceptable cause for a middle-class wife and mother concerned for the society beyond her home."[70] In Toronto, Elizabeth McMaster was president of the Ladies' Committee that established the Hospital for Sick Children in 1875.[71] Toronto's landmark hospital originally occupied a small house with six iron cots. As Judith Young notes, the Ladies' Committee maintained complete responsibility for the Hospital for Sick Children, which they ran "as a Christian household with an emphasis on loving care, nourishing food, cleanliness, and a morally uplifting environment."[72] The women dedicated themselves in particular to the care of "incurable" children, many of whom were likely suffering tuberculosis-related bone and joint disease.

By 1891, the Hospital for Sick Children had moved to College Street, housed in a substantial new building with 320 beds. Departing from its philanthropic roots, control of the hospital transitioned to a board of trustees headed by newspaper publisher John Ross Robertson.[73] By 1899, the Ladies' Committee had severed ties with the Hospital for Sick Children, refocusing their efforts instead on establishing Toronto's Home for Incurable Children;[74] the home continued in the tradition of a "small, homelike institution" for children in need of long-term care and, in later years, became Toronto's Bloorview Children's Hospital.[75] As Marcellus has argued, it was philanthropic women's groups that specialized in the care of "incurable children," particularly since emerging general hospitals were less keen to adopt this role.[76] It was precisely in this domain that the Toronto sanatorium stepped into the void to provide care for children with tuberculosis, a responsibility that came with long-term caregiving commitments, particularly for children with reactivation disease or bone and joint tuberculosis, both of which tended to be experienced as long-lasting, chronic (if not incurable) diseases.

Despite these late nineteenth-century developments, poor health continued to plague young Ontarians well into the twentieth century. Comparisons of Ontario's high infant mortality rate (for 1916, 107 infant deaths per 1,000 live births) to Great Britain (90/1,000) and New Zealand (50/1,000) suggested that social conditions needed further improvement.[77] In 1918, Alan Brown, an attending physician at the Hospital for Sick Children and the Toronto General Hospital, estimated that 30 to 50 per cent of infant deaths were preventable.[78] With the First World War, 35 to 40 per cent of young recruits failed their initial physical examinations and were rejected as unfit for service, a further reflection of the poor state of health of Canada's youth.[79] Because of these concerning findings, efforts to improve health in infancy and childhood and to protect children from infectious diseases such as tuberculosis would intensify.

In 1920 the Canadian Council on Child Welfare, a national organization that aimed to unite and professionalize child care services, was founded.[80] As Rooke and Schnell note, the transition from voluntary charitable work to professional roles in child welfare did not come easily, particularly for the "many replaced and displaced nonsalaried workers whose volunteer effort represented their self-worth and service to the broader community, and who had given a great deal of time and often money to their causes."[81] Voluntary women's groups had long been invested in the support of women and children, establishing well-baby clinics, pure milk depots, and organizations such as the Victorian Order of Nurses,[82] but the work of these women was increasingly absorbed into the domain of official public health departments.[83] In comparison to the emerging cadre of professional social workers, the older model of volunteerism came to be characterized as "middle-class matronly busybodyism," the contributions and talents of those women increasingly undervalued in comparison to the new generation of professional public health workers.[84]

Meanwhile, developments in medicine meant that physicians were achieving greater success in treating and preventing childhood illness. The introduction of diphtheria antitoxin in 1894 raised the profile of cures and prevention that could be achieved through modern medicine.[85] As the routine aspects of everyday life, including diet, fell increasingly into the domain of science and medicine, authority in health-related matters gradually shifted from parents, particularly mothers, to physicians.[86] In order to guide family homes more directly, public health and visiting nursing services evolved. The city of Toronto, for example, established a Division of Public Health Nurses in 1911. Given the financial and practical demands of public health nursing services and the problems of reaching rural and remote families,[87] other means of health education also evolved, including the Little Blue Books series of medical advice literature distributed to Canadian households free-of-charge by the federal government between 1920 and 1934.[88] Geared as they were towards the resources, values, and lifestyles of middle-class Canadians, however, poor households would find it difficult, if not impossible, to follow the home management and health advice outlined in the Blue Books.[89] The Blue Books placed responsibility for "the ultimate in a healthful living environment for the family" squarely on the shoulders of women.[90] As Dianne Dodd argues, "The Blue Books ... offered Canadians the knowledge of prevention, but failed to address social inequalities which prevented them from achieving it."[91] In effect, for families living in poverty, the advice, however well-intentioned, could be entirely "useless."[92]

Katherine Arnup examines the twentieth-century rise of "scientific motherhood" and "scientific child rearing" through a case study of Ontario's Dionne quintuplets, born in 1934.[93] It was particularly in the interwar years, Arnup argues, that mothers increasingly shared their role in child raising with medicine, child psychology, and social work. Clinics, lectures, magazines, newspapers, and advice literature were the vehicles through which "experts sought to educate women in the rules and practices of scientific motherhood," even despite the significant, lingering problem of poverty.[94] Arnup notes that children were increasingly expected to mimic an industrialized routine in life by sleeping, feeding, and undertaking bowel movements reliably, at regularly scheduled times. Healthy, robust children were believed to be the visible result of scientific child-rearing, which meant that mothers could be held to account for their purported failures if their children did not measure up. This was an unfortunate expectation, particularly in the era of tuberculosis. Though many of the rules of "scientific motherhood" aligned with the principles of resistance building, they could easily be undermined by the realities of hardship and poverty.

Poverty itself, the most direct influence on child health, was ultimately unchanged by the torrent of advice. It was one thing to be soundly schooled on the ingredients of a nutritious diet for children, but it was something else altogether to have the means to provide that diet. Persistent concerns over child health led mothers, not the unemployed, the disabled, or the elderly, to become the first group in Canada to receive provincial social assistance in the form of Mothers' Allowance.[95] At the time, however, this program was expensive and limited in funds, so only a small number of mothers would actually receive the allowance. According to Struthers, in the first mothers' allowance scheme introduced in Ontario in 1920,[96] "allowances would be restricted to needy widows with two or more children who were British subjects, owned less than $2500 in property and $350 in liquid assets, and had lived at least three years in Canada and two years in Ontario before applying for support."[97] Women whose husbands suffered medically certified total and permanent incapacitation, and deserted women whose husbands had been absent for seven or more years were the next to be brought into the scheme.[98] Struthers notes that cases granted on incapacitation of husbands accounted for "a steadily rising percentage of Mothers' Allowance families, reaching almost one-quarter of the total caseload by the late 1920s, with tuberculosis the leading cause of dependency."[99] Unquestionably, tuberculosis was an unwelcome harbinger for poor women; the disease often fragmented or incapacitated families and forced a number of women into the mothers' allowance scheme, placing limits on their independence and increasing their accountability to the moral authority of those who supervised Mothers' Allowance families.

Tuberculosis and the Sanatorium

It was within this maturing age of philanthropy, budding professionalization, medicalization, and concern for child health that the Toronto Free Hospital for Consumptives admitted its first child patient, nine-year-old Joe Hawkins, on 13 July 1905.[100] Soon after, more young tuberculosis sufferers would join Hawkins at the sanatorium in space reserved for two children's wards in the main hospital building (see figure 1.1). A fire in December 1910 disrupted the sanatorium but led to significant restructuring and improvements in its wake. A large new building exclusively for children, the Queen Mary Hospital for Consumptive Children, opened alongside the new buildings for adults (the Toronto Free Hospital

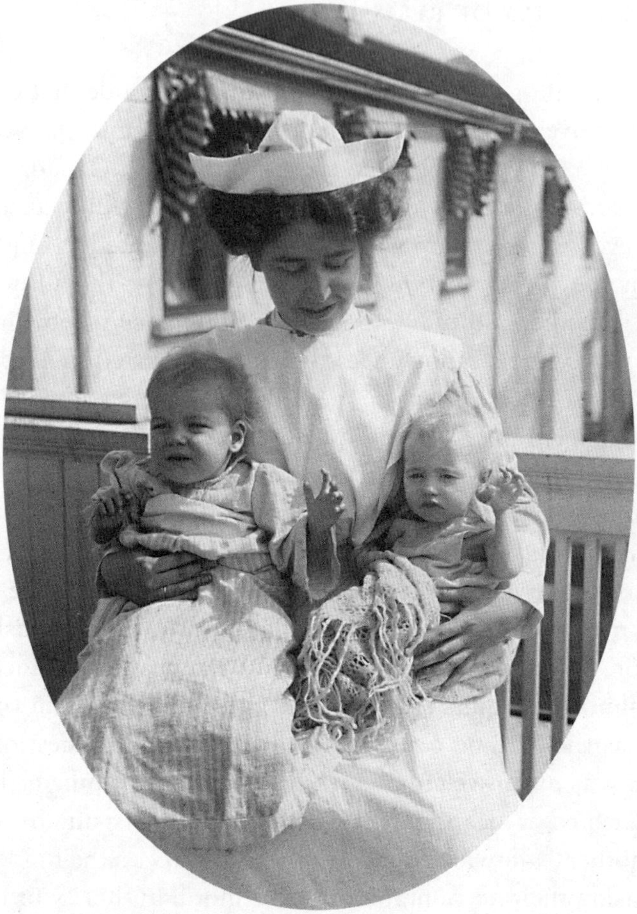

Figure 1.1 A nurse with two infant patients of the children's ward in the old Toronto Free Hospital for Consumptives before the 1910 fire.

for Consumptives and the King Edward Sanatorium) in June 1913. Though patients were housed separately (the Queen Mary for children, the King Edward for paying adults, the Free Hospital for non-paying adults), the buildings were located in close proximity on the same grounds and shared infrastructure, resources, and staff (see figure 1.2). I refer to them collectively as "the Toronto sanatorium." From its origins in 1904, the Toronto sanatorium was to provide sixty-eight years of specialized care for tuberculosis patients before the Sanatoria for Consumptives Act was repealed in 1972.[101]

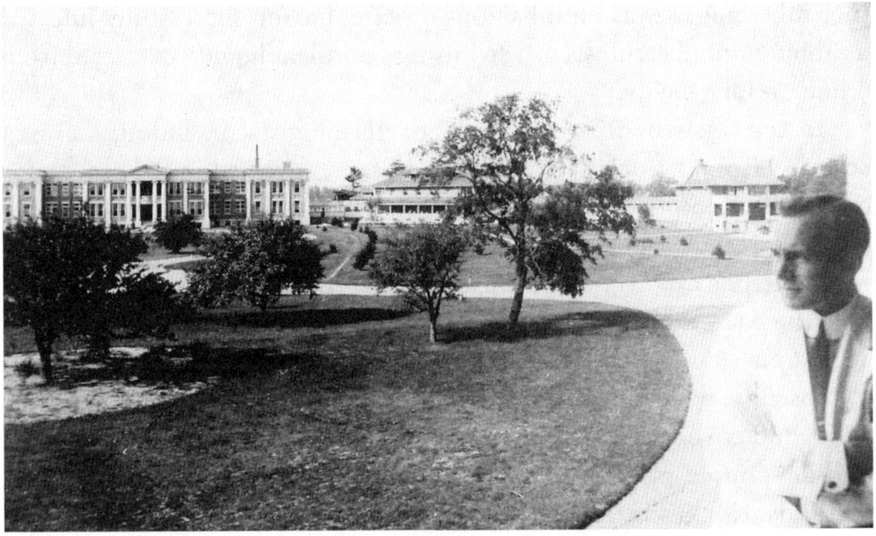

Figure 1.2 The view from the balcony of the Queen Mary Hospital for Consumptive Children. The Toronto Free Hospital for Consumptive's Main Medical (Prittie) Building (*left*), the King Edward Sanatorium (for paying patients) (*middle*), and the Administration Building (*right*).

The origins of the tuberculosis sanatorium movement have been traced to German physician Hermann Brehmer, who established the first sanatorium in Görbersdorf, Silesia, in 1854.[102] In Canada, the Toronto sanatorium was the second sanatorium complex established by the National Sanitarium Association (NSA), following the NSA's Muskoka hospitals: the Muskoka Cottage Hospital in 1897 and the Muskoka Free Hospital for Consumptives in 1902 (the NSA Muskoka sanatoria representing Canada's first movements towards hospitals for tuberculosis). When Brehmer opened his tuberculosis sanatorium in 1854 the underlying cause of tuberculosis was not known. The fact that the disease often decimated families suggested a hereditary disease, a belief popular in Northern Europe, but in Southern Europe suspicions were growing that tuberculosis might have infectious origins.[103] As early as 1790, Benjamin Marten had suggested that tuberculosis was caused by a species of "animalcula."[104] Jean-Antoine Villemin, who presented a paper at the Sorbonne in Paris in 1867, has been credited as the first to suggest explicitly that tuberculosis was an infectious disease, having successfully infected a rabbit with tuberculosis in 1865 using "purulent liquid" extracted from a human lung cavity.[105]

On the basis of these findings, bacteriologists, including German scientist Robert Koch (1843–1910), became invested in the search for evidence of pathogenic microbes.[106] In 1872, Koch's first wife, Emmy Fraatz, presented him with a microscope in celebration of his twenty-ninth birthday.[107] Making industrious use of his gift, Koch first examined the bacterium connected with anthrax disease in 1876.[108] Between 1877 and 1880, Koch developed new techniques for microbiology and microscopy, which, according to Alex Sakula, included the use of glass slides and cover slips, the fixation and staining of bacteria for contrast, and the poured-plate method of culturing bacteria.[109] In refining these methods, Koch was the first to successfully observe tuberculosis bacteria, *Mycobacterium tuberculosis*, under his microscope, firmly establishing the bacterial cause of tuberculosis in 1882.[110] The tuberculosis bacterium's outer waxy coat's resistance to typical staining methods used in the preparation of slides for microscopy had contributed to its elusiveness. Koch's staining method had met with success, but collaborator and fellow German scientist Paul Ehrlich greatly improved the technique in tuberculosis bacterium staining later in 1882 with the use of acid decolourising and heat.[111] In clinical settings, Ehrlich's staining innovations meant more ready identification of TB bacteria in patient samples and the promise of greater success in confirming tuberculosis diagnoses and states of infectiousness.[112]

Koch's findings were important in shaping a better understanding of tuberculosis, as an infectious disease, and in fuelling the public health movement to take action to reduce exposure to and transmission of tuberculosis bacteria. Clinically, however, his findings did not alter the fundamental truth that there was no cure for this infectious disease; while careful attention might reduce the risk of infection, once TB bacteria were in the body, they were most likely in the body for life. Koch isolated the tuberculosis bacterium in 1882, but it would not be until the early 1940s that promising antibiotic treatments for tuberculosis emerged. Medical historian Peter Warren has argued that very little changed in treatment during the first fifty years of the sanatorium era, from 1854 to 1904, despite the significant gain in understanding that tuberculosis was an infectious, not hereditary, disease.[113]

Even with the change in understanding, the idea of "resistance building" persevered, as relevant to building physiological resistance to a purported hereditary disease (pre-Koch) as it was to improving resistance to an infectious disease (post-Koch).[114] The absence of a cure for tuberculosis made resistance building all the more important and was a concept extended to infectious diseases more generally. In 1899, J.J. Cassidy, editor of the *Canadian Journal of Medicine and Surgery*, used the example of diphtheria to address the importance of bodily resistance to common pathogens and to emphasize the important difference between infection and disease. As Cassidy noted, "The mere existence of a germ in mucus, taken from a human throat, does not prove the existence of the disease."[115] In order for disease to manifest, "the power of resistance, naturally possessed by the individual, must first be lowered, before these microbes can penetrate the epithelium and the lymphatic glands, and elaborate their toxins."[116] Like diphtheria, in tuberculosis, infection did not equal disease, and powers of bodily resistance could mediate (or prevent altogether) the progression from infection to disease, so attention naturally turned to building those powers. The idea was particularly important in the early twentieth century, when much had come to be understood about infectious diseases, but prevention of infection was unlikely.

With tuberculosis now recognized as an infectious disease, twentieth-century attention would turn to diagnosing active cases of tuberculosis disease, and from the perspective of possible success in treatment, the earlier that a diagnosis could be confirmed, the better. The emphasis on early diagnosis would intensify over time, almost becoming the mantra of those in medicine and public health. According to medical historian Edward Shorter, new-found skills in diagnosis were an important strength in the evolving modern era of scientific medicine (represented by physicians educated at medical schools between the 1880s and 1940s).[117] Despite a growing awareness of the signs (that physicians interpreted) and symptoms (that patients experienced) of tuberculosis, however, it remained a challenging disease to diagnose. According to American TB specialist Edward Trudeau, early stages of tuberculosis disease could easily be misdiagnosed as "pleurisy, bronchitis, or malaria," most often "until hemoptysis, rapid emaciation, [and] marked hectic or cavitary signs appeared."[118] Knowledge of tuberculosis bacteria and the ability to see them in sputum samples of suspected cases via the microscope, and to see tuberculosis disease in the lungs via X-ray, were valuable technological allies assisting twentieth-century physicians in their diagnoses (with the understanding that these innovations were far from infallible, since not all tuberculosis sufferers produced bacteria-laced sputum, and X-rays could be ambiguous and misinterpreted).

In addition to the biological or technical challenges in diagnosing tuberculosis, there were a number of reasons why physicians might hesitate to pronounce a tuberculosis diagnosis, including the possibility that their patients would lose hope for recovery, and hope was a powerful emotion in the chronic disease of tuberculosis, especially in an era with no cure. Instead, physicians might choose to shroud their diagnoses in other, less frightening diseases such as bronchitis. Under those circumstances, suspicious and tuberculosis-conscious families might search in vain for physicians willing to give them a truthful diagnosis. One physician goes so far as to suggest that, "for months," ill health could linger with "cough, fever, loss of weight, the melancholy symptoms that go to make up this disease," but it was only when the situation became dire that they might "extract a confession from their physician" as to their suspected tuberculosis diagnosis.[119] Over time, this diagnostic elusiveness to spare the patient would give way to an understanding that early tuberculosis diagnoses were an advantage to patients and their families alike, enabling them to take action, perhaps to prevent the spread of infection to family members or seek earlier treatment. The evolving culture of scientific medicine would come to value the authority of "certainty"[120] in diagnoses, while patients and their families might find some modicum of comfort, not necessarily despair, in the confirmation of their tuberculosis suspicions and fears.

By the early twentieth century the tuberculosis sanatorium had entered the medical mainstream in Europe and North America and quickly gained a reputation as the most promising place for tuberculosis care and treatment. Peter Warren takes note of coverage in the *Lancet* as a measure of the rising acceptance of sanatoria.[121] A number of articles published in the *Lancet* in the first decade of the twentieth century actively encouraged new sanatorium construction through the publication of detailed architectural plans.[122] Collectively, sanatoria on both sides of the Atlantic shared an underlying goal to build patient resistance to tuberculosis through the fundamentals of fresh air and good nutrition, though particulars of the therapeutic use of bedrest and exercise could vary significantly. Warren suggests that the sanatorium's first half-century represented "one of the few times" following the rise of the germ theory "that Hygeia triumphed over Panacea in the treatment of a disease."[123] Hygeia and Panacea were the mythological daughters of Asklepios, Greek god of health and "father of medicine."[124] While Hygeia represented hygiene and disease prevention, Panacea represented cure (and cure was elusive in tuberculosis, hence Hygeia's triumph). Warren argues that early post-germ theory sanatorium treatment continued to embrace ancient principles, going back to Galen, the Roman Middle Ages physician, and his attention to "air, food and drink, rest and exercise, sleep, excretions, and state of mind" in treating disease.[125] As a result, early sanatorium treatment was slow and palliative in nature, attempting to build immunity and resistance to tuberculosis and to prevent or slow disease progression. In this way, the medical routine and rhythm of the early sanatorium era was quite different in practice, often passive in nature in contrast to the more "active" or action-oriented focus that modern medicine would come to embrace.[126] Sanatorium therapeutics did change over time, however, becoming much more action-oriented in the surgical years (as explored in chapter 6). Alongside Canadian sanatoria, public health extended resistance building into homes and communities. By 1908, there were anti-spitting by-laws, compulsory or voluntary notification of tuberculosis cases, disinfection of premises after death or removal of tuberculous sufferers, building inspections to ensure that living spaces afforded adequate light, space, and ventilation, milk inspections and the tuberculin testing of cattle herds, health inspections of school children, and the formation of local anti-tuberculosis organizations.[127]

Through these efforts, tuberculosis mortality rates declined in the first half of the twentieth century, but the reduction was complex. Changes in the overall health of bodies, nutrition, and housing, and the virulence of circulating tuberculosis bacterial strains must also be considered, as well as broad environmental changes within Canadian communities. Guy Tremblay, for example, has hypothesized that air pollution caused by coal burning (carbon monoxide) could have increased susceptibility to tuberculosis.[128] He has investigated the strong correlation between declining TB incidence and an increasing reliance on electricity, rather than polluting coal, to heat Canadian homes. In 1900, Canada's national tuberculosis mortality rate was estimated at somewhere between 180 to 200 deaths per 100,000,[129] a rate comparable to England and Wales (180.5 per 100,000) and the United States (196.9 per 100,000).[130] By 1933, well before antibiotic cures, the rate in Canada had already declined to 41.6 deaths per 100,000.[131] In the province of Ontario, the tuberculosis mortality rate had fallen further to 25 per 100,000 in 1946 (see figure 1.3) In 1924, in the midst of this decline, Toronto physician J.H. Elliott targeted the effects of public health efforts in "the improvement of living conditions, the better scale of living generally seen, better hygiene, sufficient food, [and] lessened hours of labour" bringing about "a higher degree of resistance to the disease" or lessening "the development of those conditions of debility and disease which reactivate a quiescent [latent] focus."[132] The decline of tuberculosis in Canada was uneven, however, and Indigenous communities in Canada continue to experience alarmingly high rates of infection and mortality.[133]

The focus on the home in public health work was important, since most Canadians in the early twentieth century would experience tuberculosis infection, disease, and death at home. Hospitals were still a novel phenomenon for most Canadians in the first half of the twentieth century. Smith and Nickel identify the years following the First World War as a turning point in Canadian hospital history, when deaths and births began to move into hospitals with increasing frequency, a trend that would intensify following the Second World War.[134] Sanatorium beds were severely limited in comparison to the actual number of tuberculosis sufferers, so the family home remained the principal place for the care of the tuberculous. Public health workers and a growing body of advice literature attempted to educate families on how to properly prepare for this role. *Health Knowledge: A Thorough and Concise Knowledge of the Prevention, Causes, and Treatments of Disease, Simplified for Home Use*, a 1928 American publication, offered specific advice on appointing

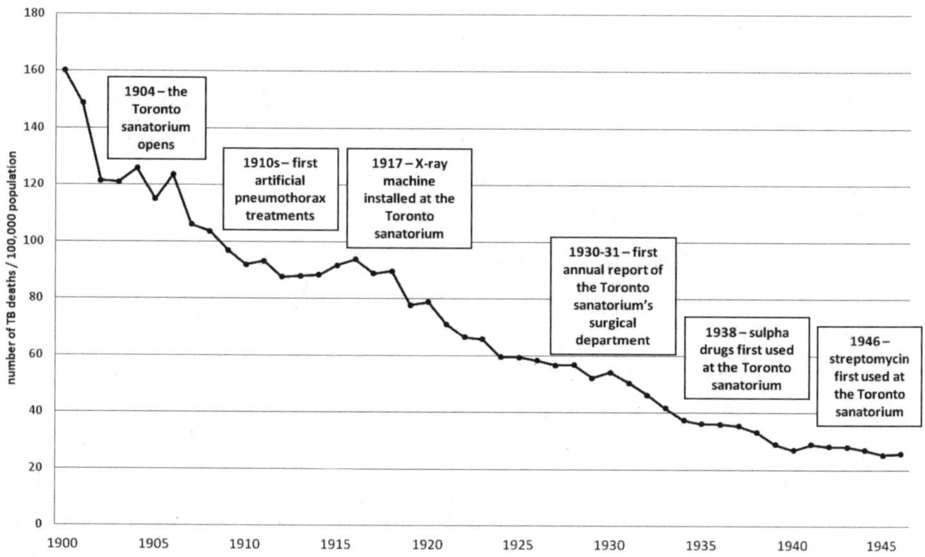

Figure 1.3 Tuberculosis mortality rate in Ontario, 1900–1946

the type of "sickroom" that tuberculosis sufferers should be provided with at home, provided the family had the means.[135] Large and sunny rooms outfitted with dark curtains or blinds were preferred. Since ventilation was important, with windows to be left open as much as possible, a coal fire was recommended to warm the sickroom (perhaps problematic, given Tremblay's perspective on the hazards of coal burning). Heavy curtains and carpeting were best avoided, since both were difficult to clean and disinfect. A long, single iron bed would suffice, best kept away from the walls so that those nursing the patient could easily access all sides of the bed.[136] Dark wallpaper or wall colourings were not recommended. Instead, a light green wall colour, believed to be the "most universally soothing colour," was advised, while red was the most objectionable. Homes were expected to stock common sickroom equipment, such as feeding-cups, thermometers, rubber sheets, air-cushions (to place under the patient's back), bed pans, and spittoons (which could be china cups with lids, or spitting flasks).

As to the actual functioning of the sickroom, *Health Knowledge* had an unambiguously gendered perspective; in home nursing, it was argued, mothers or sisters "would be best qualified to undertake the care of the invalid," since they were perceived as the ones "in the home to whom all naturally turn for the satisfaction of their most intimate personal needs," possessing "an understanding mind, a delicate and ready tact," and a "power of apprehending and supplying wants."[137] As to temperament and demeanour, home nurses were advised to "guard against noise and fuss," "move about quietly and lightly," "lift things firmly but quietly," and "speak in a quiet voice, but never in a whisper, as that is very irritating to a patient."[138] Every task in the sickroom was to be done thoroughly and punctually. Above all else, the sickroom was to be a place of utmost discretion.[139] Illness was expected in the family home, and caregivers were best to be prepared for it. In the event that sufferers died at home, as was common in the early twentieth century, *Health Knowledge* offered advice on the preparation of the body, with the understanding that "the nurse who has nursed her patient through the last illness will esteem it a privilege to perform the last simple offices."[140]

Given the shortage of beds in hospitals and sanatoria and the overwhelming number of tuberculosis sufferers, medical practitioners agreed that patients in need only of the three fundamentals (fresh air, good food, and rest) could be successfully nursed at home, particularly when family members were educated on tuberculosis, and homes were suitably appointed to support the patient and protect the health of other family members. In 1912, Toronto physician F.S. Minns provided some tuberculosis-specific home nursing advice in the medical journal *Canadian Practitioner*. He warned of the dangers of disease transmission, recommending that children not be allowed into the patient's sickroom (to protect the child from TB infection, but also to protect the patient from any infectious diseases that children might unwittingly bring into the sickroom).[141] Isolation could be achieved with a separate bedroom, an enclosed veranda, or a balcony (for examples from the city of Toronto, see figures 1.4–1.10). Though they were convenient, popular, and relatively inexpensive, Minns did not recommend the use of tents or shacks, mostly because he believed that they tended to be poorly ventilated. Nevertheless, the use of tents persisted because they were the easiest and least costly option.

In reality, most poor and working-class homes would have been challenged to provide the kind of care that TB specialists were recommending in home nursing. Limited means and overcrowding sometimes resulted in

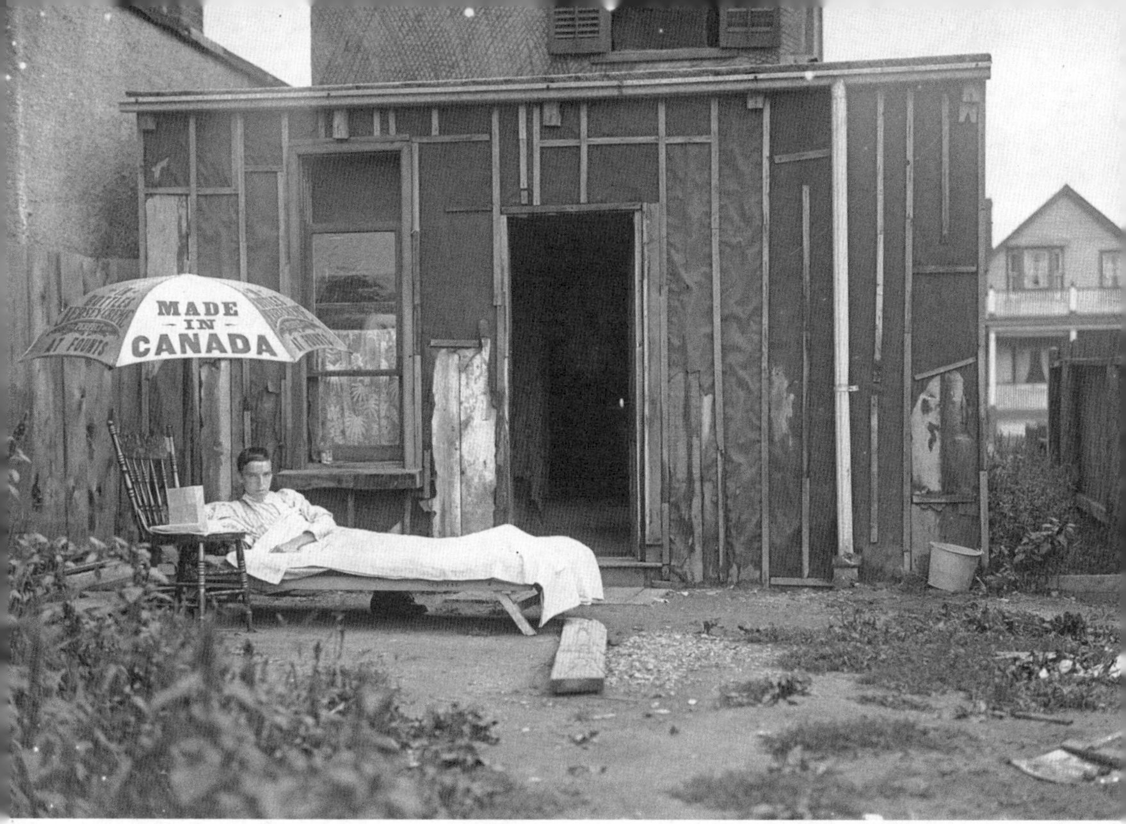

Figure 1.4 A tuberculous boy taking the cure at home in the city of Toronto because he refused admission to the sanatorium. The boy was provided with a cot and umbrella by the city's Health Department, the minimum essentials for taking rest outside in the fresh air. According to the Health Department's notation, he later died of tuberculosis at the Toronto sanatorium. The photograph is dated 6 September 1912.

communal bedrooms and bed-sharing by adults and children (see figure 1.11). As a result, simply arranging separate space for tuberculous family members would have been difficult if not impossible. In an article in *Canadian Practitioner*, the Toronto sanatorium's physician-in-chief, Dr Dobbie, advised physicians in the use of "ordinary plain food" for home-nursed tuberculosis patients, a typical daily diet for adults in 1911 consisting of six glasses of milk, six ounces of porridge, seven slices of bread and butter, nine ounces of meat, twelve ounces of soup, four ounces of potatoes, four ounces of vegetables, two ounces of milk pudding, and one cup of milk coffee.[142] Despite its simplicity, the recommended diet may well have been beyond the means of many poor and working-class families, at least with any degree of regularity. In Montreal, Poutanen and colleagues note that

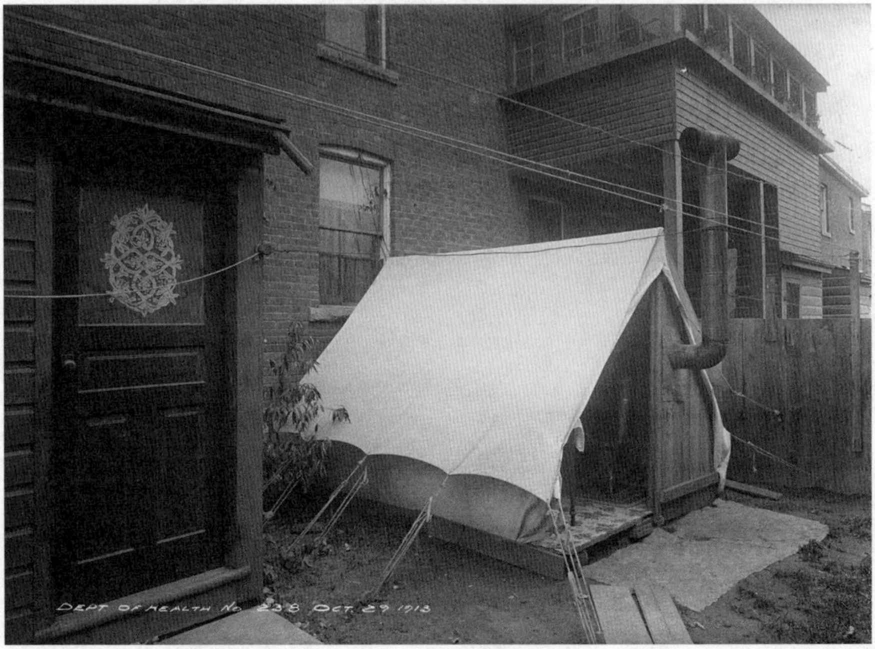

Figure 1.5 A tuberculosis sufferer's tent for fresh air and isolation at home in Toronto. The tent was equipped with a stove for heat, an electrical connection for light, and a bell to call for assistance. According to the Health Department notation, this tent was used by a former sanatorium patient. The photograph is dated 29 October 1913.

more affluent households often had domestic help, could hire home nurses, and could afford to bring their family physicians to their homes, while, on the other hand, chronically ill renters unable to hold on to a job and earn a living were vulnerable to serial evictions.[143] Even the simple recommendation to place beds close to open windows for fresh air ventilation "in a Montreal winter meant paying more for heat, clothing, blankets, and food."[144]

Worse, perhaps, than prescribing treatments or diets beyond a family's means was to experience genuinely bad advice from physicians. Among Canadian doctors, at least in the first decade or two of the twentieth century, there was great diversity in the understanding of tuberculosis and its recommended treatments, and a lack of consensus over what should be communicated to families. In her article published in the *Canadian Journal of Public Health* in 1913, Toronto tuberculosis sufferer Marion Marshall candidly recalled the treatments attempted with her tuberculous

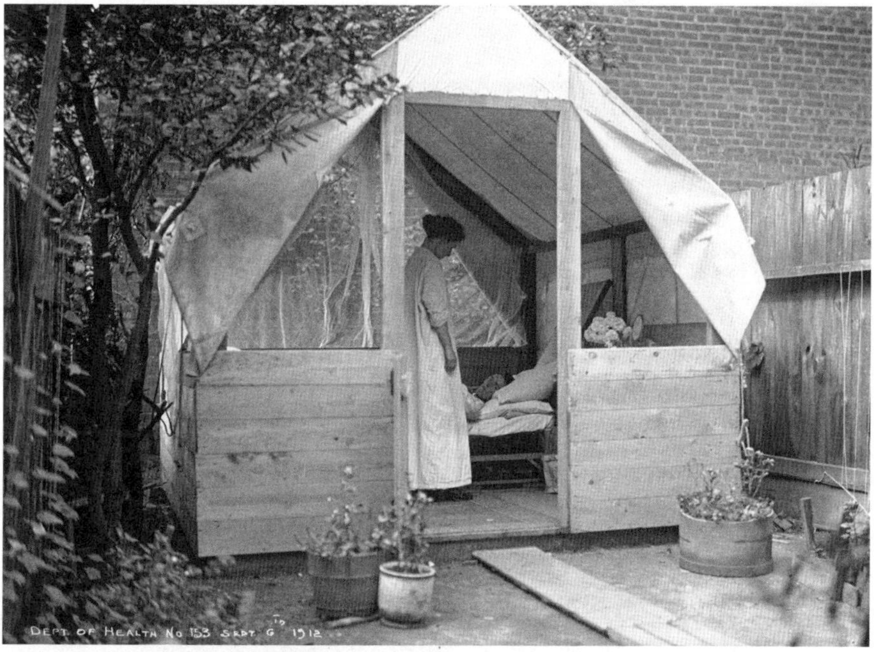

Figure 1.6 A Toronto Health Department visit with George B., a Toronto tuberculosis sufferer, in his backyard tent on 6 September 1912. This kind of tent, also known as a tent shack, was part wood and part canvas. To address ventilation concerns, the canvas could be rolled back to permit the unobstructed circulation of fresh air.

family and the lack of helpful information forthcoming from the medical professionals they had consulted.[145] In the end, she blamed her family's Toronto physician and his poor treatment choices for her family's decimation. Describing her brother's case, the doctor, in whom the family had held a "fatal confidence," had prescribed a number of "old-fashioned remedies," beginning with "gymnastic exercises for the development of the chest."[146] Her ailing brother had used "dumb-bells and clubs for some hours daily, so long as his waning strength permitted this violent and no doubt harmful exercise." Cod liver oil was prescribed "by the quart," and Marion described how her brother's digestive tract soon became "badly disordered" as a result. At the same time, however, she wrote, "Not a word was said to us, by the various doctors whom we consulted, about taking the patient's temperature or pulse, or regarding the necessity of rest in the open air." In her brother's case, "they warned us against damp air and night air," and, as a result, her brother "was

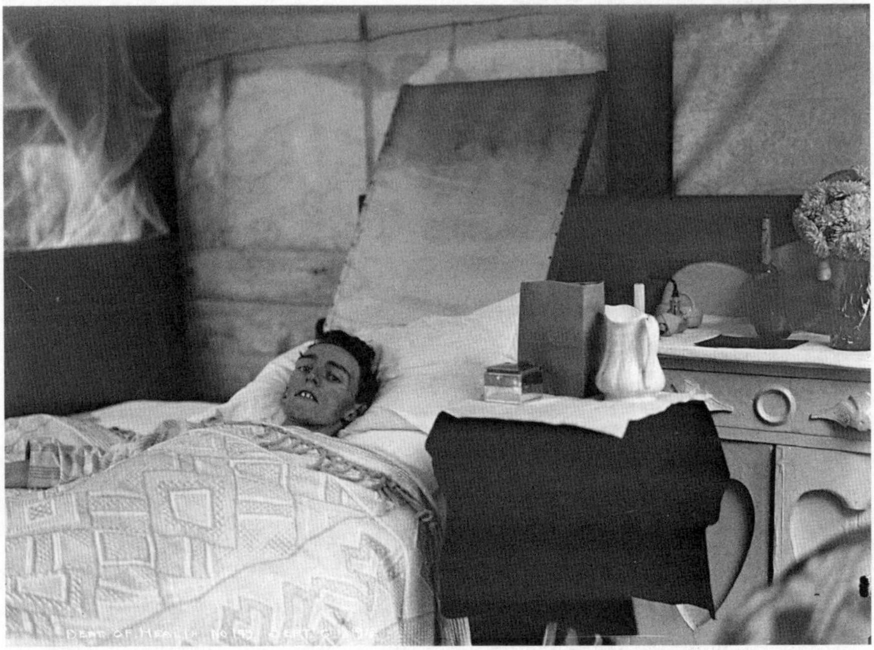

Figure 1.7 The interior of George B.'s tent, appointed with domestic comforts such as the bed, tasselled bedspread, dresser, and cut flowers in a vase. The bedside table holds a sputum cup, a paper bag for waste, and a pitcher, for water perhaps. This photograph was dated 6 September 1912. According to Toronto's death registry, B., twenty-four years old, died of tuberculosis and asthenia (extreme physical weakness) only five days later, on 11 September 1912. In this photograph, B. has the pale and emaciated appearance characteristic of advanced tuberculosis sufferers.

rarely out of doors except on fine days and then he would often walk until exhausted under the false impression that such exercise would help to restore his lessening strength."[147] Prevailing tensions in medicine concerning prescriptions of rest versus exercise, experienced first-hand by Marshall's family, are investigated further in chapter 5.

With the rise of the sanatorium era in Canada and the growing popularity of the "rest cure" in managing tuberculosis, "old-fashioned treatment by medicines" would gradually fall into disfavour.[148] As evident in Marion's brother's case, cod liver oil[149] was traditionally recommended as a treatment or cure, as was creosote,[150] whiskey, and morphine. One

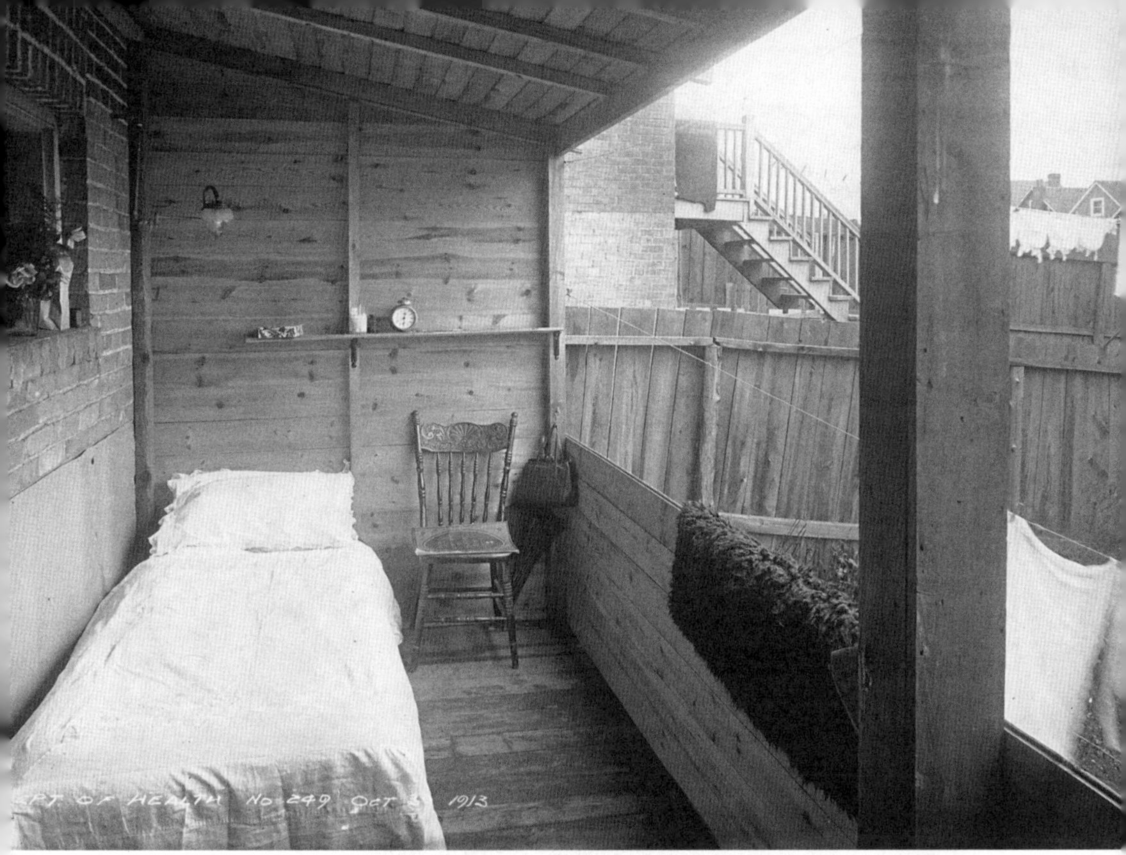

Figure 1.8 A covered porch used for fresh air resting by a tuberculosis sufferer. A clock, box of tissues, and drinking glass are positioned on the shelf above the pressed-back chair, while cut flowers in vases sit in the windowsill above the cot. The photograph is dated 3 October 1913.

early twentieth-century Canadian physician opined that he had "absolutely no faith" in any such treatments, "because I have not yet found one that did the slightest good."[151] At best, he felt, creosote, guaiacol carbonate,[152] and iodoform[153] "may do no harm," but were equally likely to cause a "fatal disturbance in the digestion, destroying the sheet anchor of our hope," food and good nutrition being "the main channel through which ... we hope to build up our patient, and so increase his resistance" to tuberculosis.[154] This particular physician really only supported of the use of strychnine (a poison), for "its tonic and stimulant action," and heroin for minimizing tuberculosis's troublesome and disturbing cough and encouraging sleep.[155]

Long walks in the open air and prescriptions for "the 'Weather-Chaser,' as the travelling invalid is called,"[156] to "Go West" or "Go

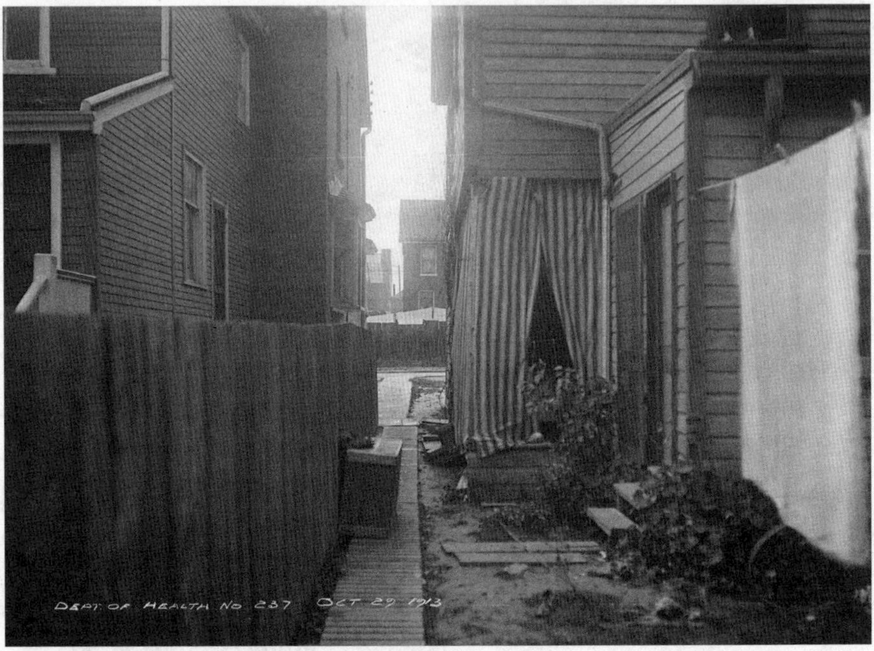

Figure 1.9 This home was photographed by Toronto's Health Department on 29 October 1913, providing an example of an improvised tent for a patient with far advanced tuberculosis who was being isolated at home.

South" (in search of more salubrious climates) was common advice provided by both physicians and home medicine texts such as *The Practical Home Physician*.[157] Sea travel, and the seasickness that came with it, was another popularly recommended treatment, borne out of traditional medicine's beliefs that vomiting (typically achieved through the use of emetics) was therapeutic because it helped to rid the body of poisons. Travel to high altitude was also recommended in tuberculosis, because of the rarity ("thinness" of oxygen), purity, and dryness of the air and its physiological stimulation of the body, encouraging chest expansion with fuller and deeper breathing.[158] In high altitude settings such as the Canadian Rockies, the climate was felt to be "stimulating," increasing appetites and weight gain, increasing "resistance to the action of micro-organisms," and, significantly, favouring an "expansion in lung capacity."[159] Always seeking a physiological explanation, one Kamloops, BC, physician argued that "for most cases altitude is highly beneficial, the rare atmosphere increasing metabolism, and calling for increased expansion of the lung tissue."[160]

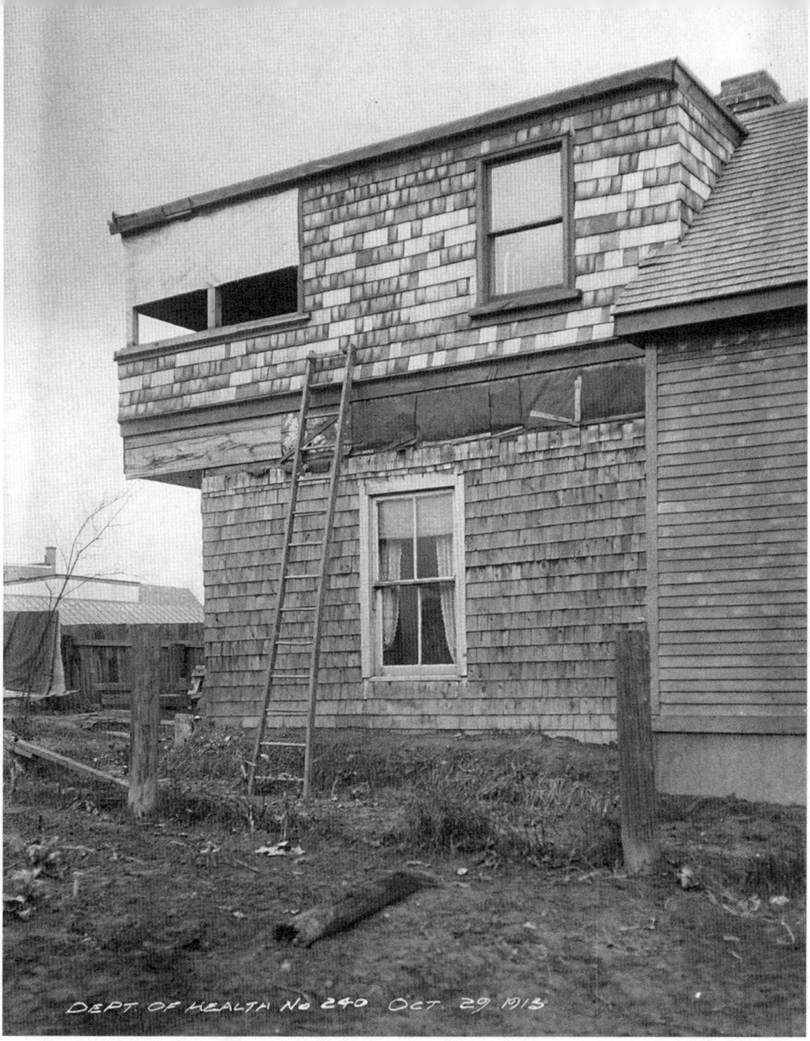

Figure 1.10 A second-floor sleeping porch built for a former sanatorium patient in the Earlscourt neighbourhood of Toronto, 29 October 1913.

While ineffective patent medicines seemed to offer fleeting hope for a few dollars, the "cure" of strict bedrest, particularly when prescribed for breadwinners and families already living in poverty, could be financially devastating, as recommendations for months (if not years) of rest seriously undermined or completely precluded the ability to work. Adults were forced to balance their limitations in illness with their responsibilities to meet family needs, and the emotional strain could be tormenting. As a "tedious"[161] or chronic disease that could stubbornly persist in an active state or threaten to reactivate at any point in life, the cure treatment exacted a heavy lifetime cost on individuals and families.

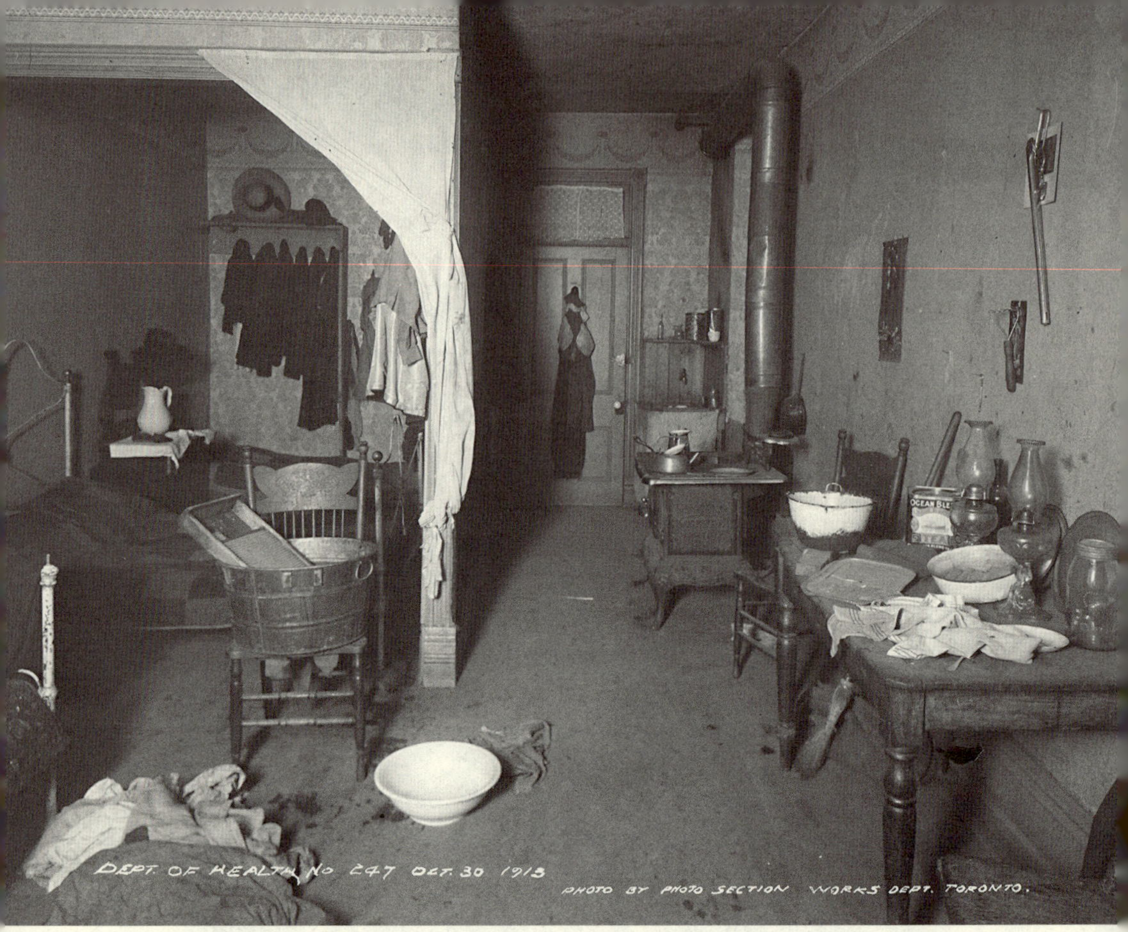

Figure 1.11 An example of a family's one-room dwelling, photographed by Toronto's Health Department in a poor Toronto neighbourhood, 30 October 1913.

What was perhaps the most distressing to Marion Marshall, however, was the fact that none of the physicians the family consulted had ever suggested anything of the infectious nature of tuberculosis. As a result, the family had not been educated on how to reduce the risks of transmission, and Marshall details the devastating result:

> The hideous disease … in ghastly succession destroyed my brother, father, mother and elder sister … we were not warned about the danger of infection, and I marvel at the fact that any members of our ill-starred family are alive, when I remember that my father was allowed to sleep with my brother almost to the end; that the sputum was not properly cared for, and that the house was never disinfected, no, not even after the various deaths which followed one another

> in a more or less rapid succession. In the light of my present knowledge of the disease, I shudder to recall that cloths used for receptacles of my brother's sputum,[162] were washed out by my mother to be ready for use again, and that for months this faithful little woman performed this loathsome task.[163]

The proper management of sputum was of particular concern in tuberculosis, since matter raised from the lungs, particularly in cavitary lung disease, was likely to contain tuberculosis bacteria. Tuberculosis patients were advised not to swallow the sputum they brought up, over concerns that this might lead to infection of their gastrointestinal tracts. Nor, of course, was the careless spitting of sputum to be tolerated. Across sanatoria and in educated homes, the use of sputum collectors became ingrained, a big part of the material culture of tuberculosis, although there was great variation in their design. Sputum collectors of a disposable variety became far more popular than handkerchiefs or other vessels that required washing, since that led to an undesirable level of exposure for caregivers (such as Marion's mother). At the sanatorium, a hinged-lid, metal frame box with a simple handle and waxed cardboard insert (that could be removed from the metal box, incinerated, and replaced with a new insert) was preferred for sputum collecting and was often referred to by patients more endearingly as a "bug box" or a "music box" (see figures 1.12a and 1.12b) The waxed paper inserts were manufactured by the "Burnitol ['Burn-it-All'] Manufacturing Co." At the Kentville sanatorium in Nova Scotia, on the other hand, Ripley recounts that "when patients were admitted to the San, the first gift presented by staff was a box of disposable tissues which they were drilled to use and discard in a paper bag pinned to their beds."[164] Ripley notes the paper bags were known as "bug bags" and were "collected daily, packed in sawdust and burned to reduce the possibility of circulating germs."

Returning to Marion's embittered experience, some physicians did not even tell patients or their families when they suspected a diagnosis of tuberculosis, let alone educate them on the dangers of transmission.[165] Barbara Bates has argued that, because of tensions within medicine, American tuberculosis specialists, in promoting their rising specialty, were sometimes critical of general practitioners for their delayed diagnoses

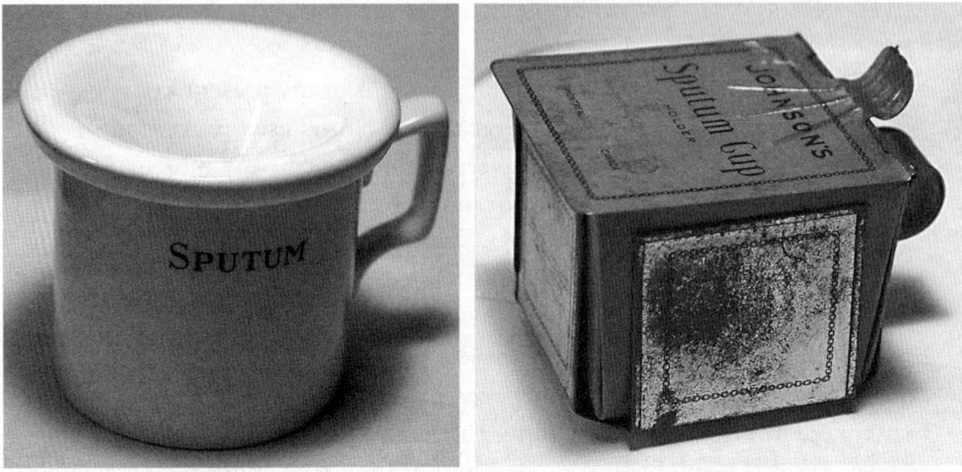

Figure 1.12 Examples of washable (*left*) and disposable (*right*) sputum cups. The disposable version was favoured at the NSA sanatoria because it minimized exposure to sputum. Photographed is Johnson's Sputum Cup Holder (manufactured by Johnson & Johnson Limited, Montreal). The front side of the cup reads, "Card with user's name may be slipped between the side grooves" so that patients could identify their own sputum cups. The cardboard insert is a no. 7 sputum cup manufactured by the Burnitol Manufacturing Co. out of Boston, Chicago, and San Francisco. "To be Certain – Burn-it-All" is inscribed on the upper margins of all four sides of the insert.

and referrals, for their prescriptions of ineffective yet costly "palliative medicines such as cough mixtures, opium, and alcohol" (lucrative for the general practitioners, since they often prepared and sold these remedies themselves),[166] and for their seeming unwillingness to embrace new scientific cures.[167] Marshall concludes that if her family had "been guided by a medical man who knew his business, all of our dear ones might be alive to-day, even … the poor, lame laddie, for he put up a good long fight under adverse circumstances."[168] Had her brother, like Marion herself, been provided with sanatorium care, she suspected, he would have had a "fine chance" of recovery. Ultimately, spreading the word about the symptoms and infectious nature of tuberculosis was not left to physicians, but was a role largely assumed in the work of the Canadian Association for the Prevention of Tuberculosis. By 1916, the association had distributed thousands of pamphlets, books, and leaflets on topics such as ventilation and treatment, and was fielding regular requests to provide tuberculosis exhibits at schools and county fairs.[169]

In comparison to the earlier and more palliative years of the sanatorium era, by the 1920s treatments were becoming increasingly medicalized. The timing is not unexpected, given the advances made in medicine in tandem with the First World War and in the years that followed. The core principles of tuberculosis care still followed along Galenic lines, but more involved interventions were also being explored. Returning to Peter Warren's symbolism, Panacea, or active attempts to cure patients of tuberculosis, became more apparent in the second half of the sanatorium era. The shift to active interventions was gradual, beginning with compression therapies such as artificial pneumothorax, Carlos Forlanini's innovation introduced to North America after 1910, but then also progressing to more active procedures such as rib removal surgeries (see chapter 6). The height of Panacea, true cure, came in the 1940s with the introduction of antibiotics intended to destroy tuberculosis bacteria, and not just mediate their activity in the body through various therapies and treatments. Because of evolving bacterial drug-resistance the victory would prove time-limited, so current attentions have now returned to the idea of strengthening the body and its immune response through immunotherapy.[170]

Up to the 1920s, both preventoria (institutions meant to build up vulnerable children who did not have active disease but were positive for TB infection) and sanatoria (for the treatment of children with active TB disease) were popular and garnered much support from physicians, especially in cases where children were living in homes with infectious adults who continued to cough or expectorate carelessly. "Sometimes the best course in such cases," suggested Dr Holbrook of the Hamilton sanatorium in 1920, "will prove to be to take the children out of the home, and for this the preventorium for purposes of protection and the children's department of the sanatorium for active disease in childhood will more and more be called into use."[171] By the 1930s, however, some debate had surfaced within the medical community regarding the merits of hospitalizing children with uncomplicated primary tuberculosis disease.[172] Primary disease was often relatively symptomless and self-limited. While children with primary disease were typically not infectious, concerns focused on the possibility that their disease might progress, and those fears would linger, as children who had experienced primary disease remained vulnerable to reactivation disease throughout their lives. Reactivation disease represents the classical picture of pulmonary tuberculosis, often with sputum raising, productive coughs, sometimes accompanied by hemorrhaging because of festering tuberculous cavities in affected lungs. As sanatorium attention began to shift away from children with uncomplicated primary disease, more beds could be freed up for a greater number of infectious reactivation disease sufferers, moving them out of their homes and communities and into sanatoria.

Around this time, as public health infrastructure in Ontario was maturing, tuberculosis specialists such as Dr Dobbie, the long-standing physician-in-chief of the Toronto sanatorium, believed that, with proper support, family homes, and not sanatoria or other institutions, were likely the best place for children with uncomplicated primary disease. Dobbie advocated greater support so that children could be cared for at home, particularly since hospitalization was a costly intervention for children who did not require specialized medical and nursing care. "If the home is satisfactory," Dobbie argued, "institutional care is not indicated. If the home is not satisfactory, is it not the duty of welfare agencies to endeavour to make it so instead of institutionalizing the children who, it is granted, are undoubtedly improved in general health after such care but on discharge return to the home in which conditions are as unsatisfactory as before the child was taken away?"[173] "The sanatoria," Dobbie concluded with certainty in 1935, "are not more important than are the homes."[174]

With the rise of antibiotic drug treatments in the 1940s and 1950s and a continuing decline in the number of TB cases reported in Ontario, other reconceptualizations of the role of sanatoria also emerged. At the origins of the rise of the sanatorium era in Ontario, sanatoria had rarely been viewed as places of quarantine. Even as early as 1873, with the passing of the first Public Health Act in Ontario, health officers and local boards of health in the province had been given the authority to remove any persons suffering from "serious contagious diseases" to hospitals.[175] Given the endemic nature of tuberculosis, however, and its widespread presence in the province, the disease was not a good candidate for quarantine, and these powers were likely more often exercised for acute, epidemic diseases such as cholera, smallpox, diphtheria, and typhoid. While there would be benefits to households if infectious members were admitted to sanatoria, hospitalization for tuberculosis at the National Sanitarium Association sanatoria had always been voluntary, with patients able to leave at any point, shedding tuberculosis bacteria or not. Furthermore, because of the nature of tuberculosis, both "common and chronic," with some sufferers experiencing a long-standing and ongoing active and infective disease process, it was well recognized by Canadian physicians that this disease, unlike other acute infectious diseases, could not be "handled" by health authorities with the use of quarantine.[176] For some, this would have meant an unimaginable lifetime of quarantine.

By 1949, however, with antibiotics, ideas on the possibilities of quarantine were changing within the context of overall declining rates of tuberculosis disease. An editorial in the *Canadian Medical Association Journal* pointed to the availability of about three to four sanatorium beds per tuberculosis death in Canada.[177] It was argued that if this number could be increased to about ten beds per death, that would make it possible to institutionally segregate "every patient in Canada with active tuberculosis," since "any patient who is expectorating tubercle bacilli is a potential hazard to his community, and under ideal conditions should certainly be segregated so that danger of his spreading the disease may be averted."[178] It appears that as tuberculosis became less common, the stigma of tuberculosis sufferers as identifiable infectious community "hazards" became more apparent and motivations towards segregation and quarantine intensified.

Science, Medicine, and the Sanatorium

As an anthropologist interested in infectious diseases and the rise of modern, scientific medicine (also known as "biomedicine"), I undertook this research to explore the experience of child tuberculosis sufferers who grew up in a time when tuberculosis was a common and familiar disease. The focus of this case study is a sample of child patients who were admitted to the Toronto sanatorium, their biographies (their lives both inside and outside of the sanatorium, as shaped by tuberculosis infection and disease), and their tuberculous bodies (as investigated, interpreted, and treated by modern medicine). Misdiagnosed cases aside for the moment, the majority of the children admitted to the sanatorium shared in the reality of tuberculosis infection, though their disease experiences could vary significantly. I try to locate their experiences outside of the sanatorium before entering the hospital, or after their discharge, provided the documentary insights exist. But, for the most part, their biographies unfold within the sanatorium, following their trials with tuberculosis, the sanatorium regimen and medical treatments, and their social relationships with staff and other patients. As much as possible, I focus on the patients' perceptions of experience, but their experiences are often understood through their connections and interactions with others, such as doctors, nurses, parents, and guardians. Many of the life stories of children who were patients in the sanatorium intersect with tuberculosis, survival, death, hospitalization, and family fragmentation or demise. Patients and families looked for "hope" at the sanatorium or, at the very least, the "truth" of the health crisis at hand. This book attempts to explore how these hopes and truths were negotiated and lived by child patients and their families.

Through this work, the exploration of patients and their interactions with modern medicine provides a means to understand why certain treatments were favoured at the sanatorium and what biological cues guided their use. The very status of patients' bodies (whether relatively healthy or not) would ultimately influence the nature of those interactions – their admissions, the length of their hospitalizations, through to the type of care and treatments they would receive at the sanatorium. Most of the children documented in this book would survive tuberculosis and live long lives, but the reality was that some would not. Understanding this context, this book embraces the diversity in their experiences and stories. In exploring the sanatorium-era medical treatments, I am interested in tracing the changing understanding of anatomy and physiology, the biologically grounded rationales for various treatments, and the explanations for treatments as provided to patients, or more often in the case of children, their families. The book is ultimately biosocial in its grounding, with a specific interest in the intertwining of social and biological dynamics in tuberculosis. The biology of the body and tuberculosis is understood via scientific principles, but there was an interpretive aspect based on experience, education, and beliefs – both among sanatorium patients (or their families) and their physicians. Since physicians were still learning about how the body functioned in variable states of health and disease, there was ample room for discussion and disagreement. The public was also learning about infectious diseases and microbes through the work of public health, visiting nurses, and family physicians. Ultimately, however, there was no simple truth, no single treatment that was unanimously upheld to successfully treat tuberculosis. Chapters 5 and 6 explore how physicians made sense of tuberculosis treatment, how they explained these treatments to their patients and families, and how and why patients, in turn, experienced the treatments.

Modern, scientific medicine (biomedicine) is embodied in the rise of the modern hospital, what van der Geest and Finkler refer to as "the premier institution of biomedicine."[179] The rise of modern hospitals and the intertwining of medicine and science in these institutions have received much attention from those interested in general hospitals, asylums, and tuberculosis sanatoria.[180] Hospitals have not always been explicitly linked with science, particularly those that existed before the twentieth century as charitable institutions, primarily for the poor or the "friendless," who had limited options for support in illness. In Toronto, this phenomenon is readily observed in the work of Elizabeth McMaster and the opening of Toronto's Hospital for Sick Children in 1875, a time "well before hospitals were transformed into institutions of medical science and became the domain of physicians."[181] The fairly recent birth of the "cultural invention" of biomedicine has been traced to nineteenth-century Germany and France as the art of medicine aligned with emerging scientific methodologies, laboratory investigation, and the rising germ theory of disease.[182] Biomedicine visibly entered into hospitals with the technological accoutrements of science, the use of antiseptics and aseptic technique, anaesthetics, and surgical refinements, building the momentum towards the modern hospital's role and reputation.[183] Certainly, by the 1920s, the transformation was evident, though the appearances of hospitals could be deceiving. According to architectural historian Annmarie Adams, Canadian hospitals built in the 1920s were "thoroughly modern," though they tended to cloak their science and "technological fetishism" outwardly in "historicist guises" in order to appeal to the familiar and soften the feel of modern medicine.[184]

As science and medicine began to align in Canada in the late 1800s, the partnership would affect the twentieth-century rise of modern hospitals that was to come. The opening of the Toronto sanatorium in 1904 is early in this transition, though it can still be firmly seated within the context of the rise of biomedicine. While the early years of the sanatorium focused on models of palliative care embracing rest, nutrition, and fresh air, the very presence of a laboratory at the Toronto sanatorium reveals its underlying biomedical orientation. According to the National Sanitarium Association's annual report for 1904–05, the Toronto sanatorium's first year of operation, laboratory supplies claimed $82.44 of the sanatorium's operating costs, an amount that certainly pales in comparison to the $4,606.67 spent on food, milk, cream, tea, and coffee, but is nonetheless significant in confirming the laboratory's existence.[185] As Godfrey Gale emphasized in his history of the Toronto sanatorium, "From its inception it was planned that the Sanatorium at Weston should provide not only good medical and nursing care, but also laboratory facilities for the scientific study of tuberculosis and for research."[186] While cures may have eluded sanatorium doctors, they could isolate and observe tuberculosis bacteria through careful laboratory investigations of patient sputum, blood, and urine samples (see figure 1.13). Guinea pigs, naturally highly susceptible to tuberculosis infection and disease, were the laboratory animals of choice and regularly inoculated with materials sampled from sanatorium patients, à la Koch and Koch's postulates, to confirm tuberculosis diagnoses.[187]

In her social history of tuberculosis in Pennsylvania, Barbara Bates notes the 1903 opening of the Phipps Institute in Philadelphia, a scientific research institute that housed a dispensary, hospital, and laboratory. The institute was intended for the study of advanced-stage tuberculosis disease, and patients admitted to the hospital provided the "materials" for laboratory investigation.[188] As Bates notes, "To the earlier goals of saving souls, relieving bodily suffering, and curing consumptives were now added the hope of conquering the disease through scientific investigation."[189] Staffing the early laboratory proved challenging, however, as

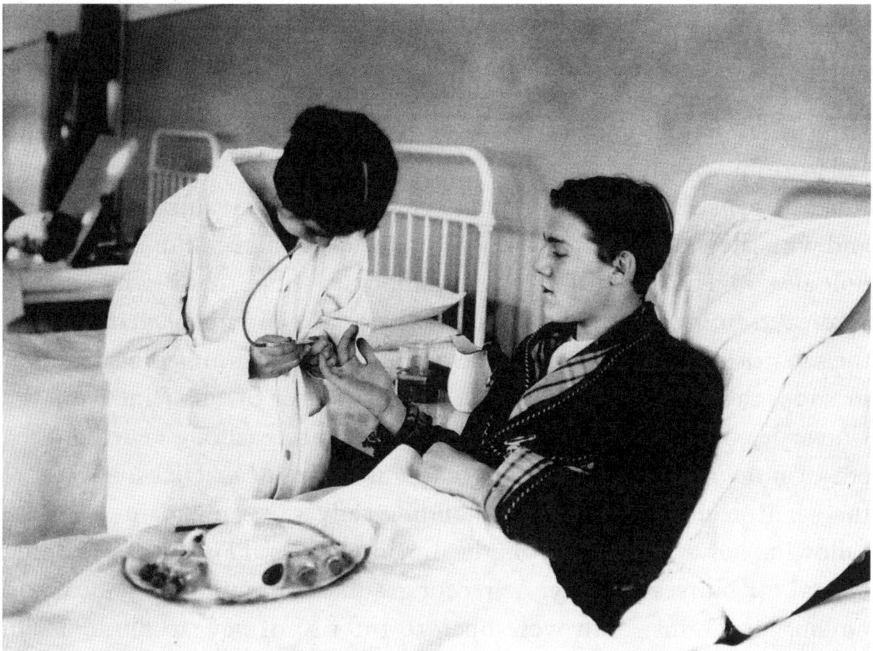

Figure 1.13 A laboratory technician on the patient ward taking a blood sample. Laboratory analysis was an important aspect of scientific medicine.

most recent physician graduates had little practical training in bacteriology and clinical pathology, at the time considered "the new laboratory sciences."[190] Autopsies were another important feature of the Phipps Institute, built into its scientific mandate, as patients would be admitted for care at the hospital only if their guardians gave consent for postmortem investigations (which, Bates notes, they could circumvent by discharging morbidly ill patients before their deaths). The Phipps Institute was meant not only to treat patients, but also to learn as much about tuberculosis disease as possible. According to Bates, autopsies were the subject of regular Monday evening meetings, requiring the attending physician "to draw on a blackboard a meticulous diagram of what he had found on physical examination." He would then have to "predict the abnormalities that the pathologist would report" and "any discrepancies between the clinical picture and the pathological findings had then to be explained by the physician."[191] This particular aspect of scientific investigation was also present at the Toronto sanatorium for, as Godfrey Gale notes, "an autopsy room was also set aside" to further the opportunities for research into the bodily effects of tuberculosis disease.[192]

From laboratory and autopsy facilities, the connections of the Toronto sanatorium with science and biomedical innovation strengthened over time, a transition reflected in the changing sanatorium architecture and with the ongoing introduction of new medical techniques and technologies.[193] This transition was undoubtedly supported by the modern medical training of the sanatorium's physicians and nurses. Dr Dobbie, the sanatorium's long-standing physician-in-chief, assumed his position in 1905, the same year that he earned his Doctor of Medicine from the University of Toronto, which places him squarely (though early) in the era of modern medical education.[194] Likewise, Miss Dickson became the sanatorium's equally long-standing lady superintendent in 1906, following her graduation from the Toronto General Hospital's Training School for Nurses in 1905. As recent graduates of modern medical and nursing programs, both were open to the rise of new technologies in medicine, ensuring the work of the sanatorium was supported and kept up-to-date with the most modern of innovations and techniques. The National Sanitarium Association's annual report for the Toronto Free Hospital for Consumptives for 1916–17 was the first to confirm via photographic evidence that medical technologies had entered the sanatorium, the captions of eight photographs reading "Patients taking ultra-violet treatment," "Apparatus for pneumothorax treatment," "Apparatus for high frequency treatment," "Examination by the fluoroscope," "Patients taking heliotherapy," "The dental room," "Taking an X-ray photograph," and "X-ray photo – normal lung and diseased lung."[195] Like the laboratory, acquiring and using the new medical technologies "emphasized the presence of science" at the sanatorium, a presence that would weave its way into the daily lives and treatment plans of patients.[196]

Biomedicine was linked to greater prestige and authority for physicians, in part because the use of all those new technologies and treatments required skilled knowledge and training typically absent from the home sickroom.[197] As a result, clear differences began to distinguish home versus sanatorium care in tuberculosis, and those differences intensified over

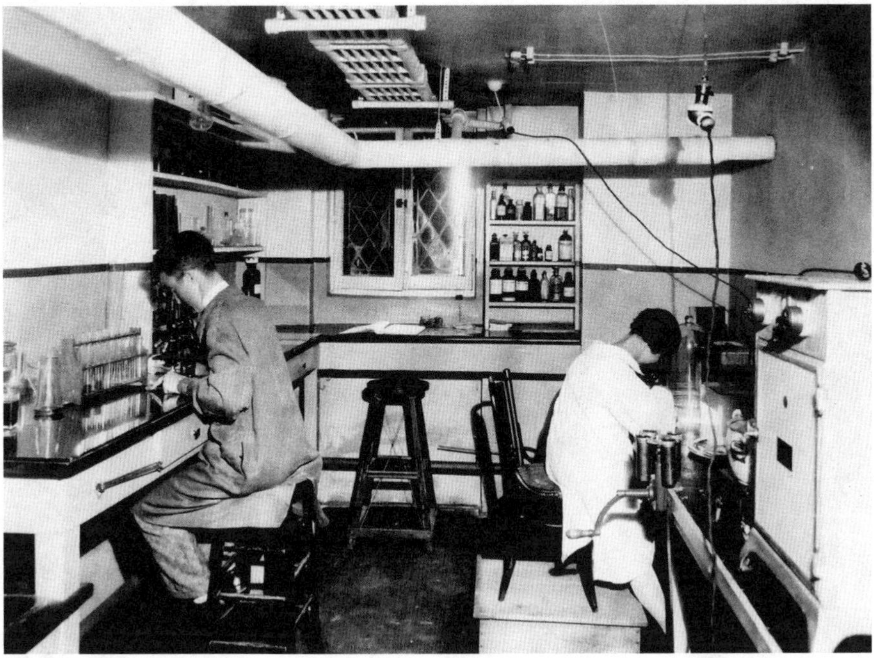

Figure 1.14 Technicians at work in one of the Toronto sanatorium's basement laboratories.

time. The National Sanitarium Association's annual report for 1926–27 was the first (and only) to feature a photograph of one of the sanatorium's basement laboratories (see figure 1.14). In the photograph, the sterilizing autoclave is located prominently in the right foreground, with a four-tube, hand-cranked centrifuge clamped to the lab bench beside it. Clear glass lab-ware, including test tubes and beakers, and glass bottles containing various solutions line the bench countertops and shelves. Two laboratory technicians, a woman in a white lab coat, and a man in a darker, perhaps brown or grey, lab coat are both looking into their microscopes as light, contrast, and magnification rendered invisible tuberculosis bacteria visible to them. By the 1930s, the sanatorium's reputation in biomedical practice was firmly ensconced with the opening of a new, dedicated surgical building, a photograph of which first appears in the 1931–32 annual report. The operating rooms were state-of-the-art and staffed with some of Toronto's leading surgeons (see figure 1.15).

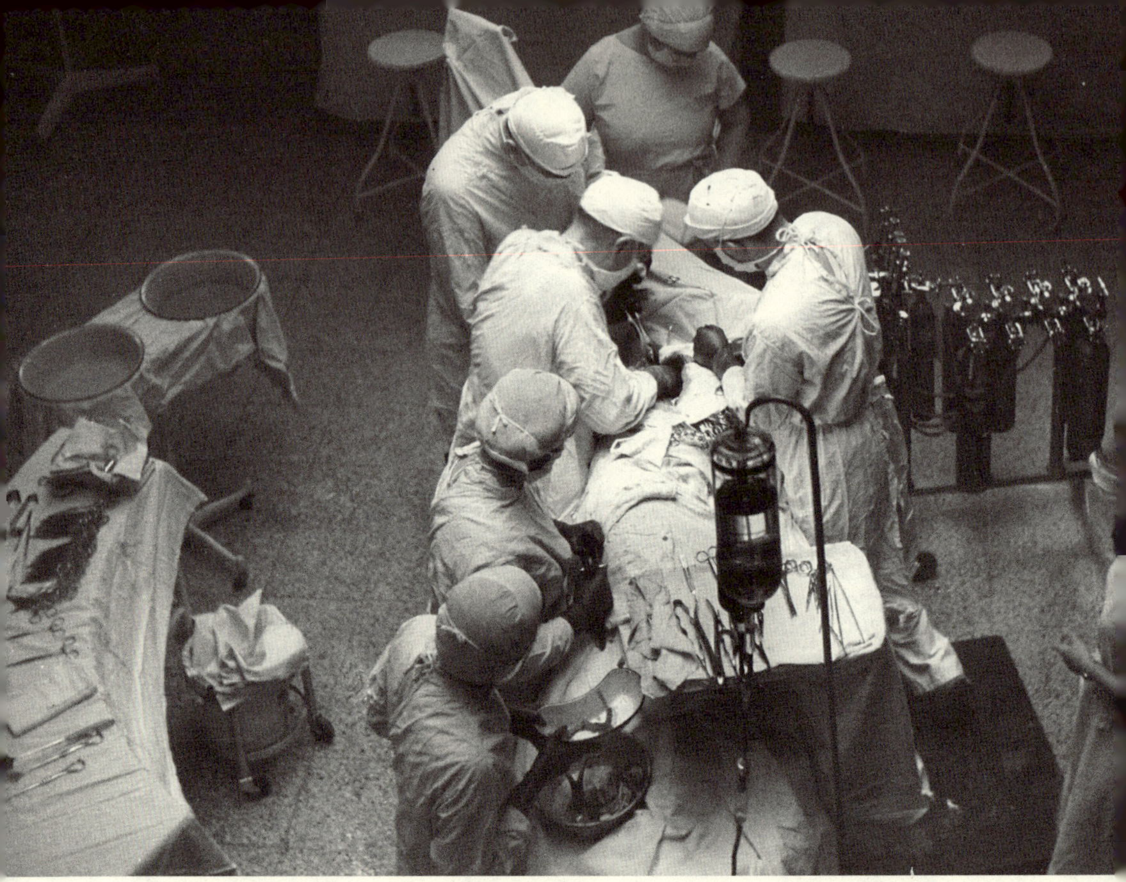

Figure 1.15 A thoracoplasty surgery in progress. This more invasive and irreversible procedure was typically reserved for active and advanced cavitary pulmonary tuberculosis. The kidney dish held by the nurse in the centre foreground of the photograph contains segments of ribs removed from the patient.

Even though modern hospitals might be united by the common language and understandings of science, van der Geest and Finkler suggest that they rarely exist as "identical clones" of biomedical practice.[198] Modern hospital cultures could vary in significant ways, even under the rubric of science. In this respect, this case study sited at the Toronto sanatorium is not intended to be representative of all early twentieth-century tuberculosis sanatoria, in Canada or elsewhere. Indeed, there is great potential for sanatoria to have varied in fundamental ways, from the type of treatments offered or favoured, to the voluntary or involuntary nature of hospitalization, the patient populations admitted, the well-funded or neglected, the rural or urban, the isolated or integrated location of the sanatorium, and so on.[199] As a result, comparative accounts are invaluable for expanding the understanding of tuberculosis hospitals. Large-scale studies of other children's sanatorium experiences are rare, but an important exception is Ann Shaw and Carole Reeves's *The Children of Craig-y-nos: Life in a Welsh Tuberculosis Sanatorium 1922–1959*. The product of an oral history project, their book documents in exquisite detail the experiences of over ninety child, adolescent, and young adult patients and former staff of the Craig-y-nos sanatorium in Wales. While the information accessed for our research projects may differ, we share an interest in reconstructing the subtleties of child patient experiences in historic tuberculosis sanatoria. Shaw and Reeves's narratives are based upon individual recollections, while my research on the Toronto sanatorium is based primarily on documentation compiled through patient chart reviews, supplemented with archival research at the West Park Healthcare Centre Archives, the City of Toronto Archives, the University of Toronto Archives, and the Archives of Ontario.

When I was conceptualizing this study in the late 1990s, "systematic use of the clinical case history" was, according to Risse and Warner, still "little cultivated."[200] In Ontario, there were some notable extant and emerging exceptions, including Cheryl Krasnick Warsh's *Moments of Unreason: The Practice of Canadian Psychiatry and the Homewood Retreat, 1883–1923* (1989), and Geoffrey Reaume's *Remembrance of Patients Past: Patient Life at the Toronto Hospital for the Insane, 1870–1940* (2000). Further insights came from Franca Iacovetta and Wendy Mitchinson's edited volume *On the Case: Explorations in Social History* (1998), which presents diverse examples of research built on case file inquiries. In the case of patient charts, Risse and Warner argue that valuable insights may be gained into various aspects of medical and hospital history, allowing researchers, amongst other things, "to draw patient profiles, to reconstruct patterns of medical practice, and to explain admission and discharge decisions,"[201] while also revealing something of "the texture of hospital life."[202] Using large collections of records, such research can shed light into an institution's "medical culture," while the individual charts can be read to understand the nature of the "clinical narrative" built on treatment options and decisions.[203] Ultimately, patient charts are "surviving artefacts of the interaction between physicians and their patients," one way, perhaps, to attempt to gain an insider's perspective on the role, function, and experience of the tuberculosis sanatorium.[204]

As much as patient charts tell us something of the patient, as Risse and Warner argue, they can also tell us something about the patients' physicians, or "why doctors did what they did, what expectations they held about their own clinical interventions, and how they explained their actions and perceived their consequences."[205] While early modern era physicians were trending towards more objective (and less subjective) evaluations of their patients, nonetheless patient charts should, according to Noll and others, be read "judiciously," since "patient files are not objective statements of clinical fact" but have the potential to reflect "the prejudices and presuppositions" of physicians and other professionals associated with medical institutions such as the sanatorium.[206] In patient charts, the physician emerges as an "observer," and the charts thus document "what the observer thought he saw, perhaps even what he wanted to see and hoped to do."[207]

I had expected some form of a standard clinical chart with uniform, abstractable data for a historical epidemiological investigation of tuberculosis sanatorium patients, but the charts had a different type of story to tell. Medicine was only in the early modern era when these charts were created, perhaps less singularly preoccupied with the large range of scientific markers and standardized data that would be routinely collected on patients in the second half of the twentieth century; instead, much more attention was devoted to detailed patient histories and overall patient constitution, rendering the charts much more of a narrative account of patients. Perhaps this is not unexpected, since Edward Shorter has argued that emerging modern doctors were meticulous history takers, genuinely interested in any and all details concerning their patients.[208] Writing in 1948, Dr Ludwig, a psychiatrist at Massachusetts General Hospital, suggested a personalizing of the professional relationship between doctors and tuberculosis patients, that by taking an interest in their personality, life situation, and emotions, physicians could reassure patients that they were still, first and foremost, viewed as "a person and not just an 'infiltrated left apex.'"[209] It was precisely this exacting focus on the patient, epitomizing the close relationships between doctors and patients in early modern medicine, that was clearly reflected in the charts, and it was an aspect that could neither be quantified nor fit into convenient categorical constructs. Far more than mere records of bodily measures, sputum analyses, and the minutiae of physical findings and medical procedures (though all of that was there), the qualitative information on patients and their lives seemed as important to collect and retain as the clinical details. In an interesting turn of events, the charts gave way to a rich, descriptive understanding of children and tuberculosis, and it was easy to feel drawn into their lives and experiences. When historian Steven Noll used patient charts in his 1914–39 case study of North Carolina's historic Caswell Training School, he also found that "the writings" in those charts "seemed more narrative than analytical and more descriptive than clinical."[210] In my own experience, this meant that the perspective and analyses would have to take a decidedly more qualitative turn, the focus much more deeply rooted in trying to understand why children and their families had the experiences that they did with tuberculosis, tuberculosis treatments, and the sanatorium.

There is much discussion amongst those invested in such studies regarding the value of clinical charts in understanding the patient's perspective and experience.[211] The patient's point of view is difficult to access historically. While it has been suggested that patient charts are more revealing of the medical perspective on patients and diseases, I have attempted, as far as possible, to also extract the patient's (or family's) perspective from these records. In this endeavour, I was greatly assisted by the regular inclusion of a large brown envelope (and its contents) in each clinical chart. The brown envelope was reserved for any and all nonmedical information pertaining to each patient, repositories of letters (incoming letters and copies of outgoing responses), conduct reports, patient report cards, notes passed between patients, and letters exchanged between patients or ex-patients and sanatorium staff members. Here is where the dialogues between patients, staff, families, and outside groups are revealed, and nothing, it seemed, was purged. Using these materials to reconstruct individual stories helps to reveal a deeper social history of childhood tuberculosis than would a purely clinical record alone. Admittedly, a private moment of anticipation surfaced each time a brown envelope was opened, particularly the thick (or even multiple) envelopes, because I knew something would soon be learned about the patient and the experience that went beyond an exclusively medical or institutional perspective. If the patient chart itself reflected the perspective of physicians and nurses, then the contents of the brown envelopes were more likely to represent the families, friends, and other non-medical persons. Unlike Noll, who found that "any information from patients themselves" was absent from the records he reviewed, occasionally I discovered material in those envelopes written by the child patients themselves.[212] Those were the truly precious finds, testament to the children's real existence amidst the wealth of medical evidence that confirmed their tuberculosis disease. It is noteworthy that as sanatorium practice became more medicalized, particularly with the introduction of antibiotics, the character of the patient chart also changed, becoming much more committed to the biomedical details and often lacking in the personal notes and correspondences that defined earlier charts. The change in the structure of the charts is intuitive, reflecting a trend towards a more exacting and objective focus on physiological and pathological details and the effects of streptomycin and other drug treatments on tuberculosis bacteria. Perhaps this makes sense, from a biomedical perspective, as attention shifted explicitly towards killing tuberculosis bacteria with antibiotics and away from broader concerns with the daily challenges and social lives of the human sufferers.

While the exacting detail of the charts reflects the attentiveness of medical and nursing staff, I believe the contents of the brown envelopes reflect their deeper interests in their patients, beyond their bodies and tuberculosis, to understand something of their home lives and struggles, their worries, fears, likes, and dislikes. For me, everything was of interest in reconstructing a child's experience with tuberculosis, from one adolescent's experience with the lung compression of artificial pneumothorax, to another's concerns that supper's potatoes had been burned. It soon became clear that researching tuberculosis and the sanatorium also meant understanding something of the nature of lives as they were lived in early twentieth-century Ontario. This is a meaningful point since tuberculosis was itself a part of that life. As a result, I quickly found myself entrenched in references to people, places, popular culture, and artifacts of the past, researching, amongst other things, celebrated hockey players, women's beauty products, and culinary delicacies like "scraped beef" and "junket." Such details explicitly connected patients with their larger world,

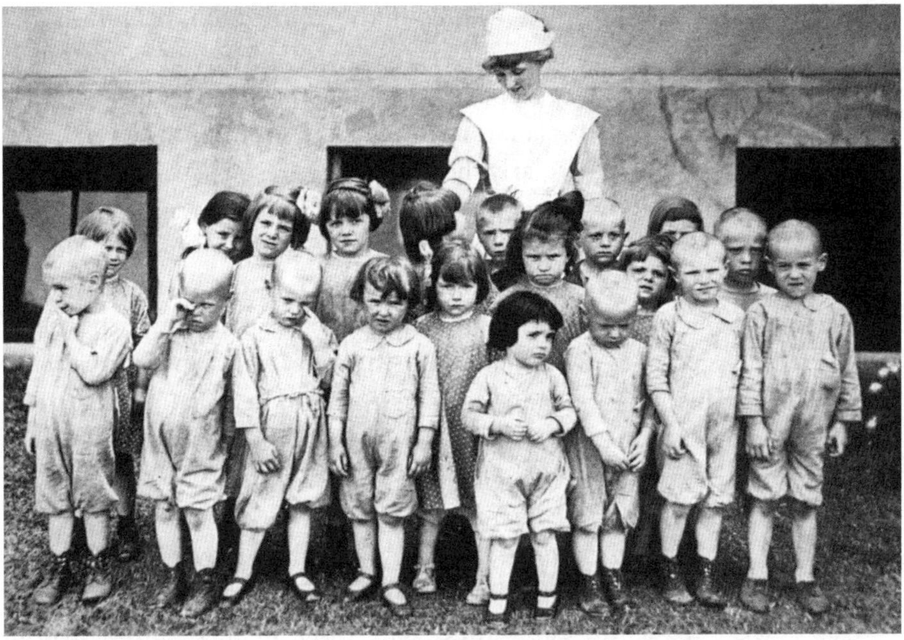

Figure 1.16 Child patients at the Queen Mary Hospital for Consumptive Children. Hair could be cropped for easier care or to control head lice. Since this photograph was selected for publication in the NSA annual report for 1916–17, the sad appearance of a number of the children could have been used to inspire "practical sympathy" (donations or other support).

not just the microcosm of the sanatorium, as do inventories of deceased patients' possessions, and the reports of home inspections for those nearing discharge.

The stories of Welsh and English children at Craig-y-nos sanatorium overlapped in many ways with those of children at the Toronto sanatorium. Shaw and Reeves noted great variability in the stories, but those admitted as older children and adolescents were generally the ones to "recall the most positive memories," some remembering their hospitalization "as one of the happiest periods of their lives."[213] Some children "were not so enthusiastic but made the best of it," while others "found it a distressing experience."[214] The sentiments were similar at the Toronto sanatorium; some children experienced the sanatorium as a foreign, rigid medical institution, but other children seemed to make the best of it, forming friendships as they shared in the journey of tuberculosis and hospitalization together (see figure 1.16) Sidney, for example, the tuberculosis orphan whose story opened this chapter, found both his health and his future wife at the sanatorium, but sanatorium life certainly did not suit all children, particularly those who were restless, overwhelmingly homesick, or bored by the daily drudgeries of bedrest. As a result, both the Craig-y-nos and Toronto sanatorium studies reinforce the understanding that there was great individual variability among children, those willing and those unwilling to cede to the sanatorium experience. Selected comparisons with Shaw and Reeves's study appear scattered throughout this book, invaluable as first-person perspectives that reinforce or add dimension to my second-hand interpretations of the Toronto sanatorium experience.

In his book, *The Changing Years: The Story of Toronto Hospital and the Fight against Tuberculosis*, Godfrey Gale has provided a detailed, chronological history of the Toronto sanatorium and how it changed over time.[215] To avoid duplicating his efforts, in this study I instead pursue a thematic analysis, more or less holding time fairly constant over the forty some years of this study, even as treatment regimens changed but the administrative roles occupied by Dobbie (the physician-in-chief) and MacPherson Dickson (the lady superintendent) remained a relative underlying constant. Admittedly, profound events occurred within these four decades – the First World War, the Great Depression, the Second World War – but it would be difficult to stratify patient stories in the context of these events, unless someone, in correspondence perhaps, explicitly made the connections. Admission to the sanatorium likely muted the impact of these events, particularly among young children who were not yet worldly enough in their perspective to appreciate the significance of what was going on outside of the sanatorium. Adding to the challenge is the fact that charts often yielded a mere snapshot of a patient's life, fragmented stories and not true longitudinal perspectives. While capturing the larger stratigraphy of social events and time is difficult, some contextualizing of the study at the sanatorium is possible. Although this is not a history of the sanatorium itself, an exploration of the nature of the institution is warranted to better understand the children's hospitalization experience. Chapter 2 provides an introduction to the social and medical world and, more broadly, the community of the sanatorium created for the patients. The idea is to situate or site this study of tuberculosis by exploring, in Megan Davies's words, "the context in which this history took place."[216]

There are already excellent, detailed national histories on Canada's struggles with tuberculosis in the early twentieth century, including George Jasper Wherrett's *The Miracle of the Empty Beds: A History of Tuberculosis in Canada* (1977) and Katherine McCuaig's *The Weariness, the Fever, and the Fret: The Campaign against Tuberculosis in Canada, 1900–1950* (1999). This book, instead, joins others that explore local case studies of Canadian sanatoria and tuberculosis experiences.[217] Unlike those studies, however, this book is built primarily on the stories of tuberculous lives as revealed through a review of patient charts. Even more explicitly, this study is focused on the lives and experiences of 822 randomly selected children who were admitted to the tuberculosis sanatorium in Toronto between 1909 and 1950. The children's archival charts were sampled from a collection preserved by West Park Healthcare Centre, the medical facility that came to replace the sanatorium when the Sanatorium Act for Consumptives was repealed in 1972. The institutional transition away from tuberculosis sanatorium had begun in 1969 when the Toronto Hospital opened a Chronic Obstructive Pulmonary Disease Unit, the revamped hospital's rising specialty in long-term care furthered in 1973 when an Amputee Program was established, and in 1974 when a Stroke/Neurological Rehabilitation Program was inaugurated.[218] Such was the reality of these historic tuberculosis sanatoria – as the disease declined in frequency, some institutional reconceptualizations were necessary if they were to remain operational medical facilities.

The approach to sampling in qualitative case studies is not even remotely analogous to the method of sampling in quantitative research. Random sampling is the "gold standard" for retrospective medical chart reviews (and most quantitative research in general) because it reduces the risk for sampling bias and allows for the generalization of study results to the larger population from which the random sample was drawn.[219] Since statistical generalizations are not the ambition of qualitative studies, however, cases are instead selected for their contributions to emerging insights. As John Creswell has noted, "I prefer to select cases that show different perspectives on the problem, process, or event I want to portray."[220] I initially randomly sampled a large enough number of cases that I was ultimately able to make targeted choices, selecting which examples would help best to flesh out the perspective on tuberculosis and children; those choices were not made in the initial random sampling of the 822 charts, but did become apparent in the analysis, interpretation, and writing. It was beneficial that the research proceeded in this manner because what I found insightful, unique, or particularly descriptive and revealing only became apparent after poring over and comparing hundreds of cases. As a result, the cases presented in this book reflect purposefully selected examples, which follow Bent Flyvbjerg's rationale on the matter, that "the typical or average case is often not the richest in information. Atypical or extreme cases often reveal more information because they activate more actors and more basic mechanisms in the situation studied."[221]

Robert Stake echoes this sentiment, expressed in another way: "The research should have a connoisseur's appetite for the best persons, places, and occasions. 'Best' usually means those that best help us to understand the case, whether typical or not."[222] I found this perspective on case selection particularly true for chapter 7, which covers more of the social lives of children in the sanatorium and includes examples of misbehaviour. Those children who misbehaved engaged more "actors" and "mechanisms," within and outside of the sanatorium. I may have created a large, random sample of 822, but to explore misbehaviour I selected examples to explore from within the data set, notably those children who had impressive or creative histories of misbehaviour. I would not venture to generalize their misbehaviour to other sanatorium populations, particularly since, at times, the misbehaviour was truly a reflection of individual characters. To dismiss them as "outliers," however, would deny their unique contributions to sanatorium life. Various researchers have extrapolated on the importance of case selection in qualitative case studies; Jack Levy notes the need to make "careful, theory-guided selection of non-random cases," all the while remaining aware of the "dangers of selection bias."[223]

At the time when this research was undertaken, the sanatorium collection had been boxed and placed in temporary storage, the sanatorium-era building in which they had long been housed scheduled for demolition.

Observing the hundreds of boxes was itself a sobering experience; the dozens of charts in each box and all of the boxes taken together were real, visual reminders of the thousands of patients hospitalized for tuberculosis in Ontario, each individual chart revealing a life story of disease and struggle. My focus was the collection's oldest (pre-1940), pre-antibiotic-era charts, filed, boxed, and stored apart from later charts. At some point historically, however, a small number of charts from 1940–50 had been filed in with this collection. If 1940–50 charts were encountered in a sampled box, they were retained in the data collection but, not unexpectedly, the overall quantity of records sampled for 1940–50 admissions is much lower than for admissions in earlier decades (see table 1.1). Substantial changes would come in tuberculosis hospitalization and treatment with the introduction of antibiotics such as streptomycin following the Second World War. While the misfiled charts offer a peek into the experience of patients who were in the sanatorium as antibiotics were being introduced in the 1940s, the study does not follow the development of those treatments further into the 1950s or beyond. As the research proceeded, boxes were sampled in the same random fashion in which they had been placed in storage, beginning with those most accessible. Because of the alphabetical (by surname) arrangement of the records, a single box might contain multiple child siblings who were admitted to the sanatorium, perhaps at the same time, but more often at different times. This aspect was invaluable for gaining a larger, familial perspective on tuberculosis, how the infection moved within families and led to sanatorium admissions.

Prior to undertaking the research, Ethics Board approvals were received. Under research agreement and ethics protocols, the study is strictly bound by privacy and confidentiality, and any descriptors that could identify individual patients, such as names, locations (including community names outside of Toronto or street addresses in the city), and specific places of employment (usually of parents) have been removed. The pseudonyms assigned to the children in this study bear no semblance to their true names. Names common to the time period under study (1909–50) were chosen from an online database of the most popular baby names by year.[224] With the use of pseudonyms, John Harley Warner notes the concerns raised that "by keeping patients anonymous while naming physicians," such research "can display an element of arrogant disrespect, or dismissal, privileging the physician … over the nameless patient."[225] This study does fall victim to this criticism, naming and even providing some biographical details about the medical and nursing staff (again with the intention of fleshing out the "site" of the study) while keeping the patients themselves "nameless." It is an absolutely necessary provision, however, ensuring the privacy of former patients and their families above and beyond all else.

Since this study is concerned with children and tuberculosis, it is important to acknowledge that there are different ways in which "childhood" may be defined. From a purely biological perspective, for example, childhood may be considered to end once puberty is reached. In the sampling of patients for this study, the definition of "childhood" borrowed a social definition linked to the age of majority. As a result, the "child" patients sampled included those of all ages from infancy up to and including seventeen years of age at the time of their admission to the sanatorium. Admittedly, adolescents sixteen to seventeen years of age may not be considered, either biologically or socially, true "children," particularly in the early twentieth century when adolescence was more likely to meld with the expectations and responsibilities of adulthood. Other studies examining tuberculosis, for example, have adopted upper ages of fourteen or fifteen years to define "children" versus "non-children," some further defining all those over ten as "adolescents."[226] Irrespective of the specifics, the majority (with a few exceptions) were dependents and were therefore not primarily responsible for maintaining homes and families (an important stressor that many adult patients experienced during their hospitalization). Further, most had parents or guardians who had vested concerns with their well-being and generated much in the way of correspondence with the sanatorium, filling all those brown envelopes.

The wide age range, spanning infancy through late adolescence, allows for a broader perspective on diversity in disease experience (e.g., primary disease versus reactivation disease, as explored in chapter 3) and hospital life prior to adulthood. Not all of the patients in this study were admitted to the children's facilities at the Toronto sanatorium (i.e., the Queen Mary Hospital for Consumptive Children and the Davies Cottage for Infants), because some of the older adolescents with reactivation-type (cavitary) tuberculosis were instead placed on the wards and in the pavilions of the Toronto Free Hospital for Consumptives, buildings typically reserved for adult patients. A broad perspective on age helps to dispel the notion that all children experienced a single type of "child-type tuberculosis," a historic diagnosis that could be contrasted to "adult-type tuberculosis." These terms appear to create a neat dichotomy in tuberculosis experience according to age. While tuberculosis did occur in childhood, age often intersected with disease insofar as "primary" and "secondary" (or reactivation) tuberculosis is concerned. Primary disease may manifest after first infection and is typically mild and self-limiting. If primary disease resolves and slips into latency, wellness is regained. After a variable period of latency, the infection may reactivate, and the secondary disease that emerges is typically associated with the more grievous symptoms of tuberculosis, such as cough, weight loss, anemia with pallor, and hemoptysis. In Canada's tuberculosis endemic years, primary infection and disease typically occurred in childhood, because the infection and its transmission were so common. Reactivation could occur at any point afterwards, but typically this was in adolescence or early adulthood. As a result, "child-type tuberculosis" really implied primary tuberculosis, with the caveat that children could also experience primary progressive or reactivation disease, particularly if they had weakened immunity. The broad age range of the children sampled highlights these variable disease experiences (both primary and secondary – or reactivation – disease) and the different medical treatments they received (with the treatments for more complex reactivation disease typically requiring greater involvement of medical and nursing staff).

The specific age breakdown of the 822 patients sampled is presented in table 1.1. Eighteen infants (under twelve months of age) (2.2% of the sample) were admitted to the sanatorium, while another thirty-one infants (3.8%) were born at the sanatorium to tuberculous mothers. None of the infants born at the sanatorium were born tuberculous, but they were nonetheless given charts so that they could be monitored and documented. Such medical documentation would have been invaluable if any cases of congenital tuberculosis (where infection passes from mother to infant via the placenta) had been diagnosed, though none ever were.

Table 1.1
Admission characteristics of the 822 child patients sampled

	n	%
Period of admission		
1909–19	258	31.4
1920–29	331	40.3
1930–39	190	23.1
1940–50	42	5.1
Not recorded in chart	1	0.1
Age of child at admission		
Infant (under 1 year)	18	2.2
1–4 years	112	13.6
5–9 years	235	28.6
10–14 years	239	29.1
15–17 years	185	22.5
Born at the sanatorium	31	3.8
Not recorded in chart	2	0.2
Gender		
Female	435	52.9
Male	378	46.0
Not recorded in chart	9	1.1
Place of residence at admission		
Toronto and surrounding area	517	62.9
Outside Toronto	264	32.1
Born at sanatorium	31	3.8
Not recorded in chart	10	1.2
Type of residence at admission		
Home	737	89.7
Institutional	44	5.4
Born at sanatorium	31	3.8
Not recorded in chart	10	1.2
Nativity		
Born in Canada	592	72.0
Born outside Canada	144	17.5
Not recorded in chart	86	10.5

Young children, between one and four years of age at admission, comprise 13.6% (n = 112) of the sample. Older children, five to nine years of age, represent 28.6% (n = 235) of the sample, while those ten to fourteen years of age, another 29.1% (n = 239). Some 22.5% (n = 185) of the patients sampled were older adolescents between fifteen and seventeen years of age at admission. In terms of gender, slightly more than half or 52.9% (n = 435) of the children sampled were female. Residents of Toronto or the surrounding area were most numerous, representing 62.9% (n = 517) of the children in the sample. Another 32.1% (n = 264) travelled to the sanatorium from more distant locales throughout Ontario. Most children (n = 737, or 89.7% of the sample) were admitted to the sanatorium from family homes, while a smaller number (n = 44, or 5.4% of the sample) came from institutions such as orphanages. The majority of child patients sampled, 592 (72.0%), had been born in Canada, and, of that number, 39 child patients were Indigenous. Another 17.5% (n = 144) of the child patients sampled were born outside of Canada and subsequently immigrated in their youth, possibly entering Canada already infected with tuberculosis, but also possibly exposed and infected after their arrival. In 10.5% (n = 86) of cases, information on place of birth was not recorded in the chart.

For the most part, children's ethnicities are not explicitly identified, but with one important exception, the identification of Indigenous patients (a collective terminology which includes First Nations, Inuit, and Métis peoples). I grappled with this decision because, on the one hand, I did not want to single out these child patients, the only culture group to be specifically identified; on the other hand, however, I did not want their specific stories and experiences to become lost in the mass of narratives. It is imperative to continue to explore the weighty impact of colonialism on the history of Indigenous peoples in Canada, and part of that history extends to interactions with colonial institutions such as hospitals and sanatoria.[227] In their interview-based study involving First Nations women and men with personal or familial experiences with now-defunct tuberculosis sanatoria, Jessica Moffatt, Maria Mayan, and Richard Long determined that experiences with hospitalization for tuberculosis could linger powerfully, far from historical, as "fear" and "mistrust" continued to shape "their feelings of today's health care system," particularly in regards to tuberculosis treatment.[228] As a result, because the legacy of sanatorium experiences continues to manifest today, it is important to explore the nature of those experiences across different Canadian tuberculosis sanatoria. The Toronto sanatorium neither segregated nor excluded Indigenous patients, though other typical challenges manifested – English was the primary language of communication, and its location near Toronto did distance some patients from their families, particularly those located on remote reserves. Since the Toronto sanatorium was a voluntary institution, patients could leave at any time, but the understanding of that right was not necessarily widely shared or known by all, particularly, it seems, among those whose interactions with the sanatorium were mediated through Indian agents. In their interviews, Moffatt and colleagues noted that respondents recalled that "traditional healing activities such as smudging, healing circles, or other group healing practices were not permitted within the sanatorium," aligned, as the sanatorium was, with the more "individualistic" type of treatment characteristic of biomedicine.[229] Further, they reported that "medical staff were often described as unfriendly" and unaware of Indigenous culture. Other patients in the sanatorium community, however, were found to be an important source of comfort and friendship.

Hospitalization for chronic tuberculosis was generally a long-term prospect; the average duration of hospitalization for the children sampled was 494 days, or about 16½ months. The shortest period of hospitalization was 1 day, while the longest was 6,657 days, which amounts to about 18 years; this latter case was somewhat unusual in that, in addition to tuberculosis, the patient also had other health-related challenges and the sanatorium effectively became both long-term home and place of employment. The average duration of hospitalization did see modest declines over time, with children admitted in the years between 1909 and 1919 remaining an average 527 days ($n = 244$), 1920–29 an average 494 days ($n = 330$), 1930–39 an average 463 days ($n = 187$), and 1940–50 an average 434 days ($n = 42$). The overall distribution of the length of hospitalization for the patients sampled is presented in table 1.2. It is noteworthy that just under one-quarter of patients sampled ($n = 185$, 22.5%)

Table 1.2
Discharge characteristics of the 822 child patients sampled

	n	%
Duration of hospitalization		
3 months and under	185	22.5
4–6 months	110	13.4
7–9 months	90	10.9
10–12 months	78	9.5
13–18 months	102	12.4
19–24 months	81	9.9
25–36 months	75	9.1
37–48 months	31	3.8
Over 48 months	51	6.2
Could not be calculated	19	2.3
Condition at end of term		
Discharged	679	82.6
Died in sanatorium	143	17.4

remained at the sanatorium for 3 months or less. On the other hand, about 6% (n = 51) of the children sampled were hospitalized for over 4 years. Almost 83% (n = 679) of the patients sampled were later discharged from the sanatorium. Discharge could be medically approved (because the patient had improved, or because the family homes were able to provide adequate home care), or undertaken for any reason against medical advice. Since hospitalization at the sanatorium was voluntary, discharges could be arranged by patients or in the case of child patients, their parents or guardians, at any point after admission. The remaining 143 (17.4%) children sampled died at the sanatorium, testament to the vulnerability of the young to tuberculosis disease and the frustrations and sorrow that sanatorium staff would face in their inability to save these "little sufferers."[230]

Through information abstracted from the medical charts of the child patients sampled for this study, situated within a larger perspective borne out of archival research and the published medical literature of the time, this book pursues an explicitly biosocial examination of the tuberculosis and sanatorium experience in childhood. The following chapters focus on different aspects of this story. Chapter 2 is intended to "site" the study, to provide a working understanding of the "place" of the sanatorium, how it was laid out and functioned, the staff who worked there, and the community and social world of patients. This understanding is critical as a reference point, a grounding for the study and the chapters that follow, but is not intended to serve as a comprehensive institutional history (for that, I would refer the reader to Godfrey Gale's history of the Toronto sanatorium). Chapter 3 examines how and why children came to be admitted into and discharged from the sanatorium and aims to embed this study of tuberculosis in the broader context of the rise of modern medicine, evolving doctor–patient relationships, and awareness of the germ theory of disease. Chapter 4 explores something of the historical epidemiology of tuberculosis, from the medical and patient/family perspectives. This chapter addresses biological and social/cultural vulnerabilities for tuberculosis infection and disease, providing examples from average Ontario households during the early twentieth-century. Both chapters 5 and 6 focus on the medical aspects of tuberculosis, including perceptions of how the disease affected the body and why certain treatment regimens became popular; since treatments were the ultimate foundation of the sanatorium experience, they were critical points of connection between patients and medical staff and it is important to consider how and why these treatments were pursued. Chapter 5 addresses the traditional therapies, while chapter 6 examines the rise of surgical treatments for tuberculosis. Attentions turn explicitly to the social world of patients in chapter 7, including observations and commentary provided by the child patients themselves. Chapter 8 explores the broader world of sanatorium patients and resistance building, including the support they received from their families and friends, as well as the support received from municipalities, the province of Ontario, and charitable organizations such as the Samaritan Club and the Weston Sanitarium Club. The final chapter summarizes major points raised in the study. Today, in Canada, the tuberculosis sanatorium lingers only as an artifact. As tuberculosis rates continued to decline and the introduction of antibiotics bolstered confidence that the disease had been conquered, the Sanatoria for Consumptives Act was repealed in 1972 and many sanatoria across the country were obliged to adapt, either by closing or repurposing, and the Toronto sanatorium was no exception.

CHAPTER 2

The Toronto Sanatorium: The Context

Sanatoriums ought to inspire hope and cheer, not sorrow and tears; to attract patients, not repel them.[1]
~ J.E. Esslemont

The origins of the sanatorium movement in Ontario can be traced to William James Gage, a Toronto entrepreneur who headed W.J. Gage and Company, a successful publishing house. Gage was born in Brampton, Ontario, in September 1849, and died in Toronto in January 1921. Industrious in his life, alongside his publishing company, Gage was also the Kinleigh Paper Company, Ltd mill owner.[2] With his great success and rising wealth, Gage's attentions turned to philanthropy. In his efforts to organize anti-tuberculosis work in Ontario, Gage was joined by a number of Toronto's leading businessmen, including agricultural industrialist Hart Massey, a fellow Methodist and philanthropist.[3] Massey had personal experience with tuberculosis, losing his son Fred Victor[4] to the disease in 1890.[5] Massey had already lost another son, Charles Albert,[6] to typhoid fever in 1884, sad proof that even great wealth could not protect against the multiple threats of infectious diseases. In 1895, Massey joined William Gage and a number of other prominent businessmen to form the National Sanitarium Association (hereafter NSA) with the intention of addressing the problem of tuberculosis in Ontario. In 1913, in recognition of his contributions to tuberculosis work, Gage was knighted by the Order of St John of Jerusalem in England.[7] Recognizing the prestigious title that came with Gage's honours, it is also important to emphasize that the NSA sanatoria represented grassroots institutions, not organized out of federal or provincial government initiatives, but under the steam and convictions of these men and the thousands of Ontarians who supported the NSA's vision philanthropically.

In the fall of 1897, the National Sanitarium Association opened the first tuberculosis sanatorium in Canada, the Muskoka Cottage Sanatorium, which, in its first year, provided thirty-five beds for paying patients, most from wealthy families.[8] This effort was soon followed with the opening of the neighbouring Muskoka Free Hospital for Consumptives, which, in its first partial year of operation, from 21 April to 30 September 1902, accommodated, on average, thirty-one patients per day.[9] The Muskoka Free Hospital was intended for patients who could not afford the full cost of hospitalization, paying either partially or not at all, their maintenance funded by their municipalities. Both sanatoria were located just outside of the town of Gravenhurst, Ontario, on a relatively isolated peninsula of land stretching into the waters of Muskoka Bay. Encouraged by the success of the Muskoka sanatoria, the National Sanitarium Association then focused attention on establishing a sanatorium closer to the city of Toronto; this sanatorium was intended primarily for Torontonians, though patients were admitted from all over the province of Ontario. Located on the outskirts of the city, in Weston, the Toronto Free Hospital for Consumptives opened as a modest 30-bed sanatorium in 1904, on the site of an old forty-acre farm and homestead.[10] At its height, the Toronto sanatorium provided 667 beds for tuberculosis patients;[11] nearby, the Hamilton Health Association's Mountain Sanatorium, which opened in May 1906, with eight patients housed in tents and a refitted barn,[12] grew to an impressive 750 beds, reputed to have become the largest tuberculosis sanatorium in the British Commonwealth.[13] While the National Sanitarium Association did intend to expand its efforts nationally, discussing the possibility of a Pacific Coast sanatorium, its efforts would remain focused on the Muskoka and Toronto sanatoria and the Gage Institute, a large diagnostic clinic located in the heart of Toronto.[14]

In its earliest incarnation, the Toronto sanatorium was somewhat ad hoc, comprising an old, repurposed stone farmhouse and additions, including ten retrofitted horse-drawn streetcars used for patient accommodation, donated by the Toronto Transit Commission after its streetcar service went electric.[15] A fire at the sanatorium in 1910[16] led to a massive rebuilding effort in its wake and, with an eye towards safety, the construction of more substantial, brick, fire-proof hospital buildings. The rebuilding was made possible by the wildly successful "Million Dollar Fund" (or the King Edward VII Memorial Fund), a fundraising campaign initiated by Gage and the National Sanitarium Association. The understanding of tuberculosis as a disease of communities, not individuals or even families, cultured a strong public commitment to tuberculosis philanthropy. The modern design of the reconstructed, post-fire sanatorium would differ significantly from its more ramshackle predecessor, housing patients in three large, independent buildings: the (new) Toronto Free Hospital for Consumptives (for non-paying patients), the King Edward Sanatorium (for paying patients), and the Queen Mary Hospital for Consumptive Children (with its associated Davies Cottage for infants). All three hospital buildings shared staff and services and were administered centrally by the physician-in-chief, William Dobbie, and the lady superintendent, Edith MacPherson Dickson.

As the sanatorium model of tuberculosis care became established, there was a quick fluorescence of sanatorium construction in Ontario (and in other Canadian provinces). In 1908, for example, there were only 250 beds available for tuberculosis patients in all of Canada, but by 1911 the number had increased to 900, and by 1916 to 2,000.[17] In addition to the NSA sanatoria in Muskoka and Toronto, by 1920 Ontario had eleven more sanatoria: Mountain Sanatorium, Hamilton (established in 1906), Minnewaska Sanatorium, Gravenhurst (1908), St Lawrence Sanatorium, Cornwall (1908), Royal Ottawa Sanatorium, Ottawa (1910), Queen Alexandra Sanatorium, London (1910), Mowat Sanatorium, Kingston (1912), St Catharines Consumptive Sanatorium, St Catharines (1912), Essex County Sanatorium, Sandwich (a historic neighbourhood of Windsor) (1913), Brant Sanatorium, Brantford (1913), Calydor Sanatorium, Gravenhurst (1916), and Freeport Sanatorium, Kitchener (1920).[18]

Built on strong community commitments to establishing sanatoria, the number of beds for tuberculosis patients (either in sanatoria or in general hospitals) also increased as a by-product of the First World War, since soldiers diagnosed with tuberculosis were admitted to sanatoria for free treatment. The care of soldiers was a federal responsibility, so new government funds were infused into the sanatorium effort in the years during and following the war. Holbrook estimates that soldier patients effectively doubled the number of beds provided by Canadian sanatoria,[19] and, once these beds were no longer required by soldiers, they became available for civilian patients. By 1939, just prior to the antibiotic revolution, there were forty-one TB sanatoria across Canada: one on Prince Edward Island (Charlottetown), three in Nova Scotia (Halifax, Kentville, Lourdes), three in New Brunswick (East Saint John, the Glades, Vallée Lourdes), eleven in Quebec (Hull, Lac Édouard, two in Montreal, Mont Joli, three in Sainte-Agathe-des-Monts, Roberval, Sainte-Foy, Trois-Rivières), thirteen in Ontario (Brantford, Cornwall, Fort William, Gravenhurst, Hamilton, Haileybury, Kingston, Kitchener, London, Ottawa, St Catharines, Weston, Windsor), five in Manitoba (Ninette, Selkirk, St Vital, two in Winnipeg), three in Saskatchewan (Fort San, Prince Albert, Saskatoon), one in Alberta (Calgary), and one in British Columbia (Kamloops) (see figure 2.1).

By 1952, the province of Ontario had fourteen privately operated sanatoria, providing 4,222 beds for tuberculosis patients, in addition to two government-operated sanatoria in Woodstock[20] (500 beds) and Moose Factory[21] (120 beds).[22] In 1953, Canada had 101 sanatoria and TB units in general hospitals, collectively providing about 19,000 beds for TB patients.[23] From the humble origins of the sanatorium movement and for much of its history, even despite the growth in the number of sanatoria in Canada, it was understood that there would never be enough beds to provide for all tuberculosis sufferers, such was the scope of the tuberculosis problem. Unlike other infectious diseases, however, the intention had never been to isolate or quarantine all active cases of tuberculosis. Instead, sanatorium care (and general hospital care of the tuberculous) would always coexist alongside much-needed homecare for this chronic disease. A reconceptualization of sanatoria and hospital care for the tuberculous would emerge with antibiotic treatments, however, as the number of TB cases declined and the possibility of hospitalizing the majority of sufferers became, for the first time in the disease's history in Canada, a possibility. It was during the rise of the antibiotic era that sanatoria began to be conceptualized as places for the isolation or quarantine of infectious tuberculosis sufferers, particularly as the endemic reality of tuberculosis began to recede. By the 1950s, in an attempt to escape the emerging stigma of sanatorium treatment, because now the sanatorium was aligned with quarantine, American sanatoria were rebranding as "chest hospitals," a terminology that one physician explained was "devoid of any stigma."[24] There were also demographic

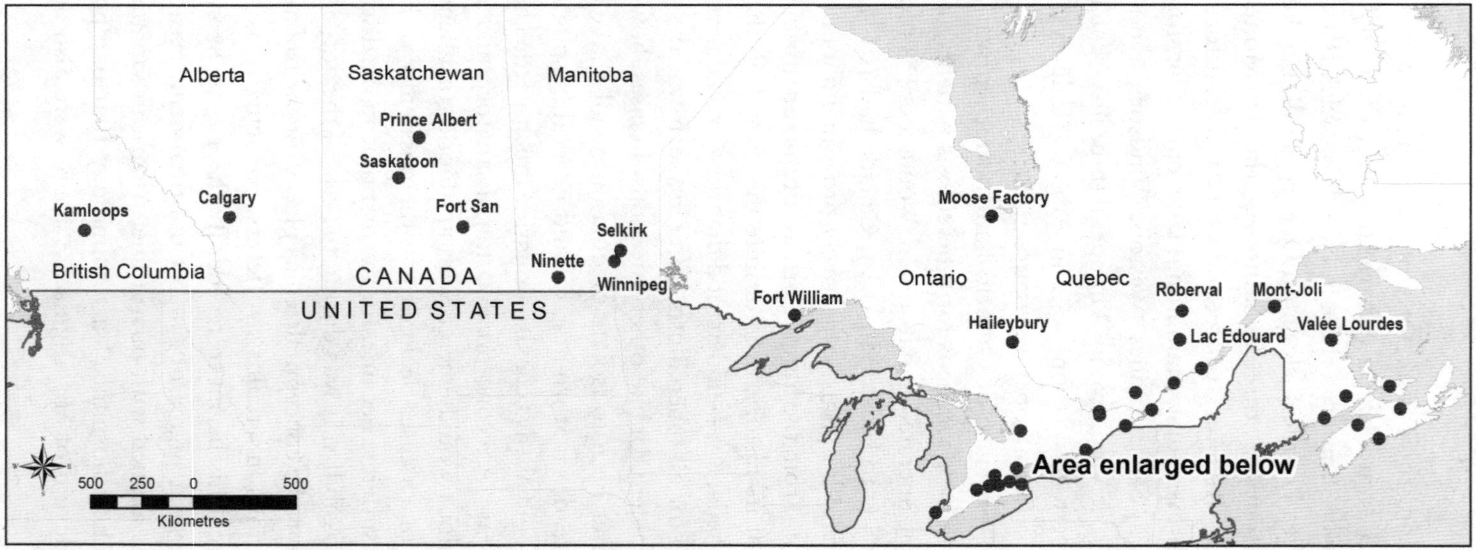

Figure 2.1 Tuberculosis sanatoria in Canada, circa 1939

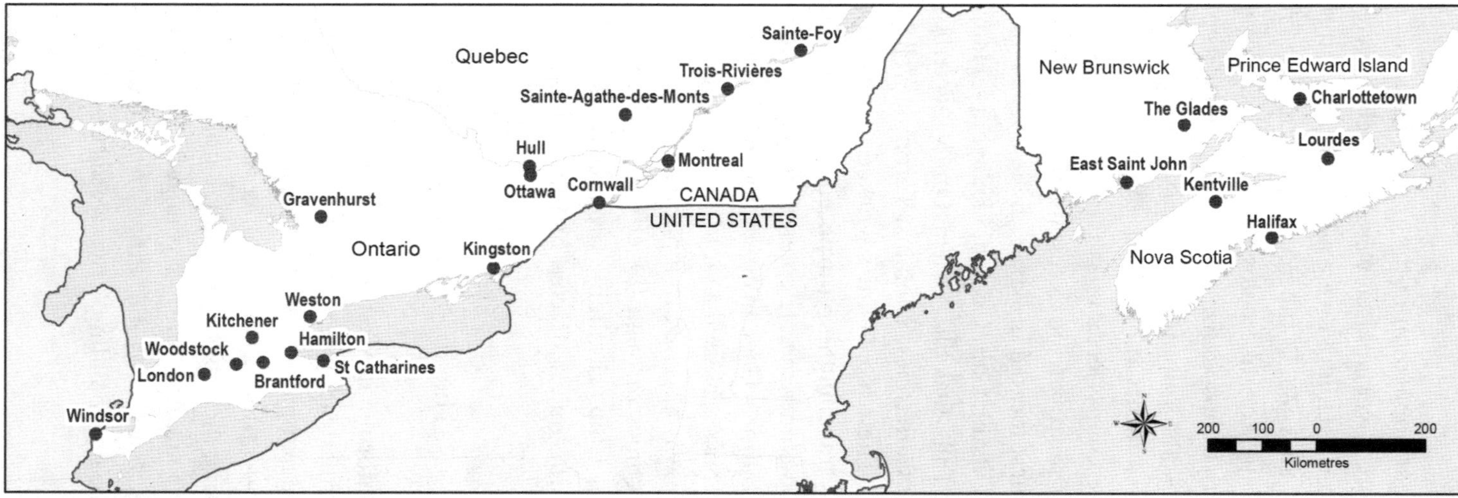
Quebec
Sainte-Foy
Trois-Rivières
Sainte-Agathe-des-Monts
Hull
Ottawa
Montreal
Cornwall
CANADA
UNITED STATES
Gravenhurst
Ontario
Kingston
Weston
Kitchener
Hamilton
Woodstock
St Catharines
London
Brantford
Windsor
New Brunswick
Prince Edward Island
Charlottetown
The Glades
Lourdes
East Saint John
Kentville
Halifax
Nova Scotia
200
100
0
200
Kilometres

shifts in the patient population in the antibiotic era; as tuberculosis became less common, fewer children were routinely infected in their youth and, as a result, fewer children were admitted to sanatoria and hospitals with tuberculosis. By 1962, as tuberculosis continued to recede, the number of beds available for tuberculosis patients had declined to 2,483.[25] The average length of hospitalization also shortened as patients typically remained in the sanatorium for about six months and then continued their antibiotic treatments at home for another eighteen months.[26]

Alongside tuberculosis beds in sanatoria and hospitals, a system of diagnostic clinics for tuberculosis testing also came to be established in Ontario, the earliest located in Barrie, Belleville, Brantford, Brockville, Chatham, Fort William, Galt, Guelph, Haileybury, Hamilton, Kitchener, London, Niagara Falls, Oakville, Orillia, Ottawa, Peterborough, Port Colborne, Simcoe, St Catharines, Timmins, Toronto, Welland, and Windsor (see figure 2.2).[27] These fixed clinics worked in concert with the mobile diagnostic clinics travelling in repurposed train cars, ships, and trailers to smaller and sometimes remote communities. In Toronto, the National Sanitarium Association's Gage Institute, located for most of its existence at 223–5 College Street, housed a large, permanent diagnostic centre for TB. This institute was also tied to a public health nursing program and offered support clinics through the efforts of the Samaritan Club and Junior Samaritan Club, charitable organizations run by middle-class women to support families affected by tuberculosis (see chapter 8).

The Toronto Sanatorium

The Toronto sanatorium in Weston opened in 1904 on the site of a forty-acre farm and homestead, just west of the junction of Weston Road and Jane Street.[28] The first patient was admitted on 2 September 1904. By its second year of operation a new building had been raised, at a cost of $20,000, increasing the capacity of the sanatorium to sixty-six beds, including beds for some of Ontario's youngest victims of tuberculosis, as described in the NSA's 1905–06 annual report where, "in one of the bright spots in the new building," two wards were reserved for children,

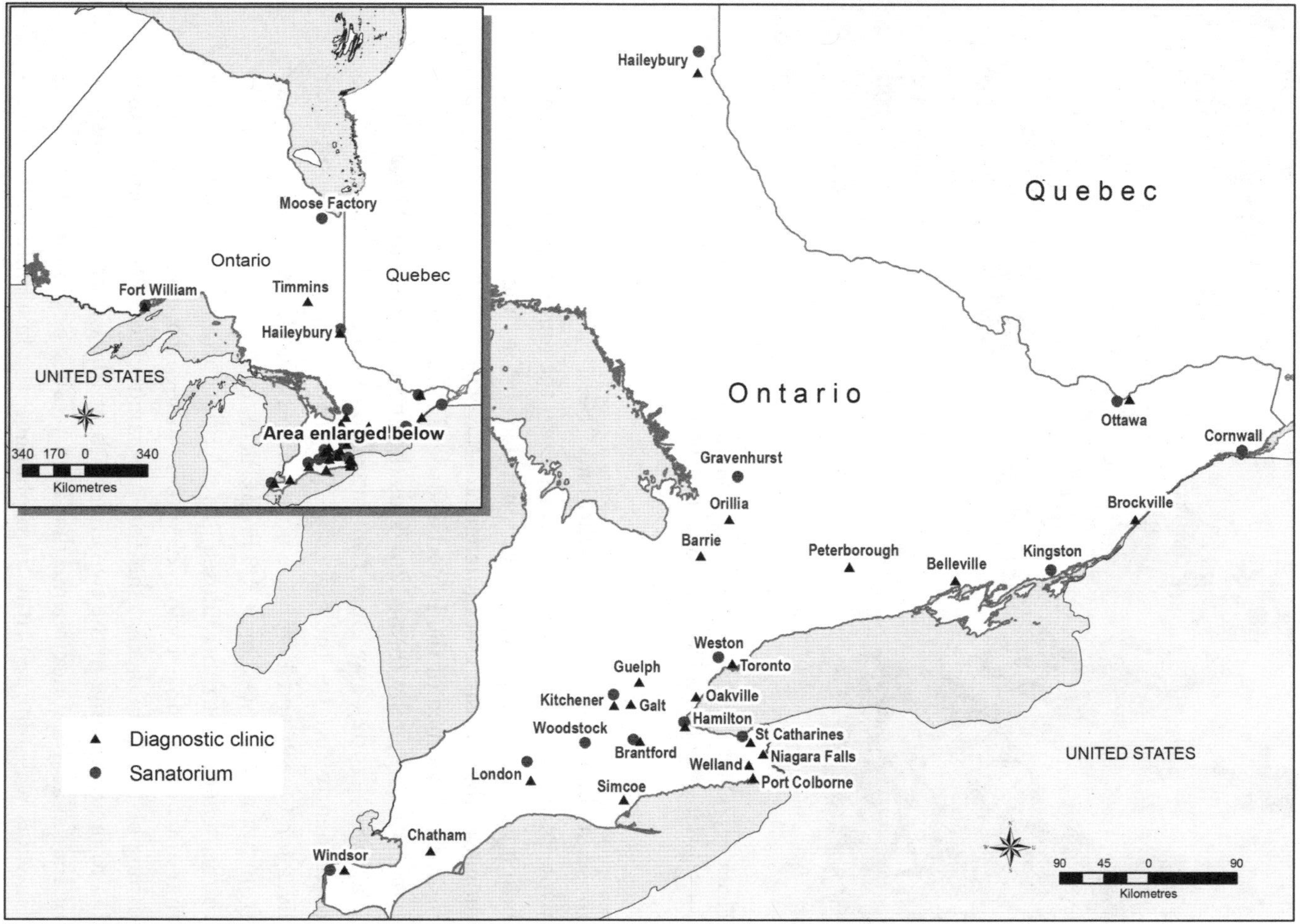

Map by Richard Maaranen, August 2015

Figure 2.2 Tuberculosis sanatoria and diagnostic clinics in Ontario, circa 1939

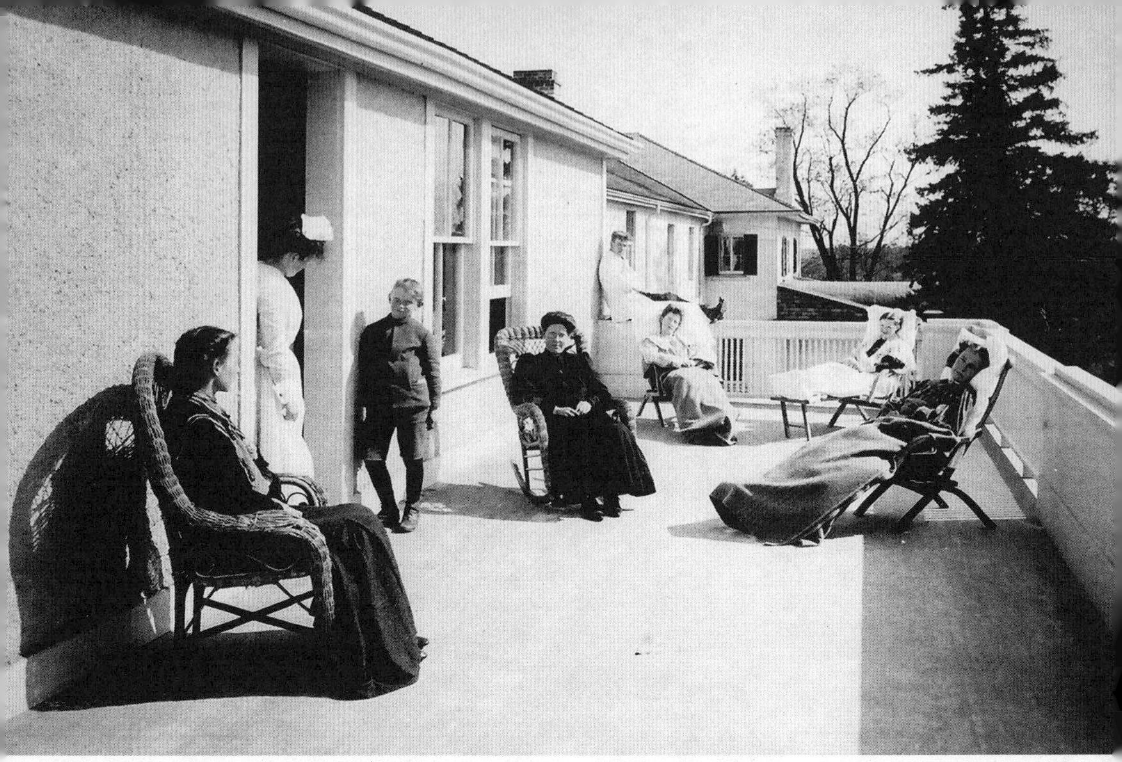

Figure 2.3 On the balcony of the old Toronto sanatorium (before the fire), with Joe Hawkins (the first child patient admitted in 1905), patients, and staff.

those in their "tender years" who had "been stricken down with the white plague."[29] At this time, according to the annual report, no other hospital in Canada provided accommodation for children suffering pulmonary tuberculosis. Once introduced, the wards were "attractively furnished" by women of the Imperial Order Daughters of the Empire. The IODE was originally formed towards the end of the South African Boer War (1899–1902), as women committed to raising the funds needed "to permanently care for the graves of our brave sons who have lost their lives for Queen and Empire, whose last resting-places are so far away from home and loved ones."[30] From there, their attentions next turned to the "enemy" of tuberculosis, "as relentless and more assiduous than that of war." In 1905, various chapters of the order led the way in establishing beds for children at the Toronto Sanatorium, a commitment that led to the furnishing of the two children's wards. Godfrey Gale's history of the sanatorium documents that on 13 July 1905, nine-year-old Joe Hawkins was admitted from an orphanage, the first child to be accommodated in the new wards (see figure 2.3).[31] Sanatorium infrastructure dedicated to children with tuberculosis would increase in Canada, alongside the introduction of preventoria and open-air schools. The women of the IODE played a role in this respect, establishing a preventorium for children (who were infected and in need of resistance building, but did not have active tuberculosis disease) on Sheldrake Avenue in Toronto in 1912.

The sanatorium continued to function in the aftermath of the 1910 fire, relying on hastily constructed pavilions to house the patients who remained. The 1911 Census of Canada includes the enumeration of the National Sanitarium and King Edward Hospital in the York South Township on the outskirts of Toronto.[32] Aside from patients (who were not considered true "residents" and therefore not documented by the census taker), forty individuals were living on site and enumerated. These included Dr Dobbie, physician-in-chief, and Miss Dickson, lady superintendent, along with one doctor,[33] thirteen nurses,[34] one stenographer, one bookkeeper, two cooks, and twenty helpers. With the post-1910 fire reconstruction, the Toronto sanatorium was formalized into three hospitals: the Toronto Free Hospital for Consumptives, the King Edward Sanatorium, and the Queen Mary Hospital for Consumptive Children (figures 2.4, 2.5). The Queen Mary Hospital represented, reputedly worldwide, the first dedicated hospital for tuberculous children,[35] its establishment affirming a strengthening commitment to children in Ontario's struggle against tuberculosis.

Construction costs for the Queen Mary were estimated at $60,000,[36] and the building was opened, with great ceremony, by Queen Mary (the spouse of King George V), on 3 June 1913; while she was not present in person, Queen Mary officially opened the doors to the Queen Mary Hospital via a telegraph switch connection with Buckingham Palace.[37] The earlier 1909 opening of Montreal's Royal Edward Institute was accompanied with similar spectacle and ceremony and remote involvement of King Edward.[38] As community achievements, the openings of tuberculosis sanatoria were generally celebrated, the buildings themselves often impressively designed and sited. Godfrey Gale describes the grandeur of the Queen Mary building as it once stood: "It was an imposing building and dominated the hospital scene for 60 years. Massive stone pillars flanked the portico which included an upstairs balcony. Inside the entrance hall corridors extended to wards on either side, while behind lay

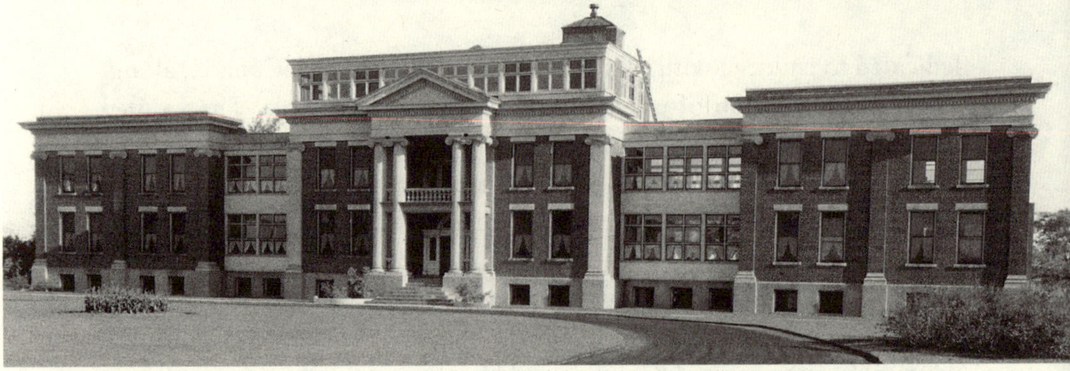

Figure 2.4 The pavilion-style Queen Mary Hospital for Consumptive Children, which opened in 1913 and was demolished in 1976. A rooftop space for fresh air and heliotherapy replaced the wide balconies and porches traditionally associated with sanatoria. Inside the building, the floorplan followed a ward-based model with some private and isolation rooms.

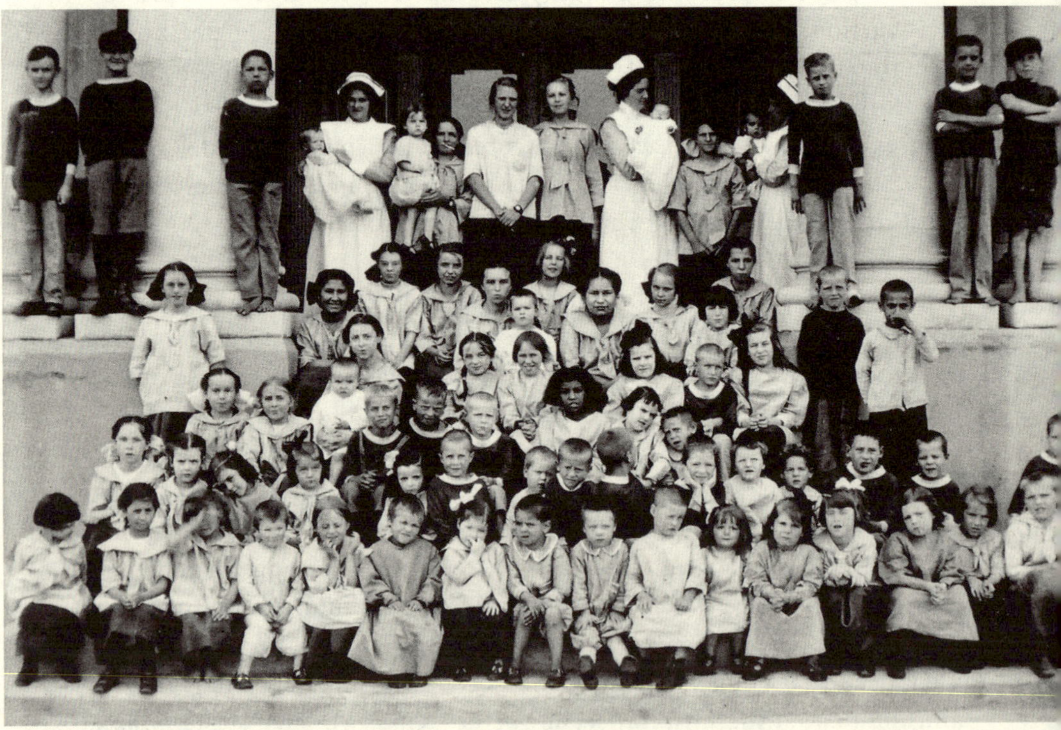

Figure 2.5 The first child patients to experience the newly opened Queen Mary Hospital, photographed on the building's front steps.

the kitchen and a bright, airy dining room. A double, curved staircase led from the hall to the upstairs wards. A penthouse on the roof contained a treatment room and play area, and later on, the X-ray and dental office."[39] The penthouse would be repurposed a number of times, at one point also providing space for the Queen Mary school. A pasteurizing and milk bottling plant was installed in the basement of the Queen Mary, which, given the dangers of bovine tuberculosis transmission through cow's milk, was an important addition to the sanatorium infrastructure in the years before commercial dairies were pasteurizing.[40] Annmarie Adams notes that pasteurization plants were scientific additions found in other early twentieth-century children's hospitals, including Toronto's Hospital for Sick Children.[41] The hospital's linen room serviced the Queen Mary, making and mending clothing for the children. Most of the hospital's needs could be met by the in-house sewing staff, but other items, such as boys' overalls, sweaters, towels, and bedspreads were typically purchased ready-made.[42]

At its height, the Queen Mary provided ninety-six beds for children.[43] The nearby Davies Cottage for Infants, a two-storey brick cottage built in 1916 with funds donated by William Davies, provided another twenty-eight beds for tuberculous infants (figure 2.6). Davies, credited as "the most important pioneer in the Canadian meat-packing industry," was born in England in 1831 and immigrated to Canada with his wife and first child in 1854.[44] By 1857 he had established William Davies and Company in Toronto, or "Hogtown," as the city came to be known via Davies's activities in the slaughter, packing, and export of cured pork (bacon), particularly to England. Described as a "lifelong and ardent Baptist," Davies had a reputation of providing generous support to churches and hospitals.[45] For the NSA, Davies had also funded the construction of the William Davies Cottage at the Muskoka Cottage Sanatorium.[46] Like Hart Massey and others, Davies's tuberculosis philanthropy was likely personally motivated, given the understanding that his two eldest sons, James and William, had both suffered the disease.

On 25 June 1917, the Toronto sanatorium was paid an "official visit of inspection" by Helen MacMurchy, government inspector of hospitals and public charities.[47] At that time, there were forty-one boys and thirty-two girls at the Queen Mary Hospital. Considering the hospital as a

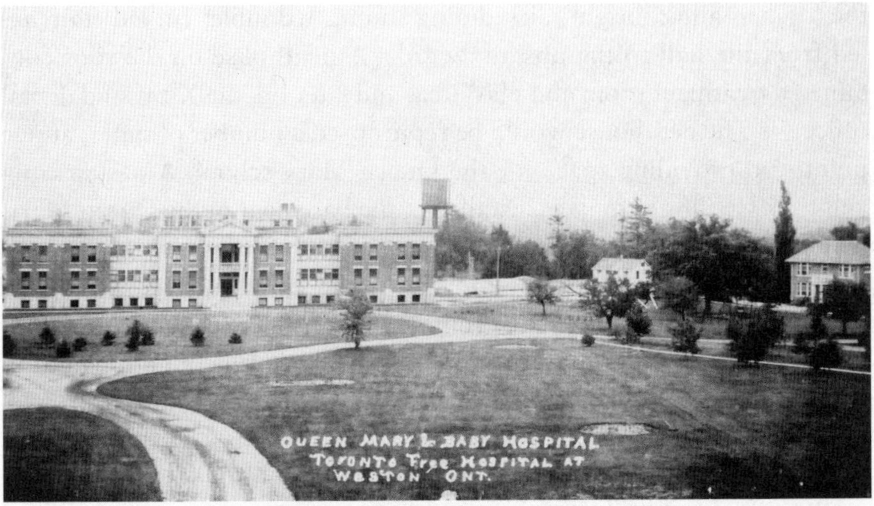
QUEEN MARY & BABY HOSPITAL
TORONTO Free HOSPITAL AT
WESTON ONT.

Figure 2.6 A view of the Queen Mary Hospital for Consumptive Children (*left*) and the brick two-storey Davies Cottage for Infants (*right*). A small playground is in the foreground between these buildings.

whole, MacMurchy described general building conditions as satisfactory. Despite war-related staff shortages[48] affecting the hospital at the time of her visit, she gave the sanatorium a good report, the beds "clean and comfortable," the grounds "in excellent order," the bathrooms "clean and properly ventilated," and the food "good and properly prepared."[49] Administratively, all was in order, with the patients "well cared for" and the staff "paying the utmost attention to their duties." MacMurchy described the Davies Cottage for Infants, opened in the year of her visit, as "well planned" and "full of sunlight," the babies "deriving great benefit from the care they [were] receiving."

Given the length of time that many children would spend in the sanatorium, it was natural that a school would be needed, and the first onsite classroom opened in 1908. By continuing their studies while hospitalized, the children, once discharged, would be better equipped to rejoin their own schools. Though children with tuberculosis may have faced an uncertain future, including the possibility of dying young, the overall positive outlook associated with most child patients reinforced the importance of continuing their education. Post-fire construction included

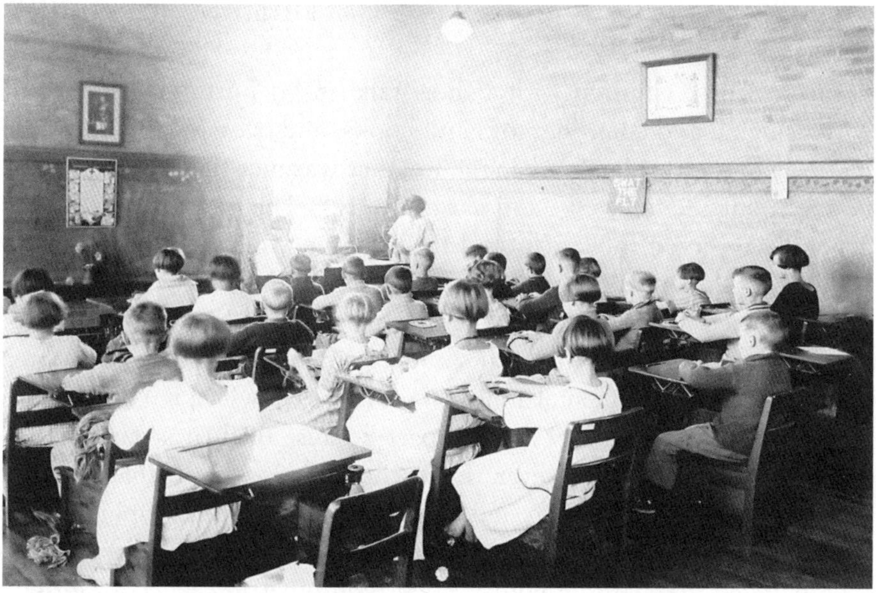

Figure 2.7 Child patients in the sanatorium schoolroom, circa 1926. A sign attached to one of the blackboards reminds the children to "Swat the Fly" (concerns over the disease-transmitting potential of houseflies was common at this time).

the opening of a new and more elaborate Queen Mary School in September 1913, considered a City of Toronto auxiliary school and providing classroom accommodation for up to twenty-nine students (figure 2.7). The number of students enrolled fluctuated because of admissions and discharges and because children could be put back on full-time bedrest if their condition declined.[50] Not all sanatoria for children were equally equipped for education. At Craig-y-nos sanatorium in Wales, for example, former child patients remembered a more haphazard system of informal bedside education.[51]

In 1915, a kindergarten was opened at the sanatorium school, the work of one of sanatorium's nursing trainees, Miss Bobette. This new class proved to be "of great value not only in training [the] small children to discipline, co-operation and occupation, but in obtaining as well a greater amount of rest and entertainment."[52] The Toronto Board of Education provided the equipment necessary for the kindergarten and, in the beginning, about twenty children were enrolled. The kindergarten ran from nine to noon, breaking for lunch and a rest period, and returning in the afternoon for another hour between three and four. The day began for these children with a short talk on "deportment," followed with "singing and counting, toys and books, and occasionally [the] dramatizing of a little play." When the weather was nice the children would be taken outside for walks and nature study.[53] The afternoon hour was generally reserved for crafts, and the children worked on raffia mats, beading, basket making, Plasticine moulding, and painting (figure 2.8).

One Queen Mary School teacher described the curriculum as "somewhat less" relative to provincial standards, mainly because of "shorter school hours and the mental ability of the children, which is a little below that of the average child," in large part because of their struggles with ill-health.[54] That said, however, the teacher did also report that the children "seem bright and interested in their work and the discipline is not hard."[55] In keeping with gender norms typical of the times, the curriculum included manual training for boys and domestic science for girls,[56] though teachers ensured that "both boys and girls have ... a practical knowledge in repairing and darning of clothing" (see figure 2.9).[57] The work of the Queen Mary girls was usually entered into the annual sewing competitions at the Canadian National Exhibition in Toronto. Over the years, many prizes were won; in 1929, for example, the Queen Mary girls were recognized with fourteen prizes for their needlework.[58]

A playground was provided for the children in the adjacent Humber Valley in May 1924. Described as "a most welcome and valuable addition to the equipment," the playground was used by the children every day during the summer. In addition to being a simple enjoyment, the playground ensured that the children spent time outside in the sunshine and fresh air. While children were regularly taken down to the Humber River to wade in the water in the summer months (figure 2.10), in 1925 a new wading pool was added to the playground, constructed with funds donated by the Young Men's Canadian Club. The sanatorium normally signed on a "director of play" to supervise the playground activities over the summer months.[59] Children were also encouraged to join in social clubs, with special divisions of the Junior Red Cross Society, Boy Scouts, and Girl Guides operating out of the sanatorium. For children, the "discipline" that came associated with Scouts and Guides, "and the Baden Powell ethos of efficiency and personal neatness," supported the sanatorium interests in cultivating the right kind of attitude that was needed in resistance building.[60]

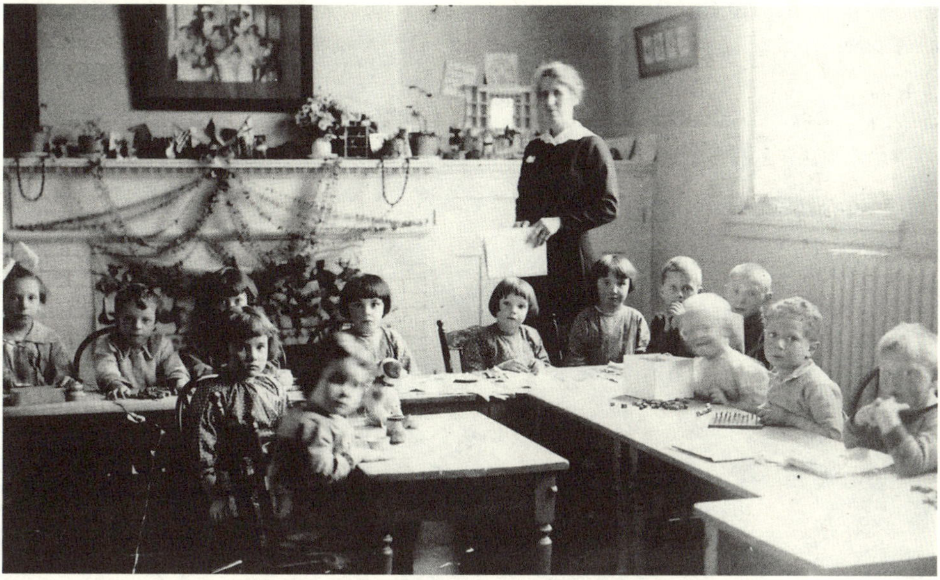

Figure 2.8 The sanatorium's kindergarten class.

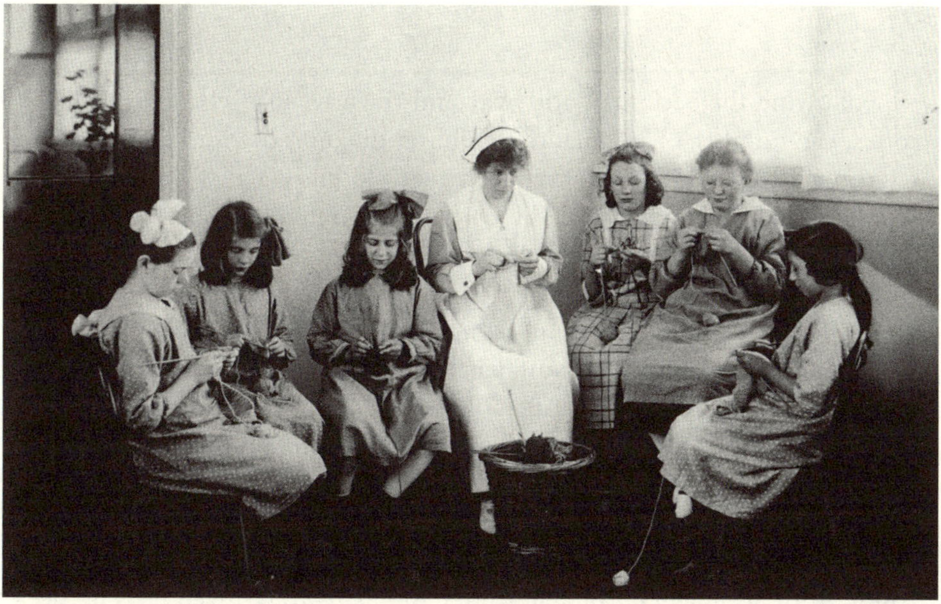

Figure 2.9 Nurse and patients knitting at the Queen Mary Hospital.

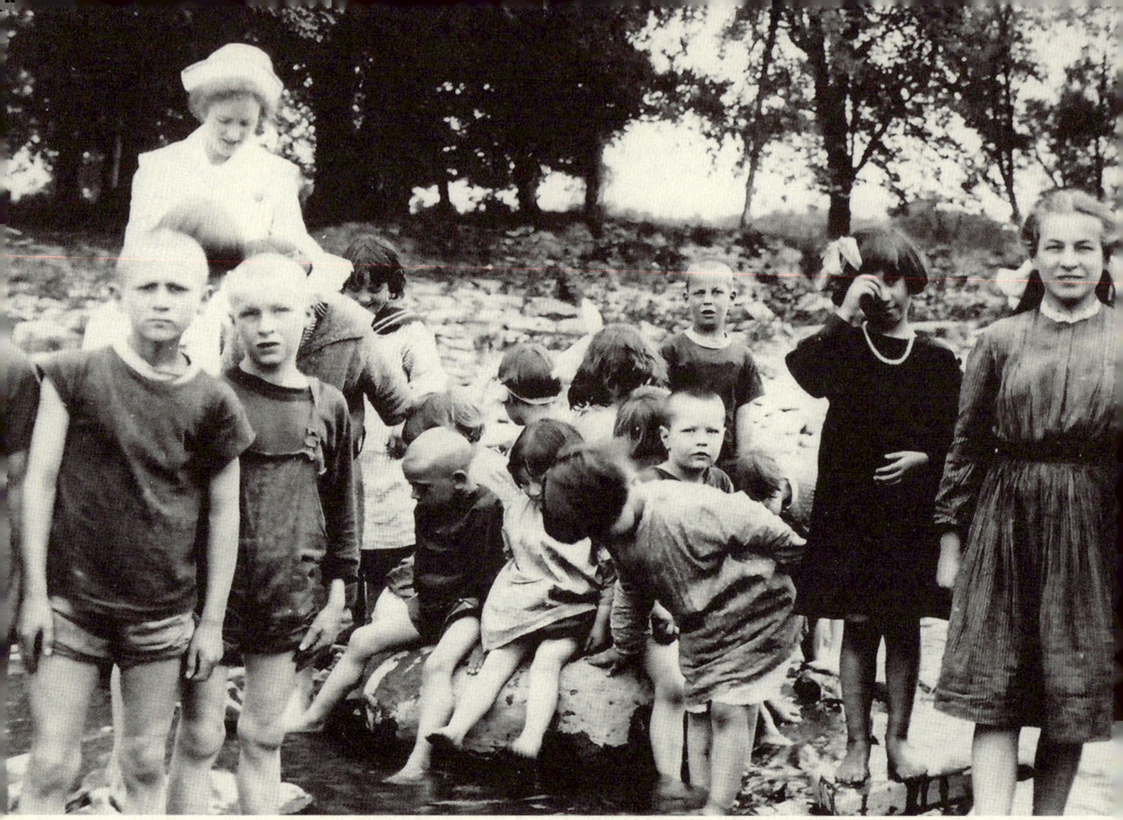

Figure 2.10 Queen Mary Hospital child patients and their nurse wade in the Humber River.

Following the Second World War and the advent of effective antibiotics, the number of infants and children diagnosed with tuberculosis continued to decline. The Davies Cottage closed in 1965, the building demolished in the same year. The Queen Mary remained open until July 1970, when the remaining children were transferred to a new pediatric ward in the main hospital buildings, and was demolished in December 1974.[61] Materially, the decommissioning and demolition of old tuberculosis sanatoria reflected the confidence in, and efficiency of, the new era of antibiotic treatments, as tuberculosis rates continued to decline and patients on drug treatments were increasingly admitted for treatment in general hospitals over shorter periods of time.

Once children were admitted, both age and disease status could influence where they were placed in the wards and buildings of the sanatorium. Adolescents, in particular, were more likely to be given beds in the adult wards instead of the Queen Mary Hospital. Many of the children sampled were admitted to the sanatorium with primary tuberculosis, a typically self-limiting disease; such children were generally not infectious because primary disease was associated with only small pulmonary lesions, low or non-existent tuberculosis bacterium in sputum (if they even raised sputum), and coughs, if present, that were minimal and not forceful enough to raise TB bacteria.[62] In comparison, adolescents were more likely to suffer reactivation disease and cavitary tuberculosis, typically associated with a high volume of TB bacteria-positive sputum and frequent, forceful coughs that were certainly capable of disseminating infection. These differences in primary and reactivation tuberculosis led to the decision to provide the children with a building of their own, though adolescents with cavitary reactivation disease could be given beds in the adult wards because of the nature of their disease and infectiousness.

Irrespective of differences in disease experience, both the children's and adults' wards in the sanatorium's pavilion-style buildings were structured around large, open ward designs with some semi-private or private rooms. The Queen Mary Hospital's Ward L for girls conforms to the arrangement of Nightingale wards outlined by Annmarie Adams for pavilion-style hospitals, with beds placed on the ward's outside walls "punctuated by a regular rhythm of large windows" to maximize fresh air circulation between patients (figure 2.11).[63] In the United States, Edward Trudeau was so convinced of the dangers of "aggregation" that, on the basis of "the new light thrown by science" on the infectious character of tuberculosis, he rejected the ward design altogether and opted for the smaller-scale segregation of the cottage plan at his Saranac Lake sanatorium.[64] As visible in the photograph, the Queen Mary's L ward is light and airy, painted a soft white or cream colour, with high coffered ceilings and pendant lights. The raised white metal beds and minimal bedding ensured that the floors could be easily accessed for regular cleaning and dusting. The Windsor chairs, wooden dressers, potted geraniums, and cut flowers in vases at the patient's bedside all help to soften the institutional feel of the ward. Adams notes that these pavilion-style wards were designed to maximize nursing supervision, since Nightingale "believed that the close surveillance of patients by nurses was essential to modern care."[65] At the far end of the ward, just beyond the third dresser in the photograph, a nurse is seated at a white table giving her a clear

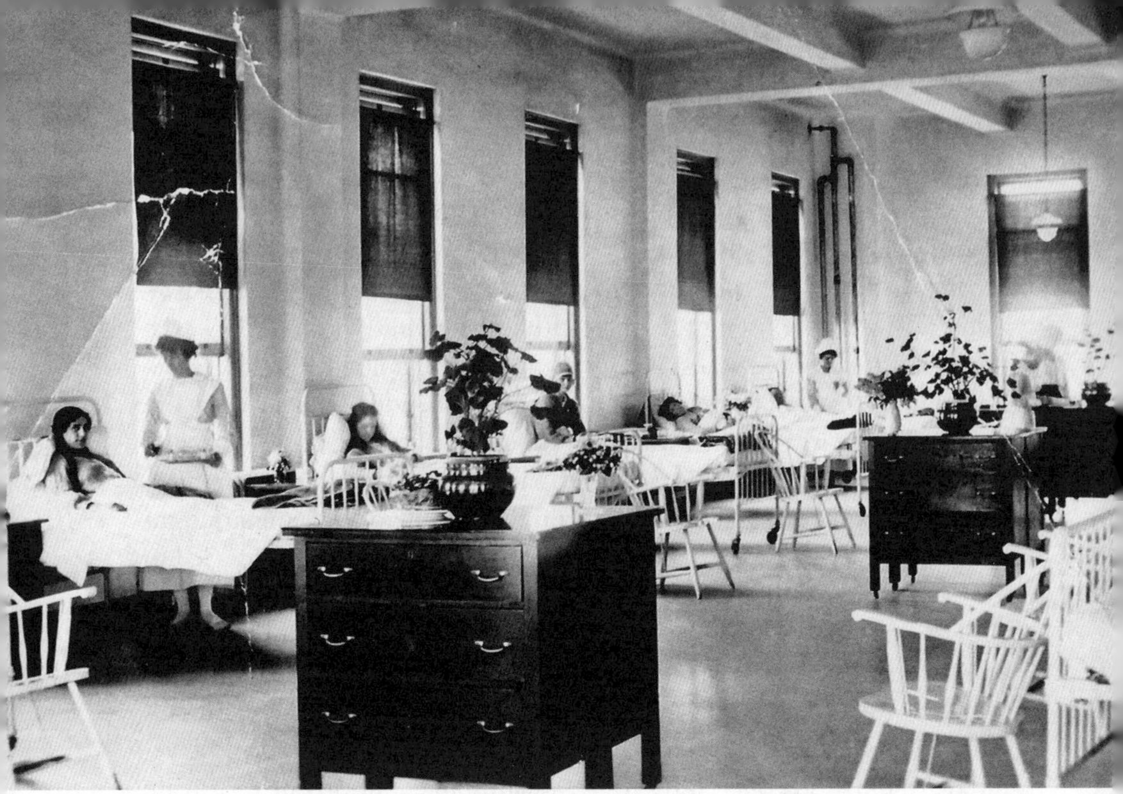

Figure 2.11 The Queen Mary Hospital's Ward L, a ground floor, twelve-bed ward for female patients, 1919.

vantage point or station from which she could monitor the ward. Two nurses attend to the patients in their beds, further reinforcing the nursing presence on the ward. This is not coincidental, since the convalescing patients typical of tuberculosis sanatoria would require substantial supportive nursing care and, as a result, the nursing staff far outnumbered the physicians.

Both children and adults were believed to benefit from the camaraderie of the ward. Since concerns of contagion were minimal for many childhood cases of tuberculosis, large wards made intuitive sense. Though adults at the sanatorium were more likely to be infectious, they were also placed on wards because staff ensured that all patients entering the sanatorium were educated on how to reduce the possibility of infecting others, learning to cover their mouths and noses, for example, to avoid disseminating tuberculosis bacteria through productive coughs and sneezes. Such was the sense of security in the education of patients that nursing and medical staff did not generally wear masks. A large number of patients would be discharged, some still producing bacteria in their sputum, and it was believed that if they did not learn how to live safely within the context of the sanatorium, they probably would not live safely back in their homes and communities.

Despite the attentions to homey comforts, child and family experiences with hospitalization could be traumatic. The Toronto sanatorium attempted to reduce the stress of hospitalization by maintaining a relatively open-door policy, allowing for regular visits on weekends. In this sense, the Toronto sanatorium was quite different from the typical experience of patients in hospitals and sanatoria in the United Kingdom, where strict rules on visiting were more common. At the Craig-y-nos sanatorium in Wales, for example, parents were restricted to one 2-hour visit per month. Many former child patients recalled being unaware of this restriction on visiting, and the limitation, paired with the inability of some parents to travel the long distance to Craig-y-nos, led some children to believe that they had simply been forgotten by their families. Decades later, the painful feelings can still be conjured, as Gareth Wyke remembered he had felt "very unloved."[66] Such was the feeling likely experienced by some of the children at the Toronto sanatorium, particularly those too young to understand the separation and why they were there in the first place.

The rising disciplines of pediatrics, psychiatry, and child psychology worked to reduce such negative hospitalization-related experiences. In this respect, the historiography of child hospitalization in the United Kingdom generally targets the 1950s as an important transition period, fuelled largely by the contributions of John Bowlby (a psychiatrist) and James Robertson (a psychiatric social worker) and those who influenced their ideas.[67] The 1959 publication of the "Platt Report" affirmed government commitment to modifying the overall culture of child hospitalization. Important changes were made as the heavily restrictive rules governing child-parent visiting were relaxed. Bowlby and Robertson's work suggested children were not as "resilient" and quick to recover, or bounce back, from stressful situations as many had once imagined, and that they could experience great anxiety and trauma through separation from their parents and assimilation to hospital culture.[68] In exploring the experience of children at the Queen Alexandra Solarium, Vancouver Island, Lenora

Marcellus uncovered a nurse's report suggesting that crying was rarely heard among the children. Marcellus argues that "the notion that small children separated from their parents rarely cried invites some speculation," particularly because of the "rigid parenting norms of the time," which "may have contributed to the nursing practice of minimizing the emotional concerns of the children."[69] It is likely that the strictness of hospitalization meshed to some extent with a greater strictness in home discipline and the rules and expectations framing child behaviour in the early twentieth century more generally.

At the Toronto sanatorium, visiting was permitted at specified hours on weekends, and each week a thousand or more visitors called upon patients. In the early days of the sanatorium few visitors had cars and relied on the Toronto Transit Commission's "old trolley" to get them out to Weston, though visitors would still have to walk the additional half mile to the sanatorium.[70] Child visitors were somewhat discouraged in order to prevent their needless exposure to TB, and to protect the health of child patients in the sanatorium from imported childhood diseases. The restrictions on visiting in England prior to the 1950s had a lot to do with concerns that "parents brought filthy germs into the wards,"[71] but also the observation that children often became upset, agitated, or sad all over again in the aftermath of visits somewhat outweighing, it was believed, the short-lived benefit of the visit. Despite the fact that the medical and nursing staff at the Toronto sanatorium remained vigilant about the possibility of imported diseases, sanatorium administrators (Dr Dobbie and Miss Dickson) did not discourage visiting, believing that visits were of tremendous emotional value to the children. For those children whose families lived close to the sanatorium and were able to visit more often, hospitalization was likely more tolerable.

Because of the hundreds of tuberculous patients, visitors could have apprehensions about entering the sanatorium. In 1913, for example, one Sunday school teacher wrote to Miss Dickson hoping to visit her student, fourteen-year-old Sarah, but unsure if a visit would pose any "danger." In her reply to the teacher, Dickson reassured her of her safety, provided visitors were "careful" in not handling anything previously handled by "careless" patients. She emphasized, however, that even after only a few weeks at the sanatorium patients had "learned to be careful," and only those patients who were not "conscientious" were potentially "dangerous to visitors." Dickson believed Sarah to be "very clean in her habits, and very teachable," and, as a result, considered it "quite safe" for the teacher and Sarah's classmates to visit. Since this exchange took place in 1913, it predated the confirmation that tuberculosis could follow an airborne route of transmission. Today, in comparison to the sanatorium era, a greater awareness of the multiple modes of tuberculosis transmission has reshaped requirements in visiting, and visitors are now provided with masks, which they wear while visiting in properly ventilated rooms.[72]

Since the sanatorium operated as a fairly open institution, in addition to regular visiting hours on weekends, patients were also permitted leaves of absence. For children, the allowance helped to protect their emotional well-being, though leaves were generally recommended only for children who were well enough. Given the large number of children admitted from the city of Toronto, a long-term agreement had been struck with the city's Department of Health permitting patients "day leave" (going and returning on the same day) or "weekend leave" (leaving on a Saturday and returning Monday) once every six weeks without the need to deduct these absences from the city's account. A slightly longer absence was granted for those approved for Christmas or New Year's leaves. Since this was a specific arrangement with the city of Toronto, however, leaves of absence for patients of other municipalities had to be arranged on a case-by-case basis, if the municipality was even open to the idea at all. For parents located outside of the city, months or years might pass before they had the opportunity to see their hospitalized children, if ever.

Sanatoria varied considerably in their relative isolation, and some of the discrepancy can be explained by the original intentions of sanatorium planners. In their study of the Westwood Sanatorium in Australia, Kirby and Madsen outline multiple unexpected effects associated with its intended geographical isolation, including the exclusion of trained nurses from professional activities, the invisibility of the hospital (leading to decreased funding and economic and infrastructural decline), and the sequestering of tuberculosis patients, not only from their families, but also society at large.[73] By the 1930s, Westwood Sanatorium, neglected and ill-funded, had become run-down. In this respect, Alice Street argues that the very qualities of hospital buildings themselves (when and where they were built, by whom, and how well they have been maintained) can engender hope or hopelessness among both patients and staff.[74] Though located on the outskirts of the city, the Toronto sanatorium benefitted from its urban connection and the firm commitment of the National Sanitarium Association to maintaining and improving it through ongoing fundraising. From its incarnation to its demise, the Toronto sanatorium never became an "out of sight, out of mind" institution, but remained visible, modern, well-staffed, comfortably appointed, and fully functional for patients and staff alike.

Because the Toronto sanatorium was open to visitors and leaves of absence, utmost importance was placed on protecting the children from additional outside diseases entering the sanatorium, balancing the emotional needs for contact with family and friends with the medical need to prevent the entry of any additional infections that could lower their resistance to tuberculosis.[75] As a result, a number of safeguards were put in place. Children who left the sanatorium on short leaves of absence, for instance, were typically put in isolation rooms off the main wards for a brief period upon their return. Despite these efforts, outbreaks of additional diseases, such as measles, chicken pox, mumps, scarlet fever, poliomyelitis, and typhoid fever seemingly could not be prevented. In 1917–18, two cases of measles appeared in the Queen Mary, one case in a little girl, and the other, a nurse. Three cases of typhoid fever involving one doctor and two nurses were also reported in the same year. Telltale symptoms of emerging disease could lead to the affected child's removal to the isolation rooms and a quarantine placed on the child's ward.

With more serious outbreaks, the whole children's hospital could be quarantined. One child who was thought to be at risk for mumps, for example, was isolated on 30 December 1927. When her mumps symptoms surfaced on 14 January 1928, the hospital was quarantined until early February. When a child admitted to the sanatorium in December 1947 developed measles, a general letter was sent out to parents advising they forego any visits prior to Christmas Day. The staff further advised that, even then, those who had never had measles should avoid the sanatorium altogether until the infection had cleared. In some cases, if necessary, a complete removal from the sanatorium could be arranged; children developing diphtheria, for example, were typically taken by ambulance to Toronto's Riverdale Isolation Hospital, a quarantine facility that had opened in the mid-1870s beside the Don Jail in Toronto. Inevitably, despite all efforts to the contrary, the Spanish influenza pandemic of 1918–19 made its way into the sanatorium, and a number of patients, as well as Dr Hayes and Dr Dobbie, became ill.[76] During this vulnerable time, visitors were severely restricted and permits, issued only under exceptional circumstances, had to be endorsed by staff in order to gain entry. Still, some patients, such as nine-year-old Gilda, struggled through multiple diseases. Gilda developed diphtheria in September 1918 and was transferred to the Riverdale Isolation Hospital. Shortly after she regained her health and returned to the Queen Mary, she became sick with Spanish influenza. Despite these serious setbacks, by May 1920 she had regained good health, having no cough, no sputum, and almost no signs of active tuberculosis.

Since secondary infections with other infectious diseases could weaken patient resistance and complicate attempts to control tuberculosis, vaccinations, if available, were used to reduce the potential for infectious diseases in the sanatorium.[77] Most children had the results of Schick and Dick testing, for diphtheria and scarlet fever exposure, respectively, in their charts. At the sanatorium, testing for these diseases became routine by 1921, and immunizations were recommended for positive reactors (a positive reaction indicating no prior exposure). Along with adult patients, all children entering the sanatorium were routinely tested for syphilis using the Kahn and Wassermann tests. Since some symptoms could overlap in TB and syphilis, such as enlargement of the cervical lymph nodes,[78] knowing whether or not patients were co-infected could be important for differentially diagnosing active tuberculosis and devising appropriate treatment plans (involving Salvarsan for treating syphilis). Routine testing for syphilis among patients at the tuberculosis sanatorium supplemented other early twentieth-century mass screening efforts, including mandatory blood tests before the issuing of marriage licences. Katherine McCuaig has described the interest in Canada in aligning tuberculosis and syphilis screening and education efforts, particularly since tuberculosis work had become quite ingrained and normalized, while syphilis remained more peripheralized and stigmatized.[79] Bundled with tuberculosis testing, the challenge of syphilis could be more effectively addressed.

Oral health was also a concern for patients in the sanatorium and, when the children's hospital opened in 1913, the "preservation of their teeth" motivated Dobbie to secure a dental chair, with all of the necessary equipment, for the sanatorium.[80] While there had always been periodic visits by dentists to the sanatorium, Dobbie wanted a more established system, where practising dentists or dental students in their final year of training could attend to the sanatorium patients regularly one or two afternoons each week. Ensuring proper care of teeth and gums was critical, since the pinkish streaks resulting from bleeding gums could easily be confused with small amounts of blood expectorated with active pulmonary tuberculosis.[81] The body's immune response to infections associated with cavities and abscesses could also result in cervical lymph node enlargement in the neck, obscuring or complicating the characteristic lymph node enlargement often associated with primary tuberculosis infection in children.[82] Bates notes that tuberculosis specialists had a particular interest in dental care, since they believed "decayed teeth" along with "infected tonsils, and even faulty vision" could all reduce bodily resistance to tuberculosis.[83] According to McCuaig, the state of children's teeth could also serve as a general indicator of relative health and tuberculosis vulnerability, because children of families with "little money for luxuries such as dentists" were often also living in under conditions of hardship and poor nutrition (figure 2.12).[84]

Along with their specialty in tuberculosis, sanatorium doctors were also required to be good medical generalists, diagnosing childhood illnesses, differentially diagnosing children who may have been admitted as TB cases, but, in fact, turned out to be non-tuberculous, and always remaining open to the idea that not all aspects of a child's condition could be linked to tuberculosis.[85] The medical staff had to be prepared to deal with complications of tuberculosis as well as conditions associated with the rundown and susceptible state of some children at admission. Diarrhea, vomiting, abscesses, non-tuberculous tonsillitis and appendicitis, poor vision, ear infections, scabies, eczema, jaundice, and anemia were all observed. Accidents happened, and the hospital's X-ray machine could be put to uses other than imaging tuberculous lungs. Such was the case for eight-year-old Claudia. To her horror, one of the Queen Mary ward

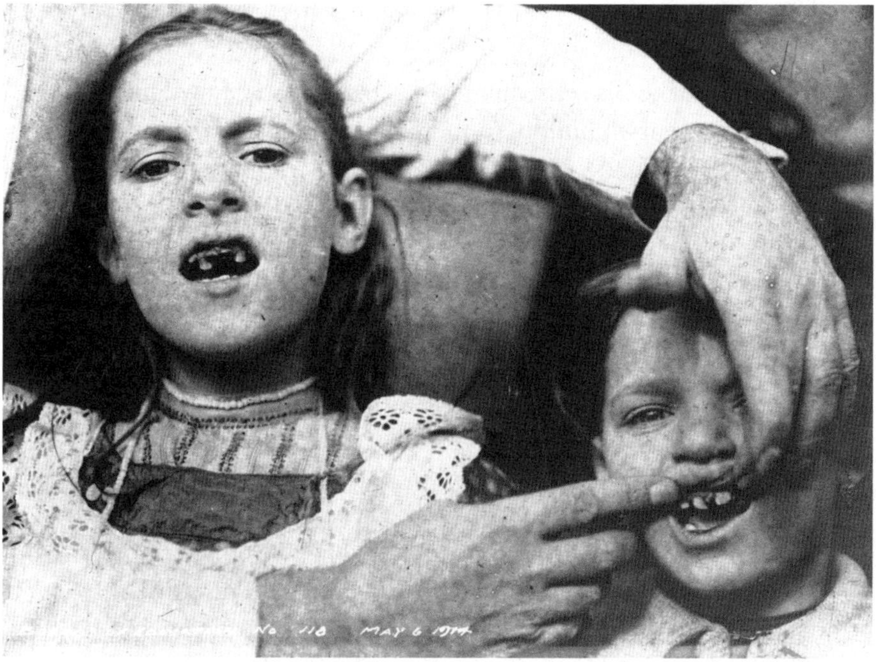

Figure 2.12 A Toronto Board of Education dental inspection revealing the state of children's teeth, 6 May 1914.

nurses discovered that Claudia had "swallowed a small lead pencil" described precisely as "1½ ins. long and about 3 mm thick (kind used on dance programs) with small white metal cap." Dr McHugh gave instructions that she be given half an ounce of "OlRicini" (castor oil, a laxative) and to watch for the passage of the pencil. Since the pencil had not made an appearance by 10 a.m. the following morning, McHugh sent Claudia over to the X-ray room and determined that the pencil, plainly visible in the X-ray, was slowly making its way through her gastrointestinal tract. Even though tuberculosis may have been their main concern, a focus on overall bodily wellness and attending to incidental complaints was important for maintaining and improving health and resistance.

Particularly after the massive post-fire reconstruction, the sanatorium took on the character of a small village, with a community of some eight hundred staff and patients, the type of facility that sociologist Erving Goffman would describe as a "total institution," self-sustaining and all-encompassing.[86] In compiling his thoughts on the early history of the sanatorium prior to his retirement in 1939, Dr Dobbie meticulously documented the extensive buildings and services found at the sanatorium:

> In this village there is to be found a butcher shop with a weekly business in meat and provisions, butter, eggs and vegetables amount to $1,000.00, a grocery store, a dry goods store, a hardware store, a paint shop, a plumbing and steamfitting shop, a drug store, a photograph gallery, a shoe shine parlor, a public health laboratory, an artificial ice factory, an electrical shop, a dressmaking establishment, a china shop, a milk depot, a baker's shop, two carpenter shops, a morgue, a postal station, a telephone office, a barber shop, a beauty parlor, a household linen workshop, an interurban cartage agency, a novelty shop, a public library, a shoe repair shop, a tuck shop, a church, a concert hall, a public school, a public playground, a greenhouse, a public radio, a water works, a steam sterilizing and disinfecting station, a sewage disposal plant, a modern central heating plant, a soap factory, a laundry,[87] five restaurants, several apartment houses, two office buildings, a public garage (accommodating nine cars), a number of private residences [including Dobbie's cottage, Glenwyld], and subsidiary industries such as market-gardening, floriculture, poultry raising, hog raising, a livery stable, without mentioning the three hospitals,[88] affording work for six physicians and 100 nurses, a village clerk, five public stenographers, a justice of the peace, several clergymen, a dentist, and numerous social workers.[89]

Unlike the NSA's tuberculosis sanatoria near Gravenhurst, the Toronto sanatorium, on the outskirts of the growing city, was not particularly isolated. Urban expansion meant that residential, commercial, and even industrial sites grew closer with each passing decade. By the 1930s, sanatorium administrators became frustrated with the noise and disturbance created by the operations of a neighbouring gravel pit, which some days persisted until midnight. Yet the sanatorium also had the acreage for gardens,[90] a hennery,[91] and a piggery,[92] and differed in this way from urban hospitals.

Endowed and Named Beds

In the early to mid-nineteenth century, Canadian hospitals were built on philanthropy and "patronized by few but the very poor."[93] These early hospitals were reputed to be places of moral reform, rather than places of true medical care or cures, focusing on vulnerabilities such as sexually transmitted diseases and alcohol-associated diseases, and the care of children born outside of marriage. Shortt notes, "Never in their wildest imaginations did the hospital's middle-class benefactors, in the early nineteenth century, imagine themselves as potential patients; they expected to receive medical care from their personal physicians in the clean comfort of their own homes."[94] But by the late nineteenth century, middle-class families began to enter hospitals. This change in attitude was encouraged by emerging medical technologies and the rising status of medicine, but was also a necessity, because the changing demography of families, particularly in urban areas, complicated the provision of adequate home care.[95]

The Toronto sanatorium presents some continuities with and departures from this broad perspective on early Canadian hospitals. The sanatorium's role intertwined with behavioural reforms, guiding people on how to live well and responsibly with a chronic infection, and was, perhaps in that respect, loosely related to the nineteenth-century lessons of moral reform imparted at the hospital. The sanatorium also reflected the expanding clientele, particularly "the affluent middle class," that characterized late nineteenth-century hospitals.[96] In fact, the first sanatorium opened by the NSA in Muskoka was for paying patients and, as affluent patients set the example and popularized hospital treatment for tuberculosis, the NSA's free Muskoka sanatorium for non-paying patients soon followed. As hospitals increasingly became known as sites of modern, scientific medicine, and much more than the custodial institutions that they had been, there was a greater willingness among all classes to use these institutions. To most, the sanatorium offered a modicum of hope in surviving tuberculosis.

The earliest tuberculosis sanatoria in Canada, those of the NSA, were made possible because of a strong culture of tuberculosis-related philanthropy, not only among wealthy Canadians, but Canadians of all economic standings. While infectious diseases were often stigmatizing and peripheralizing, the pervasive nature of tuberculosis drew communities together, encouraging citizens to help one another, at least in the earlier years of the sanatorium era. Tuberculosis had the potential to affect anyone, irrespective of wealth or social standing. Those who were or were not vulnerable to tuberculosis infection and disease could not be identified easily, and the narrower epidemiological language of "risk groups" would emerge only in the wake of antibiotics and the relative demise of tuberculosis. In TB's endemic years, it was often impossible for individuals to distance themselves, physically or psychologically, from tuberculosis, so most people shared a vested interest in controlling the disease, and it was not difficult to conjure wide-scale support, from all walks of life, for the construction and maintenance of the NSA sanatoria.

Creating unique opportunities for philanthropy, the sanatorium established a system of "endowed" and "named" beds. These beds were sponsored by individuals, estates, and organizations and represented an important source of ongoing funding (or "practical sympathy," as the sanatorium administration called it). "Endowed" beds were permanently sponsored with a one-time payment and, in 1918, a $2,000 contribution endowed a cot at the Queen Mary Hospital for Consumptive Children. Alternatively, sponsors could support the hospital with "named" beds. In 1918, a donation of $100 named a cot at the Queen Mary for one year and could be renewed. With each NSA annual report, lists of names of those supporting endowed and named beds were published. For example, from the list of nine endowed beds and twenty named beds published for the Queen Mary for 1918–19, a number of notable and affluent names can be readily identified. Because of their prominence, it was not difficult to research basic biographies in order to understand, on some level, who these philanthropists were and their possible motivations for supporting the sanatorium and sick children.

In the aftermath of the First World War, the "Victory Cot," a named bed, was sponsored by Sir Frank Baillie. Baillie, a financier and industrialist, was born in Toronto in 1875, and in his career established a brokerage company, the Canada Steel Company Limited, the Dominion Steel Foundry Company, the Canadian Cartridge Company Limited, and, in

1917, Canadian Aeroplanes Limited, which supplied the Royal Air Force with airplanes in the First World War.[97] In 1918 Baillie was knighted, but died shortly after, in January 1921 in Toronto. Though he has been described as a wealthy businessman with "little interest in charity," his wife, Edith, appeared to be the family philanthropist, serving as a board member for Toronto's Home for Incurable Children and likely responsible for the cot sponsorship.[98] The Sternberg Recital Cot, another named bed, was funded by Amy Sternberg, proprietor of the Sternberg Studio of Dancing in Toronto. An unmarried entrepreneur who reportedly "led an unorthodox life," Sternberg taught the art of dance to the children of some of Toronto's wealthiest families.[99] Those children would play a role in Sternberg's philanthropy, dancing in her annual recitals in support of hospital charities, including an extravaganza in 1915 to benefit the wartime efforts of the Red Cross. Sternberg's declining health and economic troubles led her to close her dance studio in 1929, and, in 1935, at fifty-four years of age, she died.[100] The J. Frater Taylor named bed (figure 2.13) was supported by James Frater Taylor, a Scottish businessman of modest public school education who had come to Canada in 1909 when he was thirty-six years of age, "on behalf of London capitalists who had invested millions" in the northern Ontario industrial centre of Sault Ste Marie.[101] Taylor was appointed president of the Lake Superior Corporation in the "Soo," to reinvigorate the corporation, which, under his direction, grew to include a steel mill, a rail mill (for manufacturing railway track), a railway, a power plant, and seventeen subsidiary companies (including limestone quarries, coal mines, and pulp and paper mills). Taylor was also a financier in the Canadian Nickel Corporation, which purchased the Murray Mine near Sudbury in 1913.[102] He involved himself in hospital work in Sault Ste Marie, in 1912 chairing the Special Finance Committee, which was formed under his direction to raise much-needed revenue for the Sault Ste Marie General Hospital.[103]

While much of the sanatorium's obvious (named) philanthropy could read like a "Who's Who" of Canadian society, contributions also came from community- or industry-related organizations, including the City Dairy Employees. That is an interesting point, given the tensions over milk management (ultimately leading to compulsory pasteurization of milk) and the likely presence of children in the sanatorium who were infected

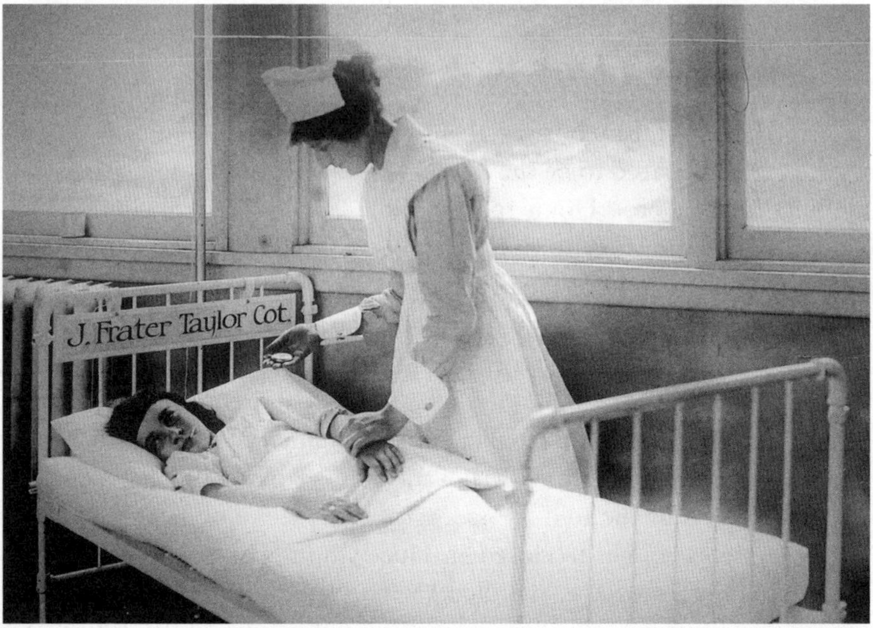

Figure 2.13 A child patient in the J. Frator Taylor named bed. The child has a thermometer in her mouth, which the nurse will read in order to determine whether or not she has a fever. Meanwhile, with pocket watch in hand, the nurse is measuring the girl's pulse rate. These were two routine health indicators recorded regularly in patient charts.

with milk from tuberculous cows. However, the sanatorium movement would not have been so successful in raising the funds needed to support these hospitals without the contributions of thousands of Ontarians, most of whom remain unnamed, but whose ongoing one-, two-, or five-dollar donations made campaigns such as the National Sanitarium Association's "Million Dollar Fund" (and the post-fire reconstruction) possible.

In recognition of cot sponsorship, a brass sign, engraved according to the sponsor's wishes, hung prominently at the head of each endowed bed; less expensive wooden signs were used for the named beds. In order to encourage their ongoing support, notes on each child's progress were provided each year, at Christmas, to cot sponsors and included a photograph of the child resting in or sitting on the bed with the cot sign prominently featured. The cot notes must be read cautiously, since these were intended as a type of public presentation of the children to their cot sponsors. As a result, the featured patients were described endearingly, in the best light, so that all of the positive feelings associated with philanthropy would be reinforced, the innocent child patients clearly "deserving" of the support. In their attempts to personalize these short stories, staff (most likely ward nurses) reflected on each child's character and often detailed the hardships that the child patients had faced in their short lives – their perseverance through tuberculosis, their improvements or losses over the previous year, and their industriousness in making the best of their time at the sanatorium. Such was the case for Edward, who occupied the Freemasons' Queen City Lodge 552 named cot. In one year, Edward's cot note reported, "Another year has passed and poor Ed is still confined to his Ward. He is such a patient little fellow that he really should have better luck. His brothers, in the Babies Section, have been improving daily giving promise of complete recovery." By the following year, Edward had come to terms with the restrictions of bedrest: "Ed is still confined to bed but since he gets so much enjoyment from reading he does not fuss about his lot. At Hallowe'en he had the most attractive Ward, the decorations having been provided by his 'Cot Sign Friends' as Ed calls his benefactors." Members of the Toronto branch of the Dickens' Fellowship, a global fellowship for Charles Dickens aficionados, had funded a cot occupied by eleven-year-old Nellie. Nellie's first cot note was written five months after she had arrived at the sanatorium; despite the fact that she was still considered "under weight," she had been reclassified as an "up patient" and was much happier at the sanatorium because she had been able to begin attending school. Her trajectory as a good patient and pupil was emphasized in her cot note the following year: "The child who occupies this cot is a thin tall girl of twelve years – Nellie – Her father is dead, and her mother is a patient in another Sanitorium. Nellie loves 'dressing up,' and spends many hours in the land of make-believe. She is very artistic and enjoys directing little plays in which she is the principal actress. She reads a great deal especially fairy stories, and has also proved a good pupil at school." Her last cot note described Nellie's "steady progress toward better health," even though she needed her strength of character "to fight at times to maintain progress." Nellie had continued to define herself as a good student, and her cot sponsors were apprised of her growing fondness for the pianoforte, receiving some instruction from the nursing staff, and her hopes "to continue with her music when she is discharged."

The connections established through cot notes sometimes inspired cot sponsors to do more for the children occupying their beds than just provide sponsorship payments. Some cot sponsors visited the children they funded. In Edward's case, cot sponsors sent Hallowe'en decorations to liven up his ward, and at Easter in 1935, the Gooderham Chapter IODE presented their "cot child" with a large Easter egg and some clothing. Thoughtfully, they also sent along a package of smaller eggs to be given out to the other children on the ward. Six-year-old Marie's Christmas note sent to her "J.B. Martin Cot" patron in December 1935, described her as a very neat little girl who liked to play with dolls and help to look after the younger children on her ward. Marie, in turn, received a letter from Martin himself, who wrote, "I have just learned that you occupy the J.B. Martin Cot and the management tells me that you are such a good little girl." He praised her for being "neat and orderly," making her own bed, and helping staff with the children. "Now that is surely worth something," Martin surmised, "and if I had known sooner about you, Santa would have brought you this little gift." The family of Jesse Bauman Martin (1897–1974) was part of the Old Order Mennonite congregation located near Waterloo, Ontario. Ordained in 1925, at the time when he wrote this letter to Marie, he was pastor of the Erb Street Mennonite congregation in Waterloo and married to Naomi Collier Martin, both noted for their lifelong charitable work.[104] The nurse who delivered Martin's Christmas gift noted that he had sent Marie "a very beautiful doll."

Overall, endowed cots worked quite favourably to support the sanatorium and the children who occupied those cots, but there were occasional complications, including an incident where cot sponsors decided to publish the progress note and photograph of their cot child in a widely circulated local entertainment magazine. In that note, it was mentioned that the little girl in question had immigrated to Ontario with her foster parents. The parents objected strongly to this publication, disappointed that their daughter had learned that she was not their biological child in this manner. Dobbie tried to remedy the situation, telling the girl that there had been mistakes in her write-up and not to pay any attention to what was written on account of those mistakes. Unfortunately, Dobbie understood that the "other children in the Queen Mary" had been "painfully frank in telling her what foster-parents are," and, understandably, the girl had become quite upset.

The Toronto Sanatorium Staff

The Toronto sanatorium was part of Toronto's larger medical landscape, interconnected with the city's other main medical institutions, including the Toronto General Hospital, the Hospital for Sick Children,[105] Toronto Western Hospital, and Women's College Hospital, with children regularly transferred to the sanatorium when tuberculosis became the suspected cause of their ill-health. The opening of the Queen Mary marked a significant moment in Canadian history, providing the first specialized institution for the full-time care of tuberculous children, complementing the work of other local hospitals and the IODE Preventorium in Toronto. The Toronto sanatorium gained a reputation for its specialized care of infants, children, and pregnant (and tuberculous) women, and its growing surgical repertoire kept the sanatorium connected with physicians and surgeons from the city's other medical institutions. The sanatorium quickly earned its place in nursing and medical training, where professional lives could be nurtured, for some for the length of their careers. Over the majority of this study, there was administrative continuity at the sanatorium as both Dr Dobbie and Miss Dickson, fresh out of their medical and nursing training, assumed their roles and remained in their positions for decades until their retirements.

William James Dobbie

William Dobbie was born in Guelph, Ontario, on 20 April 1873, son of James Dobbie, a carpenter and millwright, and Elizabeth "Lizzie" Dobbie (Edmondson). Less than three years later, on 20 March 1876, William's forty-year-old father died of heart disease.[106] At the time of the 1881 census of Canada, eight-year-old William was living in his thirty-three-year-old widowed mother's home with his two sisters, Isabella, ten, and

Jemina, five, and his six-year-old brother, John. William's mother had been born in Ireland and immigrated to Canada as an infant in 1849. William and his siblings were all born in Ontario, identified by Scottish ancestry (after their deceased father) and Presbyterian in religion. After the death of her husband, Lizzie became a shopkeeper in Guelph, evidently able to support her family, since both her sons would go on to become university-educated and successful professionals in medicine.

William Dobbie's career in medicine materialized after a winding journey. As a student, Dobbie attended Guelph Public School and Guelph's Collegiate Institute for his primary and secondary education.[107] By the 1890s, Dobbie had relocated to Toronto, where he earned a bachelor of arts at the University of Toronto in 1897, followed by a master of arts in 1899.[108] From there, he returned to Guelph and taught at the Guelph Collegiate Institute. The 1901 census finds him, at twenty-seven years of age, living in his mother's nine-room home/store rental on Cork Street in Guelph. By this time, fifty-six-year-old Elizabeth was no longer working, but her son was earning $850 a year as a teacher.

Dobbie would leave teaching and subsequently return to Toronto to begin studies at Trinity Medical College in 1902, receiving a First Scholarship in his first year and a First Medallist distinction in his second year. According to his University of Toronto yearbook entry, "as a practical man he is unexcelled and scholastically his course has been a brilliant one."[109] Dobbie received his doctor of medicine, master in surgery accreditation in 1905, when he was thirty-two years of age. By this time Trinity Medical College had become part of the University of Toronto. Dobbie's younger brother, John A. Dobbie, also completed medical training and later served as medical superintendent of the Ottawa General Hospital.[110] The Dobbie brothers would qualify as "modern" doctors under Edward Shorter's classification, the era representing physicians who graduated from medical school between 1880 and 1950, benefitting from the insights of the germ theory and microbiology and schooled in the science of anatomy (both pathological and microscopic), chemistry, and physiology.[111] Shorter argues that medicine's deepening connections with science had profound effects on the doctor–patient relationship of the modern era, patients increasingly "willing to submit to the doctor because they saw him bathed in the particular glow of science."[112] Earlier, traditional era physicians, on the other hand, did not necessarily conjure such respect, possibly because they came to be perceived as "largely uneducated" and "hopelessly overnumerous" "meddlars" who possessed an "almost maniacally perverse therapeutic philosophy."[113] As medical schools restructured and the profession became more restricted, the number of physicians declined, while their education and their social status, reflected in their income, homes, cars, and community work, increased.[114] The modern physician's knowledge of science and improved status may have attracted patients to them for diagnoses and treatments, but one great strength that modern physicians possessed was their attention to, and interest in, their patients. Shorter argues that the close doctor–patient relationship of the modern era could be therapeutic in itself, where doctors expressed true interest in their patients, and the "good chat" of the consultation provided enormous psychological value in healing.[115] As a result, in Canada, the tuberculosis sanatorium arose in an era ripe for medical authority grounded in science and strong emotional influence in illness.

Dobbie assumed the position of physician-in-chief of the Toronto Sanatorium shortly after earning his MD in October 1905. Because Dobbie was not yet fully licensed to practise medicine, Allan Adams, the outgoing physician-in-chief who had tendered his resignation in July 1905, continued to visit the sanatorium two days a week.[116] At the time of his appointment, Dobbie earned a salary of $25 per month.[117] For almost thirty-four years, Dobbie remained physician-in-chief, until his retirement in 1939 (figure 2.14), when he was succeeded by Dr McHugh (who had been responsible for the Queen Mary Hospital). Dobbie continued in tuberculosis work even after his retirement, overseeing the operations of the NSA's Gage Institute in Toronto and the examination of more than ten thousand clinic patients per year. He also continued to lecture to student nurses at the sanatorium and advise the sanatorium's Board of Trustees, representing the board at the meetings of the Canadian Hospital Association and other professional associations.[118]

In his administrative role as physician-in-chief of the Toronto sanatorium, Dobbie spent considerable time on correspondence, judging by the volume of incoming and outgoing letters in the records. One woman who worked as Dobbie's secretary in the 1930s recalled him as "a quiet man,

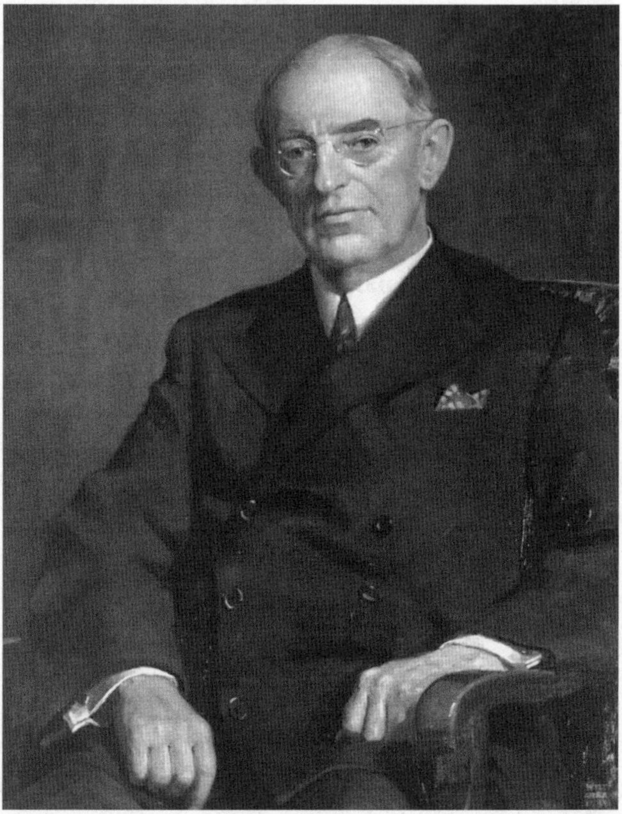

Figure 2.14 W.J. Dobbie's portrait painted on the occasion of his retirement in 1939.

reserved, not much conversation, pleasant."[119] As she took dictation, "there would be very little conversation other than any instructions that he might want to give me ... he was very pleasant and he was approachable." Dobbie appeared efficient, professional, and diligent in his role as physician-in-chief. Correspondence, particularly with family members, never seemed cursory; indeed, as the primary means by which Dobbie communicated with families, the content and detail of his letters were critical. In addition to medical matters, Dobbie also attempted, to the extent possible, to support families emotionally during periods of hospitalization and separation.

The typical long-term nature of hospitalization and the daily medical and social interactions between patients and staff led some patients to foster significant emotional connections with the sanatorium, even after they were discharged, as judged by the volume of correspondence that was maintained between staff and ex-patients (or their families), often to update on the progress of their lives, the status of their tuberculosis, to celebrate accomplishments, or to mourn passings. This was not a phenomenon unique to the Toronto sanatorium. When he was medical superintendent of the Ninette sanatorium in Manitoba, Alfred Paine mailed out an annual Christmas newsletter to all ex-patients and staff who sent holiday cards, often four hundred or so.[120] In a late 1960s study of an Ontario sanatorium in the midst of its functional transition away from tuberculosis, one interviewed nurse "recalled the 'good old days,' when the patients developed a loyalty to the sanatorium. Even after being released, they would come back for holidays and special occasions which were viewed as reunions."[121]

Since multiple cases of TB were often found in single households, parents and children could be hospitalized at the same time (figure 2.15). Sometimes family members were sent to the same sanatorium, but at other times they were separated by admissions to different sanatoria and often looked to Dobbie to bridge the gap with his letters. One mother wrote to Dobbie in 1931, seeking information on her daughters, Kate and Miranda, gently chastising her husband, who had "all a man's evasion of details, and you know how a Mother is." She could not visit her girls, and it had been well over two months since she had seen them because she was hospitalized at another Ontario sanatorium, but she wrote to Dobbie for an update, suspecting he understood "how a Mother longs to hear of her babies." She wanted to know about her youngest, Miranda, how much she weighed and if she seemed strong. She had seen pictures of Kate and noted, "She seems to be thriving, thanks to your care," but also wanted to know her weight. More importantly, she wanted Dobbie to know that "it has taken a load of care off my mind to know the children are in such good hands." She was "trying not to worry" and she was "feeling a lot better," but, she confided, "a Mother's heart is with her children," so the more she knew of them, the better. It was through correspondence that she would weather the separation from her daughters, as all three worked to build their tuberculosis resistance.

In another instance, a father, prepared for the worst, wrote to Dobbie "man to man" in 1925, to determine the "real condition" of his young son and Dobbie's medical "opinion" of his case. His son had been at the

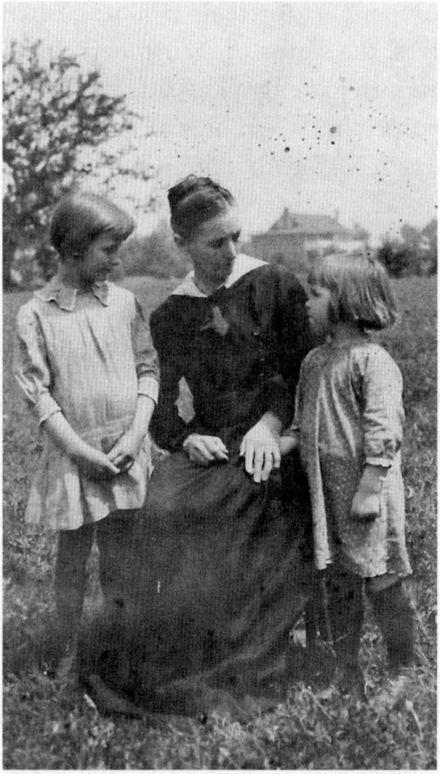

Figure 2.15 A mother and her daughters, all found to be tuberculous and admitted to the Toronto sanatorium. Medical staff must have been confident that this mother was no longer infectious, as direct contact between infectious parents and their children at the sanatorium was generally discouraged.

Toronto sanatorium for five weeks and, as he explained, he was seeking some ease for his worrying mind: "I can assure you that the absence or separation from this boy is affecting my brain which is none too strong due to War disability. I don't have to tell you any more except that lack of information is worrying me, you will understand, the worst I am prepared for[,] the best would do me a world of good. I am asking you because a manly confidence would be better by far than a once a week look at my son and the rest of the week a cloud of doubt." Another father hospitalized far away in another sanatorium wrote to Dobbie in November 1920, seeking any information on his infant daughter, Sophia. "I don't know her condition at all," he wrote, "only that if I don't soon come to see her that I shall never see her again." Believing that knowing something of his daughter's condition would give him "some satisfaction," he appealed to Dobbie for occasional communications. "Doing satisfactorily" in his own treatment, Sophia's father was a strict bed patient and expected to remain in bed for at least two months, unable to visit his daughter in person. In this instance, Dobbie's work in filling the space of separation between parent and child was critical as, true to his understanding, this father would never see his daughter again. Sophie's father never recovered and he died in the sanatorium, sometime around June 1921. As a result, Dobbie's letters really were his last connections with his infant daughter.

Though Dobbie's correspondence with families was often medical, it was not always so. Lucy was just under two years of age when she was admitted to the sanatorium in 1933. At the time of her admission, Lucy's father was already a patient at the Muskoka sanatorium and her mother was in the process of being admitted. About a year after his daughter was admitted to the Toronto sanatorium, Lucy's father wrote to Dobbie asking for information on her progress and if it would "be possible to get a lady who is in touch with the children to write a few lines each month concerning Lucy's advance in talking, playing, play things," and so forth. He explained that his wife was "among other married women" at the Muskoka sanatorium and that "very often the topic of conversation is their children and what they have done." As a result, "hearing others talk like this and not even knowing those little things about her child is rather discouraging causing her to fret and lose confidence in others." This was the sad reality for parents unable to visit their children, not knowing "those little things." In his reply, Dobbie provided Lucy's mother with a wealth of information to share with the other women on her ward, including a report written by one of Lucy's nurses most involved with her care:

> For her age ... she appears to be a child of the average intelligence, is very observant and her talking ability quite up to the average standard. She forms sentences very clearly and she is easily understood.
>
> On returning from the Surgical Building [where she had been for a few days to have a gland incised and drained] a few days ago she showed great interest in recognizing the children she had left the week before, calling all by name. She was very interested in watching their play and seemed very happy to be with them again.

> Lucy was very pleased in receiving a toy elephant sent to her from her mother a few weeks ago. She is very fond of dolls or any toy; books especially give her a great deal of pleasure.
>
> She is a very dainty little girl, loves to get dressed up, asks for her skirt and sweater which we dress her in frequently. A little rose pull over sweater is her favourite, and another favourite is a light green dress.

The nurse had taken special care in writing her report, trying to capture "those little things," the quirks and preferences that render children unique and adorable. It is easy to imagine Lucy's mother's gratitude for these words, making her daughter once again real in her imagination, a kind and friendly girl who liked toy elephants, books, pink sweaters, and green dresses. Dobbie agreed to send along monthly updates on Lucy, more for her social development, since it was unlikely that her tuberculous condition would change markedly over such short periods of time. Lucy's mother likely revelled in these details that she could share, with all of a mother's pride, with the other women on her ward. Eventually, Lucy's condition did improve and her disease was latent by the time she was discharged at six years of age. Over four years may have passed, but at last Lucy was reunited with her parents and taken home.

In his capacity, Dobbie was unlikely to have as much day-to-day contact with patients as the nursing and medical staff, but he did make regular rounds on the wards and could be called in to help manage various troubles. In his autobiography, Sidney Hobbs described Dobbie as "the autocratic Dr Dobbie, the Chief Administrator," though this may have had something to do with the nature of their meeting, as Hobbs was recalling the time he was reprimanded by Dobbie for being found on the women's ward (which was most explicitly against the rules).[122] On the other hand, a former child patient at the Queen Mary recalled that Dobbie often dressed up to play the role of Santa Claus at Christmas and that, each week, he made a point of visiting the children at the Queen Mary, sitting and talking with them, and making the effort to know each child by name.[123] Former student nurses described Dobbie as "fatherly" and somewhat prone to rambling in his regular two-hour evening nursing school lectures,[124] with a voice described as hypnotic: "He … spoke …

just ... like ... this..."[125] One former nursing student remembered of the lectures, "You almost had to have a dinner bell ringing in your ear all the time to keep you awake because [of] that sing-song voice; you'd be asleep before you knew it." He was also known to have a somewhat sarcastic sense of humour, and he expected nothing less than good work and discipline, so if nurses nodded off at his evening lectures, he might make fun of them, or, if they made mistakes, "he'd tell us to go back to Woolworth's and sell pins and needles."[126] Interestingly, these descriptions of Dobbie mesh with Linda Bryder's insights into how British sanatorium administrators were viewed, as "strict disciplinarians," yet "kind" and "sincere," as "fathers," and as "benevolent autocrats."[127] "The ideal superintendent," wrote one British physician in 1911, "must ... be more than a keen and vigorous physician. His relations with his patients are more intimate and his control over them more absolute than is the case with the ordinary practitioner. He supervises every detail of their lives, their rest and exercise, their work and play, their eating and drinking – even, to some extent, their intercourse and conversation. To wield such ample powers wisely and well, so as to promote not only the health but the happiness of patients, is by no means an easy task, and calls for a happy combination of geniality, tact, and discretion."[128] Superintendents had the power to influence the quality of the patient experience at sanatoria, shaping the institutional character and inner workings. On a daily basis, however, it was the ward staff, the physicians, but the nurses in particular, who had the greatest contact with patients.

In his personal life, William Dobbie married Mabel James. The couple had married at St Anne's Church, in Toronto, on 2 June 1908, when William was thirty-five and Mabel was thirty years of age. William was listed as a "bachelor" and "physician" at the time of the marriage, a few years into his sanatorium appointment; for Mabel, born in 1877 in York, it was also her first marriage. Some years earlier, at the time of the 1901 census, Mabel had been living with her widowed mother, Milbro (Carruthers) James, and working as a schoolteacher. When alive, Mabel's father, Robert James, had been a farmer. Like many middle-class women of her time, Mabel gave up employment when she married William, though the couple did not have children.[129] For the duration of his career, William and Mabel lived on site in a cottage named "Glenwyld" and, as a result, Dobbie never really lived apart from his work at the sanatorium. Interviews conducted in Godfrey Gale's oral history project suggest that sanatorium staff rarely saw Mrs Dobbie, perhaps at the odd social occasion for honoured visitors. Mabel was, however, active in the arts, hosting an event for the Outdoor Sketch Club of the Women's Art Association at Glenwyld in 1915.[130] She had also been a lifetime member of the Canadian Field Naturalist Association. When William retired, he and Mabel moved out of their cottage at the sanatorium and relocated to a home on Eglinton Avenue West. Within just three years of his retirement, "apparently in the best of health when he retired [for the] night, Dr Dobbie was fatally stricken soon after rising," and died on the morning of 20 April 1942.[131]

Miss Edith MacPherson Dickson

Edith MacPherson Dickson was appointed lady superintendent of the Toronto sanatorium in January 1906, following the departure of Miss Tuck, the sanatorium's first head nurse who had worked with Dr Adams, physician-in-chief.[132] In this position, she was responsible for overseeing the nursing staff and managing all aspects of the daily care of hundreds of patients, many of whom were on full bedrest, and the diet and food orders for both patients and staff at the hospital. In connection with patient care, Dickson, like Dobbie, maintained correspondence with families and friends, and also coordinated services with charitable and government organizations such as the Sanitarium Club and Children's Aid. In total, Dickson was lady superintendent and director of nursing at the Toronto sanatorium from 1906 until her retirement in 1934.[133]

In 1871, William Dickson and Rubina (MacPherson) Dickson, Edith Dickson's parents, were living in the Ontario district of South Simcoe, Tecumseth. At that time, the couple had one child, four-month-old George. William and Rubina had both been born in Ontario, were of Scottish ancestry, and were listed as Presbyterian. At twenty-two years of age, William worked as a merchant, while Rubina, then eighteen years of age, raised their young son. Five years later, in 1876, Edith was born. The 1881 census enumeration finds five-year-old Edith living in the Tecumseth home shared with her mother and father, now ten-year-old George, seven-year old John, and younger brother Frank, then one year of age. At this time, William was employed as a dry goods clerk. By the next census, ten years later, the family had moved to the Toronto area, occupying a home in the census district of York West. The family had grown and fourteen-year-old Edith now had six siblings, the inter-census arrivals including eight-year-old William, six-year-old Jessie, and two-year-old Rubina. Brother George, now twenty years of age, worked as a clerk in an insurance office, while seventeen-year-old John was employed as a dry goods clerk. Edith's father, now forty-two, had become a real estate agent. This growing, middle-class family had hired a live-in domestic, thirty-one-year-old Rachel Fiddes, a native of Scotland.

Following the family through to the 1901 census finds them living in a leased home on Avenue Road in Toronto's Ward 4. The home had nine rooms for the seven family members still living in the household, another child, nine-year-old Gladys, arriving in the inter-census period. Younger daughters, Jessie (sixteen years), Rubina (twelve years), and Gladys were all in school full time for ten months of the year, while son George (thirty years) was employed and earning $650 a year. William continued to work as an estate agent, earning $800 per year. Active in her church, Dickson (now twenty-four years) was a soprano soloist in Chalmers' Presbyterian Church choir in Toronto.[134] Living in a middle-class family with opportunities for completing her education, Edith fit the ideal demographic at that time for entry into the rising profession of modern, scientific trained nursing.

The Toronto General Hospital Training School for Nurses was established in 1881; Dickson was one of fifteen graduates in 1905, earning her certification in October of that year.[135] At this time, the school offered a three-year program, which means that Dickson was about twenty-six years of age at admission if she entered the training school in 1902. In 1902 alone, there was an impressive 658 applicants to the program, but just 29 applicants were admitted on probation and, of those, only 19 continued on after probation.[136] If, as Jardine has described, the TGH School for Nurses was looking to produce the new generation of professionalized nurses for leadership, then it certainly found success in Dickson, who not only became lady superintendent at the Toronto sanatorium in the year that she graduated, but also became actively involved in the development of Canadian nursing.[137] In her career, Dickson's work would reach beyond the sanatorium as she became involved in the much wider world of Canadian nursing. From 1920 to 1922 Dickson served as president of the Canadian National Association of Trained Nurses (which would become the Canadian Nurses Association), earning the distinction of being the first Canadian-trained nurse to hold the position.[138] Throughout her career, Dickson pursued issues in nursing education and professionalization, both within Ontario and nationally.[139] Her involvement took her to international conferences, such as the International Council of Nurses congress in Helsinki, in 1925, where she served as a discussant on the topic of nursing legislation.[140] At fifty-eight years of age, Dickson retired from the sanatorium and relocated to a farm in Clarkson, Ontario (now part of the city of Mississauga).[141] Dickson was recognized for her work and contributions in 1936, with the Mary Agnes Snively[142] Memorial Medal and again in 1958 when she was bestowed with an honorary membership in the Canadian Nurses Association.[143] Dickson died in 1966, then ninety years of age.

Industrious from the start, shortly after her appointment as lady superintendent in 1906, Dickson established a nursing school at the sanatorium (figure 2.16).[144] According to Dobbie, following the end of the sanatorium's first year of operation, Dr Adams, the first physician-in-chief, had noted difficulties "in securing nurses who were willing to undertake the work of caring for consumptive patients."[145] On a practical level, opening a nursing school staffed the wards with trainees, and some of the graduate nurses were subsequently hired for permanent positions. A large and efficient nursing staff was critical to the sanatorium, and the number of nurses far outweighed the number of doctors, a necessity because hundreds of patients at the sanatorium would be undertaking complete bedrest and require substantial bedside supportive care. Recruiting nurses was not a problem unique to the Toronto sanatorium. In Britain, nurses who worked with tuberculosis patients were perceived as offering merely custodial nursing care, lacking somewhat in the more prestigious appointments expected among the new generation of professionalized nurses.[146] At the Westwood tuberculosis sanatorium in Australia, Kirby and Madsen noted difficulties in maintaining an adequate nursing staff, in part because of the hospital's isolation.[147] The problem was pervasive

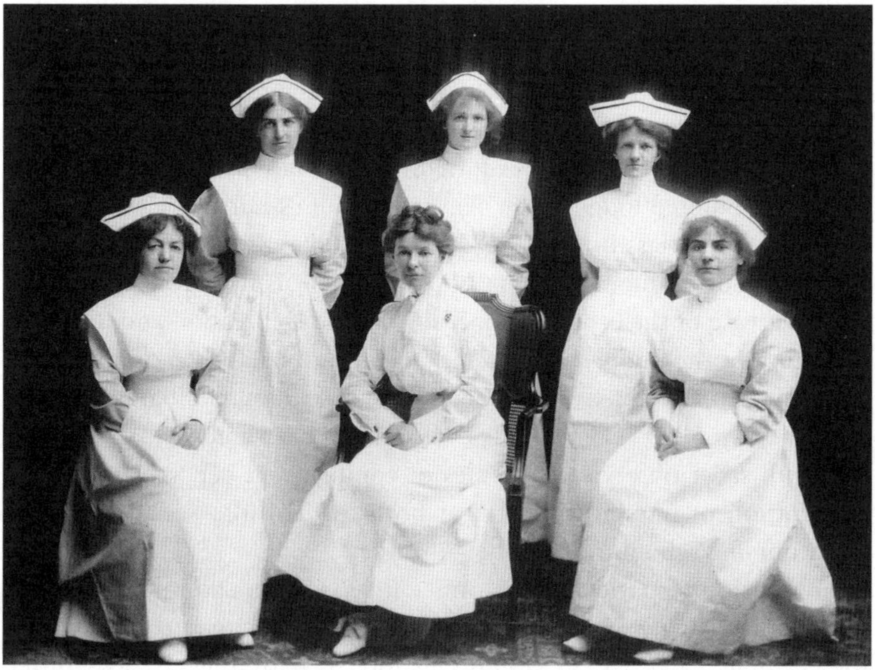

Figure 2.16 Miss Dickson (*centre*), lady superintendent, with the 1916 graduates of the sanatorium nursing school.

and, writing on British sanatoria in 1911, Esslemont describes how understaffing ultimately affected the quality of patient care in tuberculosis sanatoria: "Patients who ought to be having complete rest must fetch and carry for themselves, or else remain in discomfort – suffering, it may be, from cold feet for want of a hot-water bottle, or sleepless and keeping others from sleep owing to a cough which a glass of hot milk would speedily allay."[148] In addition to supporting patients, attracting the new class of modern trained nurse was important, for as Jardine argues, their education and efficiency tended to improve the reputation of hospitals as "safer and more attractive" institutions.[149]

The sanatorium's nursing school began graduating nurses from its program in 1908. With the rebuilding in the aftermath of the 1910 fire, trainees had been provided with a new and much-improved nurses' residence. The buildings that housed the Connaught Home for Nurses and Connaught School for Nurses were officially opened in 1914 by the Duke of Connaught, governor general of Canada.[150] As Jardine has noted in relation to the Toronto General Hospital School for Nurses, it was critical to have a well-appointed residence, since "daughters of the middle class," the demographic typically admitted into nursing schools, would not be drawn to, or perhaps even permitted by their families to live in, inadequately appointed lodgings.[151] The sanatorium's nursing school saw its last graduating class in 1936, two years following Dickson's retirement; it was one of a number of small nursing schools in Toronto forced to close because of the economic hardship of the Depression and a general reduction in the number of nursing positions available to graduates.[152] According to Gale, between 1908 and 1936, 262 nurses had graduated from the school.[153] Like Dobbie, Dickson had been a notable disciplinarian, with strict observance of rules of conduct and deportment a basic expectation of nursing trainees, at both the Toronto sanatorium and other nursing schools in the city.[154]

In addition to patient care, trainee nurses were also involved in the more utilitarian aspects of ward management. Every two to three weeks, for example, each patient would be supplied with a new straw-stuffed mattress. As one former trainee recalled, the old "straw mattress was taken outside. All the old straw pulled out of it. The mattress put with the laundry. We got a new stick, a new bale of hay and we filled the mattress."[155] Before placing a freshly stuffed mattress back on a patient's bed, nursing trainees would fill a pail with water and Lysol and carefully wash the springs, the bed frame, the windowsill closest to the patient, and any other washable surfaces. A large sheet of rubber would be placed over top of the mattress to prevent the spikes of the springs from poking up through the straw. Another graduate recalled that, as a nursing student, she was responsible for cleaning the patients' bathrooms. One day, she and another student nurse had rolled up their sleeves to scrub a bathtub, "stiff cuffs we wore in those days, about four or five inches deep, so we had taken our cuffs off, [and] rolled our sleeves up." Mid-conversation, "all of a sudden there was dead silence ... and when I looked around, Miss MacPherson Dickson," who was in the midst of making her rounds. "She asked us to roll our sleeves down and put on our cuffs and then she would show us how to clean a bathtub without splashing our cuffs," but not before dryly commenting that they "looked like a pair of char women."[156] In keeping with the times, and grounded in her own training at the Toronto General Hospital, Dickson would have also been judged as much on her "character refinement" as her "academic achievement,"[157] lessons that she would pass along to the sanatorium's nursing students.

A former Toronto sanatorium nursing trainee of the 1920s remembered the rules and regulations for nurses in training had been "quite strict" and that some of the young trainees had resisted conformity.[158] Trainees could be dismissed for myriad reasons, if they cut their hair too short, for example, or if they were caught smoking or consuming alcohol. The trainees worked long hours, typically twelve hours per day, not unlike the nursing school at the Toronto General Hospital where trainees "did little else but work, eat, and sleep."[159] The day began at 5 a.m. with a bath, followed by the morning's school parade and inspection. As one former trainee remembered, "You couldn't have a strand of hair out of place; it was two hairnets. And your blue dress and your white apron had to be exactly together. If anything was amiss at all, if there was a little run in your stocking or a little dirty place on your shoe, you lost your two to seven time off for that week."[160] Dobbie's two-hour lectures for nursing trainees began precisely at seven each evening, so trainees valued those five short hours between the end of the workday and the beginning of the evening lecture.

In the matter of patient care, at the very least, "every patient had to be thoroughly bathed every day" and "they had to have a back rub at least three times a day from the day staff."[161] Following the morning preparations, nurses accompanied physicians on their rounds: "We had an armful of charts and we gave the doctor the chart for the patient he was talking to. On that chart had to be every last little detail, exactly when the last pill was given, exactly when, if the patient was hemorrhaging, what quantity, and so on. A very exacting chart was kept for each patient at all times."[162] The charts reflected the scientific practice of medicine at this time, detailed with minutiae and exactness. With the focus placed on "good, nourishing food," mealtimes also placed demands on the nurses. One former trainee remembered the routine well: "One big tray, fully set, on each hand and, if you spilled a drop of milk or soup or anything, you had to go back to the kitchen again and clean it up. You couldn't put a tray down in front of a patient that wasn't 'A1.'"[163]

Miss Wilkinson

When Miss Dickson retired in 1934, Miss Maude Wilkinson was hired to take her place as lady superintendent; Wilkinson remained in this position until 1942.[164] Wilkinson had been a nurse in the First World War and continued to work for the Department of Soldiers' Civil Re-establishment after the war ended. Wilkinson stayed with the department for four years, then accepted a position as director of the Red Cross Outpost Hospital Service in Ontario. In this role, Wilkinson was responsible for establishing and visiting outpost hospitals and nursing stations in rural and remote Ontario. After a time, however, Wilkinson began to feel that "the life of a traveling salesman was no job for an old lady of 52,"[165] so she accepted an offer for the position of lady superintendent at the Toronto sanatorium. Not well versed in the specialties of tuberculosis nursing, Wilkinson was awarded a scholarship for a placement in southern Tennessee, where she could shadow tuberculosis field nurses. When she returned to Toronto, she moved into the lady superintendent's residence at the sanatorium. She was pleased with her accommodations: "There were two bedrooms with a connecting bathroom and at the end of the living room there was a completely equipped kitchenette. It was an apartment designed for a Lady." But there was a drawback, as she soon discovered "the Lady had no time to enjoy it."[166] After Wilkinson retired from the sanatorium she rented a large Toronto residence and established her own private nursing home with eighteen patient beds and a small staff.

The Medical Staff

The medical staff employed at the sanatorium comprised medical interns, resident physicians, staff physicians, and specialists. Medical students were hired as interns in the summer months to fill vacation-related staffing shortages. In the 1930s, graduates of the University of Toronto's

Gallie Course in surgery[167] assisted the sanatorium's surgical staff in what was viewed as a "most useful arrangement."[168] Resident physicians typically held one-year appointments at the sanatorium, working under the supervision of licensed physicians, to fulfil post-medical degree residency training in tuberculosis. In the early 1940s, the year of "intensive study" began with a three -month focus on the diagnosis and treatment of pulmonary tuberculosis, followed by three months devoted to radiology, including technique and interpretation. The third quarter was reserved for genitourinary tuberculosis, laryngology, and bronchoscopy, while the fourth quarter rounded out the experience with a focus on bone and joint tuberculosis, and other forms of extra-pulmonary tuberculosis. Resident physicians were encouraged to avail themselves of the sanatorium's extensive library holdings, the large patient population for observation and practice, and other staff members who would be "only too willing to offer facilities and assistance as may be required."[169]

Resident physicians employed by the sanatorium were provided with board (meals and lodging), laundry, and a salary. In exchange, it was expected that they would not take on any outside medical or surgical work (except in cases of emergency) and that they would not receive any financial compensation from patients for medical services rendered. Hired as members of the Medical Department, resident physicians were advised that they had no authority over the running of the Nursing, Domestic, or other ancillary departments and should, therefore, "be as tactful as may be" in any contacts or connections they had with those departments.[170] This meant that physicians were not to give orders directly to nursing staff. Instead, to promote a spirit of cooperation, any medical orders were written in Order Books and the head of the Nursing Department decided when, how, and by whom those orders were to be carried out.

Physicians were expected to see the patients assigned to their wards immediately upon admission and prescribe any temporary treatments needed until more comprehensive initial examinations could be undertaken. Within twenty-four hours of admission, physicians were expected to have collected detailed patient histories and to have secured samples of sputum, urine, and blood for analysis. Each month after admission, patients were subject to complete physical examinations. Physicians were reminded that tuberculosis patients could also suffer other medical conditions, that "every symptom is not due to Tuberculosis," and to "be careful to diagnose and treat accordingly."[171] A full set of X-rays and laboratory tests were ordered routinely every six months, though additional tests could be undertaken at any time, as needed.[172] Physicians were expected to closely monitor their patients' conditions and maintain a "List of Serious Patients" for those on their wards. Dobbie advised physicians to "see that names are put on this list *in good time*" so that family and friends could be notified and so that the charge nurse on the ward would know to monitor those patients more closely. Dobbie believed that "it is much better that the friends of a patient should be warned *too* soon, or *too* often than that they should not be warned at all." He did not believe that this responsibility should fall to the nurses, though he acknowledged that they would "gladly give every cooperation if encouraged to do so."[173]

In terms of daily routine, physicians on day schedules were typically expected to be on duty by 9 a.m. each day in order to make their rounds or commence the treatments outlined in their daily schedules.[174] Physicians on night duty worked from 5 p.m. to 9 a.m. the next day. Like staff physicians, resident physicians were also scheduled to work at the Gage Institute outpatient clinics held at the College Street building on Tuesdays, 2–5 p.m., Fridays 2–5 p.m. and 6:30–8:00 p.m., and every second Monday of each month.[175] Living on-site at the sanatorium, physicians were able to entertain friends, but were requested to do so in their own apartments.[176] Tobacco use was permitted among physicians, though they were asked to refrain from smoking on the wards, preferably limiting their smoking to their own rooms.[177]

Most staff physicians were hired early on in their medical careers, since appointments were generally made at the junior level with only, according to Dobbie, "merely nominal" salaries. According to his 1921 census listing, Dobbie himself made $8,000/year as physician-in-chief, while staff physicians Omer Hagur (twenty-six years) and Michael McHugh (twenty-seven years) earned $1,200/year. Dr Charles Bood (twenty-seven years) earned $1,800/year, while X-ray specialist Dr Frank Pepperdene (sixty-five years) earned $2,000/year. Nurses' wages varied considerably, some earning $800/year, others, likely trainees, as little as

$120/year. Helpers' wages also varied, but many earned about $360/year. Dr Roy Garrett joined the medical staff in 1930, fresh out of an internship. At that time, about 450 patients were under treatment at the sanatorium. From Garrett's perspective, coming from an internship that paid $25 per month, his starting salary of $150 per month with board was most impressive.[178] Following the completion of his first year, Garrett's salary increased to $175, and when he married in 1932, his salary increased further to $225 per month, though board was now provided to him only when he worked nights or weekends. The increase in salary was meant to offset the average cost of an apartment in Toronto in the early 1930s; a one-bedroom apartment could be rented at that time for about $45 per month (and, for his commute to work, Garrett noted that the luxury of a Ford Model A Coupe with rumble seat could be purchased for as little as $700). From his own experience, Garrett supported the sanatorium's salary-based system, believing that it placed patient care at the forefront: "To my mind, working for a salary is an excellent way to practice medicine. The relationship between physician and patient is on a medical basis only. The matter of payment does not arise. The patient receives whatever treatment is necessary and the physician can certainly never be accused of lining his pockets at the expense of the patient."[179] The ward placed under Garrett's charge was located on the top floor of the Prittie (Main Medical) Building, providing beds for about seventy adult patients. The ward had recently been opened and was still not completely painted when he joined the staff. As Garrett recalled, "The floor had been filled with the most seriously ill from other hospitals and, as a result, the mortality rate at first was very high." In his first three months of work on the ward, twenty-seven patients died.[180] To place this number in context, when he started at the sanatorium in 1930, the overall mortality rate for tuberculosis in Ontario was about fifty-four deaths per 100,000 in the population.[181]

Another long-term physician at the sanatorium, Michael J. McHugh received his medical degree from the University of Toronto in 1921,[182] but had already started working at the Toronto sanatorium in 1920,[183] presumably as an intern. In 1929, Dr McHugh's assignment was to the Queen Mary Hospital and Davies Cottage (120 beds) and Wards F, G, and H of the Prittie (Main Medical) Building (60 beds).[184] His workday typically ran from 8:30 a.m. to 5:00 p.m., with a lunch break between 12:30 and 1:30 p.m. McHugh's work was diverse, ranging from patient rounds, throat and nose clinics, pneumothorax and special procedures (tuberculin, vaccination, antitoxin, heliotherapy) clinics, progress examinations, X-ray examinations, and other special examinations and treatments, as assigned. McHugh's schedule had him off-duty on Saturday afternoons and evenings and off on alternate Sunday afternoons and evenings.

In his years of employment at the sanatorium, McHugh had become an associate member of the medical staff and, upon Dobbie's retirement in 1939, he was appointed the new physician-in-chief. According to Gale's biography, McHugh remained in this position until 1947 when, on account of ill health, he was forced to retire.[185] McHugh died the following year, in 1948. McHugh was married, his wife a concert singer and contralto soloist at Toronto's Yorkminster (Park) Baptist Church.[186] Described variously as "impressive," "business-like," "a perfect gentleman," "very kind," and "pleasant," McHugh was well liked by patients and staff.[187] A former staff dining room employee noted, "He was quite a happy Irishman. He did love his baked potatoes ... when I used to serve, I gave him the largest baked potato."[188] One of the former sanatorium nurses recalled his compassionate character: "I never knew him to turn anybody down if they had a problem ... I think he was one of the [most] ideal doctors I ever met."[189]

As therapeutic measures at the sanatorium evolved in the first half of the twentieth century, so, too, did the cadre of medical specialists. Dr Frank Simpson Pepperdene was the sanatorium's long-standing X-ray specialist. According to Gale's history, the new X-ray technology that had been developed by pioneers such as Röntgen and Crookes in Europe was slowly incorporated into medical facilities in Canada.[190] In 1914, both the new Gage Institute building on College Street, Toronto, and the NSA's Muskoka sanatorium were equipped with X-ray machines. The Toronto sanatorium would have its own X-ray machine installed in 1917. As medical historian J.T.H. Connor notes, most Ontario hospitals had X-ray machines by the late 1920s, the "new photography" marking "the beginning of the fusion of medicine with high-technology – a combination that contemporary Ontarians eagerly embraced and soundly supported."[191] Early X-ray technologies were crude, however, with films developed onto sheets of glass measuring a substantial 14 × 17 inches in size, the images offering only a poor contrast of light and shadow. As a result, early X-rays may have been an aid in determining the extent of tuberculosis disease, but could not replace the value in a physician's careful physical examination of the chest using both ear and stethoscope.[192]

Dr Pepperdene received his doctor of science and doctor of medicine degrees from Oxford University. According to Gale, Pepperdene arrived in Canada in 1911 and began working for the National Sanitarium Association in 1915, living in a cottage on site at the Toronto sanatorium. Pepperdene had sustained significant radiation exposure-related trauma, eventually cancer, in his training with Crookes and Röntgen, and, by the early 1930s, was quite debilitated.[193] One former nurse in the last stretch of her nursing training, just prior to graduation, had studied with Dr Pepperdene in the Radiology Department. Undaunted by his injuries, she recalled telling him that she wanted to sign up to work with him as an X-ray technician, "but he was very sweet and very kind and said that they didn't know enough about X-ray yet for young ladies to be taking part, and that he thought I'd do very, very well just to go look after the sick people."[194] By this time, Pepperdene's declining condition was readily apparent, one of his arms completely paralyzed, the other destined for the same fate. She remembered, "When he put the machine on, sometimes his two arms would flap like wings. I'd run to him and put my arms around him as tightly as I could to try to keep the arms quiet and that's how we got along for a long time."[195] Pepperdene retired from the sanatorium and NSA work in 1933, and died of cancer (due to his history of massive radiation exposure) within the year.[196]

Other specialists were hired over time to staff the sanatorium's growing surgical department, a strong indication of the trend towards more medicalized tuberculosis care that emerged in Canada, particularly in the interwar period. In the 1930s, the Toronto sanatorium's older "cure" approach to tuberculosis (fresh air, good nutrition, rest) was increasingly supplemented with surgical interventions, where appropriate (see chapter 6). As Grzybowski and Allen note, "The efficacy of surgery alone between 1930 and 1948 may have been considerable. It seemed to hasten recovery, it produced some cures, and it relieved pain and various anatomic obstructions."[197] In 1931, R.I. Harris, bone and joint surgeon, completed a successful bone graft on a tuberculous spine at the Toronto sanatorium, and, in 1933, J.G. McClelland, genitourinary or renal surgeon, performed the first nephrectomy, the surgical removal of a tuberculous kidney.[198] Both the surgical staff and expertise at the sanatorium would grow over time, including the arrival, in 1929, of Dr Hugh Coulthard, who initially worked under Dr Harris, but would later become chief resident surgeon. Much to the surprise of patients, Coulthard was fluent in Mandarin, having been born in China to missionary parents, and studying medicine in England before arriving in Canada.[199] When Dr Harris joined the armed forces in the Second World War, Drs Coulthard and Garrett worked together to continue the surgeries, performing spinal fusions and knee excisions, but referring more complex cases, such as tuberculosis of the hip joint, to the Toronto General Hospital. As Garrett reflected back, he admitted, "During this period, I spent some of the most enjoyable afternoons in my entire stay at the hospital when I assisted Hugh Coulthard in spinal fusions."[200] R.M. Janes was appointed as the first thoracic (chest) surgeon, eventually undertaking more complex thoracoplasty surgeries as the surgical facilities expanded, particularly with the opening of the sanatorium's A.E. Ames (surgical) Building in 1933.[201]

The Nursing Staff and Trainees

Sanatorium nurses could find their day-to-day work "psychologically and emotionally demanding," at times overtly "depressing"[202] because, according to one former Toronto sanatorium nurse, over long periods of hospitalization, the nurses got to know their patients and understood that "many of them weren't going to get well."[203] Strong nurse-patient connections were characteristic of long-term care institutions such as the sanatorium. Lenora Marcellus's study of nurses who worked at the Queen Alexandra Solarium for Crippled Children on Vancouver Island suggested close, almost parental relationships between nurses and child patients.[204] Nurses recognized that child patients could experience fears upon admission, not only concerning their "health and chances for a good recovery," but also because of the "new and unknown environment" of the hospital, the treatments that might be undertaken, and the separation from their families.[205]

One former student at the Toronto sanatorium's Connaught School for Nurses in the 1920s recalled that in addition to the training and lectures they received at the sanatorium, the nursing students also did ten-month placements at Fordham General Hospital in New York to gain wider experience in general medicine, surgery, pediatrics, and obstetrics.[206] Arguably, however, according to one former trainee, the sanatorium itself offered diverse experiences, "the whole picture," with opportunities in pediatrics, obstetrics, and surgery in addition to the more typical tuberculosis work. For those pursuing public health and family nursing work, "we had the experience of seeing what [tuberculosis] did to a man, what it did to a woman, and what it did to the children."[207] In their training, the sanatorium nurses also benefitted from a further two months' affiliation at Toronto's Riverdale Isolation Hospital (which specialized in infectious diseases other than tuberculosis). With the economic difficulties arising from the Great Depression, rotations to New York were discontinued in the 1930s, replaced instead with general hospital training at the Toronto General Hospital.[208] The close relationship with the Toronto General Hospital persisted well beyond the closing of the sanatorium nursing school in 1936.

Staff Conduct and Infection Control

While strict behavioural expectations were placed on patients, a feature commonly shared by diverse sanatoria in North America,[209] so, too, were staff expected to follow specific rules and codes of conduct to ensure safety in their work at the sanatorium amidst all of those confirmed and infectious cases. Over the years, Dobbie issued various memoranda outlining his expectations of staff and their conduct. In 1929, for example, he instructed staff on ten best practices to be followed to reduce the risk of tuberculosis transmission from patients. Two of the rules concerned clothing, Dobbie advising that those coming into close contact with patients should wear washable clothes that could be "frequently and easily cleaned." The cuffs and aprons worn by nurses and the coats worn by physicians[210] and employees were to be carefully removed when going off duty. Employees were to have their own, individual drinking glasses and were advised to "use no other." The mouth was to be carefully guarded, intended for food and drink, but not as "a receptacle for fingers, pins, pencils," and so forth. Three of Dobbie's rules concerned patients, with employees instructed to avoid patients sneezing or coughing in their faces, to never eat anything given to them by patients, and to never allow patients to touch their person or their belongings unnecessarily. The remaining three rules explicitly addressed handwashing: "Wash the hands *frequently*, and *always* before meals," "Don't touch the face, head, or anything else after handling a patient until you have washed your hands," and "*Wash your hands, wash your hands again, and then wash them some more.*"[211] Evidently, hands were of particular concern in tuberculosis transmission.

Staff could follow these rules faithfully and consistently, yet also discretely and kindly. Glenys Jones (Davies), a former nurse at the Craig-y-nos sanatorium in Wales, recalled, "If you were speaking to a patient who was coughing, you'd turn your head a little, not to make it obvious to the patient. If a patient offered you a sweet, you took it but said that you couldn't put it in your mouth because you were busy."[212] While some of Dobbie's rules may seem harsh, almost stigmatizing to patients, it must be understood that staff generally did not routinely wear the "personal protective equipment," the masks, gloves, and gowns so common in medical practice today. Contemporary research suggests that while this equipment protects staff from infection, it may also strain relationships and communication between health care providers and patients, with patient emotions ranging from feeling "unclean" or "dirty," to anxiety, depression, loneliness, or even anger.[213] In the sanatorium era, as staff typically interacted directly with patients, many of whom unquestionably infectious, they relied on their application of these rules of comportment, not protective equipment, to reduce the risk of their own infection. Undoubtedly, however, this increased the vulnerability of staff to infection.

Adding to the vulnerability was the lack of awareness of TB's airborne capabilities. As a result, Dobbie's rules addressed the risk of contact – direct contact (with touch, and with hands, particularly hand-to-mouth), indirect contact (proximity to the potentially bacteria-laden mucus and sputum liberated with coughs and sneezes), and fomite contamination (of aprons, coats, pencils, and drinking glasses) – but not contamination of the air itself. One Toronto General Hospital nursing trainee on placement at the sanatorium from September to December 1939 recalled "eagerly anticipating" her affiliation with the sanatorium, her first nursing experience outside of the Toronto General Hospital. She had looked forward to it with "both anticipation and fear," largely because of the fact that TB, "at that time, a very serious disease, had really no specific treatment or cure."[214] As a modern nursing trainee learning about infection-control techniques at the Toronto General Hospital, she had fully expected to wear a mask on the wards, but "this wasn't the case at that time. The policy was, surgical patients who were very ill, patients who were so ill that they couldn't control their coughing, and a new patient wore masks."[215]

Upholding his belief in the protection afforded by rules and regimen, Dobbie shifted responsibility back to staff, suggesting that "for a physician or nurse to contract a communicable disease from a patient is a dire reflection on their carefulness and their ability to carry out efficiently the principles of asepsis."[216] Staff took Dobbie's memos to heart. The nursing trainee on placement from the Toronto General Hospital in 1939 recalled, "We were frightened to death to eat anything without washing our hands and washing our hands and washing our hands."[217] As she described it, upon entering the staff dining room for meals, "we always took off our aprons, we had Hoover aprons, and then we washed our hands [in] an old, round basin with the foot pedals."[218] Ideally, only nurses and nursing trainees who skin-tested positive for tuberculosis infection were accepted to work at the sanatorium, and they received regular chest X-rays, about every six months, to ensure that they were not experiencing unnoticed TB disease activity.[219] Infection of staff was a very real possibility in the sanatorium era, but the risk was hotly debated. Ongoing longitudinal studies of nurses and medical students that began in the 1930s and 1940s eventually consolidated understandings of the potential danger of occupational exposures and tuberculosis infection in the 1950s.[220] Those understandings were fuelled by a new awareness of the role of airborne transmission of tuberculosis bacteria. Even the most dedicated and rigorous of handwashing regimes would be no match for the airborne transmission of tuberculosis bacteria, and the typical lack of masks among staff and patients only aggravated the risk. William Wells, researching tuberculosis in the 1930s, had suggested that tuberculosis bacteria carried on tiny droplet nuclei had airborne capabilities.[221] Even before Wells, some believed tuberculosis to be a "crowd-poison," transmitted by "substances" present in air exhaled from tuberculosis patients.[222] It would not be until the 1950s, however, that a series of carefully designed experiments (involving guinea pigs placed in hospital rooftop chambers and delivered with treated and untreated tuberculosis ward air) undertaken by Wells's student, Richard Riley,[223] would conclusively establish the airborne transmission of tuberculosis.[224] By the 1960s, the risk of occupational infections "was acknowledged as [a] simple, self-evident truth."[225] In response, new technological innovations, including the use of ultraviolet germicidal irradiation air disinfection systems, upper-room ultraviolet light, and negative air ionization, have been put into use to reduce the possibility of transmission within hospitals.[226] In contrast to the early sanatorium era, staff and visitors coming into contact with infectious tuberculosis patients in medical settings today may be required to wear masks.

For their part, sanatorium designers also tried to reduce transmission risks in the sanatorium.[227] Richard Hobday notes that the vulnerability of tuberculosis bacteria to sunlight had long been known, with Robert Koch demonstrating the lethal relationship in 1890; as a result, windows became prominent in sanatorium designs in order to admit an abundance of bacteria-killing UV light.[228] The accumulation of dust was another hazard, since it was widely believed that tuberculosis bacteria expelled from bodies could settle in dust on floors and surfaces, and, if disturbed, lead to transmission. Over time, in design, sanatoria would avoid dust-collecting surfaces such as door and window mouldings, baseboards, and chair rails; even the tops of large cabinets were angled in order to minimize dust collection.[229]

With emphasis upon the importance of order and cleanliness, the sanatorium staff who lived on-site, physicians and nurses included, were expected to follow specific rules in their residences and in their manner. In this way, staff, like patients, were moderated in their lives and work at the sanatorium. In September 1915, for example, Dr Dobbie circulated the "Rules for Employees' Quarters," instructing employees that their personal belongings should be "kept tidy" and that "personal cleanliness" should always be given "careful attention."[230] Walls and woodwork were not to be used for striking matches, and no litter (such as paper, matches, cigarette stubs) was to be thrown on the floors. "Intoxicating liquors" were not permitted in the employees' quarters,[231] and "profane and obscene language" would not be tolerated. Random inspections could be undertaken at any time in order to certify cleanliness and the absence of unpermitted goods. Overall, Dobbie noted, "general good conduct is desirable, and all employees are expected to co-operate towards this end." Further to behavioural expectations, also in September 1915, a notice was circulated to all employees reminding them that "working hours" ran 7:30 a.m. to 12 noon, and then again from 1:00 to 5:30 p.m. each day and that "STRICT OBSERVANCE WILL BE EXPECTED." Further, the meal hours for employees included breakfast at 7:00 a.m., dinner at 12:15 p.m., and tea at 5:45 p.m., with "10 MINUTES GRACE *ONLY* ALLOWED ON THESE HOURS, EXCEPT TO ORDERLIES AND MEN ENGAGED ON SPECIAL WORK." Presumably, the ten minutes' grace would allow staff to get all necessary handwashing out of the way before eating. Employees were also expected to follow rules governing the communal dining room: to be prompt for mealtimes and to take their places in a quiet and orderly manner, to avoid "boisterous conduct such as shouting, whistling, singing, [and] loud talking," to (again) avoid the use of "profane or obscene language," and, for men, to display "gentlemanly conduct." In the event that any employees violated the dining room rules, the waiters were instructed to report persistent offenders.[232]

A former nurse at the Welsh sanatorium Craig-y-nos, Valerie Brent (Price) recalled that staff mealtimes were important, and nurses were encouraged to consume some 4,500 calories every day. As nurses, they put themselves in a "vulnerable position" for tuberculosis disease, and "had to keep [their] immune system as healthy as possible;"[233] well supplied with nutritious food and ample calories, it was also through diet that sanatorium administrators tried to offset the occupational risks of infection and disease. Diet was important for building resistance, not only among patients, but also staff. The sanatorium was a large hospital that relied on orderly, disciplined behaviour. Staff, like patients, were expected to conform to the rules and regimen. However, staff found precious moments to break the tension and gravity of their role in caring for patients (figure 2.17).

Conclusions

While wealthy businessmen organized the first gatherings to establish tuberculosis sanatoria in Canada, the effort was widely embraced and supported through philanthropy. The rise of the tuberculosis sanatorium acknowledged the widespread risk of tuberculosis infection and disease, and the attempt to effectively treat tuberculosis in specialized hospitals, or at the very least to push active disease into latency. The sanatorium was conceptualized as a place for resistance building, where patients might spend months or years with the benefit of nutritious diets, rest, fresh air, and sunshine. Ultimately, for the children in this study, the sanatorium was the "site" of their experience, where medical care, illness, and recovery or death played out.

The sanatorium became its own little self-sufficient community within the local area of Weston and the larger city of Toronto. Aside from the large contingent of medical and nursing staff, there were other employees who contributed to the functioning of the sanatorium community, such as schoolteachers, trade and maintenance workers, and clerical and catering staff. While the hospital was equipped to function as an independent entity, patients were not restricted from interacting with the larger community, able to receive visitors and take needed leaves of absence away from the sanatorium.

The medical and nursing staff working under Dobbie and Dickson's long administrative reign embraced the principles and practice of modern, scientific medicine. Many of the original staff were physicians and nurses early in their careers, sometimes hired fresh out of medical and nursing school or internships. To meet a general tuberculosis nursing shortage, the sanatorium introduced its own nursing school from which much-needed nursing staff could be recruited. Not only were the medical and nursing staff themselves the product of recent, modern education, but they also played a role in the ongoing training of new physicians and nurses

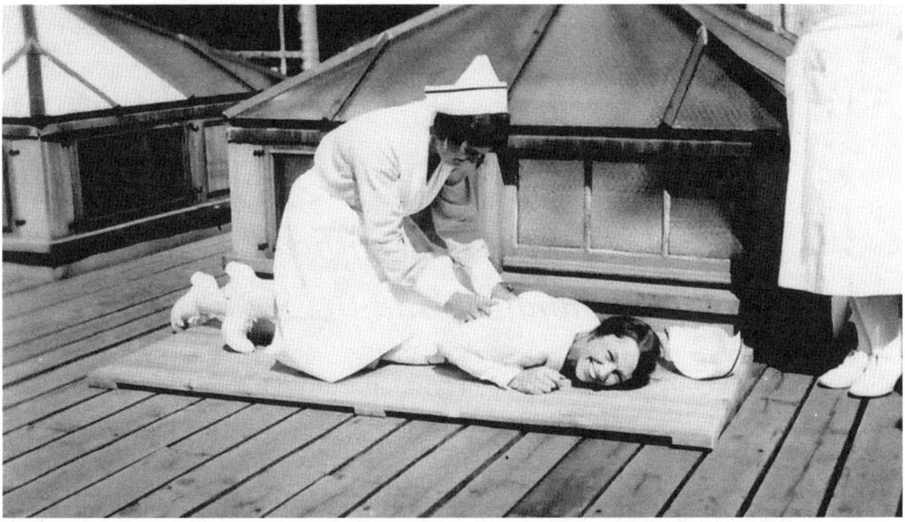

Figure 2.17 Two nurses enjoy a moment of lightheartedness and laughter.

specializing in tuberculosis. Considering the length of time that some staff were employed at the sanatorium, it seems that both physicians and nurses valued their work at the sanatorium, even despite the relatively low pay, the hard work, the absence of fast cures, and the sadness of the reality that a large number of patients would not survive tuberculosis.

The staff were expected to adhere to firm rules regarding their work and comportment, imparting a sensibility that paralleled the regimented lives expected of patients in the institution. Infection was always a risk in the sanatorium's pre-antibiotic era, but the administration believed in the power of discipline and diet to protect staff from infection and disease. If, as will be explored in further chapters, patients were required to follow the rules to reduce the risk of tuberculosis transmission and to speed their own recovery from the disease, staff were also counted on to follow a strict, rule-defined existence in their professional and personal lives within the sanatorium community.

CHAPTER 3

Guarded Hopes and Difficult Truths: Children, Families, and the Sanatorium

> Prognosis in tuberculosis is fraught with difficulty. One patient, diagnosed early and treated promptly and skillfully under the best conditions, may go steadily downhill, while another makes uninterrupted improvement, despite every unfavourable circumstance.[1]
>
> ~ W. Stobie

Discoveries in science and medicine would play a powerful role in shaping public perceptions of disease and disease risk. According to historian Nancy Tomes, by the early twentieth century, the germ theory of disease had inspired a whole new phenomenon of "germ consciousness," a public awareness of the hidden microbial world and the diseases that could come with it.[2] According to Tomes, the rising "consciousness" would feed the anxieties of "germ panic" and, with that, the "germ sell" as industry attracted consumers in the sale of everything from toilets and vacuum cleaners to soap and refrigerators. Armed with knowledge and technology, attempts to mitigate the suffering and loss of infectious disease were heightened and optimism underscored beliefs that medicine and public health could triumph over germs and disease. Tuberculosis bacteria occupied a special place in this emerging awareness, made profoundly personal with the advent of tuberculin testing. Both the Mantoux and Pirquet tests were simple enough, but their revelations of infected bodies had significant implications for both individual and population-level understandings of tuberculosis and its wide dissemination. "Germ consciousness" reached new, lofty heights as routine tuberculin testing and X-ray surveys rendered the hidden scope of tuberculosis bacteria and their effects on the body visible, emphasizing the very real risk of transmission within families and communities.

Tuberculin had been another Koch innovation, prepared through successive cultivations of tuberculosis bacteria in his laboratory.[3] Koch's aim to find a cure for tuberculosis in this work may have ultimately failed, but tuberculin proved invaluable as a diagnostic agent, using solutions of Old Tuberculin[4] to identify individuals with histories of tuberculosis bacterial infection. The Mantoux test involved an injection of Old Tuberculin into the uppermost layers of the skin via a needle placed almost parallel to the skin surface. For children or parents apprehensive of needles and injections, there was also the Pirquet test where a needle or scarifier was used to abrade the skin surface upon which a drop of undiluted Old Tuberculin was then placed.[5] Positive reactions to either of these tests were strongly suggestive of infection, useful in determining if disease symptoms in an unwell child could be attributed to tuberculosis by first establishing whether or not the child had been infected. Typically, tuberculin testing could be effective at detecting infection beginning anywhere from three to seven weeks after infection.[6] While the method of tuberculin testing was not itself complicated, interpreting the results was neither straightforward nor infallible. Physicians soon realized that false-negatives could result if patients were tested while they had a fever.[7] It was for this reason that some children were given a succession of tuberculin tests when they presented as TB suspects. An interwar handbook by the Canadian Tuberculosis Association also explains that tuberculin testing "tells whether or not tuberculosis germs have entered the body. But it tells only that and no more."[8] Tuberculin testing was not useful in determining if that infection was active or latent. As a result, in the case of a positive tuberculin reaction, the next step might be a chest X-ray to determine "if any damage to the lung has already been done," with serial X-rays used to track any changes in disease activity.[9] Until the 1930s, it was not uncommon for North American physicians to view a positive tuberculin test in childhood as "an asset," even "desirable," providing evidence that a child had been infected with, overcame (if no disease emerged), and potentially gained some immunity to tuberculosis.[10] Increasingly, however, it was understood that in later years, some of these children would be returning to their physicians, now as young adults with more grievous reactivation disease capable of spreading the infection to others.[11]

Tuberculin testing permitted the first large-scale (population or community) screenings and assessments, providing powerful confirmation of just how widespread tuberculosis infection could be. Within this context, the reality of germ consciousness became acute. In 1924, J.H. Elliott, an Ontario physician and tuberculosis specialist, reviewed two Canadian tuberculin surveys of children ten to fourteen years of age, one a 1922 survey of 800 children in Saskatchewan, the other an early 1920s survey of 540 children living in "rural and small town" Ontario. In the Saskatchewan study, 57 per cent of the children reacted positively, confirming that their bodies were host to TB bacteria, while in Ontario 41 per cent were positive reactors. The high percentages were alarming and suggested the need for much more preventive work in Canada to ease the spread of TB bacteria between bodies and to protect vulnerable children from infection.[12] Even more worrying, other infection estimates were far less conservative, as Dobbie suggested that the proportion of children infected gradually increased with age "until at fifteen years it reaches about 90 per cent."[13] Ronald Bayne, a physician reflecting on the problem of tuberculosis, wrote in 1998 that when he "was growing up in Québec over 50 years ago, tuberculosis was common, even among young people. A positive Mantoux test was just a sign of maturity."[14] As Bayne suggests, there was an expectation that many Canadians would be infected with tuberculosis bacteria early in life, so common that it was like a rite of passage to adulthood. The scope of infection declined dramatically, however, as the century progressed. By 1969, with at least two decades of effective antibiotic treatments in place, it was estimated that only about 4 per cent of Canadian children would experience tuberculosis infection by the time they were of school-leaving age.[15] It was through this dramatic decline that endemic TB would lose its grip in Canada.

The large, population-based results of tuberculin surveys furthered ideas and understandings about the natural resistance of infected bodies against active TB disease. Biologically, tuberculosis bacteria have exceptional capabilities to establish high levels of population infection (as revealed in the surveys), but, as good as tuberculosis bacteria are at moving between bodies, Gagneux notes that only about 10 per cent of those infected will go on to develop active disease, suggesting that tuberculosis bacteria are not "particularly good" at causing disease once in the body.[16]

It was precisely this observation, the large numbers infected but the much smaller proportion actually developing active disease, that encouraged physicians to continue investing in the idea of resistance building, both in family homes and at the sanatorium. Since the body was equipped with a natural ability to resist tuberculosis bacteria by pushing the infection into latency, some bodies might benefit from a little assistance in finding that resistance.

Understanding that widespread infection was a given in Canada's endemic age, public health attention shifted to identifying those suffering active tuberculosis disease through mass chest X-ray surveys. The findings could prove unnerving, demonstrated in a number of child patients sampled whose tuberculosis was discovered incidentally upon mass X-ray screenings arranged through their schools at diagnostic clinics like the Gage Institute in Toronto. In those surveys, invariably there were seemingly healthy children discovered to have evidence of tuberculous cavities (or other tuberculosis-related pathologies) in their lungs. For these children, this was the first uncovering of their disease and, in the aftermath of such chest X-rays, a sense of vulnerability could surface. If "illness" was typically identified by "experiences judged serious enough to warrant seeking formal medical advice,"[17] then the chance discovery of tuberculous pathologies among children taking part in routine chest X-ray surveys meant that the "illness" label would come suddenly, without warning, preparation, or outwardly apparent or concerning bodily symptoms. Physicians, nurses, and public health workers alike became quite familiar with this scenario, understanding that tuberculosis disease could begin its ravaging of the body well before any disease symptoms became apparent (in the same stealthy way that cancer can manifest). Waiting on the appearance of symptoms to diagnose tuberculosis typically meant diagnosing a case that was already in a relatively advanced state, so chest X-rays, like cancer screening today, were meant to identify tuberculosis cases at the earliest stage possible when any resistance-building efforts would be most effective. J.E. Esslemont, writing in 1911, stressed the urgency of early tuberculosis diagnoses, noting that otherwise a whole cascade of "too lates" would likely culminate in death: "Too late ... is the trouble diagnosed; too late is the patient sent to a sanatorium; too late are money and devotion lavished on him by anxious friends, and these fate-fraught words, 'too late,' pursue him to the inevitable end, dog him until a merciful death ensues."[18]

To avoid the shock of "too late," in the early decades of the twentieth-century public health encouraged a mindful attentiveness to the body, educating the masses for better recognition of the early symptoms of tuberculosis. The general sensitivities of germ consciousness positioned amidst the mass tuberculin screenings and chest X-ray surveys ensured that tuberculosis consciousness matured as people invested greater attention in their bodies. Historian Edward Shorter argues that in the first half of the twentieth century people became more likely to perceive and interrogate the potential symptoms of ill-health, reflecting a changing bodily awareness in patients as medicine expanded into its scientific era.[19] Whereas earlier nineteenth-century "traditional" patients may have sought out physicians only for the most "alarming" or "disabling" symptoms (such as coughing up blood or broken bones), Shorter argues that modern patients became much more sensitive to the subtler symptoms of their potential unwellness.[20] In the case of tuberculosis, downplaying, denying, or ignoring symptoms might only delay diagnosis and treatment, so physicians could guide patients and their understandings of what should be considered "concerning" or not. Shorter suggests that, in the modern era, patient sensitivities were heightened when it came to the respiratory tract, with its associated "runny nose," "cough,"[21] and "sore throat" attracting particular concern.[22] The ongoing challenge of tuberculosis, along with crises such as the 1918–19 influenza pandemic, further sharpened attention to the deadly potential of these seemingly mundane symptoms.[23] Paul Starr's characterization of modern medicine's "emotional" function meant that people sought out physicians "not just for remedies, but also for clarification of the nature and meaning of their internal experience. 'Am I sick?' we ask. 'Is what I feel significant, or should I ignore it?'"[24] Patients sought clarity and reassurance from their physicians. Though equipped with "a greater sensitivity to the body's internal state,"[25] patients were perhaps less confident in their abilities to distinguish between what should be concerning and what should not. While most would understand that the "churchyard cough" of tuberculosis was an "inevitable prelude to the grave,"[26] often well beyond physicians' help, the more mild or vague symptoms of loss of appetite, fatigue, or night sweats could reasonably be attributed to other conditions. Physicians in the modern era were ideally positioned to address this dilemma, as their modern training in science meant that they had become more expert symptom interpreters and diagnosticians than their nineteenth-century colleagues, exhibiting skills that also improved their ability to provide patients with reasonable prognoses.[27]

Within the context of this growing tuberculosis consciousness, important questions emerge about what was happening within families. How did children come to be diagnosed with TB, and under what conditions were their admissions to the sanatorium negotiated? How willing were parents to send children to the sanatorium, and did they have a choice in the matter? As sanatoria emerged, what was their benefit over home care? How did parents and children weather the separation of hospitalization? What did families want from the sanatorium? Cure certainly would have been the ideal, but, as a start, parents often just wanted "the truth." Appeals for the "truth" surfaced regularly in the letters that parents and guardians wrote to Dobbie and Dickson and were really questions about a child's prognosis. With a prognosis, at least, families could either hope that a child would survive tuberculosis, or could prepare for the worst, a child's likely death. Requests for "the truth" were so common that I gained the impression that prognoses might well have been elusive, that families either did not receive or did not trust their physicians' prognoses, or that they believed that the best truths would come from the tuberculosis specialists at the sanatorium.

Strength and confidence in "the truth" would rise as physicians gained new understanding of tuberculosis and became more skilled diagnosticians in the modern period of medicine.[28] The great emphasis that modern medicine placed on careful observation and documentation is evident in the patient charts, where detailed daily evaluations of patients traced the tendencies in patient trajectories of improvement or decline through changes in the signs and symptoms of tuberculosis, such as fever, weight loss (or gain), and anemia. Gifted with a greater knowledge about the body and its workings, and assisted by powerful medical technologies such as the microscope and X-ray, doctors seemingly "had the power to see the future."[29] Despite the fact that sanatorium physicians could offer a prognosis, any long-term, reassuring quality of that prognosis was problematic. In this matter, English physician Samuel Gee (1839–1911) offered an aphorism to his fellow physicians: "Never give a definite opinion as to how long a patient suffering from phthisis will live, for the only certainty is that – if you do – you will be wrong."[30] Tuberculosis was rife with uncertainty, as both disease and prognosis could shift dramatically and frequently, even oscillating between activity and latency, influenced by the body's variable state of resistance. One benefit of sanatorium care, therefore, was the constant reappraisal of patients' prognoses, perhaps even daily.

Aside from the prognosis, parents and guardians were also invested in the treatments available at the sanatorium; though some doubted the curative potential of bedrest, more were impressed with the rise of artificial pneumothorax and other tuberculosis-related surgeries. If families were not convinced that "something was being done" actively to assist their children in overcoming the disease,[31] it would be difficult to accept the painful separation of hospitalization and children could be discharged in frustration. While some parents, guardians, or patients might have doubted the sanatorium, others did not, and the overall willingness of the public to invest philanthropically in the sanatorium's construction and maintenance are perhaps symbolic of the confidence in the institution, its work, and its staff of tuberculosis experts. Belief in the institution and continued success in fundraising contributed to the visibility and budding authority of TB specialists at the sanatorium. Anxieties surrounding the expanding tuberculosis consciousness helped to situate and solidify the role of the sanatorium, but the family home was also ultimately an important site for TB experiences for many children in this study, before and after their hospitalization at the sanatorium. As a result, this chapter explores some of the home dynamics surrounding TB among family members, before turning attention explicitly to the sanatorium. Before admission, children's home lives were often influenced by tuberculosis, a feature that could play an important role in how they perceived and received their admission to the sanatorium. The chapter considers some of the overarching issues surrounding the admission of children to the Toronto sanatorium, how and why those admissions were sought out and negotiated, and why they were sometimes resisted by children and/or their families. The chapter then considers how those children who were admitted were evaluated to inform and guide treatment decisions. Patient experiences and outcomes, ranging from death to discharge, are also explored. Death was the most feared consequence of tuberculosis disease, the grief and loss often exacerbated by the physical separation of hospitalization. The events leading to death in tuberculosis could vary considerably, from the long, chronic, wasting demise classically associated with tuberculosis, to acute and sudden deaths, sometimes connected with additional stressors, such as influenza. The majority of the children sampled in this study would survive both hospitalization and tuberculosis. For them, the chapter examines their experiences with discharge. While some children (or their families) sought early discharge against medical advice, others waited patiently, perhaps for months or years, until their physical condition suggested that it was time to be discharged. Memories or perceptions of past tuberculosis sanatoria often conjure suffering, sadness, resignation, and the abandonment and isolation of the sick and infectious. But at the time when they were in use, sanatoria offered hope, "where before there was only despair"[32] borne out of the "age-long fatalism"[33] traditionally associated with tuberculosis diagnoses. It was this hope that filled the beds at the Toronto sanatorium to capacity, forcing others onto wait lists for admission.

Facing Disease: Tuberculosis in the Home

Families and homes were not immune to the anxieties that tuberculosis inspired. While losing family members to tuberculosis was not uncommon, as a typically long, chronic disease, families also coped with the daily struggles of poor health and illness. The stressor of tuberculosis ultimately affected personal and familial relationships within the home, the wake of disease and death sometimes far-reaching. Common as it was, tuberculosis could become the very focal point around which family relations were negotiated, affecting parents and children alike, and exerting the melancholy, weathering effects of long-term poor health. In her study of nineteenth-century New Englander Deborah Vinal Fiske, Sheila Rothman reveals how Deborah, described as an "invalid" with tuberculosis, resignedly yet practically prepared her daughters not only to become orphans, but also successful boarders in the new homes to which they would surely be sent upon her death, just as she had been boarded out following her own mother's death.[34] Deborah ensured that her daughters acquired the refinements, such as sewing skills and respectful characters, that would render them desirable for adoption into new homes.

While some tuberculous fathers and mothers such as Deborah may have responsibly prepared for their deaths, others laboured under the restricting physical effects of the disease. Tuberculosis could easily interfere with child–parent relationships through frightening symptoms such as physical weakness, laboured breathing, hoarseness, coughing, and, perhaps the worst, hemorrhaging. Prescriptions for extended bedrest redefined the role of tuberculous mothers and fathers, often placing them outside regular family life and emotionally distancing them from their children. Hurt's examination of a tuberculous woman's diary from the 1940s reveals her concerns about the effect that the rest cure had on her relationship with her young son. She wrote, "Mark already ignores me. I think it is because I am in bed and I am a 'stationary' object."[35] In his book *Working-Class Childhood* (1982), Jeremy Seabrook interviewed a number of women and men on their English working-class childhoods. Miss Renshaw, born in the early 1890s, was ninety when she reflected on her childhood. Renshaw's mother had been an "invalid" with "consumption" and, as a result, her father played a prominent role in her childhood.[36] Miss Renshaw recalled, "My mother was always apart from us. I grew up knowing she hadn't long to live. Of course, nowadays, they would never have dreamed of having six children, with her suffering like that. I never felt close to her as I did to my father. She sat on an old sofa, whipcord, hard horsehair, and she coughed and she was always dreadfully pale, poor thing. She always seemed to have the mark of death on her. I know it sounds dreadful, but I was afraid of her. I used to avoid her."[37] She had good memories of her father, "a beautiful person" who had treated her mother "tenderly" and "waited on her." She had not shared her father's love of her mother, however, reasoning, "I think children work things out. I knew it was no good letting myself grow too attached to her, because I always knew I would lose her."[38] Sure enough, Miss Renshaw's mother had died when she was twelve years old and, because she was the eldest child, the loss would come with new responsibilities, as she left school, took on work, and helped her father run the household.

Because of disease transmission concerns and the recommended isolation of the sickroom (or the solitary backyard tent), there could be a real physical distancing of tuberculous parents. A 1949 American publication by Nurse Dorothy Deming, *Home Care of Tuberculosis: A Guide for the Family*, advised that infants and children should never be allowed to play in the sickroom, though older children could stand in the doorway, a small concession perhaps but still unlikely to foster close emotional connections.[39] If at all possible, Deming suggested, children should be sent away to live elsewhere until family physicians felt confident about their safe return. In France, as early as 1903, this approach was institutionalized with the introduction of the Grancher system, wherein children were separated from their older, tuberculous family members and sent to the countryside to take up residence with farming families, preferably those without children or with adult children who had already left home; while the Grancher system stirred up some interest in the province of Quebec, the system was not adopted in Canada.[40] If children remained in the home, then Deming was firm on her prohibitions against kissing, advising physicians that their patients "must understand that the family's love is shown in other ways while [they are] sick, and the family must take individual responsibility for keeping the rule: No Kissing." While Deming acknowledged that "these rules may seem hard, especially if it is mother who is sick," she believed "the best sign of affection" was "to protect loved ones from a dangerous, catching disease."[41]

Former child patients at the Welsh sanatorium at Craig-y-nos reflected on how their family relationships were changed by tuberculosis and hospitalization. Many of those interviewed for Ann Shaw and Carole Reeves's *The Children of Craig-y-nos: Life in a Welsh Tuberculosis Sanatorium 1922–1959* felt more self-reliant upon their return home.[42] Gwyn Thomas, admitted to the sanatorium at six years of age in 1942, reported, "The Craig-y-nos experience did me no harm – it made me tough as nails."[43] Vanessa Dodd was only two years old when she was admitted to the Craig-y-nos sanatorium in 1953. Dodd describes how tuberculosis persisted in shaping her family's relationship at home, once she was discharged and over the course of her childhood, as the family "bonded perhaps dysfunctionally, through numerous jaunts to hospitals for X-rays and appointments with chest consultants."[44] Other former Craig-y-nos child patients recalled alienation upon their return home. Gareth Wyke, for example, remembered that when he returned home at ten years of age after about five years at the sanatorium, he had a new sister who did not know him and rejected him as her brother.[45] Undoubtedly, returning home could be a trauma unto itself, as children had to come to terms with how both they and their families had changed in the time they spent apart.

Entering the Toronto Sanatorium

Families had various reasons for wanting (or not wanting) their children admitted to the sanatorium. Among the Toronto patients sampled, parents who perceived the sanatorium as a place for dying (and not of hope) were less willing to have their children admitted, and apparently this was not a feeling unique in Ontario. Gwyn, the former child patient at Craig-y-nos, remembered that her mother had been very reluctant to have her daughter admitted, "because she believed that everybody who went there died."[46] Yet parents also recognized that the best chances for their children's survival might be found at the sanatorium, where children would be more likely, willing, or encouraged by example to follow the rules surrounding the regimen of resistance building and healing. In this instance, parents were more willing to pass authority over their children to the medical and nursing staff at the sanatorium, a significant concession undoubtedly made in response to the seriousness of the situation at hand. According to Ripley's history of Nova Scotia's Kentville sanatorium, thirteen-year-old Victor Cleyle was admitted on these grounds, once Victor's physician had diagnosed tuberculosis, because "asking him to be quiet and rest his barewire electric energy was akin to putting an elevator spring in a soup can. His failure to master the cure at home came as no surprise and it was decided that the regime of the sanatorium would suit his illness best."[47] Parents' fears that children would not respect home discipline to "faithfully take the rest cure" were also found in the Toronto sanatorium narratives. The sentiment seems to have resonated widely, for Bashford also notes that a key role of the sanatorium in Australia was to provide patients with support to cultivate the "self-discipline" that they would need inside and outside, once they were discharged.[48] A long-term discipline to follow the rest cure was essential, since if improvement materialized, it would typically progress slowly, and physicians could not assure with any certainty that the effort would lead to cure. If cure was elusive (and true cures typically were), then at the very least patients learned, through discipline, how to reduce the "danger" of infecting others. According to Bashford, once patients traded in their own will for that of the institutional or medical will, they were ready to learn "a new way of being" and take the steps to "cultivate a new consumptive self."[49] These ideas of resignation and redefinition of self under the weight of tuberculosis are powerful reminders of how the chronic infection of tuberculosis required a mindful consciousness to minimize the ongoing bodily risks.

In Ontario, family physicians or physicians working out of diagnostic clinics such as the Gage Institute typically negotiated sanatorium admissions on behalf of families, writing to Dobbie directly in seeking the admission of their patients to the sanatorium. More urgent requests were made in cases of failing health, in instances where transmission within the home was apparent, and where the risks of infecting young children were most real. Upon such enquiries, Dobbie mailed out a standard physical examination report, to be completed by family or clinic physicians. In many instances, physicians were certain of their tuberculosis diagnoses, given physical findings and, most tellingly, a family history of the disease. Other times, a diagnosis of TB seemed most likely, but for one reason or another, could not be confirmed absolutely. As noted by one physician, "It has been said for many years that any disease can mimic tuberculosis and tuberculosis can mimic any disease."[50]

Charlotte's physician wrote to Dobbie in August 1933, seeking her admission to the sanatorium. He noted that this thirteen-year-old schoolgirl had a very bad family history of tuberculosis, as he had personally witnessed the deaths of Charlotte's father, mother, sister, and brother to tuberculosis over the previous six years; her elder brother Carl had already been admitted to the Toronto sanatorium. Following the deaths of her parents, Charlotte had been taken in by an aunt, and when Charlotte's tuberculosis symptoms became apparent, confirmed by a positive sputum sample, she was living with three young cousins. Because of the vulnerability of those children to infection, Charlotte's physician wanted her admitted "as soon as possible." Bed shortages and waiting lists were common, however, and over two months passed and Charlotte still had not been admitted. Concerned with his sister's condition and pressured by the fact that his aunt wanted "to get her into the Queen Mary as soon as possible," Carl, while still a patient at the sanatorium, wrote to Dr Coulthard (his physician at the sanatorium) directly, "worrying" and personally requesting his sister's admission. Thirteen days after Coulthard received this note, Charlotte was admitted to the Toronto sanatorium, in November 1933. The admission was prudent, as the sanatorium physician who examined Charlotte upon her arrival found her to be suffering advanced pulmonary tuberculosis with signs of cavitation in her left lung. Both Charlotte's positive sputum and her lung cavitation suggested that that the risk of infecting her young cousins had been quite real, or perhaps by that time, a reality. While taking in orphaned children was a widely embraced family responsibility, the action itself could propel tuberculosis infection from one household into another.

In an attempt to close the cavities in her lung, an artificial pneumothorax (or therapeutic compression of her lung – see chapter 6) had been attempted in the month that Charlotte was admitted, but, despite the procedure, staff noted she remained "a very sick girl." By May 1934 it was determined that Charlotte's infection had spread to her right lung. In the meantime, Carl had been discharged into the care of his grandmother, but he remained in contact with Coulthard and wrote to him in August 1934. As an ex-sanatorium patient himself, Charlotte's brother had his own ideas and expectations about how his younger sister should look after ten months at the sanatorium, and after visiting with her on a number of occasions, he did not "think she looks very good." While his grandmother was "very anxious to know how she really is," Carl did not want to tell her that his sister was not good because he did not know "for sure." According to his letter, Carl himself had been "getting along fine" since his discharge, gaining four or five pounds and feeling "real good." His grandmother had provided him with a little cabin all to himself, although he ate his meals with the rest of the family in the farmhouse. His only immediate worry was the arrival of winter, dreading the cold. Sadly, however, Carl's intuition had been correct, as Dr Coulthard wrote him, "Charlotte is not as well as she was a few months ago. Her cough and sputum remain just as they have been since her admittance to hospital. Her temperature is still elevated at times." The artificial pneumothorax had failed to close the three cavities in Charlotte's left lung and, more seriously, her "good lung" was getting worse. In the end, despite the attempts to save Charlotte, she died at the hospital in May 1935, the fifth member of her family to succumb to tuberculosis.

In the same way that Charlotte's aunt feared for the health of her young children, Nora's father and stepmother had also come to view her as a risk in the family home. A schoolgirl living in rural Ontario, Nora had lost her mother to TB a number of years before she was admitted to the Toronto sanatorium in March 1918. Her father, described as a poor factory labourer, had remarried, and while he and his new wife were both healthy, they suspected that eight-year-old Nora, "tubercular for some years," was the reason that their home continued to struggle with tuberculosis. The family had ultimately turned to their church's pastor, who, in January 1918, wrote to Dobbie, appealing to have Nora admitted on compassionate grounds, explaining that Nora's father and stepmother had already lost two infants to tuberculosis. According to the pastor, Nora's stepmother was due to "give birth to another in April and would certainly not be able to look after this child then." He emphasized that "she had it hard enough the last time," losing her infant, and he, in his role, had ultimately "buried the babe." The pastor wanted "to see that the little one" due to arrive was "given every chance" to survive, but felt that would be possible only if Nora's "contamination [of] the home" was addressed. As in Charlotte's case, Nora's situation highlights the tensions that could surface in caring for tuberculous children at home. Parents generally expressed reluctance or regret in sending their children away to the sanatorium, but often had to consider, very pragmatically, the quality of care that they could provide and the potential risk of tuberculosis taking hold of other children at home. The zeal of public health efforts to educate families on tuberculosis likely fostered this dynamic, stirring up apprehensions over infection risks, or "contamination," as the situation was described in Nora's case. Nora's stepmother anticipated the struggles she would face in caring for both Nora and the infant due in a few months' time, her angst growing because of the two infants she had already buried. Nora was admitted in early March 1918, but she never did return home, because her condition continued to decline and she died at the sanatorium some nine months later.

While parents may have been conflicted in sending their children away to the sanatorium, many understood the rationale for hospitalization. For children with uncomplicated primary tuberculosis, supportive care, nutritious food, and the balancing of rest and exercise were meant to build resistance to disease; for children with reactivation tuberculosis these measures, supplemented with medical or surgical treatments, were intended to build resistance and reduce destructive disease progression. Parents of children with primary disease may have felt confident that they could provide adequate care at home, especially in well-appointed, comfortable, middle-class or wealthy homes (figure 3.1). For parents in poor homes, however, meeting even the basics of care could be difficult, if not impossible.

Such was the case for one mother from northern Ontario who wanted her seemingly perpetually sick children admitted to an institution, be it a sanatorium or a preventorium, so that they might build up their health in general and their resistance to tuberculosis in particular. Estelle, a forty-one-year-old mother and homemaker, had "been coughing for almost five years" when she was admitted to the Toronto sanatorium in 1939. She despaired at having to leave her children, who remained at home with their father, but worried in particular about the health of her three youngest (who were ten, six, and four years of age). For several years her children had been plagued with ill-health, suffering "repeated attacks of tonsillitis, running ears and terrible coughs," followed by measles in 1938, which had left her ten-year-old daughter with "a pain in her side, sore eyes and a dry hard cough." She described her children as underweight, all with bad tonsils. She was particularly concerned that they had been unnecessarily exposed to tuberculosis, her family doctor having allowed her children to share her bed to the point at which she "took seriously ill" and was shortly thereafter admitted to the sanatorium.[51]

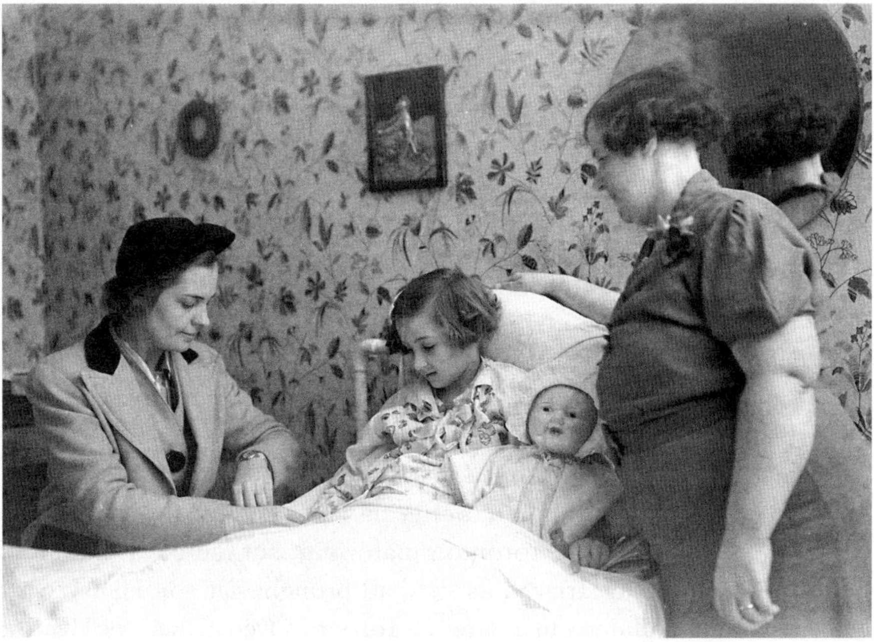

Figure 3.1 A city of Toronto public health nurse measuring a child's pulse rate in her home, circa 1940. The home is well-appointed for home nursing in illness. The child is in her own wallpapered bedroom, tucked into a bed with clean linens and a doll by her side.

Estelle's husband worked hard to support the family, employed steadily and earning a wage of $22 per week, but the cost of living in northern Ontario was crushing, in part because of the poor-quality farmland. She readily admitted, "We can't afford to buy the children milk or fruit and very little vegetables, so they are very undernourished." She could not even encourage her children outside for fresh air in the summer because the air was often thick with mosquitoes and blackflies from June to September each year. While she knew a screened-in veranda would be helpful, money was too scarce for such luxuries. Recognizing that home conditions were not ideal for her vulnerable children, and "afraid of T.B. getting a hold of the children if they are not taken care of," from her bed at the Toronto sanatorium, Estelle wrote to both the Gage Institute and the IODE preventorium in Toronto to see what could be done for them. It is easy to see how Estelle's sense of family responsibility did not end when she was admitted to the sanatorium and encouraged to rest in an effort to gain control over her tuberculosis. Rather than focus on healing,

Estelle understandably remained distractedly worried about the well-being of her children, and this was the experience for many adults admitted to the sanatorium who were racked with guilt over the families they had left behind. Within a couple of months, however, Estelle received word that the preventorium would accept her three youngest, the superintendent promising that they would do their best "to build them up and make them happy."

Other mothers were also confronted with difficult decisions upon their admissions to the sanatorium. Alma, a young mother from a community in northern Ontario, was recommended for immediate sanatorium care in the late 1920s. Alma's husband had died after an accident, leaving her alone to care for their children. Suffering from advanced tuberculosis, Alma was admitted to the Toronto sanatorium, but there was an unexpected twist upon her arrival, as she had brought her son Henry with her. As Dobbie explained in a letter to Toronto's Department of Health, Henry had fallen ill ten days before Alma was set to leave for the sanatorium, and since "there was no one with whom she could leave the child" and no doctor available to give Henry "any care," she felt she had little choice other than to bring him along. Upon examination, Alma's two-year-old son was found to be suffering from acute bronchopneumonia with a fever that, on some days, was as high as 105°F. Feeling that Henry was seriously ill and quite possibly tuberculous because of his close contact with his mother, Dobbie opted to keep him at the sanatorium for observation and treatment. After six months, he was progressing reasonably well, though prone to fluctuations in temperature and a slight cough with expectoration. Henry's mother had made more substantial improvement during this time, gaining thirty-four pounds, establishing a normal temperature, and showing no signs of either cough or sputum. No doubt Alma was motivated to leave the sanatorium as quickly as possible, given that she had left her other young children behind in the care of friends when she was admitted. When Alma left, she took Henry back home with her, though Dobbie would have preferred that he stay longer.

It is not surprising that some parents resisted sending their children to the sanatorium "under the care of strangers," especially those parents who lived far from the city and would seldom have the opportunity to visit the sanatorium or meet the staff in person. Sadie and Faye's father had been hesitant to send his daughters to the sanatorium. Apparently, in July 1921, Moro tests[52] confirmed their tuberculosis infection, and "these little ones were advised [for] Hospital treatment, but the father refused to part with them." In the meantime, while trying to convince him of the importance of hospitalization, home conditions and the girls' health were monitored through periodic visits by public health nurses. On 12 August, the visiting nurse reported that the children were "having breakfast while I visited, which consisted of porridge, bread and butter, tomatoes and milk." The "children [were] clean and tidy" and "home conditions fair." At that time, Sadie and Faye's mother reiterated that she "does not want them to go to Hospital." Another visit on 20 September confirmed that the girls "seem to be gaining in weight" and that the home was "clean and neat" with "a good supply of food." The children were put to bed at eight each night and "live out of doors." Sadie and Faye's admission note indicated that the girls' father "continued to send them to school until finally they became so run down in health that he ultimately consented to their removal from home." While the father was gently criticized for the "whole year of valuable time [that] had been lost," his resistance could have been grounded in any number of reasons, including the worry that he was potentially sending his children away to die alone in the sanatorium. He did eventually consent to their admission in June 1922, and in just under a year of hospitalization, both Sadie and Faye had made good progress, each gaining about seven pounds in weight before they were discharged back home to their seemingly anxious father at his request.

In addition to their parents' reservations and hesitations, children themselves could also resist the prospect of hospitalization. Mattie, fifteen years old and living in Toronto when she was diagnosed with tuberculosis, is a case in point. Mattie had been recommended for a comprehensive examination at the Gage Institute in Toronto in June 1921, after two of her sputum samples returned positive for tuberculosis bacteria. In a note that she brought to her Gage Institute appointment, Mattie's physician explained that she was willing, grudgingly, but at his request, to enter a sanatorium for a period of time "for educational purposes." Because Mattie's TB-positive sputum suggested that she was most likely infectious, she caught the attention of Toronto's Public Health Department. According to the case notes of a city public health nurse, despite the physician's confidence that he had convinced Mattie of the importance of entering the sanatorium for treatment, Mattie quite emphatically did not want to go the Toronto sanatorium, as her 18 June visit noted, "She does not want to go to Weston." Then again, on 7 July, the nurse reported, "Refuses to go to Weston." By 10 August, however, the nurse noted Mattie was "anxious to be admitted" to the Muskoka Free Hospital for Consumptives "for treatment," likely because she had "not been feeling well." Mattie's preference for the Muskoka sanatorium was not uncommon. Located on a lake in the heart of Ontario's burgeoning cottage country, Muskoka was appealing because of its cottage-like ambiance. Many tuberculosis sufferers, on the other hand, believed that the Toronto sanatorium was the final place for hopeless cases. To Mattie, Muskoka's attraction outweighed the advantage of being hospitalized at a sanatorium closer to her family in Toronto. Ultimately, however, Mattie's condition declined further and, on 17 August, the nurse noted that she had "become quite ill" and was admitted to a Toronto hospital. Despite her aversions, her tuberculosis diagnosis resulted in her subsequent transfer to the Toronto sanatorium.

Tuberculosis was a difficult disease experience, characterized by great variation in how the illness presented and the tendency to shift between latency and progression. As a result, prognoses were usually uncertain at best. In his 1930s text *Tuberculosis among Children and Young Adults*, Myers offered pointed advice to physicians negotiating the diagnosis and management of tuberculosis, particularly among adolescents, who were more likely than younger children to be aware of the significance of their tuberculous condition.[53] Adolescents, he noted, were often concerned about exactly how long they would have to spend in bedrest. Despite a poor physical condition and tangible evidence of poor health, some young patients found it difficult to commit to the restrictions of bedrest and their separation from family and home. Mattie, for example, was finally admitted to the Toronto sanatorium in September 1921. At that time, her condition was grave and she suffered a notable cough, filling one-eighth of a sputum box each day, at times with blood-streaked sputum. Despite all the efforts to get Mattie into the sanatorium for treatment, however, she could not be convinced to remain. Forty-two days after her admission, a very short period by sanatorium standards, especially given the seriousness of her condition, she was taken home by her mother and father.

Because of the many uncertainties of tuberculosis, Myers suggested, "the physician is wise who does not definitely commit himself" to answering questions about length of treatment and bedrest because, "in reality, he does not know."[54] Undoubtedly, physicians' ambiguity could stoke anxieties or irritation among their patients. On the other hand, "many a patient has refused treatment and has continued to disseminate tubercle bacilli to his associates and eventually lost his life because his physician stated that one or more years of strict bedrest would be necessary to bring the disease under control."[55] If adolescents were recommended for sanatorium treatment and asked, "How long will I be away?," physicians were advised to "be extremely cautious in answering the question."[56] Myers suggested physicians buy time and flexibility, telling their patients "to plan on at least a few months," following which their condition would be re-evaluated by sanatorium staff.[57]

Staging Disease: The Classification of Patients

Given the complexities of tuberculosis, its ability to be latent, active, advanced, incipient, or fluctuating between classifications, physicians first tried to determine disease status among incoming patients, typically within a few days after admission, with a comprehensive physical examination. This examination would provide an important comparison to the family physician's provisional diagnosis, outlining the nature and extent of the disease and establishing the baselines from which the children's progress at the sanatorium could be measured. Any complications were also noted at this time and decisions made regarding treatment options. When a child was admitted, "the minimum requirements" involved a physical examination using the "four classical procedures:" inspection (a visual assessment), palpation (an exploration by touch), percussion (tapping the body surfaces to evaluate underlying structure and constitution), and auscultation (listening to the sounds of the body, with or without a stethoscope), with particular emphasis on the two latter procedures.[58] For children with primary disease, however, the four procedures proved of "almost no value," since primary disease typically "produced little or no change in [these] signs."[59] Depending on the technology available to the medical staff, the examination may have been supplemented with X-ray or fluoroscopic imaging (figure 3.2). Physicians were encouraged to trust their own senses in the examination and then compare their assessments with X-ray findings. It was strongly recommended not to begin an examination with X-rays; to do so was likened to "reading the final chapter of a book first instead of commencing at the beginning," and valuable insights gained from the classical examination could be missed.[60] The physician's findings were annotated using medical shorthand on standardized pages, providing a blank outline of the front and rear views of a torso (see, for example, figure 3.3). Most children had consecutives pages in their charts representing the results of their periodic reassessments.

For office examinations, Dr F.S. Minns offered some advice in a 1912 publication in *Canadian Practitioner*. To begin, he recommended to physicians, "never do the examination if you are in a hurry," because at least an hour would be required for a truly thorough investigation.[61] Physicians were instructed to direct patients to remove all layers of clothing covering the chest, to sit up, even if they were bed patients, and to cover their mouths and noses with folded cheesecloth or gauze handkerchiefs. In order to avoid the undue influence of the patient's own perception of his or her condition, physicians were advised to do a complete examination before taking the patient's history. Chest, eyes, ears, nose, throat, abdomen, and any other relevant organs or tissues of interest could be included in the physical examination. After the examination, as patients dressed, physicians were advised to make a written record of all findings and observations. Depending on the laboratory facilities available, they could sample secretions, sputum, blood, urine, or tissues for testing. A tuberculin test was strongly recommended, if only to confirm infection, as well as a chest X-ray and guinea pig inoculation, if possible.

Minns recommended multiple chest examinations, on different days and at different hours, in order to control for variability in the patient's condition and to gain a better sense of the disease's eccentricities. Physicians were advised, "Do not commit yourself to a diagnosis unless you are absolutely sure of your findings," and, if tuberculosis was identified, to wait at least one month (during which time repeated examinations could be undertaken) before attempting to make any sort of prognosis and, even then, "with reserve," since tuberculosis was often difficult to

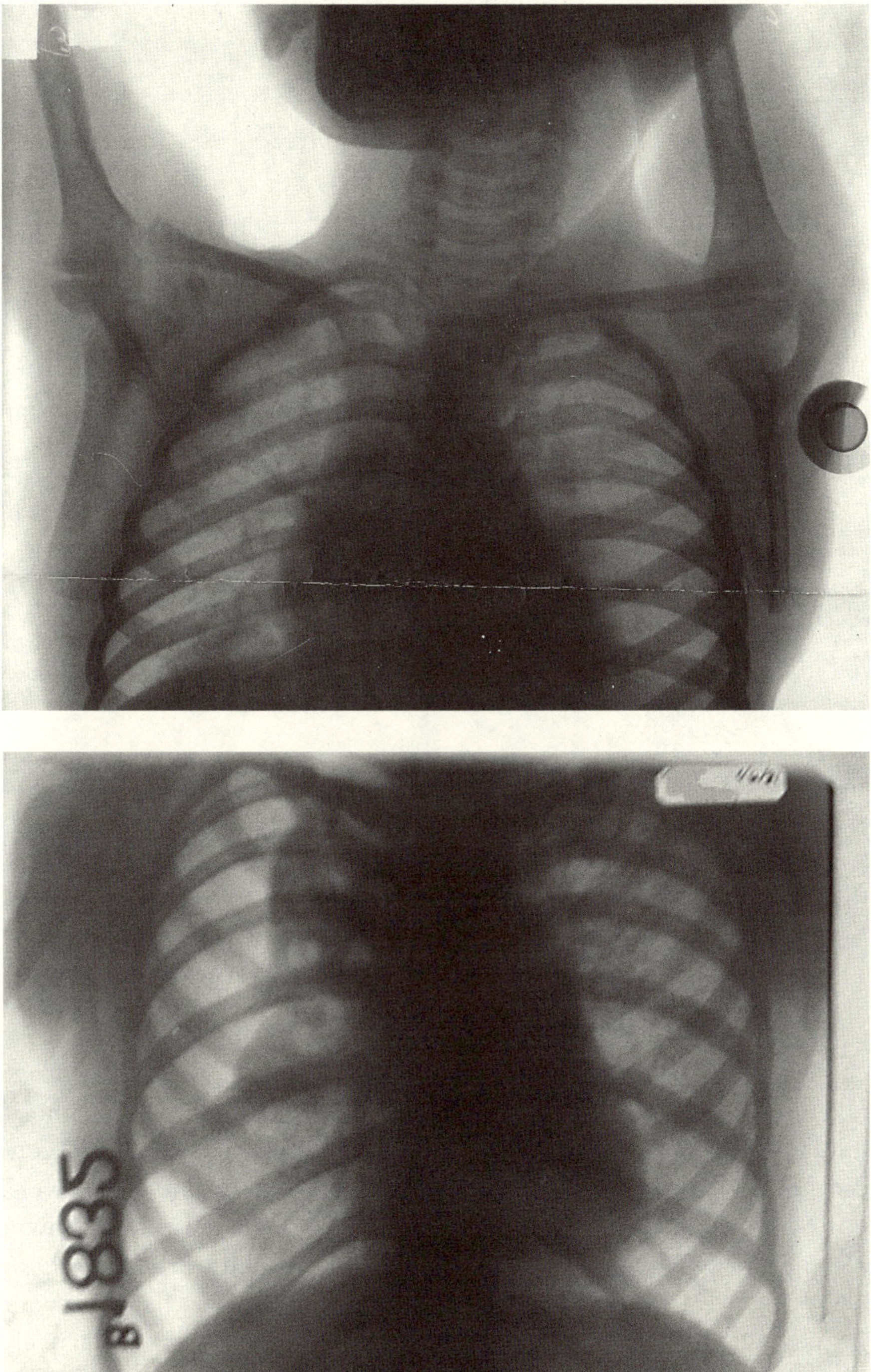

Figure 3.2 Chest X-rays for two children. On the top, a five-year-old boy with hilar tuberculosis and, on the bottom, a fourteen-year-old girl with advanced pulmonary tuberculosis.

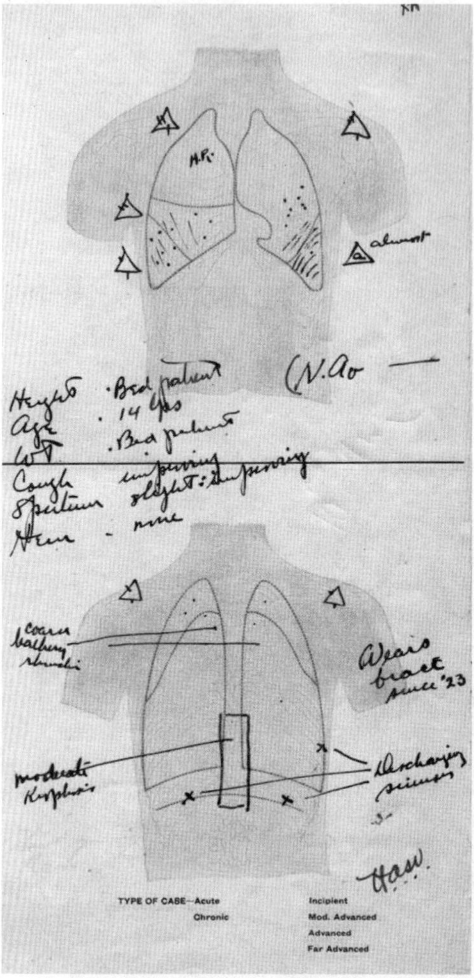

Figure 3.3 Physical examination findings for a fourteen-year-old child with lung and spine involvement. The spine has a "moderate kyphosis" and "discharging sinuses." The child wore a brace and was a bed patient so height and weight could not be measured. Cough was recorded as "improving," and sputum was "slight and improving." The child did not suffer hemorrhages.

characterize in terms of expected outcomes.[62] Some physicians may have taken this too far, conservatively holding off on a tuberculosis diagnosis until it was evident even to the patient, perhaps out of kindness and concern, or perhaps because of worries over their own diagnostic prowess. For Minns, moderation was key, and he recommended neither downplaying a patient's condition, "Oh, you only have a little bronchitis," nor delivering a fatal prognosis, "There is not a ghost of a chance of your getting better."[63] Finally, Minns also suggested that physicians actively involve their patients in assessing their own health, advising that patients carry with them small notebooks in which they could record health-related details, such as sputum quantity, fever, and weight changes. In the spirit of sharing information with patients and educating them (and, by extension, their families and other associates), and not excluding them with overly scientific medical jargon, Minns advised, "When explaining things to patients, make your language as simple as possible; don't talk over his head; don't be too technical; never be mysterious. Explain germs; what they are; how they grow; how they are carried from one place to another; how to destroy them."[64] At the Toronto sanatorium, this sentiment was expressed over and over again, with Dobbie's carefully worded and detailed correspondences with patients and their families. It would be of little benefit to complicate tuberculosis; for public welfare and prevention, the more that everybody understood about the bacterial infection of tuberculosis, the better.

Professional courtesies guided Dobbie in sending out reports of the sanatorium's initial findings to referring family physicians. Through these reports, physicians could assess their own diagnostic abilities, learning through comparisons of their diagnoses and sanatorium findings. In turn, by keeping them informed and involved, family physicians could act as liaisons with parents or guardians, providing them with updates on each child's progress at the sanatorium. Dobbie's 1928 letter to twelve-year-old Violet's family physician provides a good example of a typical initial examination summary:

> I beg to advise in connection with your patient, Violet, who was admitted to this institution on the 21st inst., that our examination indicates that she is a moderately advanced case of tuberculosis with involvement of both lungs, extending from the hilum upwards. Family history is negative, except that the mother is subject to asthma. The child's height is 4'10-¾"; weight 71½ lbs. She has slight cough, occasionally some expectoration, and some shortness of breath. There is a slight degree of cyanosis [a bluish skin colour caused by oxygen deprivation]; appetite only fair. Temperature 98-4/5°, pulse 108, blood pressure 90/65. The Wassermann [test for syphilis infection] was negative. Physical signs were dullness on either side of the sternum, extending upwards towards the apices. The X-ray plate shows dense hila, especially on the left; few enlarged lymph nodes, and lack of brilliancy in the middle third of each lung.

Overall, Violet's physical findings suggested she was suffering primary tuberculosis disease with a focus in her lung's hilar lymph nodes. Fever was a common symptom, but Violet's temperature fell just short of the concern-raising cut-off of 99.4° for females (99° for males).[65] Like elevations in temperature, a patient's pulse rate (the number of times the heart beats in a minute) was also used as a barometer of disease activity that guided recommended activity: "Under 100, no restriction; from 100 to 120 no work or exercise; over 120, rest in bed."[66] Violet's pulse rate and other symptoms placed her in the "no work or exercise" category and, perhaps because of the limitations placed on her activity, Violet's parents believed she was "not particularly happy" at the sanatorium. Despite the poor evaluation of her health, just over a month after being admitted and with Dobbie's support, she was taken back home by her mother.

Once the nature and extent of disease could be evaluated, children were classified according to advisable levels of activity, though, in reality, most children (and adults) began their lives at the sanatorium as strict bed patients, a practice that was a major source of discontentment for many, including Violet. At the Toronto sanatorium, from "bed patient," children could move through the classification scheme to "ambulatory patient," and "working patient" (among children, "work" in the form of attending the sanatorium school, craft work, or perhaps tending the sanatorium gardens). Twelve stages – three bed, seven ambulatory, and three working – defined how much rest patients required in their treatment. The culture of treatment at the Toronto sanatorium departed from the "graduated labour" schemes popular in England. Unlike English sanatoria, the focus at the Toronto sanatorium was really on how much *rest* was needed, and not on how much *work* or *exercise* was associated with treatment and patient rehabilitation (for more on this, see chapter 5). Bed patients classed as C3-0, for example, had no out-of-bed privileges, not even toilet or bathroom visits. By class C1-2, "some occupation in bed" might be permitted. The class B, or ambulatory, status was the most drawn out, with patients moving slowly between eating one meal in the dining room, to all three meals, making their own beds, and being granted occasional leave permits for sojourns outside the sanatorium. Working (class A) patients varied between "some light work" assigned for no more than one hour each half day, up to "some regular work" for more than two hours each half day.

In practice, children learned the everyday vocabulary of this classification. A former child patient remembered beginning her hospitalization as a "blanket patient," which she came to understand meant that "you could get dressed but you had to stay in your bed most of the day, [and] your meals were brought to you."[67] She next became an "up-patient," which meant that she could go to the dining room for meals. Before leaving the sanatorium, she had graduated to a "full-time patient," a classification that allowed her to "get up and go to school, go out into the yard and play, and things like that."[68] The classification scheme was carefully managed by sanatorium staff and, even if patients regained their health enough to be upwardly mobile, they were moved, nevertheless, through the levels slowly and cautiously. Perhaps the most difficult cases involved patients on total bedrest (C3-0 patients) because they lacked even bathroom and toilet privileges. All patients began their life at the sanatorium in this stage, at least until the exact nature of their disease and their resistance to it could be determined. Children and adults alike struggled with the limitations placed on bed patients, including the discomfort and embarrassment of sponge-baths and bed pans. At Craig-y-nos Douglas Herbert remembered being given a bedpan each morning: "They woke you up at six o'clock and you didn't get breakfast until you used it."[69]

Violet's parents felt that the bedrest restrictions were responsible for her unhappiness at the sanatorium and led to their decision to discharge her, even though Dobbie had tried to explain to the family's physician why she was being kept in bed. "Because she feels so well," Dobbie wrote in his letter, "she may not like the idea of being confined to bed, but it has been explained to her that she must remain in bed until her temperature has been normal for some time." It appears that how patients such as Violet felt and what they wrote in letters home was sometimes at odds with what they were willing to tell the sanatorium staff. Dobbie understood that, when asked, Violet "denied being discontented," and staff who worked with her reported "she appears to be quite happy," her bed located "in one of the brightest rooms in the hospital" that she shared "with two other little girls." It was quickly realized that such discrepancies could be intentional, one means perhaps for homesick patients to play on family sympathies and earn their discharges back home. On another occasion, Dobbie wrote to a mother who also had concerns that her daughter was being kept in bed. He reassured her, "It is not necessary to be alarmed when children are put to bed as they are put to bed to give them more rest so that they will perhaps gain more weight when it is needed or that temperature or pulse rate may be better controlled." If a patient's condition progressed favourably, their status could be upgraded, allowing them increasing privileges, but these privileges could also be taken away if their condition took a turn for the worse. Overall, the amount of bedrest prescribed often served as a good measure of perceived disease activity.

One former child patient revealed that, at the sanatorium, "time really didn't mean that much to us,"[70] likely because of all the time spent resting and relatively disconnected from the realities of the outside world. Yet the sanatorium did attempt to instil the kind of orderly routine that defined the typical daily lives of schoolchildren. Children who were not bed patients were up at seven each morning, responsible for brushing their teeth, combing their hair, making their beds, tidying their rooms, and making their way to the children's dining room for breakfast at their assigned tables (figure 3.4). From there, the children would then begin their day's lessons at the school. At the Queen Mary Hospital, in 1939, all children were called in by seven in the evening, the doors were locked, the children were settled into their beds for the evening in comparative quiet, and the lights were turned out by nine. A ward aide was left to supervise the first floor (and main doors) continuously until 11:30 each night. While the staff maintained this orderly routine, however, children sometimes covertly adopted their own night-time rituals, the stories of which are detailed in chapter 7.

Older adolescents were often accommodated in the adult wards at the Toronto sanatorium, perhaps even in the informal and less supervised pavilions if their status was good and their disease well controlled. In his autobiography, Sidney Hobbs, fifteen years of age when he entered the Toronto sanatorium in 1931, recalled the morning routine of the pavilions, or the "shacks" as he called them (figure 3.5). By 8:30 each morning patients had to be up and dressed (which they did in the heated bathrooms), beds had to be made, and dressers tidied and dusted.[71] The windows of the pavilions would then be closed and the "steam" (from radiators)

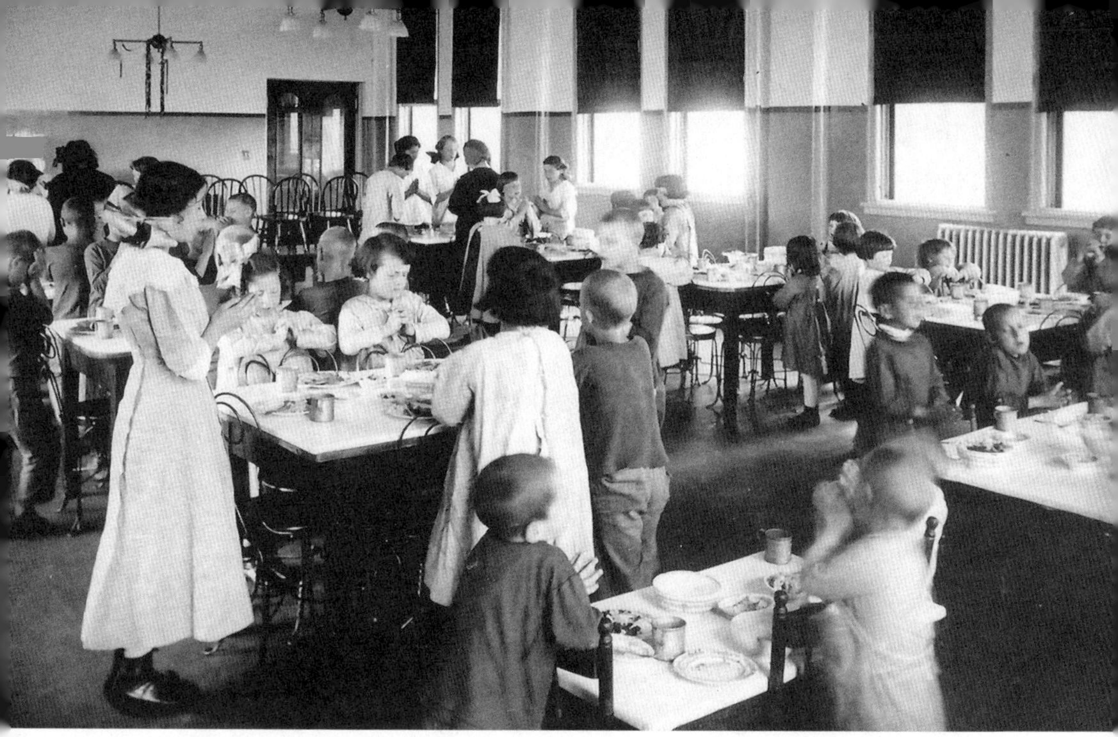

Figure 3.4 The dining room at the Queen Mary Hospital where the children stand to give thanks and say grace before their meal. Full dining room privileges would be granted only to children in good health, otherwise meals would be taken in bed. A similar photograph featured in a commemorative booklet celebrating the opening of the Queen Mary is entitled "Grace before Meat at the Queen Mary Hospital" and details the words of the prayer spoken by the children: "Be present at our table, Lord, / Be here and everywhere adored, / Thy children bless, / and grant that we / May dwell in paradise with Thee."

turned on as patients left the pavilions for breakfast in the dining room with the hope that they would return to reasonably warm beds. Patients in the pavilions, adults and adolescents, had relatively more freedom, since they were apart from the surveillance of the main hospital buildings. Hobbs took advantage of the latitude to earn some pocket money (he said, for soft drinks, candy, and movies) by doing other patients' laundry: "Pyjamas washed and ironed for 10 cents, shirts washed and ironed and collar starched using milk for stiffener, washing in the basins in the washroom and hanging there to dry out of sight of the authorities," and ironing on top of his dresser using newspapers, a blanket, and a sheet to protect its surface. He was later casually employed as a sanatorium switchboard operator and tuck shop delivery man, the latter position he particularly enjoyed since he was able to meet new patients on the wards while

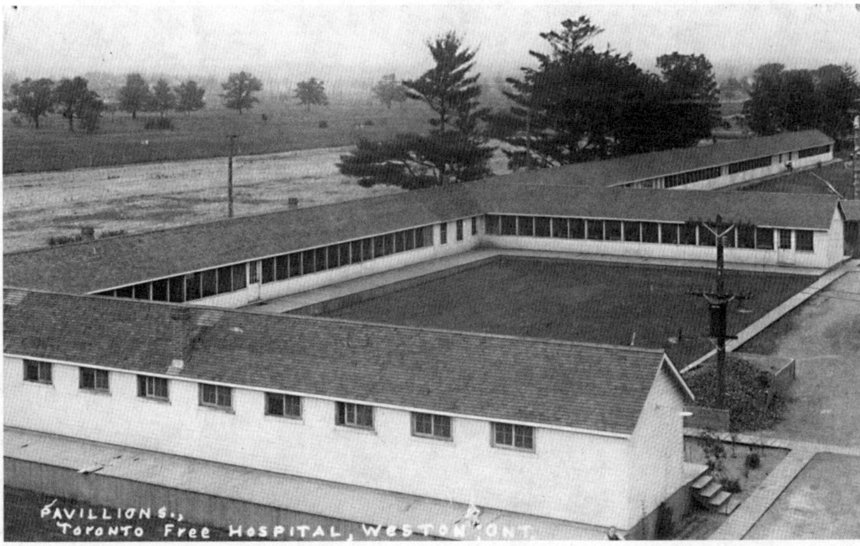

Figure 3.5 The pavilions at the Toronto sanatorium. Some of the older adolescents sufficiently improved in health could be transferred from the main hospital buildings to the pavilions. Here, they would enjoy less supervision. The pavilions provided emergency shelter to patients displaced by the 1910 fire and were then expanded and improved to provide more beds for patients.

earning better hourly pay. Patients such as Sidney exemplified industriousness, attempting to make the best of their hospitalization. But then again, Sidney had been orphaned by tuberculosis, so perhaps he was motivated to make the best of his difficult position.

Not only was the Toronto sanatorium the first institution in Canada specialized in the care of tuberculous infants and children, it was also the preferred place for pregnant tuberculous women to have their babies. Pregnant women admitted to the Muskoka sanatorium were often transferred to Toronto as their anticipated day of confinement grew closer. Congenital tuberculosis among babies, where infection passes via the placenta from infected mothers to their infants in utero, is exceedingly rare and only a few hundred cases have ever been reported around the world.[72] No instances of congenital tuberculosis were documented in the 822 cases sampled, though all infants born at the sanatorium were carefully examined and observed. A former staff physician who began work at the sanatorium in 1930 reported that he had never observed a single case of congenital tuberculosis.[73]

In the early years of the Toronto sanatorium, newborns were discharged as quickly as arrangements could be made for their care, the intention being to get them out of the sanatorium and prevent their needless exposure to tuberculosis. Celia, for example, was born at the Toronto sanatorium in 1915. Her father was listed in her chart as "unknown" and her mother, a patient at the sanatorium, suffered from active tuberculosis. In order to protect her health, Celia had been separated from her mother at birth and fed a diet that included formulas of "albumin water" (raw egg whites and water) and an ambiguous "milk mist" (perhaps cow's milk diluted with water). When Celia was about four months old Miss Dickson began to look for suitable accommodations so that she might be discharged. One possibility was Toronto's Infants' Home and Infirmary, founded at 21 Mary Street in 1875 by a group of Toronto women, and one of the few charitable institutions in the city prepared and willing to accept infants. The home had a particular interest in the support and "rehabilitation" of unmarried mothers and their infants.[74] Where possible, the home encouraged both mothers and their infants to be brought into the institution together so that the babies could be breastfed.[75] The home, in turn, received provincial funding covering the daily maintenance costs of not only the infants, but also the mothers under its care. According to Neff, the government supported this dual responsibility, largely because of the significantly lower infant mortality rates at this home in comparison to others that relied on formula feeding alone.[76]

When Miss Dickson wrote to the home looking to admit Celia, the superintendent replied that the home could not accept the infant since it was understood that she had a mother and "whether [the] babe is nursing or not, we do not take them from the mother." There was an added provision to her letter, however, that if this was a case requiring special consideration, the matter could be taken to the home's managers for appeal. With Celia's admission still a possibility, Miss Dickson elaborated, "I may say that this baby's mother is tuberculous, and for that reason it is necessary for the infant and the mother to be separated. This baby has not been handled by the mother since birth, and is in good condition, taking its food well, and is in every way apparently a normal baby." Dickson emphasized that staff did not think it "wise to retain this child for a greater length of time, because in a short time it will be handling things that our tuberculous children are playing with,[77] and that would not be a wise procedure." Miss Dickson wrote of their difficulties in keeping the infant safe from infection, since the "little tots suffering from tuberculosis sometimes go to her crib and play with her." The infants' home agreed to admit Celia, provided the sanatorium guarantee in writing that, should she show any hint of tuberculosis, she would be quickly transferred back to the sanatorium. The home's concern over disease was well founded, since such institutions were periodically plagued with disease outbreaks. Just two years earlier in 1913, for example, the home had admitted a child who, after admission, developed measles and diphtheria.[78] The infections quickly circulated and were ultimately responsible for twenty-five child deaths. The circumstances under which Celia was to be admitted to the home were not uncommon for the times. Considering some two thousand Toronto children were placed in orphanages in 1918 alone, James Struthers has noted, "One-half were there because of the illness or desertion of a parent, one-quarter because of the death of a parent, and less than 10 percent because of emotional or physical neglect. Only 1 percent were true orphans."[79] Charlotte Neff's study of the Toronto Girls' Home suggests that these charitable institutions had a preference for providing temporary respite care for children from families struggling under the weight of poverty or sickness.[80] As a result, orphanages such as the infants' home functioned as part of the supportive network for families under stress.

Celia was one of a number of infants born at the sanatorium and, over time, protocols shifted towards keeping them at the sanatorium longer, even despite their apparent health. Though never explicitly stated, it seems likely that because infants are so susceptible to infection in their first vulnerable year of life, they were kept at the sanatorium in order to protect them from possible exposure upon discharge to their family homes (or potentially hazardous environments, such as orphanages). Since these infants born at the sanatorium clearly had mothers who suffered active tuberculosis, it was most probable that there were others in the family home, fathers or siblings, who were also infected and perhaps not as careful or educated as patients in the sanatorium in protecting against transmission. The reality was that infants would likely face their biggest infection challenges upon their return to homes that had already yielded cases of tuberculosis,[81] so keeping them at the sanatorium in their most vulnerable first months of life seemed to make sense.

When Oliver was born at the Toronto sanatorium in 1936, he was assessed as a healthy, six-pound baby who had experienced a normal but relatively quick birth. Oliver's mother had been transferred from the Muskoka sanatorium when she was seven months pregnant, her physicians not confident that she would even live long enough to deliver her baby. She persevered, however, and experienced the birth of her son, but ultimately died only twelve days after his delivery. To safeguard Oliver's health and prevent infection, he had been separated from his mother at birth and fed on formula. For the time that Oliver would remain at the sanatorium, no physical signs of TB were ever noted and, with the exception of a bout of diarrhea in the summer of 1936 when he lost six pounds, his general condition always remained good.

Oliver was left alone at the sanatorium after his mother's death, though he did have family. Oliver's eldest sister wrote to a patient at the sanatorium whom her mother, prior to her death, had appointed as Oliver's godmother, explaining their situation. Oliver's sister and the rest of his family were living in northern Ontario, and both the distance to the sanatorium and the hazardous or impassable roads in winter had prevented the family from visiting him. As Oliver's sister explained to his godmother, she was hesitant to have him discharged because, in the absence of her mother, she did not have confidence in her abilities to care for her infant brother: "It is a long time since we haven't heard [about] him but it wasn't because we had forgotten him. We always think about him and often desire to have him with us but as it is kind of difficult for me to take care of him when he was so young. I think it wouldn't be so bad when he has done two months or so and when you see fine weather coming it doesn't seem as bad." As the letter continued, it became apparent that the family was not entirely sure if they were even allowed to bring Oliver home, his sister explicitly writing to the godmother, "I would be glad to know if we may have the child and bring him home with the rest of the family." She continued, "Some people have been telling us that if we wanted him we would be able to get him any time." And again, "It may not be right away but we thought it would be better to make sure whether we could get him or not." It is unclear why Oliver's sister and the rest of the family felt they could not simply take Oliver home. It may have been that they believed Oliver, like his mother, was tuberculous and that he would have to remain in the sanatorium. Yet Oliver's sister had also written to Dobbie, explicitly asking him if Oliver had become "property of the hospital" because he had been left there for so long. In his reply, Dobbie reassured her that this had never been the case and once the weather improved, almost a year after his birth at the sanatorium, Oliver's father and sister arrived to meet him and take him home. Eleven years later, a follow-up report confirmed that Oliver was alive and well with his family, having never shown any signs or suggestions of tuberculosis.

Deaths in the Sanatorium

Ultimately, it was a sad reality that not all child patients would survive tuberculosis, even with the support of sanatorium care. The National Sanitarium Association's annual report for 1936 was the last year to provide tables summarizing the disease status (apparently arrested, disease quiescent, improved, stationary, failed, and died) of patients discharged. Of the 1,537 child cases discharged from the Queen Mary Hospital in the twenty-four years since its opening in 1913, 223 (14.5 per cent) had died at the sanatorium.[82] Adding in the 37 deaths among the 155 child patients at the sanatorium before the opening of the Queen Mary,[83] some 260 (15.3 per cent) of 1,692 child patients died at the sanatorium between 1904 and 1936. Of the 822 children sampled in this study, 143 (17.4 per cent) died at the sanatorium (see table 3.1), though the numbers are not directly comparable to the annual report figures because the sample includes adolescent patients who were placed in beds in the adult wards (not just the children in the Queen Mary Hospital). Overall, the proportion of patients from the adult wards who died at the sanatorium was much higher, a reflection of the dangers of more aggressive reactivation disease and the possibility that, among adults, those suffering the most severe cases of disease ended up at the sanatorium. Of the 9,258

Table 3.1
Distribution of deaths and discharges according to age

Age at admission	Number (*n*) of cases	Discharged % (*n*)	Died % (*n*)
Born at sanatorium	31	80.6 (25)	19.4 (6)
Less than 1 year	18	55.6 (10)	44.4 (8)*
1–4 years	112	91.1 (102)*	8.9 (10)
5–9 years	235	91.9 (216)*	8.1 (19)
10–14 years	239	83.3 (199)	16.7 (40)
15–17 years	185	67.6 (125)	32.4 (60)*
Total	820[a]	82.6 (677)	17.4 (143)

$\chi^2 = 58.079$, 5 *df*, $p < .001$; * = a significant excess, according to the distribution of observed and expected cases in chi-square analysis.
[a] Total does not add up to 822, because of missing age information for two cases.

adult patients discharged in the thirty-two years between 1904 and 1936, 3,981 (43.0 per cent) were reported to have died at the sanatorium.[84]

In an era when there was no certain cure for tuberculosis, dying at the sanatorium was always a possibility and, for parents, this reality likely played into the apprehensions they experienced upon sending their children away. This concern was not unique to the sanatorium, as Julie-Marie Strange describes a strong culture of home death, with "the vigilance of friends and the familiar environment of the home" to "ease the distress of impending death," fuelling a general "obstinacy" of parents to hospitalize sick children "for fear of them dying alone and in unfamiliar surroundings."[85] Yet, with tuberculosis, hopes for improvement at the sanatorium always lingered, even though the unpredictability of the disease, its twists and turns through progress and decline, may have guarded those hopes. As indicated in table 3.1, there was a significant association between the age of child patients sampled and the distribution of deaths. Particularly vulnerable to dying of tuberculosis were infants under one year of age (44 per cent of sampled infants admitted to the sanatorium died at the sanatorium) and older adolescents fifteen to seventeen years of age (32 per cent of these older adolescents sampled died at the sanatorium). These findings are neither surprising nor unexpected. In the case of infants, poorly developed immune function can be linked to their vulnerability to primary progressive disease following infection, while older adolescents likely succumbed to more aggressive reactivation disease. The younger children sampled (particularly those between one and nine years of age) were probably less likely to die of tuberculosis in the sanatorium because this age group was being treated most commonly for uncomplicated primary disease, which, with adequate immune function, is more often self-limiting in its expression. For this reason, some tuberculosis experts identified the ages between five and fifteen, or two to three and ten to eleven as the "golden years" of lower tuberculosis morbidity and mortality.[86] The effect would wane as children moved into adolescence and the risk of reactivation disease became a reality. A common statistic posits that about 10 per cent of infected children would experience reactivation by the time they reached adulthood.[87]

The sample numbers underestimate the true burdens of tuberculosis mortality, given the understanding that, when possible, parents discharged their morbidly ill children so that they could die at home, in the company of their families.[88] This was the experience for Cora, seventeen years old when she was admitted in September 1929 with advanced and bilateral (affecting both lungs) pulmonary tuberculosis. The doctors at the sanatorium realized that Cora's prognosis was not overwhelmingly good, and though she had held steady for many months, by 1931 her health began to fail dramatically. Ultimately, they felt, she would most likely die. When Dobbie wrote to Cora's mother with this regrettable news, she immediately wrote back, absolutely certain that if her daughter was going to die, then she wanted her to die at home:

> Doc Doby – Dear sir I am writing to you about Cora in regards to bringing her home as I think now it is the best place for her as I feel you all have done your best for her to regain her health but she has failed so fast in the past month or so and is home sick and wants to come home and I know she will not be contented there now for she

> feels she is not going to get better and wants to come home to me and I want her home so I have a tent pitched in the lawn for her where she can be comfortable and I know happy with me and I would be more happy to as she is all I have to live for and she is very dear to me.

While Dobbie agreed that it made the most sense for Cora to return home, they faced problems arranging her transportation. Cora was a "stretcher case," too weak to get out of bed, and certainly unable to weather travel by train. Her mother did the best she could in finding transportation for Cora, writing Dobbie that she would secure the services of an undertaker's car "so as she can come comfortably." In fairness to Cora's mother, the station wagon-like vehicles used as ambulances and hearses at the time were fairly interchangeable in their design, and funeral homes were sometimes called upon to provide their hearses for private ambulance services.[89] Despite the practicality, however, it is difficult to imagine how Cora would have felt travelling back home from the sanatorium in a hearse, ultimately failed in her battle with tuberculosis and awaiting the sureness of death. Perhaps the reassurance of returning home to her mother's care would have been enough to outweigh these anxieties. It is hard to know, but such was the sobering reality of tuberculosis.

At the Toronto sanatorium, deaths among child patients were more likely to occur if children entered the sanatorium in late, advanced stages of the disease, when complications arose, or if the disease progressed quickly or dangerously, as in the case of TB meningitis (affecting the brain) and disseminated miliary TB (in the bloodstream).[90] In urgent cases, when it became clear that a child was failing, parents or guardians were contacted but, unlike Cora's mother, it was often difficult, if not impossible, for those who lived far away from Toronto to either see their children or bring them home before they died. In the event that a child did die suddenly, parents or guardians were notified by mail, telegraph, telephone, or the closest police office. Even then, it was sometimes impossible to reach parents if they lived far-removed from settlements or if their occupations took them into remote areas, as was particularly the case for a number of Indigenous parents who were involved in seasonal hunting and trapping. Sometimes, when parents or guardians were reached by telephone or telegraph they asked the sanatorium staff to pass along final words to their children or to arrange appropriate spiritual guidance for critically ill children. The sanatorium staff were sensitive in these matters. When one Roman Catholic child passed away alone in his bed of sudden heart failure in the early 1920s, the night nurse on duty immediately sought out a well-versed Catholic patient to see if the boy could still be given last rites[91] even after his death. In documentation concerning the case, it was reported that the nurse became visibly distressed when she was advised that, in this child's case, the opportunity for last rites had quickly come and gone.

In a disease as unpredictable as tuberculosis, the timing of end-of-life rituals such as last rites could be difficult to negotiate. When Maxine, a thirteen-year-old school girl, was admitted to the Queen Mary in May 1928, her prognosis was determined to be "poor." Both of Maxine's lungs showed signs of advanced disease, two-thirds of her left lung and one-half of the right. In August 1928, Dobbie wrote to Maxine's father with devastating news: "Very sorry … to report that there [had been] no improvement" in Maxine's condition and that he did "not feel that there is going to be any improvement in her condition." Believing that she was "gradually failing," Dobbie noted that "as a precaution we have had the last rites of the Roman Catholic church administered to her," though "just how long she may live" he was "unable to say." As it was, Maxine went on to live for almost two more months, surely believing that, having been given last rites, nobody really expected her to recover.

Undoubtedly, parents suffered emotionally when they received such news from the sanatorium, but ultimately and pragmatically, they also had to make some difficult decisions regarding the handling of their children's bodies. Vivian was seventeen years old and living in northern Ontario when she was admitted to the sanatorium in February 1931. Her mother had died twelve years earlier in the Spanish influenza epidemic of 1918–19 and her father passed away four years earlier from complications arising from a leg abscess. He had remarried after Vivian's mother's death and Vivian and her siblings, from each of her father's first and second marriages, lived together with her stepmother, who was alive and well. Vivian had entered the sanatorium in a very serious condition, showing signs typical of advanced, bilateral pulmonary disease, a case of reactivation tuberculosis that likely stemmed from a primary infection earlier in her life. Vivian was believed to have acquired that infection from a neighbouring family, making friends with a girl her own age who, it turned out, had active tuberculosis. Vivian's family doctor wrote to Dobbie in January 1931, describing Vivian's disease as "moderate in extent," but "quite rapid" in its progression. He felt that her right lung was more affected and that Vivian was "already having some pleurisy," since her disease first manifested eight to ten weeks earlier, and strongly urged her admission to the sanatorium.

Once she was admitted, in an attempt to stop the spread of the disease, an artificial pneumothorax was induced on Vivian's right lung. On 16 June, however, it was noted that Vivian was failing, her uncollapsed lung rapidly becoming diseased. In October, Dobbie wrote to Vivian's stepmother, advising her that her daughter would likely die. Since Vivian's stepmother could not read or write, she relied on her town's postmaster to help her with her correspondence with Dobbie. It is evident that she had accepted the inevitable death of her daughter and wanted to plan accordingly, as explained by the postmaster: "Mrs —— of this place has shown me your letter in which you inform her of the serious condition of her daughter Vivian. As you are no doubt aware, Mrs —— is at present in very poor circumstances, being dependant only on the allowance which she receives from The Mother's Allowance Board. As the father of Vivian is buried at ——, Ontario, a few miles from here, it is the wish of Mrs —— that Vivian would be buried beside him." The postmaster's letter continued, as he requested advice on "what is usually done by the Government to prepare the body for burial. If there is a coffin supplied or is this done by relatives? I have no knowledge of anything like this and Mrs. ——, being unable to write herself, has asked me for this information." In closing his letter, he requested that "in the event of Vivian being critical or dying" that Dobbie telegram Vivian's mother and "hold body for instructions." This letter was written the very day that Vivian died in the sanatorium. Vivian had been admitted as a free (non-paying) patient, her hospitalization costs covered by her municipality. In cases such as Vivian's, where death occurred, municipalities were responsible for all burial costs, but those responsibilities extended only to arranging for local (in the Toronto area) and inexpensive burials. The "social inequities of disease did not end with death," Esyllt Jones has argued, "but extended to the fate of the corpse."[92] In her study of Winnipeggers caught in the grips of the 1918–19 influenza pandemic, Jones determined that working-class and immigrant families had struggled with the escalating costs to provide decent and culturally appropriate burials.[93] In the same sense, poor and working-class Ontarians were relatively powerless to have the bodies of their children shipped home from the sanatorium and buried in meaningful places. In Vivian's case, given her stepmother's financial hardship, and despite her wishes, it is likely that Vivian's body was never shipped home nor laid to rest beside her father. This is significant since, as Julie-Marie Strange has suggested, "the rituals associated with caring for, and disposing of, the corpse illustrates the use of rites as symbolic languages for grief, sympathy and condolence."[94] These lonely, disconnected burials far from home and family only reinforced, in the long term, the ongoing feelings of separation and loss, and the inability to fully mourn the passing of children.

Undoubtedly, difficult living conditions and the regular presence of sickness and death could dull or harden emotional responses to tuberculosis in its endemic age, particularly if families had already experienced loss as a result of the disease. Sisters Ellie, twenty years of age, and Sarah, thirteen years of age, were admitted to the sanatorium in 1929. Residing in northern Ontario, the district's public health nurse had a very difficult time convincing the poor family that the sisters needed to be sent south to the sanatorium as soon as possible. Ellie and Sarah were living in a small home with their mother, father, and four siblings. Four other siblings had already died, two where the cause of death was confirmed as tuberculosis. The nurse wrote to Dobbie in August 1929, seeking a place for Ellie and Sarah in the sanatorium, both of whom, she felt, were "suffering from an advanced condition of pulmonary tuberculosis" disease. "It is urgent," she argued, "that these older girls be removed from the [four] younger children as a means of discontinuing the source of infection." Her attentions focused on the home, she suggested "very careful supervision" and "frequent examination" would be needed to ensure that those vulnerable children "receive attention should any active condition develop." As residents of an unorganized territory in Ontario, the nurse reassured Dobbie "the Government[95] would pay for their maintenance" at the sanatorium if their parents could not afford to do so.

Once Dobbie confirmed that placements had been arranged for Ellie and Sarah, the nurse again wrote to him, two weeks later, indicating that the girls, delayed in their arrival, were on their way. She explained, "We have had great difficulty trying to persuade the family to send these girls away." Noting the bad family history, "in that two sisters died in 1928 with tuberculosis and there are four smaller children at home who are contacts," nonetheless, she felt, "the parents seem very indifferent about the two who are sick." Though Sarah initially improved at the sanatorium, gaining nine pounds by December 1929, both sisters ultimately died within days of each other in March 1930. Their parents were notified of the girls' deaths, to which their father responded with a brief telegram, stating simply: "You can bury Ellie and Sarah as you like. I cannot give any financial help and I cannot come there." His message seems resigned and dispassionate, almost as if the family had lost hope for Ellie and Sarah the day they left for the sanatorium, as was understandable in light of the fact that they had already buried four children. But as Julie-Marie Strange has argued, such stoic responses to death did not mean that people were "devoid of emotion," but that for working-class or poor families "their circumstances blunted its expression: love and grief were like life – unextravagant."[96]

According to protocols, when children died at the sanatorium, an inventory was taken of their possessions, and families either claimed those items or donated them for hospital use. Many parents made requests for specific items, typically small keepsakes of their lost children. Some children entered the sanatorium with virtually no possessions, often the case for those children who came from very poor homes, or orphanages and other institutions. Other children had many possessions. Minnie was six years old when she was admitted in April 1925. Her mother had died of TB four years earlier, when Minnie was only two years old. Prior to her admission to the sanatorium, the child had already suffered through measles, chicken pox, whooping cough, pneumonia, and bronchitis, her resistance to disease in general quite poor. When she was admitted, her prognosis was not good. Minnie had a slight cough and moist rales, sounds of a "bubbling character" caused by fluid in her lungs.[97] Even at her young age, she typically filled one-quarter of a sputum box each day. After three years of struggling against tuberculosis, Minnie died at the sanatorium in November 1928, succumbing to advanced pulmonary tuberculosis. She left behind her father and a brother. Both her father and her late mother's sister (Minnie's aunt) had remained vigilant over the child during her long hospitalization, often surprising her with gifts and distractions. As a result, compared to other children sampled, Minnie's documented inventory of possessions was quite lengthy:

> 2 jars of cream, 1 mirror, 1 hand lotion, 1 bottle perfume, 2 writing pads, 1 glass mug, 1 jar, 1 soap box, 1 jack in box, 1 doll bed, 4 dolls, 1 spoon, 1 magnifying glass, 1 box containing train and dishes, 1 box doll dishes, 2 boxes paints, 1 toy candy store, 1 doll basket, 1 bottle bath salts, 1 bible, 2 strings beads, 2 balls wool, 1 bundle cards, 1 pr scissors, 6 story books, 1 puzzle game, 1 comb set, 1 pipette, 1 bottle oil, 1 tooth brush in case, 1 box powder, 1 bead bag, 1 doll carriage, 1 glass cup, 1 ring, 1 bracelet, 1 purse containing 3 cents; clothing: 1 bed jacket, 1 bedroom slippers, 1 pr garters, 1 pr stockings, 1 laundry bag, 2 petticoats, 1 pr drawers, 5 prs bloomers, 3 dresses, 1 sweater, 1 pr shoes, 1 hat, 1 nightgown, 2 vests, 2 handkerchiefs, 1 kimona, 1 cushion.

On the basis of her inventory, Minnie seemed as interested in her dolls and crafts as she was in the perfumes, creams, powders, and other fascinations of a young girl growing up, a transition never fully completed because of her untimely death.

Inevitably, children at the sanatorium also experienced the loss, sometimes sudden and unexpected, of their friends and ward mates at the sanatorium. One woman who entered the Queen Mary Hospital as a child in the late 1920s remembered, decades later, the death of a fellow patient, Martha, whom she had befriended at the sanatorium. "There were four of us in this ward," she recalled, "and we were doing dolls, bed dolls. We used to make them out of crèpe paper with a Kewpie doll in the centre and we used to sell all these things to Eaton's." The four girls had been sitting on their beds, working on their dolls, when Martha, who had been suffering a bit of a cold, "gave a very bad cough and she died right there in front of us. It was just one of those very unfortunate things and we were all very, very sad."[98] Ex-patients of the Craig-y-nos sanatorium in Wales who were hospitalized as children also remembered the experience of death. Rose Pugh (Hunt) recalled, "The nurses used to say, 'Oh she died in her sleep,'" so Pugh (Hunt), who did not want to die, "would struggle to keep awake."[99] Children quickly learned the significance of waking up to find an "empty unmade bed" on their wards.[100]

Tuberculosis was such an unpredictable disease that outward symptoms sometimes did nothing to suggest the gravity of a child's condition. While some children, such as Martha, succumbed to tuberculosis and its complications quite suddenly, other children had more variable disease experiences, moving liminally between poor prognoses and improvement. Such was the case for ten-year-old Suzanne, admitted to the Toronto sanatorium in March 1918, and by July in serious condition and "failing rapidly." Suzanne had "rallied," actually improving between August and October, but she ultimately died in early November 1918, her struggle for health fatally compromised by Spanish influenza. Even though the sanatorium had instituted more restrictive rules on visiting in 1918 and 1919, during the Spanish influenza pandemic, the regular movement of staff between home and sanatorium and the ongoing admission of tuberculosis patients during the crisis represented serious vulnerabilities for the ingress of the influenza virus. Upon being informed of her daughter's death, Suzanne's stepmother wrote to Miss Dickson in late November 1918, clearly in shock over her sudden passing. "I am writing to thank you also the doctors and Nurses of the Queen Mary Hospital for the kindness and attention you extended our little girl Suzanne during her time at the Hospital," she wrote, "but we do wish you had let us know that she was worse," because "we feel dreadfully bad to think no one of us were with her at the last." She was regretful, "not even know[ing] she had got the 'Flu,'" and she had questions: "Did she ask for any one or any thing? Was any one with her when she passed away? Did she suffer at all?" The letter was referred to Dobbie and, upon enquiring on the conditions surrounding Suzanne's death from the ward nurses who had looked after her, he replied to Suzanne's stepmother, understanding her grief that she had not been with her daughter "at the end." Dobbie explained the suddenness of Suzanne's death, her influenza symptoms not "unusual," but ultimately, "her strength … was not sufficient to withstand the additional trouble and her heart failed very rapidly." Furthermore, Dobbie reassured her that "one of the nurses was with her constantly and at the end. She did not appear to suffer and she passed away very quietly. On many occasions she spoke of her Mother but she did not make any requests. During her long illness the nurses endeavoured to do all they could to make her comfortable and happy and I feel that their efforts were very successful." Choosing his words with care, Dobbie had attempted to spare Suzanne's stepmother any further grief for not being there to comfort her daughter. According to the attending nurse's report submitted to Dobbie, it was clear that Suzanne, before of her death, "was asking for her mother."

Like Suzanne's mother, when four-year-old Rose was admitted to the sanatorium in July 1921, her mother held out hope for her young daughter's recovery. On 3 August, Rose's mother wrote an optimistic letter to Dobbie inquiring, "How is Rose getting along," and if there was anything she should provide for her daughter while she was in the sanatorium. "Is there any thing particular I can send her to eat," she asked, "as I don't want to send her stuff and she is not allowed to eat it. Like chocolates[,] oranges or things like that." She closed her letter, thankful to the sanatorium and the staff, "God Bless yous and help yous in your work," requesting, "kiss her for me." Despite her mother's hopefulness, Dobbie was in an unfortunate position, having to respond with a report that Rose's condition had declined quickly since her admission. By 15 August, Rose's health had deteriorated further and Dobbie was compelled to send an urgent telegram to her mother: "Rose much worse, ~~have no hope~~. Condition now very serious." The telegram that was sent out did not include the dire warning that Dobbie had ultimately chosen to omit from the draft. Rose's mother received the news and immediately wrote back to Dobbie on the same day, "Telegram received. Needless to say sorry for such a report. Let me know further how she is as it is very inconvenient for me to come down unless really necessary. As two have the whooping cough and I cannot leave baby very handy as he is nursing and he has it also. Hope news will be better next time." Understandably, Rose's mother was in a most difficult position, trying to manage whooping cough and three sick children at home. It would not be easy for her to put all of this aside and rush to the sanatorium. Unfortunately, Rose died in the sanatorium on the day of this exchange. It is hard to imagine the grief and guilt that Rose's mother would experience in the aftermath. Staff worked hard in their attempts to reunite parents and their dying children, but death could come unexpectedly and quickly. As it was, Rose's mother would be reunited with her daughter only after her death, as her body was shipped home to her mother the day after she died for funeral preparations and burial. Undoubtedly, any parents who were considering admitting their children to the sanatorium were well aware of these stories of unexpected deaths. Despite the hope the sanatorium offered, the choice to hospitalize children could come with deep anxiety.

Preparing to Leave: Indications for Discharge

Despite the stories of passings and losses, most of the children sampled did well at the sanatorium and would be discharged. Physicians looked to a number of physiological cues to help determine when a child was best suited for release, including the absence of fever, a transition to bacterium-negative sputum (or, better yet, the absence of sputum altogether), and weight gain. Since tuberculosis infection was forever, discharged patients were advised to report periodically for follow-ups at chest clinics where X-rays could be taken at regular intervals to monitor any changes in health status. Clinics were available throughout Ontario, though remote areas would be served only by the periodic visits of travelling clinics, if at all. Large urban areas often benefitted from year-round, fixed clinics, such as the Gage Institute in Toronto. Continued vigilance over tuberculosis was recommended, even among children who were discharged with latent tuberculosis, because of the lingering life-long possibility of disease reactivation.

Some children left the sanatorium before achieving the physiological landmarks of improvement typically associated with discharges, much to Dobbie's disappointment, but such was the reality of a voluntary institution. Douglas, for example, was a fifteen-year old schoolboy living with his family on the outskirts of Toronto when he was admitted to the sanatorium in October 1935. On the day before his admission Douglas had expectorated a whole cupful of blood, a rather alarming indication of the advanced and serious nature of his disease. Douglas was started on artificial pneumothorax treatment in the month that he was admitted. By March 1936, however, Douglas's homesickness became overwhelming and his father wrote to Dobbie asking if his son might return home for the summer. He promised to ensure his son's commitment to rest and to pitch a tent in the backyard so that Douglas could sleep outside and get as much fresh air as possible. Dobbie was not convinced that a summer leave was in Douglas's best interest because his resistance to the disease had been so poor, as evidenced by the fact that, despite all the regular sanatorium measures, his disease had continued to progress since his admission. Leaving the hospital for a visit at home would also place Douglas's regular schedule of pneumothorax refills in jeopardy. All of this was considered in light of the fact that he still had some cough and was producing about half a box of sputum per day. Douglas's father persisted, however, probably encouraged by his son's insistence, and Douglas was granted a weekend leave at home late in May.

By August, Douglas's father was once again writing Dobbie to see if his son might have a week's leave so that he could celebrate his birthday at home with his family. And, once again, Dobbie did not recommend a leave for Douglas since, he argued, "going out now would give him a set back, from which it would take some months to recover." Douglas had overcome his cough, but still produced four ounces (about eight tablespoons) of sputum per day; his artificial pneumothorax was retaining good compression and Dobbie did not want to risk all the progress that they were seeing in his case. Douglas's father persisted and, about a week later, wrote an apologetic letter to Dobbie indicating that he had decided to permanently discharge his son "owing to his leave being refused." He felt that Douglas had "worked himself up into such a state of mind that if I do not take him out he will walk out and make his way home the best way he can." Rather than "risk that or try and keep him there" in that "state of mind," Douglas's father felt it was time for Douglas to come home, weighing in that "trying to make him stay … against his will" was likely a greater "danger to his health" than attempting to do the "very best for him at home." The challenge, however, would be in continuing Douglas's regular artificial pneumothorax treatments, since

Douglas's father felt he would risk his job if he had to transport Douglas to the sanatorium during working hours, so he enquired about the possibility of evening or Sunday morning appointments. Dobbie wrote back to Douglas's father, disappointed with the decision, believing that Douglas should have been old enough "to regard medical advice more seriously." He informed Douglas's father that it would be possible to get the pneumothorax refills at the sanatorium, but that the only time for pneumothorax procedures was at 10:30 each weekday morning, without exception. For individuals who were not patients in the sanatorium, there was also a $2 charge for each treatment. Satisfied he could make it work, Douglas's father went ahead with the discharge, his son leaving the sanatorium only some ten months after he was admitted as an advanced and serious case. Perhaps surprising all involved, after his discharge Douglas did remain faithful to his refills, receiving 500 cc of air each time at the sanatorium clinic dependably every fourteen days until October 1937. True to his father's promise, Douglas had progressed well at his parents' house, leading a "sedentary" life with them, and an X-ray taken in 1937 failed to show any signs of active disease progression.

Like Douglas, there were many other children who found it difficult to settle into life at the sanatorium. Curtis, a ten-year old Indigenous child from southern Ontario, was admitted to the Queen Mary in January 1917. Over three years later, in March 1920, he was discharged from the hospital for reasons of "French leave," which was sanatorium vernacular for "ran away." A day after disappearing from the sanatorium, Curtis arrived back home at his parents' house. His father wrote to Dobbie immediately, on the day of Curtis's unexpected arrival, informing him "that my son Curtis arrived home this morning" and "sorry that he came away without letting you know." While Curtis's father had been surprised to find his son back home, he did not "think it would be wise now to send him back as he would probably not stay there again," so he suggested that Dobbie "give him leave of absence for an indefinite time." Curtis's father intended to report his son's discharge to his Indian agent, who would, he understood, make a report to the Indian Department in Ottawa. Despite his son's unexpected arrival back home, Curtis's father was "glad that he looks well" and thanked Dobbie "for the attention you have given him," only regretting that Curtis had run away from the sanatorium. Ultimately, Curtis's father "would [have liked] to have him stay there till he [was] discharged." Dobbie replied, "Sorry that he was so unwise to leave the institution the way that he did." Dobbie felt that Curtis's physical condition was sufficiently good that, with adequate care, rest, and nourishment, he would probably continue to do well at home. He admitted, "It is a little difficult to deal with a boy of his age in an institution of this kind. He is beginning to feel that he wants certain liberties which is not always possible for us to let him have." Curtis had been granted many leaves of absence during his time at the sanatorium, taking day trips to the Canadian National Exhibition in Toronto, going home for Christmas, and spending the summer of 1919 with his family. Even despite these allowances, however, Curtis had grown increasingly impatient with the routine of sanatorium life, and all appeared to agree that, given his conviction to leave, he would probably do best at home.

Not all parents, however, wanted their children discharged, perhaps recognizing that they may have been better off remaining at the sanatorium. As a case in point, when Lucy's mother learned that her daughter would be discharged in March 1931, she wrote to Dobbie to ask if she could get Lucy's hospitalization extended, the problem being that she was "handicapped in regards to sleeping accommodations." She was seeking an extension of Lucy's hospitalization over the summer months so that she could find a bigger home to adequately accommodate her daughter. "It is not that I do not want her at home," she explained, "but I do want to do the best thing possible for her health." Lucy's mother was ultimately concerned that if home conditions were not adequate, her daughter would suffer. As she understood, "some of the young ones seem to be going home only to have to return [to the sanatorium] soon again," and she was sure, "I do not want that to happen to her." Lucy, however, had been in the sanatorium for a number of years, admitted in March 1925, at ten years of age. She had been placed in the hospital by City Order (meaning the city of Toronto paid her hospitalization costs), and Dobbie doubted that the city would be willing to extend her stay any longer if, medically, she was found fit for discharge. All of the signs pointed to her readiness. Lucy did not have a temperature, cough, or sputum, she had gained over thirty pounds in weight, and her general condition was good. Despite her mother's insistence that she could not provide adequate accommodations for her now sixteen-year-old daughter, Lucy was discharged in April 1931.

When fourteen-year-old Daniel was being considered for early discharge in 1925 because of his persistent misconduct, his mother gently protested. Sickness and poverty rendered his family unable to provide the kind of care and nutrition that Daniel would need to maintain his resistance to tuberculosis. Daniel's mother provided a lengthy explanation of the family's difficult situation in a letter to Dobbie, "lest you should think we were merely trying to shift the worry and trouble of my dear little boy into your hands." Daniel's mother explained that he was the eldest of her seven living children, the eighth, a daughter, had been "born dead" during the influenza pandemic in 1918. Daniel's father, "normally healthy when married," had suffered pneumonia, congestion of the lungs, and tuberculosis for some years but, under treatment, "for the past three years has not grown worse." Daniel's father had a poor family history, and five of his eight siblings had died "after manhood and womanhood" of tuberculosis or anemia. "Being delicate," Daniel's father did not have "a large salary which prevents us securing many nourishing things to help our little ones to health," Daniel's mother explained. She, herself, had been quite ill since the recent birth of her last baby; without a doctor or nurse in attendance at the delivery she had taken "a chill from exposure and for five days I had such a high temperature and two hemorrhages that the doctor ordered me to the hospital and after two weeks in bed I am allowed up but am very weak and suffer from chills and night sweats which worry the doctor considerably." During her complicated post-partum recovery, her mother, Daniel's grandmother, came to help the family, but fell ill and had been sick in bed for two weeks with tonsillitis and a neck abscess, which would be opened by a doctor and drained. "As she is elderly and in poor health and refuses to go to the hospital," she explained, "I also have the care of her and will have for a few weeks yet." Understandably, "having all the housework, washing and cooking as well as the care of six little ones," in addition to her own mother, she felt, "I am in no condition to give Daniel the care and training, nor the nourishing food he has been receiving under your supervision, nor have we the money to secure the comforts he requires." Daniel's mother was desperate to prolong her son's stay at the sanatorium, and for good reason, as this family was clearly struggling. Daniel's mother had already seen her fair share of misery with a tuberculous and "delicate" husband, a tuberculous son, a stillborn infant, her own post-partum illness and debility, and an elderly, unwell mother, in addition to her six children at home. Given the hardships this family was facing, it is understandable why Daniel's mother felt his best prospects for recovery lay at the sanatorium, emphasizing to Dobbie in the letter that "at every visit he praises his doctor and nurse[,] seems so pleased with his food and care[,] and really seems to be improving in health and looks so much brighter and more contented."

In her desperation and scrambling to prevent his discharge, Daniel's mother reassured Dobbie that she would be writing to her son and that her husband had "talked very fiercely and seriously of the consequences of his disobedience" with him at his last visit. She asked if her son could be given another chance at the sanatorium. She freely admitted that Daniel could be hard to handle, recognizing that he had a "bad temper," and was devastated that he could not be brought under control. As she wrote to Dobbie, "You who are so clever and gifted and with such skill as to be in charge of so many doomed lives will surely, in this instance, realize how heart-broken and discouraged I am at the prospect of his only chance of attaining health being sacrificed through his own fault." From his mother's perspective, Daniel would have to find a way to reign in his wilful disobedience if he had any hopes of recovering from tuberculosis. Sympathetic to the family's situation, Dobbie had allowed Daniel to remain at the sanatorium for two additional months, though Daniel's discharge was eventually arranged because of his continuing "disobedience," "untruthfulness," and "destruction of hospital property."

The issue of home conditions arose in both Lucy's and Daniel's mothers' letters and was a matter that would receive greater attention. Sanatorium physicians believed that children returning to poor living conditions would have to be more robust than those who returned to better circumstances. The quality of nutrition, access to medical care, and ability to provide sundries such as clothing would all be considered, as well as the nature of the home environment. When seven-year-old Lester was admitted to the sanatorium in 1924, his father was already a patient in the adult wards. In March 1927, the clerk of the municipal council responsible for Lester's maintenance costs wrote to Dobbie asking how much longer he thought Lester would need to stay at the sanatorium. Dobbie responded that Lester had made great improvements while at the sanatorium and that his length of stay would really depend "on the conditions in which it will be necessary for him to live after he goes out." During Lester's hospitalization, his mother had relocated the family to Toronto, so Julia Stewart, one of the National Sanitarium Association's visiting nurses, was sent out in March 1927, to evaluate the family's Toronto residence and Lester's mother's ability to provide for him (and his three siblings at home). Stewart noted that Lester's mother rented a house for $45 per month, but, by taking in roomers, she was able to bring in $45.50 per month. The Mothers' Allowance Commission provided her with $45 per month, though the amount would be increased to $50 if Lester was discharged. Lester's eldest brother also contributed another $5 per week to the household through his earnings. The cost of coal was "a large item," but also gas and electricity, particularly when there were roomers in the home. Stewart noted, "Living space for family is limited," with Lester's mother and fourteen-year-old sister sharing the single bedroom. Lester's two brothers slept on a couch in the dining room. Lester would have to be accommodated with a cot in his mother's bedroom. Though short on sleeping space, Stewart noted that Lester's mother "is quite willing to have him home" if Dobbie considered "it advisable under these conditions." Other than the crowding, which was not uncommon in Toronto homes, conditions appeared acceptable and Lester was taken home by his elder sister a few weeks later in April 1927.

Outside of the city, inspections revealed variation in the character of family homes. Gilbert was admitted to the sanatorium in 1924, at the age of seven, from a family home in small-town Ontario. Gilbert had four siblings, and all of them, in addition to his parents, were alive. Gilbert's mother's tuberculin test had been positive for tuberculosis infection, although she did not appear to suffer active disease. When Gilbert was considered for discharge in 1927, an inspector from the Children's Aid Society evaluated the living conditions to which Gilbert and his brother, also at the sanatorium, would return. The inspector arrived at the family's six-room, wood frame bungalow, unannounced, one day in May 1927. He noted the home to be "of good appearance," "spotlessly clean," and "well furnished," with "screen doors and windows." Particular attention was directed at the bedrooms, in which "each boy will sleep separate." Each bedroom had a bed equipped with "a comfortable spring mattress, and clean linen, and nice bed spread," and a washstand and dresser. The bedrooms were of generous dimensions, measuring twelve feet by ten with ceilings eight feet high. Focusing on the home more generally, the inspector also noted that it was provided with "a good well" and a "vegetable garden," and was located close to both church and school on the banks of a river. Since the inspector's visit was unexpected, it was all the more impressive that "the appearance of the home" suggested Gilbert's mother was "a very capable housekeeper." The inspector recommended the return of the children to this home and was prepared to keep it "under supervision for a time to watch and advise the parents." Over time, the discharge protocol became more detailed, with parents or guardians asked to provide written answers to a questionnaire concerning the ability to provide transportation home, adequate room and board, clothing, and any necessary medical care. Increasing attention to aftercare was fuelled by an understanding that the weeks, months, or years that children spent at the sanatorium building resistance and improving their health to the point of discharge could easily be undone if proper care was not taken to ensure a suitable environment for them at home.

When it came to the subject of discharges, children who had immigrated to Canada experienced even more scrutiny. For some children, the prospect of discharge from the sanatorium came associated with possible deportation from Canada. In the early twentieth century, any immigrants struck down by tuberculosis and becoming public charges in hospitals or sanatoria within five years of their arrival faced mandatory deportation back to their countries of origin. For example, fourteen-year-old Alma had sailed from Scotland to Canada in 1913. The intention was that Alma would take up residence with her father in Toronto because her mother, "an invalid," had been hospitalized in Edinburgh (possibly with tuberculosis). According to the letter that Alma's father wrote to Dobbie, his daughter had become quite ill during her transatlantic journey, "during her passage across which was a very bad one she became very sick and ill and unable to eat and when she arrived in Toronto I found her so ill that I call in a Doctor who says she has a touch of Tuberculosis and order her to your institution." Trusting that Dobbie would "do all in your power for my dear daughter," Alma's father reassured him, "if you will advise me to do any thing for her good I will gladly do." Facing tuberculosis, it is clear that Alma's father understood the seriousness of the situation at hand, writing Dobbie, "Doctor it would be an awful thing to loose such a sweet little girl at her age and she is the only one we have. Trusting God will give you power to restore my daughter to health." It appears that the Toronto physician who had made the original diagnosis had underestimated Alma's condition, suggesting to her father that she had a "touch of Tuberculosis." Alma would almost certainly have been ordered for deportation, but as it was her tuberculosis was so far advanced that she died only three months after her admission to the sanatorium. The responsibility fell to sanatorium administrators, such as Dr Dobbie, to report any cases of recent immigrants entering the sanatorium as indigent patients. At the Toronto sanatorium, even when deportation orders were drafted for patients by the federal government, only Dobbie had the power to approve their removal from the sanatorium, and only at a time when their discharge would jeopardize neither their own health, nor the health of others. Piles of paperwork ensued, with immigration officials writing to Dobbie with repeated enquiries to determine if patients scheduled for deportation were yet "fit to travel." Adult patients likely understood the situation and undoubtedly also knew when they were nearing a good physical condition for discharge. As a result, there were occasions when such patients simply up and left the sanatorium, providing no contact information or forwarding addresses, just vanishing into the expanse of Canada. Other acutely ill patients, such as Alma, died in the sanatorium, forever evading their deportation orders. For some patients, however, deportation actually did become a reality.

A Newfoundland family's deportation in the early 1920s attests to the difficulties and anxieties surrounding the process. Both husband and wife had been patients at the National Sanitarium Association's Muskoka sanatorium, while their two-year-old son, Joseph, had been separated from them and admitted to the Davies Cottage at the Toronto sanatorium. As Joseph's father's letter to Miss Dickson, lady superintendent, suggests, they were becoming increasingly anxious about Joseph's health. "When you have a moment to spare," he wrote, "I would be deeply grateful to you if you would drop me a line and tell me how my little baby boy is progressing in health and general condition." During their time in Ontario, another son had died in a Toronto hospital, and Joseph's father was frustrated because they could not "get any satisfaction as to what was the cause of his death," nor did they even know where he had been buried. "This life is so full of hard luck and misfortunes," he explained, "that I am tempted to make the best of it and go back to work again." In the meantime, having been "taken" from the Muskoka sanatorium and "detained" under poor conditions at a facility in Quebec, they awaited their deportation, held up because of a delay in Joseph's discharge from the Toronto sanatorium. They had already spent four weeks at the immigration detention centre and were anxious to return to Newfoundland. Joseph's father wrote to Dobbie, "in the interest of humanity," to determine how long it would be until his son was fit to join them. "You know Dr Dobbie," he wrote, "this place where we are at present located is by no means suited to our condition for the food and accommodation is of the poorest description." He did not consider it "just" to be kept there "any longer than absolutely necessary." Joseph's discharge was delayed by almost a month because, in addition to tuberculosis, he had contracted scarlet fever and whooping cough and placed under a mandatory six-week quarantine. Once this period had passed, Joseph was reunited with his parents in Quebec. From there, the family would continue back to Newfoundland.

There was diversity among the hospitalized children who had migrated, some arriving in Canada with their families, others travelling alone or in the care of an agency. One of the largest agencies involved in bringing children to Canada was Dr Barnardo's Homes, which ran a shelter on Jarvis Street in Toronto. According to Jacalyn Duffin, in response to a growing number of orphans in London, England, Thomas Barnardo had initiated a scheme in 1868 "to export these children to families or labour situations in Canada."[101] Duffin estimates that by 1925, when the practice was abolished, some thirty thousand "Barnardo boys" and "Barnardo girls" had entered Canada. Eleanor, eleven years of age, was one such girl. Eleanor was admitted to the sanatorium from the Jarvis Street shelter in July 1923. In a letter to the shelter's physician, Dobbie indicated that upon examination Eleanor was found to suffer from "extensive involvement of the whole of the left lung and scattered areas throughout the right." Even despite the "extensive lesion," Eleanor was found to be in "very good condition but has frequent cough." At the time of Eleanor's admission, the Toronto shelter superintendents had been away in England. Upon their return, the lady superintendent of Dr Bernardo's Homes in Toronto wrote to Dobbie in July 1923, "distressed to learn that our little girl Eleanor has developed consumption and that it has been necessary to place her in hospital." Agency administrators were well aware of the implications of tuberculosis diagnoses among the children they brought over and were already prepared to make the arrangements for her return voyage "to the Old Country" within two weeks, so long as Dobbie approved her discharge, without discussion or protest. Eleanor left the sanatorium in August 1923, stopping first at the shelter in Toronto, before boarding a ship with two Barnardo staff members for her ultimate return to England.

Because of the problems associated with diagnosing tuberculosis, there was ample room for contentious deportations. Thirteen-year-old Richard, born in England and another Barnardo child, entered the Toronto sanatorium in late April 1924. Just over two months later, in July 1924, he was discharged and deported back to England. Less than a month after Richard left Canada, Dobbie received a letter from a clearly displeased medical director of Dr Barnardo's Homes in London, suggesting, "You may perhaps remember that one of our boys, Richard by name, was by you recommended for deportation as suffering from consumption, on the strength probably of an X-ray examination." The medical director noted that upon his return to England he was admitted to hospital and, upon examination, he was found to have "no cough, the chest is normal, and he is quite well, with normal temperature and pulse." Discerning no evidence of active tuberculosis, the director continued, "We sent him to the London Hospital to be X-rayed, and the report there was that there was nothing wrong with the lung tissue, but there was a little prominence of the hilum – shadows and a few glands on each side, with a little peribronchial fibrosis." The results of the examination suggested "no evidence of lung infection other than the slight hilum trouble which had apparently subsided by the time he arrived home." The director then made it personal, writing Dobbie, "I thought you would be interested to hear this, as it was on the strength of your report that he was deported. P.S. He is clamouring to be allowed to go out [to Canada] again, but this of course is impossible." The postscript in the director's letter is the clincher, undoubtedly intended to weigh on Dobbie's conscience for the role he had played in Richard's deportation. Despite his fervent wishes, Richard's tuberculosis diagnosis ensured he would never return to live in Canada. The description of the boy's chest X-ray in London strongly suggests that he had probably experienced primary tuberculosis disease in Canada (he may even have been first infected in Canada), evident in the attention to the hilar lymph nodes in his lungs. The director's account suggests that Richard's primary disease had gone latent by the time of his return to London. Dobbie, however, was well aware of Richard's condition, recognizing that even if his tuberculous infection had gone latent, it still represented a chronic, lifelong infection vulnerable to reactivation and that Richard was unlikely "ever to become normal in health and strength and earning capacity." On the basis of that realization, in local follow-up correspondence, Dobbie argued that deporting Richard seemed to be "the desirable thing to do." From Richard's story, it appears that even the possibility of future tuberculosis disease carried enough weight to influence orders of deportation. If the intention of the five-year rule was to exclude immigrants who came to Canada ill and unable to productively contribute to society, then there was a serious flaw, since healthy, uninfected children who arrived in Canada would have to continue to evade tuberculosis infection for a solid five years, a highly unlikely reality given the extent of infection circulating in the country. The reality is that many immigrant children would likely be infected in Canada, but if they were not diagnosed and they were not admitted to a sanatorium, and if they were fortunate enough to experience primary infection as a fairly benign and overlooked event, then they would not attract the attention of the deportation authorities.

Conclusion

In the age of endemic TB, public health and medicine encouraged a mindful attentiveness to the body, and to be watchful for early symptoms of tuberculosis, both in seeming wellness and in apparent illness. The real and tangible threat of tuberculosis, weighty in its presence, cultured a particular vigilance over the body, as every cough, fever, night sweat, and pound of weight lost suggested tuberculosis, especially among those who knew, via tuberculin testing, that their bodies already harboured tuberculosis bacteria. Even among those whose tuberculosis had gone latent, a bodily self-consciousness could linger because of the very real possibility of reactivation. Former sanatorium patients were encouraged to be "watchful" over their bodies. If illness threatened, the Canadian Tuberculosis Association advised, "Do not lightly blame other diseases, such as influenza or 'cold,' for symptoms and signs which may be caused by tuberculous relapse. Do not neglect 'pink' streaks in your sputum and imagine they come from your gums or throat. Report them to your doctor and let him decide where the blood came from."[102] Ultimately, it seems likely that the more people knew about tuberculosis and how common the infection was in early twentieth-century Canada, the more they cultured the tuberculosis consciousness. This new awareness likely helped to drive patients to physicians and to the sanatorium in larger numbers, seeking assurance, relief, and treatment. In its endemic age, the effects of tuberculosis were visible, from the long-term wasting effects on bodies to the decimation of families and orphaned children.

From the time of tuberculin surveys to the rise of antibiotic treatments in the 1940s, the sanatorium offered the greatest hope in overcoming tuberculosis. In Canada, the Toronto sanatorium was a modern and dynamic institution, scientific in its grounding, and, as a result, treatments changed as more was learned of tuberculosis and its effects on the body. Most parents who sent their children to the sanatorium did so for the promise of a firm diagnosis, a realistic prognosis, and access to the most modern of tuberculosis treatments. Cure was not necessarily an inherent expectation at a time when much was understood about bacteria and infectious diseases, yet only a handful of diseases could be reliably controlled, prevented, or cured; those few cures and palliatives were enough, however, to conjure patient respect for the modern doctor's science, skills, and understanding of the body, galvanizing a wider acceptance of emerging "medical authority."[103] While patients and their families placed faith in the early sanatorium treatment models of rest, fresh air, and diet, undoubtedly, as the sanatorium era progressed, even more assurance would be found in the emerging, active, and invasive surgical treatments for tuberculosis that provided such clear evidence that "something was being done." Though patients did die at the Toronto sanatorium, the institution was never intended to specialize exclusively in care of the dying. People were confident that modern medicine would find a cure for tuberculosis and, if that were to happen, places like the Toronto sanatorium would be the most likely sites of those miracles. As a result, there was strong support for the sanatorium, and people invested in it as a place of hope and healing.

CHAPTER 4

Tuberculosis and the Body: Biology, Beliefs, and Experience

Now we know that once the primary complex has been allowed to develop, as manifested by a positive tuberculin reaction, there is no treatment of any avail; that is, the condition is beyond recall. Immunity does not develop sufficiently to destroy the tubercle bacilli.[1]

~ J. Arthur Myers et al.

More than a little ominous sounding, as American physician Arthur Myers warned in 1938, before antibiotics, there was a permanence associated with tuberculosis infection that, for most individuals, would last a lifetime. In chronic infections such as tuberculosis the aptitudes and vulnerabilities of pathogen and immune system may, together, influence how those infections are experienced by the body. Shaped by variable biologies, the tuberculosis experience could vary greatly among and between individuals. As a result, and as a starting point in exploring those variable tuberculosis experiences, it is important to understand something of the biological underpinnings of tuberculosis and the body – why, in the years before antibiotics, tuberculosis infection could be latent or active, and why tuberculosis disease could be acute, but more often chronic, in its manifestation. Only then is it possible to fully understand why some sufferers experienced mild versus devastating disease, and why some fell victim to rampant, "galloping" tuberculosis disease and death, while others were tormented by a slow, chronic, wasting disease. Biologies may influence how tuberculosis bacteria exist in the body, sometimes dormant and sometimes active, depending on the power of host resistance and the particular infecting strains of tuberculosis bacteria. All of the children sampled in this study may have shared in the experience of infection, but, from that common point, their stories could be quite different.

At times, this chapter moves outside the sanatorium, into family and community spaces, to consider the question of infection, or the manner in which children came to be infected with tuberculosis. Infection and primary tuberculosis disease were common occurrences in childhood, but epidemiological studies suggest a more general tendency towards resistance to tuberculosis bacteria. While most infected children could contain latent tuberculosis bacteria in their bodies, it has been estimated that between 5 and 10 per cent of those with latent infection would go on to develop active tuberculosis disease at any point (or even at various points) in their lifetime, the risk varying by factors such as age and health status.[2] Active disease emerging after a period of latency was known as "reactivation disease." The focus on biologies does not suggest, however, that social contexts will be forgotten. While human immune defences are built on biological foundations, laid in place by genes inherited from biological parents and their links to deeper evolutionary histories of interactions with tuberculosis bacteria, immune function is ultimately entrenched in bodies that occupy social worlds. Those experiencing social inequalities, living in poverty or under oppression, may encounter the greatest challenges in expressing strong, resilient immune function against pathogens such as *Mycobacterium tuberculosis*.[3] As one physician argued, many Canadian children in the sanatorium era had low resistance to tuberculosis, their bodies, because of poverty, denied a healthful standard of living and therefore offering a suitable "soil" for the "growth" of tuberculosis bacteria. "Too often," Cassidy argued, "their early lives are passed in crowded, unclean, damp houses; their food is insufficient or unnutritious; their surroundings are most hurtful and anti-hygienic, so that it is no wonder if they become rachitic, scrofulous, anemic ... Their emaciated and weakened bodies, wanting in proper vitality, form a favorable and fruitful soil for the propagation of the dreaded bacillus, of which they ultimately become the victims."[4] Given the complexities of tuberculosis infection, the sanatorium played two key roles: to assist children with primary disease to build up their resistance, contain TB bacteria, and coax the disease into a latent state, and to actively support children experiencing primary progressive disease or reactivation disease in managing their symptoms and slowing or preventing further disease progression. Neither was easy, given the fact that early- to mid-sanatorium-era patients would not benefit from the effective antibiotic treatments, such as streptomycin, which would come later.

Encouraged by the potential of natural immunity to tuberculosis, staff at the Toronto sanatorium aimed to build resistance among the children admitted, but differences ultimately manifested. This chapter explores the diversity of disease states (primary versus reactivation disease) observed among the children admitted to the Toronto sanatorium, exploring the different ways in which tuberculosis affected their bodies (the sites of infection and disease) and compromised their well-being, and the prevailing beliefs concerning tuberculosis risks that framed lay perceptions of how children came to be infected. The chapter also addresses the medical difficulties in establishing a tuberculosis diagnosis, often the result of confusion created by the complexities of the larger disease environment, and the difficulties encountered in building resistance, given the impact of social circumstances and evolutionary legacies in shaping individual- and population-level differences in bodily resistance and susceptibility. The chapter concludes by considering the lingering impact of chronic infection, the lived experience of that biological permanence emphasized by Myers (in the introductory quote), as interpreted by those experiencing tuberculosis, and their families and communities.

Primary Tuberculosis

Despite attempts to protect children against tuberculosis infection, the disease was common and rife, and, as outlined in chapter 3, a rising tuberculosis consciousness was fuelled by the belief that infection in youth was inescapable. Not all tuberculosis exposures led automatically to infection, however, particularly, as Kline and Lorin note, if inhaled droplet nuclei fell on the ciliated epithelium of the upper respiratory tract, where tuberculosis bacteria could be swept away before being given the opportunity to colonize and multiply.[5] If, however, inhaled droplet nuclei were drawn deeper into the airway, beyond the ciliated epithelium, and into the bronchioles or alveoli of the lungs, then a successful infection became more likely.[6] According to Jackson and McLeod, the body initially offers no immune response, and TB bacteria are able to multiply at a rate of one division every eighteen to twenty-four hours.[7] As intracellular pathogens, tuberculosis bacteria trigger the immune cells involved in cell-mediated immunity (also known as Th1, or T helper 1, type immunity), which includes the important work of macrophages and lysosomes (the alternative is humoral or Th2 immunity and the work of antibodies).[8] Macrophages are phagocytes, cells that seek out and swallow up tuberculosis bacteria in an attempt to prevent their dissemination in the body. However, tuberculosis bacteria have adapted to this type of containment and can remain viable, even multiplying inside the macrophages that consume them.[9] Classic research by Armstrong and Hart, published in 1971, examined two important steps in cell-mediated immunity, first, when macrophages consume tuberculosis bacteria and trap them within phagosomes (membrane-bound vesicles within the macrophages), and second, the subsequent fusion of phagosomes with organelles known as lysosomes.[10] Lysosomes work cooperatively to deliver enzymes to the phagosome in order to digest engulfed pathogens and complete the steps required to successfully manage bacterial infection. Through their experiments, Armstrong and Hart observed that phagosomes containing live and viable TB bacteria did not fuse with lysosomes. As a result, despite intended defences, macrophages become host and home to tuberculosis bacteria. When lysosome fusion fails, macrophages may follow an alternate or secondary line of defence, joining with other immune cells (e.g., lymphocytes) to form solid-walled granulomas to capture and contain TB bacteria. The granulomas fibrose and then calcify, limiting tuberculosis bacteria to the confines of the granuloma. This approach may be less effective from a long-term perspective, since anything disrupting the integrity of the prison-like granuloma would free live, viable tuberculosis bacteria from the granuloma. The body resorts to this secondary strategy to contain TB bacteria, but it cannot kill them by this means. The live bacteria held within the granulomas may become the source of endogenous reactivation (reactivation disease), a concept explored in the next section, should the granulomas fail to keep them contained.

In the body, the location of pathological changes and the nature of the immune response vary, depending on the route of infection. If tuberculosis bacteria are inhaled, the lung tissue (or parenchyma) may be home to the initial site of infection (known as the "Ghon focus"). Because the lungs are supplied with a complex network of vessels from both the blood supply and lymphatic systems, they are ultimately linked with other organs and tissues of the body through these systems. It is via these linkages, in what is known as "lymphohematogenous" (*lympho* = lymphatic; *hemato* = blood) dissemination, that tuberculosis bacteria are able to migrate from the lungs to other organs and tissues, such as the regional lymph nodes in primary disease, or perhaps the brain, the kidneys, and bones and joints in primary progressive and reactivation disease.[11]

Lymph nodes serve as the sentinels of tuberculosis infection, becoming swollen and enlarged as the immune system detects and engages with tuberculosis bacteria that have entered the body. Enlarged regional lymph nodes became the hallmark of primary infection and disease in children historically,[12] but the response was non-specific, since lymph nodes can enlarge for a variety of reasons. Because of the lymph node response, primary tuberculosis was also known commonly as "glandular tuberculosis" (lymph nodes being glands). The seeding of regional lymph nodes with tuberculosis bacteria typically takes place during the two- to ten-week period of incubation after infection as they travel, contained in macrophages, the lymphatic system.[13] In respiratory infection, tuberculosis bacteria may travel from the original site of infection in the lungs (the Ghon focus) into the lymphatic system and to local lymph nodes. Children with primary tuberculosis typically experienced hilar, mediastinal, or cervical lymphadenopathy (swollen or enlarged lymph nodes).[14] When the primary focus of infection is established via the respiratory route, the hilar (in the hilar region of the lungs) and mediastinal (associated with the esophagus and trachea) lymph nodes are commonly affected, often with little or no involvement of the lung parenchyma beyond the Ghon focus, the original site of infection.[15] If the focus of primary infection is established in the upper respiratory tract, then cervical lymph nodes in the neck can become swollen in primary disease;[16] alternatively, cervical lymph nodes may also swell following a secondary hematogenous or lymphatic dissemination from the lungs.[17] If tuberculosis bacteria are consumed by mouth, they may seed the cervical lymph nodes or a number of different organs or tissues along the gastrointestinal tract. Jadvar and colleagues describe presentations of tuberculous forms of peritonitis (TB of the peritoneum, a membrane that lines the abdominal and pelvic cavities), lymphadenitis of the abdominal lymph nodes (including the mesenteric, omental, and peripancreatic lymph nodes), gastritis and duodenitis, enteritis, appendicitis, and ileocecal, colonic, hepatosplenic, and pancreatic tuberculosis.[18]

Primary disease of the lymph nodes does not produce the classic symptoms of pulmonary tuberculosis (such as cough and haemoptysis, the spitting or coughing up of blood or blood-streaked sputum). Instead, many children with uncomplicated primary tuberculosis disease affecting their lymph nodes often presented in a "below par" state, "not well and yet not really ill."[19] Primary disease was most often self-limited, the body's immune response guiding the formation of granulomas to contain the tuberculosis bacteria, the granulomas then consolidating through fibrosis and calcification.[20] As Kline and Lorin note, as consolidation, fibrosis, and calcification proceed at the localized site of the Ghon focus in the lungs, "lymphohematogenous spread stops, and regional lymph nodes stabilize," while TB bacteria that had "been seeded during early lymphohematogenous spread either are destroyed or remain dormant, alive but controlled."[21] The body's tendency to resolve the first interaction with tuberculosis bacteria contributed to the perception of "childhood tuberculosis" as a relatively minor illness, more concerning as a foreshadower of reactivation disease that might come later in life.

While primary disease may have typically been a minor, self-limiting disease for many children, for other children primary lymph node involvement could become complicated and progressive, particularly if lymph nodes became caseous ("cheeselike") and necrotic. According to a 1923 article published by Isaac Erb, then a pathologist at Toronto's Hospital for Sick Children, caseating mediastinal lymph nodes could erode to the extent that they ruptured into adjacent blood vessels, the thoracic duct, or a bronchus, causing complications of tuberculous meningitis, miliary tuberculosis, or, in the case of erosion into the bronchus, pneumonia.[22] Kline and Lorin note that in a small number of children the complications of primary progressive disease develop, particularly in malnourished children, children less than three years of age, or immunosuppressed children; progressive disease can lead to the "overt clinical manifestations" of tuberculosis.[23]

Among infected children who resolved primary infection and moved into a state of latent infection, there was always a risk in future that calcified granulomas could break down and release viable TB bacteria. This is known as "endogenous reactivation," as the bacteria already contained within the body are released, erupting into active infection all over again. With respect to primary disease, the role of the sanatorium was to build up resistance, coax the infection into a latent state and prevent primary progressive disease, and build resistance to prevent future disease reactivation through the best possible resolution of the primary disease. While the sanatorium provided regimen and therapeutics, in the absence of antibiotics it was ultimately the children's own immune function that would ensure recovery from tuberculosis disease.

Virgil, a fifteen-year old Indigenous child, was admitted to the sanatorium in June 1938, possibly tuberculous, though this was difficult to confirm, because Virgil was also suffering the more immediate effects of bronchopneumonia. Virgil had developed a "cold" in April 1938, at which time he was kept home from school at the request of an anxious teacher concerned about the health of the other students in Virgil's classroom. With tuberculosis suspected, a number of chest X-rays were undertaken, and on the basis of pathological findings he was admitted to the sanatorium. Virgil's clinical notes suggest that his condition had improved in his first three months of bedrest at the sanatorium: "The diagnosis was broncho-pneumonia of the base of the left lung; etiology was undetermined. At the time of admission the right hilum was heavy and there were a number of heavy, patchy markings in a triangular area running downwards from the left hilum to the diaphragm ... After three months of bed rest, the right hilum had cleared considerably and there was no vestige of the lesion previously seen at the left base. Temperature remained normal except during one or two colds." Virgil presented a classical picture of "hilar tuberculosis," or tuberculosis of the hilar lymph nodes. Dobbie explained the hilar involvement in a letter to Virgil's mother as "tuberculosis of the glands at the root of the lungs." Both the left and right lungs have a "hilum," a wedge-shaped area located centrally in each lung and home to the hilar lymph nodes. The hilum is a dynamic location, because this is where "the bronchus, blood-vessels, nerves and lymphatics enter or leave" the lungs.[24] Virgil's tuberculin skin test was strongly positive, convincing evidence of his tuberculosis infection, but laboratory cultures of his sputum samples always remained negative for tuberculosis bacteria. This finding was typical of primary disease, however, since primary disease did not produce the type of destructive lung cavities that teemed with tuberculosis bacteria. It is for this reason that children with primary disease were typically not capable of infecting others.

Cervical adenitis (also known as "scrofula"[25]) involves either the cervical or supraclavicular lymph nodes, which become inflamed by bacterial infection.[26] One woman who was at the Queen Mary Hospital as a child in the late 1920s remembered that a little girl whom she had befriended suffered greatly because of the swollen lymph nodes in her neck. She recalled that her friend's glands "hurt her all the time," and, in pain, "she would roll her head back and forth" on her pillow.[27] Enlarged cervical lymph nodes were a vastly non-specific sign of tuberculosis, however, and could also be triggered by conditions as diverse as diseased teeth, diseased tonsils, acute upper respiratory tract infections, Hodgkin's disease, and syphilis.[28] While TB-related cervical lymph node inflammation did not require any particular treatments (because primary disease typically ran a self-limited course), suppurating (oozing or discharging pus) lymph nodes could be treated with heliotherapy (exposure to the sun or ultraviolet light) and X-ray therapy (now commonly referred to as "radiation therapy" when used in the treatment of cancers).[29] Physicians were anxious about actively incising and draining, or in any way tampering with abscessed and suppurating lymph nodes because of fears that the wound would be opportunistically colonized by other bacteria, particularly staphylococcus or streptococcus bacteria, and a dangerous septic sinus would then have to be dealt with.[30]

As tuberculosis rates declined in Ontario, the disease gradually lost its widespread, endemic dissemination, particularly after the introduction of antibiotic treatments. This meant that children were less likely to encounter tuberculosis bacteria, and, as a result, the average ages at which children were first infected, if at all, began to rise. Oliver, for example, was seventeen years old when he was admitted in 1947 with signs of primary disease. He first became aware of a tender swelling on the right side of his neck in January 1947. In May 1947 the admitting physician noted Oliver's swollen cervical lymph nodes. Oliver's initial chest X-ray appeared to be clear of any tuberculosis-related pathologies, indicating that his lungs were not affected. In July, it was documented that a small sinus had developed in the area of Oliver's lymph node and discharged a small amount of pus. A sample of the pus was collected and laboratory analysis confirmed the presence of tuberculosis bacteria. A subsequent chest X-ray revealed the appearance of a "suspicious area" in the apex of Oliver's left lung. The last X-ray taken before Oliver's discharge in 1949 showed an improvement in his chest condition and the beginning of calcification in the area of his cervical lymph nodes, now swollen on both sides of his neck. Marais and colleagues' review of the pre-antibiotic tuberculosis literature suggests that the granulomas marking the sites of primary disease would typically calcify anywhere from one to three years after primary infection.[31] By the time calcification appeared, the danger of progressive disease was believed to have passed, though subsequent breakdown of the calcified granuloma and reactivation could occur at any point later in life.[32] When Oliver was discharged in 1949, however, his primary disease was determined to be soundly latent.

Secondary Tuberculosis: Reactivation Disease

Endogenous reactivation tuberculosis occurs when an earlier primary infection gone latent resurges into active disease. If the latent period is short, it can be difficult to make sharp distinctions between progressive primary disease, or a continuation of the disease process from the time of primary infection, and reactivation disease.[33] Among the children sampled, it was often older children, particularly adolescents, who were admitted with reactivation tuberculosis. Reactivation can be linked to changes in immune function and an inability to continue to contain viable tuberculosis bacteria lingering in the body. Reactivation risks were embedded in the realities of early twentieth-century life, including the physiological challenges of other infectious and non-infectious diseases, poor nutrition, and hard living and working conditions, stressors typically borne by the poor and working class in Ontario, but really anyone was vulnerable.

When Ruby, a seventeen-year-old office clerk, was admitted to the sanatorium in February 1948, she had all the symptoms characteristic of reactivation tuberculosis, including lung cavitation, weight loss, and a sputum-raising cough. Ruby's physician documented the effects of her active tuberculous disease on the basis of her chronology of examinations and chest X-rays:

> In November, 1947, Ruby suffered an attack of flu, subsequently had a mild persistent cough, without sputum. January 5, 1948 pain on her right side, mid-axillary line, below the 9th rib on getting up in the morning which prevented her from taking a deep breath but subsided by noon. She saw her doctor who said it was muscular but put her to bed for 2 weeks and referred her to the Gage [Institute] where routine [miniature] film was taken. February 2nd called back to the Gage for repeat full sized film and tuberculin test was done which was strongly positive. On the 7th of February she was told she should come to sanatorium and has been in bed since at home. She was not working from the 1st to the 7th of February and stayed at home awaiting Gage report. Since October, 1947 she has lost 12 lbs. Present weight 120 lbs. She has been feeling feverish in the evenings. Considerable cough and sputum in January, yellow, one dram [about ¾ teaspoon] per day. She now has no sputum and very little cough. Since she has been in bed for the past 2 weeks her appetite has improved. She knows of no contact with tuberculosis.

It is perhaps no wonder that Ruby could not pinpoint her "contact with tuberculosis," since she was likely experiencing reactivation tuberculosis stemming from an undetected primary infection earlier in her life. At the time of her admission to the sanatorium, Ruby was diagnosed with active pulmonary tuberculosis. Despite the seemingly mild or inconsistent symptoms (her cough coming and going, for example), her disease was defined as far advanced, and chest X-rays revealed a large cavity in her right lung in the area of her third rib. Clinically, "the tuberculous cavity" is considered "the lethal lesion,"[34] and patients would often experience disconcerting symptoms associated with it: furious coughing, sputum production, and, perhaps the worst, raising blood from the site of tissue destruction in their lungs.

Variability in the expression of signs and symptoms and the skills of physicians to interpret them sometimes led to delayed diagnoses until the decidedly more unambiguous advanced stages of reactivation disease. Despite alarming symptoms, children or their families might still resist suggestions for sanatorium treatment and, even if convinced of the importance of treatment, the destructive effects of tuberculosis on their bodies could sometimes become too far advanced for any hope of effective resistance building. When fourteen-year old Alec was examined at a northern Ontario chest clinic in 1934, he was found to be tuberculous. The child's family history was negative for tuberculosis and there was no suspected contact with outside cases. Alec's medical history indicated that he had suffered pleurisy with effusion affecting his left lung back in 1929. Pleurisy involves an inflammation of the pleura, the membrane that envelopes the lungs and lines the walls of the thoracic cavity.[35] "With effusion" means that the inflammation is accompanied by fluid accumulation in the intrapleural space between the lungs and the outer wall of the chest cavity. On the basis of their review of the pre-antibiotic literature, Marais and colleagues note that pleural effusions were likely to occur in children over five years of age approximately three to seven months after a primary tuberculosis infection.[36] Alec's pleural effusion, therefore, may have suggested something about the timing of his initial primary disease, some years earlier in 1929. At the chest clinic the physician determined that Alec had been "fairly well" since his pleural effusion until about 1933, "when he developed a cough and noticed some fatigue. He spat up some blood at this time following which he spent four months in bed." He gained some weight on bedrest and his cough became less frequent. The physician's "general impression of patient," however, was only "fair." Now that he was suffering definitive reactivation disease, it was felt that Alec would need a long period of strict bedrest.

Because Alec was producing tuberculosis bacteria in his sputum (and was therefore infectious), hospitalization was strongly encouraged in order to protect the health of his siblings at home. It was also advised that Alec's entire family travel to a neighbouring town for tuberculin testing and chest X-rays while the mobile clinic was still in their area. Despite the strong consensus that Alec should be admitted to a sanatorium, he staunchly refused to leave home. In fact, he had held out for two more years until his condition worsened to such an extent that, at seventeen years of age, he came to accept the idea of hospitalization. He was admitted to the Toronto sanatorium in 1936. Unfortunately, his tuberculosis had become far advanced by that time, and Alec died at the sanatorium in January 1937, less than a year after he was admitted. It is impossible to know whether an earlier admittance, and the benefits of improved diet, rest, or perhaps any of the evolving surgical therapies, would have ultimately saved Alec.

When seventeen-year-old Felton was admitted to the sanatorium in December 1947, there had been no suspicions that he was tuberculous, he was simply picked up by a routine tuberculin skin testing clinic held at his Toronto school in October 1947; in the 1940s, as tuberculosis rates continued to decline, tuberculin results became more meaningful in locating the decreasing body of people who were infected. When his test returned positive, Felton was recommended for a chest X-ray at Toronto's Gage Institute and, on the basis of the picture of his lungs, sanatorium care was advised. On admission, Felton appeared to be in fairly good physical condition, the only hint of disease being his slight pallor and the fact that he had lost seven pounds over the previous six months. Another chest X-ray taken at his admission revealed minor but definite changes in the apical region of his left lung in the area above the clavicle (collarbone) and in the first interspace (or intercostal space) which falls between the clavicle and the uppermost first rib. This was very concerning, since pathological changes in the apical area of the lungs were strongly associated with reactivation tuberculosis.[37]

Felton provided both blood and gastric (stomach) contents samples for laboratory analysis. The blood sample was used to test his sedimentation rate,[38] a relatively simple laboratory test requiring a blood sample, a tall, thin vertical tube, and about an hour's time. The test relies on the natural tendency for whole blood to separate, where lighter plasma ascends to the top of the tube and heavier red blood cells descend to form a sediment at the bottom of the tube. The test measures the amount of clear plasma present in the top portion of the tube after an hour's separation time.[39] The rationale is that increased protein concentrations in the blood resulting from immune system activity cause red blood cells to descend the tube more rapidly, and, the faster the fall, the more clear plasma at the top of the tube after an hour. While the sedimentation rate was interpreted as a barometer of immune system activity, the test was non-specific in the sense that it could not identify the root cause of immune stimulation, but for most children admitted to the sanatorium, tuberculosis was the common suspected culprit. In the sanatorium era Myers argued that "the sedimentation rate is a much more delicate indication of changes in the lesion than symptoms, physical examination or X-ray film."[40] Felton's sedimentation rate was evaluated as 3 mm/hr, a value that fell into a normal or unremarkable range.

Felton was neither coughing nor producing sputum, so the search for active tuberculosis bacteria in his body focused on sampling his gastric contents, the idea being that he may have swallowed respiratory tract secretions, along with tuberculosis bacteria. Like Felton, children seldom had sputum-raising coughs and tended to be paucibacillary (meaning that they were host to only small numbers of TB bacteria[41]), so this test of gastric contents was fairly common among child patients. Gastric contents were sampled through fluid aspiration where, via a rubber tube, saline was introduced into the stomach and the contents then suctioned out for analysis. A routine procedure perhaps, but the process of getting the tube past the back of the mouth (and the strong gag reflex), down the throat, and into the stomach could be quite traumatic. Roy Harry, a former child patient at the Craig-y-nos sanatorium in Wales, specifically recalled his resistance to the procedure, trying to evade the tube by shaking his head, kicking out his feet, and sliding down the chair.[42] For Felton, his gastric contents culture returned positive, confirming that he had swallowed[43] sputum with tuberculosis bacteria. This test provided the first clear evidence that Felton's tuberculosis infection was active.

Despite all of the familiarity with TB and the advances made in diagnosing the disease, when Beverly was admitted in 1948, sanatorium physicians were not entirely convinced that she suffered any ongoing disease activity, though she was provisionally diagnosed with minimal pulmonary tuberculosis. In the summer of 1948, feeling entirely well, sixteen-year-old Beverly had received a chest X-ray as part of a routine survey. The X-ray suggested some "abnormal" findings and she was referred to the Gage Institute for follow-up. The abnormality was described as "a small rather soft appearing lesion in the [lung] parenchyma of the right 1st interspace" (in the area of her right lung's apex). Since two of Beverly's brothers had been patients at the Toronto sanatorium, the likely route of her exposure seemed evident; Beverly herself had been admitted to a preventorium for a period of resistance building some years earlier when she was nine years old. Sanatorium physicians carefully monitored Beverly, employing the classical array of diagnostic tests to assess whether or not her infection was active:

> When she arrived here, the sedimentation rate was 6. Six fasting gastric contents cultured for tubercle bacilli during her stay here, have all been negative. The tuberculin test was positive. Her sedimentation rate was normal throughout her stay here except on the 20th of September, 1949, it was 22, at which time she had a cold and sore throat. In January 1949, she was allowed up to one meal daily. The lesion in her right first interspace looks now very much the same as it did when she arrived. Medical conference agreed that she ought to remain here for approximately one year. Her latest X-ray film taken on the 20th of September, shows no change from her previous films. Planograms taken in January 1949 revealed no definite evidence of cavitation.

Beverly's normal sedimentation rate and her negative tuberculosis bacteria culturing results were encouraging, but counterbalanced by the lesion that was plainly evident in the apex of her right lung. The lesion, however, did not appear to change over time and, on the basis of that observation, Beverly's disease was determined to be latent, the non-cavitary lesion viewed as a remnant of past disease activity. Her immune system had apparently contained the infection, at least for the year that she had been in the sanatorium. Her post-discharge advice still recommended that she live cautiously, resting at least fourteen hours every day until her scheduled check-up two months after discharge. Follow-ups continued until almost seven and a half years after her discharge, at which time it was determined that her infection remained consistently inactive.

Sites of Tuberculosis Infection and Disease in Children

In addition to the complexities of primary and secondary disease, children also experienced variation in the sites of infection and disease in their bodies, further shaping their diverse tuberculosis experiences. Pulmonary infection includes disease of the lungs and the hilar lymph nodes associated with the lungs, but tuberculosis is entirely capable of establishing infection outside of the lungs, in other tissues and organs of the body. One estimate suggests that about 30 per cent of children with tuberculosis will experience extra-pulmonary (outside of the lung) forms of disease.[44] Extra-pulmonary forms of tuberculosis may arise directly (e.g., colonization of the gastrointestinal tract following consumption of tuberculous cow's milk), or secondary to pulmonary infection via lymphohematogenous dissemination (i.e., dissemination from the lungs by either the lymphatic or blood supply systems). Pleural tuberculosis (or "tuberculous pleurisy," characterized by a tuberculous pleural effusion,[45] or the accumulation of fluid in the pleural cavity[46]) and tuberculous adenitis (known as "scrofula" when the cervical lymph nodes in the neck are involved), mentioned earlier in the chapter, are two of the more common extra-pulmonary forms of tuberculosis, followed by genitourinary tuberculosis, miliary tuberculosis (an infection of the bloodstream, resulting from either respiratory or digestive tract infection, which can disseminate and seed various tissues and organs of the body[47]), tuberculosis of the bones and joints, and tuberculous meningitis (infection of the brain).[48] In Toronto, and North America more generally, the number of cases of extra-pulmonary forms of tuberculosis caused by *Mycobacterium bovis* and the ingestion of infected cow's milk and meat, particularly TB of the mesenteric glands (associated with the digestive tract), cervical glands ("scrofula"), and bone and joint tuberculosis, decreased significantly with the introduction of routine cattle inspection and the pasteurization of milk (figures 4.1, 4.2).[49]

Alternatively, extra-pulmonary forms of disease could arise secondary to pulmonary infection,[50] particularly when a poor host immune response (or low resistance) enabled the escape of tuberculosis bacteria from the lungs.[51] Since the sanatorium era, more recent research has also discovered that, in addition to variations in individual immune resistance, different infecting strains of *Mycobacterium tuberculosis* can influence the

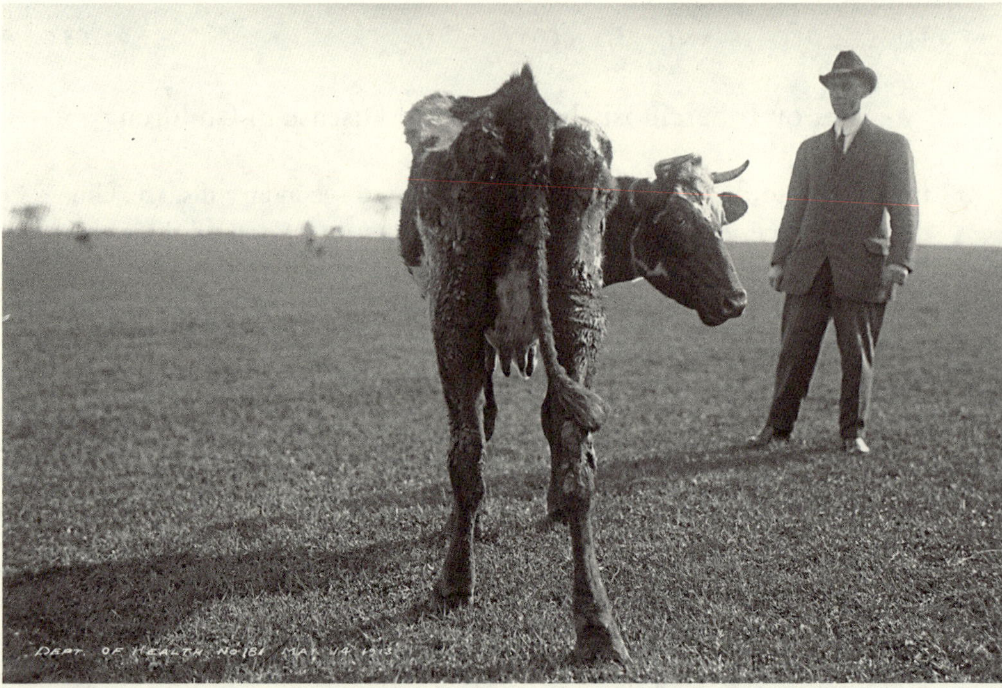

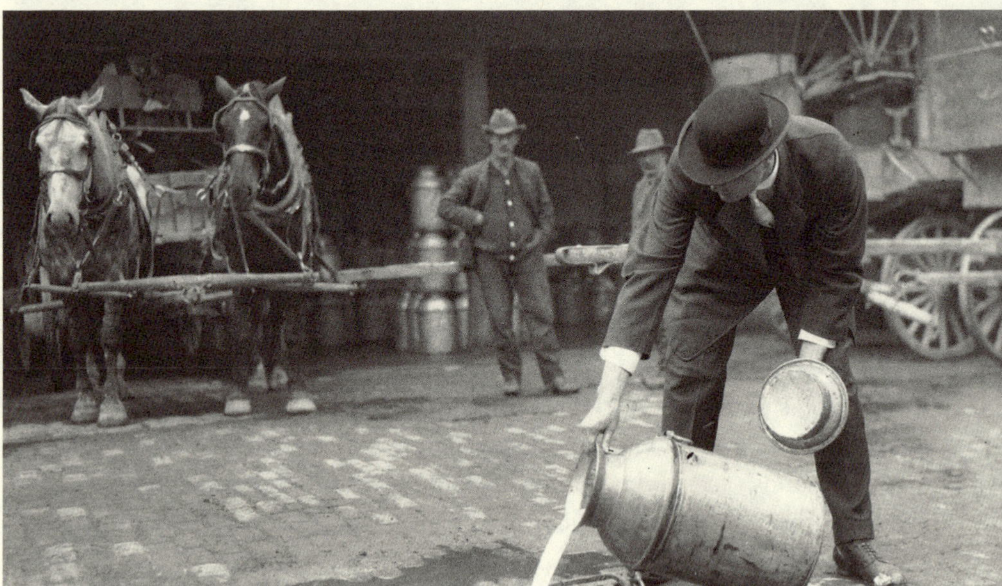

Figure 4.1 Top Inspection of an emaciated dairy cow, possibly tuberculous, her wasting mirroring the type of weight loss experienced by human sufferers with advanced tuberculosis, 14 May 1913.

Figure 4.2 Bottom A Toronto milk inspector destroys contaminated milk, May 1913. In the handling of milk, pasteurization would reduce the need to destroy tainted supplies.

site or sites of disease within the body, with some strains more likely to result in extra-pulmonary disease. According to Hesseling and colleagues, those strains of *Mycobacterium tuberculosis* that lead to extra-pulmonary infection may do so because they parasitize macrophages more "efficiently," overcoming host defences and spreading infection past initial sites in the lung and local lymph nodes.[52] Hesseling and colleagues note that two different strains of tuberculosis bacteria, those of the Beijing and S genotypes, are more often associated with extra-pulmonary disease than strains of the LAM genotype, perhaps indicating that strains of the LAM genotype are less effective disseminators.[53] Their findings point to the varying abilities of different strains of tuberculosis bacteria and the understanding that disease expression is mediated not only by the status of the immune system, but also by characteristics of tuberculosis bacteria themselves.

Some of the children sampled at the Toronto sanatorium suffered bone and joint tuberculosis. In their review of the literature, Aufderheide and Rodriguez-Martin conclude that spinal tuberculosis (also known as "Pott's disease"[54]) is the most common form of skeletal lesion caused by tuberculosis, representing some 50 per cent of all cases of skeletal involvement, and often affecting the lower spine from the eighth thoracic vertebra down through to the fourth lumbar vertebra.[55] Overall, thoracic, lumbar, and lumbrosacral regions are most often affected, followed by the cervical (neck) vertebrae.[56] This particular distribution of spinal tuberculosis is shaped, in part, by the arterial blood supply to the spinal column, since infection of vertebrae occurs typically (though not exclusively) via a secondary spread of TB bacteria from a primary focus in the lungs or other organs via the blood supply (i.e., a "hematogenous" spread).[57] The highly vascularized trabecular bone of the vertebral bodies, rich in blood supply and oxygen (tuberculosis bacteria are aerobic, meaning they require oxygen), is particularly vulnerable to tuberculosis, as are the intervertebral disks lying in between adjacent vertebra. In the individual, spinal tuberculosis is not typically widespread, as tuberculous pathologies tend to localize to no more than one to four vertebrae (of the thirty-three vertebrae that typically make up the spine).[58] While children more often experienced disease in the upper thoracic spine, spinal TB in adults frequently manifested lower down the thoracolumbar spine.[59] Spinal tuberculosis

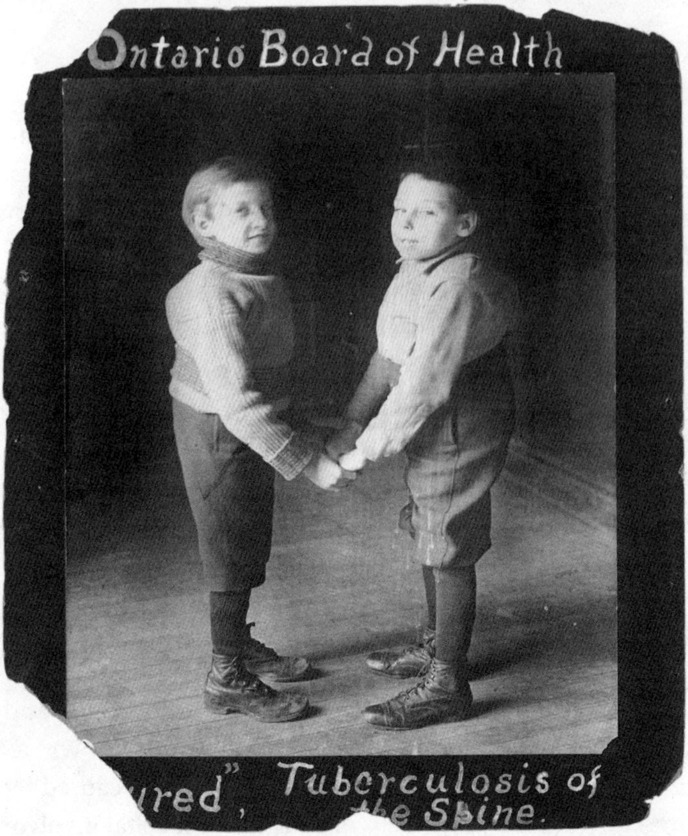

Figure 4.3 Two boys with spinal tuberculosis ("Pott's disease"), which has caused destruction and collapse of vertebrae resulting in characteristic kyphosis. The introduction of surgical treatments (especially spinal fusions) at the Toronto Sanatorium was intended to stop disease progression and strengthen the spine to prevent further collapse.

results in destruction of vertebral bodies, causing the spine to lose its structure and collapse.[60] The bone destruction associated with tuberculosis cannot be reversed, leading to long-lasting sequelae, such as spinal instability and deformity, the most notable of which is kyphosis, an atypical angulation of the spine leading to a "humpback" appearance (see figure 4.3).[61] Aside from the spine, other common sites of skeletal tuberculosis are the hip (the femoral head and pelvis) and the knee. Like the vertebral bodies, the femoral head and the patella are also composed of highly vascularized trabecular bone, providing both the means for infection via the blood supply and the oxygen-rich environment favoured by tuberculosis bacteria.

Bone and joint tuberculosis could strike children at any age, even the very youngest. Baby Lila was admitted to the Davies Cottage in January 1923, when she was nineteen months old, at least nine pounds underweight, and suffering from both pulmonary tuberculosis and tuberculosis of the hip. Given her young age, Lila's tuberculosis disease was likely due to primary progressive disease, though she may have experienced a brief latent period followed by reactivation disease. In either case, while she was at the sanatorium, Lila's condition improved. A stubborn pathological draining sinus in the area of her hip joint eventually healed and, by December 1923, her weight had increased to twenty-five pounds. She was so excited by Christmas preparations that year, and so energetic in general, that staff found it difficult to photograph Lila for her cot patron "as she constantly danced on her mattress." Over time, however, tuberculosis proved itself an unpredictable disease, able to linger and strike fresh, particularly among very young and vulnerable children with poorly developed immune function. Despite the optimism of her initial advances, Lila ultimately succumbed to tuberculosis almost two years later, in November 1925, while she was still a patient at the sanatorium. Since the whereabouts of her mother were not known and there was no father listed on her admission record, Lila's burial was charitably arranged by the Children's Aid Society.

Perceptions of Exposure and Infection

The question of exposure and transmission of tuberculosis is important, especially among children who represent, in an epidemiological sense, the next potential generation of tuberculosis hosts in a population. Studies suggest that there are age-related features underlying exposure and transmission risks, such that most tuberculosis transmission to young children, specifically those less than three years of age, is likely to occur within the family home.[62] Tuberculosis has been described as "the quintessential family disease," an infection that passed through generations as tuberculosis bacteria moved from the bodies of infectious adults to their susceptible children.[63] Walter B. Kendall, physician-in-chief of the National Sanitarium Association's Muskoka sanatorium, described tuberculosis as a "house disease," where one member "sow[s] the seed" and all present "[take] part in the harvest."[64] According to an interwar handbook produced by the Canadian Tuberculosis Association, in cases of childhood infection, "often there are older persons in the household – relatives, boarders, servants – who have chronic tuberculosis and don't even know it. They may believe they are suffering from bronchitis or asthma or heart disease. Such people are especially dangerous to others because usually they take no care to protect others from the sickness."[65] In a 1920 publication, John Howard Holbrook, Hamilton's Mountain Sanatorium's physician-in-chief, wrote that the "transmission from an open adult case to the child may be considered the most frequent manner in which the disease is spread."[66]

Questions about routes of exposure and infection were often impossible to answer with any degree of certainty, but were routinely asked when documenting the medical histories for each child. A large proportion of the children sampled came from households affected by tuberculosis (see table 4.1). As recorded in their medical histories, with information provided by either the children or their parents or guardians, about 38 per cent (n = 315) of the children sampled had both parents alive and well. Among another 20 per cent (n = 168) of the child patients sampled, both parents were known to be alive, though one or both of them suffered from tuberculosis. In another 240 cases (29 per cent), only one parent was known to be alive, the other parent deceased, not present (in some cases, due to desertion), or otherwise not known. In 155 of those cases, only the mother was alive or known, but about one-fifth of them were suffering from tuberculosis. For the other 85 children, only the father was alive or known, and of that number, 7 fathers had active tuberculosis. In the majority of these latter cases, the mothers had died, either due to tuberculosis or some other cause. Forty-two (5 per cent) of the children in the sample had lost both of their parents, either due to death or abandonment. In those 42 cases, at least 28 children were known to have lost one or both parents to tuberculosis. The specifics of the numbers are less important that the overall understanding that only just over a third (38 per cent) of the children sampled had both parents alive and well, the remainder of the children having experienced disease or loss of parents due to one cause or another.

Table 4.1
Status of parents of admitted children

Status of parents	*n*	%
Both parents alive, present and known	*483*	*58.8*
Both alive and well	315	38.3
Father alive and well, mother alive but has TB	108	13.1
Mother alive and well, father alive but has TB	48	5.8
Both alive, but both have TB	12	1.5
Neither parent alive, present, or known	*42*	*5.1*
Both parents died TB	10	1.2
Mother died TB, father died (not TB)	11	1.3
Mother died TB, father's status not known	5	0.6
Father died TB, mother died cause not known	1	0.1
Father died TB, mother's status not known	1	0.1
Mother died cause not known, father's status not known	3	0.4
Both parents died, both causes not known	11	1.3
Only mother alive, present, or known	*155*	*18.9*
Mother alive and well, father died TB	41	5.0
Mother alive and well, father died cause not known	61	7.4
Mother alive and well, father's status not known	20	2.4
Mother alive but has TB, father died TB	12	1.5
Mother alive but has TB, father died (not TB)	9	1.1
Mother alive but has TB, father's status not known	12	1.5
Only father alive, present, or known	*85*	*10.3*
Father alive and well, mother died TB	55	6.7
Father alive and well, mother died (not TB)	23	2.8
Father alive but has TB, mother died TB	3	0.4
Father alive but has TB, mother died (not TB)	1	0.1
Father alive but has TB, mother's status not known	3	0.4
Missing information	*57*	*6.9*

Table 4.2
Perceived source of exposure to tuberculosis infection

Perceived exposure to infection	*n*	%
Mother	168	20.4
Father	80	9.7
Sibling(s)	61	7.4
Combined immediate family	89	10.8
Other family	19	2.3
Household visitors, boarders, neighbours	22	2.7
Institution life (school, camp, hospital)	11	1.3
Milk consumption	3	0.4
Job-related	2	0.2
Not known or missing in chart	366	44.5

When a child was admitted and the child's history was taken, either the child or the adult accompanying the child (usually a parent or guardian) was asked to comment on how he or she believed infection had occurred. The asking was part of the standard medical history though, as Jonathan Gillis suggests, "the patient story was described as important, but at the same time flawed – full of exaggeration, verbosity, and irrelevancy," perhaps even incorporating "incorrect words and ideas."[67] Physicians would ask the question about infection and record the answer, but that did not mean physicians necessarily believed it to be accurate or correct. Even if that is the case, however, these answers are intriguing because they reflect people's perceptions concerning routes of infection. Most importantly, in almost half of the cases sampled (45 per cent, or 366 cases), a specific or likely source of infection could not be identified (see table 4.2). This finding weighs in on the insidious nature of tuberculosis, springing up in cases where people were genuinely baffled about how infection could have occurred, particularly in cases where there was no family history of the disease. Among the remaining 456 children, some attempt was made to account for the likely mechanism or manner of tuberculosis infection.

The responses to this question were themed and will be reviewed in terms of the percentages of various responses, but it is important to note that while they are insightful for understanding perceptions, the answers should not be taken to reflect any exacting or absolute epidemiological reality, because most people were probably guessing.

As detailed in table 4.2, among 168 of the children (20 per cent of the sample), the mother was suspected as the source of infection, followed by exposure to an infectious father among 80 children (10 per cent of the sample) (figures 4.4, 4.5). Relative to fathers, mothers were perhaps a more intuitive source of infection, since typical early to mid-twentieth-century gender roles placed mothers, more often than fathers, in the family home and raising children. The closer, more intensive, and longer duration contact between mothers and children may have resulted in greater dangers of large-dose or massive infection of children if mothers had active disease and were infectious. In a 1923 publication, Dr Harold Parsons (of the Toronto Hospital for Sick Children's Chest Clinic) reviewed five hundred case histories of children with tuberculosis and he found that fathers and mothers were identified as the "infecting agents" in 36 per cent and 27 per cent of cases, respectively.[68] Parsons admits that the impact of tuberculous fathers on the infection of children in the household was much greater than he had expected, given his impression that mothers were the more "natural" source of infection. In his interpretation, he suggests that men may have been more careless with their sputum. Parsons was not alone in his findings, as other studies also found that exposure to tuberculous fathers, compared to tuberculous mothers, was linked to a higher incidence of infection among children, though higher tuberculosis mortality among children was found among those with tuberculous mothers.[69]

There were many instances documented in the cases sampled of infants and children having been separated from their mothers and fathers because of tuberculosis illness or death. Maggie, a one-year-old when she was admitted to the Davies Cottage in 1936, entered the hospital from her grandparents' home, since both of her parents had been hospitalized at the Muskoka sanatorium. On admission, Maggie was found to be "exceedingly anaemic and water-logged from having been kept on a diet of milk until she was 13 months of age." The staff placed her on a "well

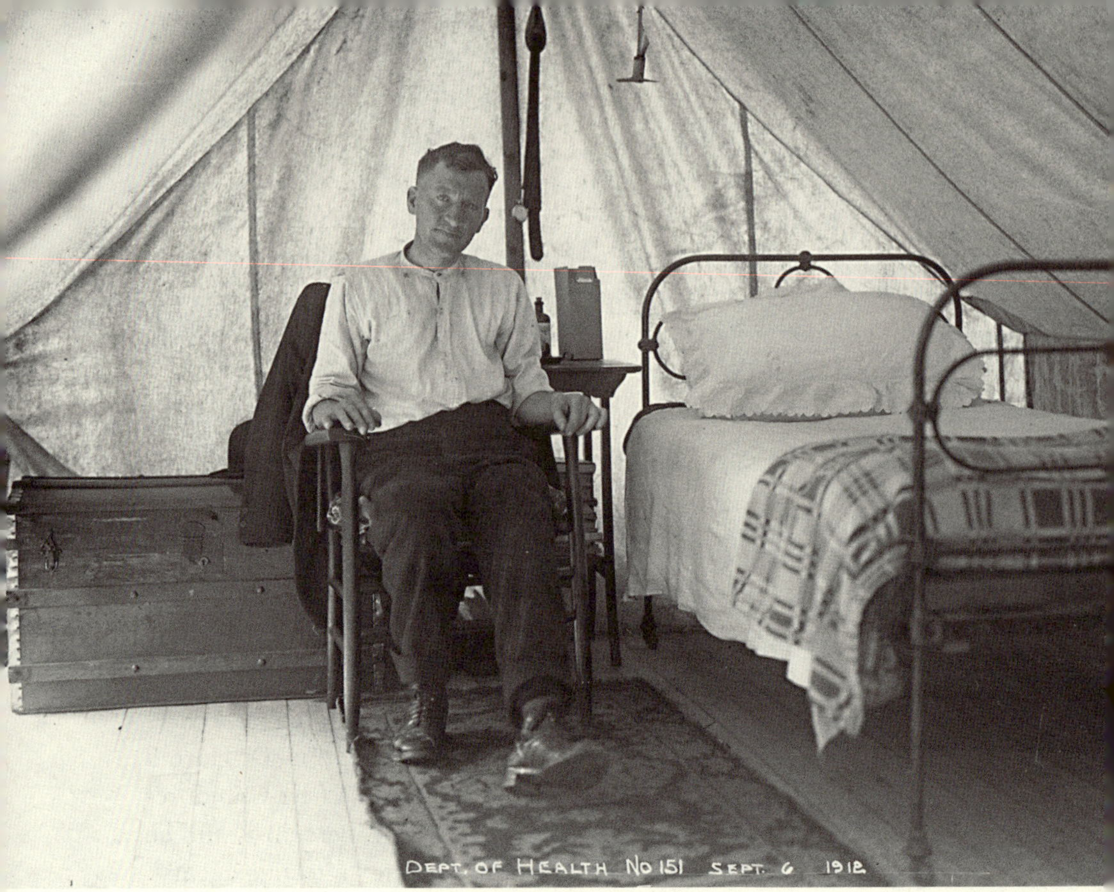
DEPT. OF HEALTH No 151 SEPT. 6 1912

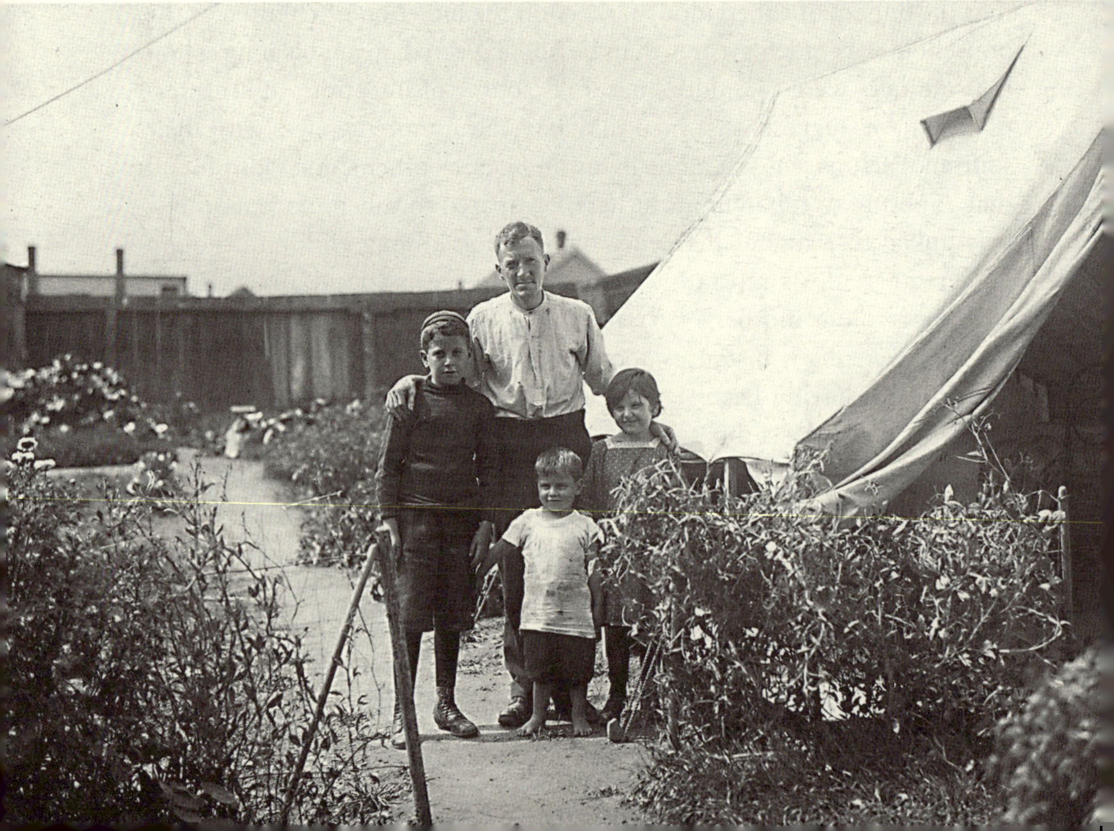

balanced" diet, her health evidently quickly improving and her anemia disappearing. At the time of her discharge, a pulmonary lesion that had been found in the lower lobe of her right lung was in the process of calcifying, indicating that her body was healing through the process of sequestering TB bacteria in granulomas. During her stay in the sanatorium, Maggie's father wrote many letters to Dobbie enquiring about her health; even as he faced his own tuberculosis struggles, he remained focused on his child. Dobbie also received correspondence from Maggie's aunt (her mother's sister) who had promised Maggie's mother that she would ensure her niece was always "comfortably dressed." She had meant to send Maggie some toys for Christmas, but the family was "heart broken and grief stricken" by the sudden passing of another of Maggie's aunts, only fourteen years of age, at the Muskoka sanatorium, their attentions then focusing on Maggie's mother, whose "condition is such that she may go any minute." Maggie's aunt was a registered nurse working in the United States and, in her letter to Dobbie, she delivered a stinging indictment of Maggie's family's physician, whom she ultimately held responsible for the "tragedy of it all," because he had taken care of Maggie's mother for a

Figure 4.4 Opposite top The interior of David C.'s backyard tent, as photographed by Toronto's Health Department, 6 September 1912. The sparsely appointed tent provides a single-sized iron bed, a side table (with a stack of books on the lower shelf, and a corked glass bottle, perhaps containing a patent medicine, resting on top alongside a small candlestick), a chair, a trunk for storage, and a carpet runner. To keep track of time, a pocket watch hangs from the rear tent pole, while a sticky stretch of flypaper hangs above the bed (likely to reduce the nuisance and disease-transmitting potential of houseflies).

Figure 4.5 Opposite bottom Toronto's Health Department provided David C. with his backyard tent and noted, 6 September 1912, "Although a chronic consumptive, [C.] is making a brave fight for improvement in the garden of his home. In the summer he raises all the vegetables and fruits required by his family, while the wife necessarily the wage-earner of the family, is employed at the City Hall." An examination of Toronto's death registry reveals that David took a turn for the worse. Less than three years after this photograph was taken with his children, thirty-nine-year-old David died of pulmonary tuberculosis at the Toronto sanatorium in May 1915.

full year, never recognizing or diagnosing tuberculosis. Because of his failings, she argued, the family had not taken any precautions to protect their children, including Maggie, from infection. "It makes me very sad and bitter," wrote Maggie's aunt, "when in this day and age so much can be done." For Maggie, the effects would be everlasting, as her mother died at the Muskoka sanatorium in 1937, almost six months before she was discharged from the Toronto sanatorium. Like Maggie, many other children would experience the loss of their mothers to tuberculosis.

The loss of parents to tuberculosis was sometimes implicated in the "moral ruin" of the children who were left motherless, fatherless, or orphaned. Such was the case for fifteen-year-old Carolyn, who was transferred to the sanatorium from a Toronto hospital in February 1931. It was reported that Carolyn had been deeply affected by the death of her mother a few years earlier and, as the result of a troubled home life, she had been placed in an industrial school in an effort to improve her behaviour. Charlotte Neff notes that industrial schools, while originally intended under Ontario's 1874 Act respecting Industrial Schools to provide education to a wide range of children (including orphans, children whose parents were imprisoned, children reliant upon charity, children who could not be controlled by their parents, or parents who neglected their children), had, by 1884, come to include as potential students children found guilty of petty crimes. As a result of this addition, according to Neff, the industrial schools "became effectively reformatories focusing on the wrongdoing of children rather than that of their parents."[70] Likely because of the reputation of industrial schools, upon Carolyn's admission Dobbie wrote to the Department of Health, wanting to clarify if there were any issues with her behaviour. The reply he received explained Carolyn's circumstances, that she had been admitted to the school about two months earlier "because of lack of discipline in the home." As the eldest child in her family, upon her mother's death, Carolyn had been "left to care for the home and younger children" and, "consequently, due to too much responsibility and lack of proper supervision, the child got in with bad companions and she was placed in the School for proper discipline." The department felt that because Carolyn was so ill, she was unlikely to present any behavioural problems at the sanatorium.

Dobbie also received a letter from the superintendent of the industrial school, clearly supportive of Carolyn, and explaining her background further: "We are very much interested in this poor girl. She comes of a good family, but her mother died something over a year ago, and this girl was left in charge of the home, without sufficient parental control – the father I judge being rather easygoing. The result was moral disaster. I am informed by those who knew the family, that the girl's mother was of the 'salt of the earth,' which makes it especially pitiful to find her daughter in such sad condition." While sanatorium physicians were still trying to narrow down the extent of Carolyn's tuberculous involvement, they were also treating her for chronic peritonitis. The cause of the peritonitis was traced to an undiagnosed gonorrheal infection, presumably some sexual activity being part of the "moral disaster" that had led to her admission to the industrial school. Despite all the correspondence, concern, and attempts to help Carolyn, however, her tuberculosis was so far advanced that she died in the sanatorium just over a month after her admission.

Not only parents, but also siblings who suffered cavitary tuberculosis could represent sources of infection for children in the family home. In the sample of sanatorium children, tuberculous siblings were suggested as the route of exposure and infection in sixty-one cases (7 per cent of the sample). Parsons's estimates on data from the Hospital for Sick Children's Chest Clinic identify sisters and brothers in about 20 and 11 per cent of infections among children assessed at the clinic, respectively.[71] Marshall was twelve years old when he was admitted to the Toronto sanatorium in January 1916. Marshall's father was known to have a troublesome sputum-raising morning cough, but showed no evidence of any weight loss. Marshall's mother appeared healthy, with no cough, though in her interactions with sanatorium staff, she was apparently found to "talk a great deal." Marshall had one sister, who was healthy, and two living brothers, one healthy and the other a less robust "TB suspect." It was Marshall's eldest brother, nineteen-year-old Douglas, who had died of tuberculosis in 1915. Douglas had suffered active tuberculosis for at least a year preceding his death, and though he had been admitted to the Toronto sanatorium, he had remained for only about three weeks. Following his departure from the sanatorium, Douglas and his wife, Grace, moved in with his parents and siblings. Not long after settling into the family home, Douglas and Grace celebrated the arrival of their first child, healthy at birth, but the infant died within three months of tuberculous meningitis. Feeling unwell with a slight cough and weight loss, Grace then underwent an examination at the Gage Institute. She was examined by Dr Dobbie, who found no clear physical signs pointing to tuberculosis. Some weeks later, Grace was admitted to a local hospital and underwent surgery for a suspected tuberculous abscess. In the aftermath of that surgery, Grace died. Douglas, Grace, the baby, and Marshall all shared a home and in tuberculosis infection. Of the four, only Marshall would survive tuberculosis, spending a year and a half at the sanatorium before he was taken home by his parents in September 1917. The gross misfortune of this family details how easily the infection could circulate within a family and the particular vulnerability of infants. Marshall's brother may have been the source of his infection, or perhaps his sister-in-law. No one individual family member could be identified as the source of his infection, and this was also true of eighty-nine (11 per cent) of the children sampled in this study who came from homes where multiple family members suffered tuberculosis.

In nineteen cases (2 per cent of the sample), other family members beyond the immediate family were identified as sources of infection. This was the case for Lyle, an infant admitted to the Davies Cottage in 1931. He had three siblings, and all had been admitted to the IODE Preventorium in Toronto. In this instance, Lyle's tuberculous grandfather was identified as the most likely source of infection. Gloria, "a sweet little girl of six years," was admitted to the sanatorium in March 1940 and remained for ten months. Her patron's cot note described her as a child with "a happy smile, winning the hearts of those who know her, although very quiet at times." She reportedly enjoyed attending the hospital school and learning her A-B-Cs. Gloria's grandfather, who lived with the family, had been found to be tuberculous in August 1939. In another case, when eight-year-old Enid was admitted in 1927, it was noted that her mother, hospitalized for illness, had been away from the home "for some considerable time" and that, as a result, Enid had "not had much intelligent care." As to exposure, it was noted that "an Uncle died of Tuberculosis in her home when Enid was a wee child so no doubt this [was] the source of infection." Outside of the immediate and extended family, visitors, boarders, and neighbours were believed to account for another twenty-two cases (3 per cent) of infection among the children sampled. Generally, the fear of tuberculosis cultivated anxieties over anyone with "suspicious coughs" entering the family home. Eleven cases of infection (1 per cent of the sample) involved children who had been admitted from institutions such as hospitals, industrial schools, and orphanages.

Consumption of infected milk (from cows infected with *Mycobacterium bovis*) was identified as the source of infection among three children (0.4 per cent) in the sample. This number underestimates the true impact of this source of infection. In 1918, Dr C.J. Hastings, of Toronto, estimated that an overwhelming 26 per cent of all cases of tuberculosis in children could be attributed to infection, via the milk supply, with *Mycobacterium bovis*.[72] The dangers of bovine-human transmission had long been understood in the province. As early as 1895, not long after Koch's discovery of the tuberculosis bacterium, and despite his own conviction that *Mycobacterium bovis* posed little risk to humans,[73] Ontario had passed legislation for the tuberculin testing of cattle.[74] The import and export of cattle was dutifully monitored by the Canadian federal government. In 1908, if cattle were imported from the United States or Mexico without satisfactory tuberculin testing charts, they were quarantined and tested. In Canada, tests were often undertaken by municipal veterinarians, who were supplied with free tuberculin. Cattle testing positive for tuberculosis infection were not necessarily destroyed, but permanently identified with a capital *T* cut out of their right ears.[75]

Given a large number of childhood tuberculosis infections attributed to bovine origins surfacing well into the first few decades of the twentieth century, the rigour of this testing can be surmised to have been weak at best. In 1912, Charles Hodgetts, former chief medical officer of health for Ontario, acknowledged the presence of bovine tuberculosis in Canada and the fact that milk from tuberculous cows continued to be sold. As "the artificial food of too many Canadian babies," he argued it "essential that the provincial government should by statutory enactment provide the means by which city and town authorities have the power of the inspection of dairies and dairy cattle from which the milk is sold – this should include the power to license after inspection and the tubercular testing of all such cattle."[76] Even as late as 1920, Dr Holbrook, physician-in-chief of the Mountain Sanatorium in Hamilton, was certain that since "no individual in a democracy can have the right to destroy another either by quick or slow methods," dairy farmers should not be permitted to sell raw (unpasteurized) milk from potentially tuberculous cows.[77] While countries would establish their own protocols and timelines for milk pasteurization, it is notable that in Ireland, for example, the pasteurization of milk extended beyond milk intended for human consumption, as pasteurized milk was also returned to farms for the feeding of calves in attempts to break chains of tuberculosis transmission across generations of cattle.[78]

Katherine McCuaig's history of tuberculosis in Canada reveals that Ontario was the first province to pass compulsory milk pasteurization law under Premier Mitch Hepburn (1934–42).[79] While farm lobbyists attempted to derail compulsory pasteurization, attention turned to Ontario's children, who were viewed as the true victims of those protests. A National Research Council report provided to Hepburn indicated "that over 10 percent of the 490 children at the [Hospital for Sick Children] suffered from bovine tuberculosis acquired from raw milk."[80] McCuaig reports that Hepburn was profoundly influenced by a hospital tour, where he encountered "two long rows of cots filled with bovine TB patients."[81] Through Hepburn's efforts (and despite the risk that he could lose the votes of farmers), compulsory milk pasteurization was first introduced to cities and towns, and subsequently extended to rural areas, such that "by 1941 over 98 percent of the milk sold in Ontario in fluid form was pasteurized."[82] Early on, it was determined that pasteurization was preferred over destroying diseased cattle, since late-1920s estimates suggested that 35–50 per cent of cattle were likely infected with tuberculosis, and destroying those cattle would come at great economic disadvantage and possibly jeopardize the province's milk supply.[83]

While compulsory pasteurization tended to milk sold commercially, farming families could still opt to use raw milk from their own cows. The story of nine-year-old Harvey, which came to Dobbie's attention in 1930, documents the risks of bovine tuberculosis and childhood infection. The family doctor who had examined Harvey and recommended him for sanatorium treatment wrote to Dobbie that, in his opinion, "the disease was from milk from a tubercular cow." The cow had lived on Harvey's family's farm, described as a "great pet" of Harvey's, so it was believed that he had been at risk for contracting bovine tuberculosis not only by drinking infected milk, but also through his regular care and handling of the cow. Prior to Harvey's admission to the sanatorium, the family's physician had conducted a laparotomy, which involved making a small incision in Harvey's abdomen so that he could have a closer look at what was happing inside of Harvey's body. He believed Harvey to be suffering abdominal tuberculosis, but this was a difficult diagnosis, because his symptoms could easily be attributed to any number of conditions, ranging from an intestinal obstruction or a strangulated hernia, to appendicitis or typhoid fever.[84] Staff at the sanatorium also surmised that Harvey was suffering "tuberculous peritonitis," however, effectively confirming the family physician's diagnosis.

Harvey's family had been placed on a farm in northern Ontario in the 1920s under a federal resettlement scheme. Harvey's father maintained a lengthy correspondence with Dobbie, documenting how the family had expected they would be placed on a farm that provided "proper housing and stabling," but since most of the properties available under the scheme were abandoned farms, reality did not meet with the family's expectations. As Harvey's father described to Dobbie, "On arrival ... the whole family were placed in an old log hut 16 ft by 24 ft which previous to this had for 5 years been housing pigs and had been done up at the expence of $143 for our reception." The tight confines of the log hut meant that the family of eight was obliged to share one "community bedroom," the space of which he likened to the size of one horse stall. Only making matters worse, the log hut had a tendency to flood in spring, and one morning in 1928, the family woke to find two feet of water in their home, forcing them to move their sleeping quarters into a neighbouring tool shed.

In addition to the troubles the family faced in farming the land, which Harvey's father described as "an unfenced weed patch," the family had been provided with animals upon their arrival, but, according to Harvey's father, these were mostly older cows and horses. Harvey's father suspected that the cattle had not been tuberculin tested, and one cow, Harvey's "pet," subsequently died of tuberculosis. Paralleling the family's struggle with poor housing, the farm animals were also inadequately stabled, as described by Harvey's father: "As regards stabling for horses and cows nothing existed except a partly built up place at one end of the barn ... Now the 'Freeze up' came and the only surprising thing was, that I didn't lose my entire stock ... I might mention here that it was the middle of the next winter before I got the material to fix up a log hut for a byre" (a cow barn, or shed). Harvey's father reported that altogether he had lost three cows and four horses. In addition to Harvey's cow that died of tuberculosis, the other two cows "died practically due to ... exposure ... owing to bad stabling ... One of the cows[,] had it lived a month more[,] would have been 19 years old." Two of the horses, both over twenty years of age, "died through chills contracted through bad stabling." Many of the same mechanisms associated with the transmission of *Mycobacterium tuberculosis* in people are responsible for the spread of *Mycobacterium bovis* in cattle, including crowding (for easing transmission) and poor maintenance or nutrition (for compromising immune function and resistance). Harvey's father knew that he needed to provision his animals as best he could if they were to survive the hardships of poor stabling in a northern Ontario winter, for, as he wrote, "as anyone knows[,] a cold stable calls for more feed and extra rations." Yet a meagre yield from the poor-quality farm land meant extra rations were hard to come by, and the animals suffered as a result.

Harvey's father's concerns regarding the stabling of his animals were very much in keeping with official recommendations for management of cattle and the risks of bovine tuberculosis. Decades earlier, at a meeting of the International Commission on the Control of Bovine Tuberculosis in Ottawa in 1910, the commission recommended not only routine tuberculin testing and the slaughter of infected cattle to prevent exposure, but also attention to conditions in which cattle were living with an eye towards (like humans) building up their resistance to infection: "This can be done by stabling them in clean, disinfected, and properly lighted and ventilated barns, giving them abundant clean water and nutritious food, and a sufficient amount of daily exercise in the open air, and attending generally to those conditions which are known to contribute to the health of animals."[85] Harvey's father fully believed that the cow responsible for Harvey's infection had been weakened through poor stabling, the cow as vulnerable to the bad conditions on the farm as Harvey's family. As Merrill Singer has noted, "The health of animals, both domestic and wild, is significantly impacted by human activity and human social structures. Domestic animals owned by the rich, for example, are likely to be fed better, housed better, and receive better veterinary care than animals belonging to the poor."[86] In this way, the poor health of Harvey's cow was a reflection of both the family's difficult living situation and Harvey's poor health. More than anything else, Harvey's father wanted somebody to take responsibility for his son's tuberculosis, knowing full well that his son had not simply been randomly infected, though he would never find satisfactory resolution along those lines. In the end, after Harvey's tuberculosis diagnosis and admission to the sanatorium, the family had abandoned the hated farm.

Returning to table 4.2 and perceived routes of infection, work-related exposures were suspected for two children (0.2 per cent of the sample). Hannah was one of those cases, admitted to the sanatorium in November 1915. For much of 1915, nine-year-old Hannah had worked carrying and emptying the sputum cups for tuberculosis patients, a staggeringly risky responsibility for a child of her age. The sanatorium's examining physician suspected this as the most likely route of Hannah's exposure and infection. If not the contents of the sputum cups themselves, then Hannah's close association with the infectious adults who were producing the sputum could have certainly accounted for her infection. If not those adults, then Hannah's own mother had died of TB at age thirty, about eight years prior to the Hannah's admission to the Toronto sanatorium. And, if not her mother, then Hannah also had an elder brother with tuberculosis who suffered both cough and sputum production. Over the course of her short nine years, Hannah had been virtually surrounded by tuberculosis, emphasizing the sense of "inescapability" surrounding tuberculosis infection in Canada's endemic years.

Precisely this reality resulted in almost 45 per cent (n = 344) of the children sampled having no idea of how or why they had been exposed and infected. As children aged, the sense of inescapability extended beyond the family home as children become more integrated with their larger communities.[87] The more time spent in the community, the more likely it was that exposure and transmission could occur outside the family home, perhaps in places like schools, public transportation vehicles, churches, dance halls, health clinics, and doctor's office waiting rooms.[88] Outside the home, the disease was rife and the infection was circulating, and chances were that, sooner or later, children would encounter tuberculosis, even if they had managed to escape it in their homes. In November 1939, four-year-old Eliza was admitted to the sanatorium. Her infection presented as a mystery, since there were no other reported cases of TB in Eliza's family, and her mother, father, and all of her siblings were alive and well. Even a healthy family did not ensure freedom from infection in TB's endemic years, however, and in Eliza's case, the only possible opportunity for exposure that her parents could fathom was her regular visits to the local country store. The store had been a popular gathering spot for a group of men, many of them apparently suffering "suspicious coughs."

Eliza's infection was aggressive and progressive, diagnosed as miliary TB, which meant that tuberculosis bacteria were travelling widely and dangerously through her bloodstream. Her condition rapidly declined and she was admitted to the sanatorium in a very bad state. In late November, only a few weeks after her admission, Eliza's father received a letter from the sanatorium informing him that his daughter had developed complications over the previous day or two. The laboratory had been sent a sample of her spinal fluid, and the findings confirmed the diagnosis of tuberculous meningitis, noted in the letter to be a "fairly common complication of miliary tuberculosis," which meant that tuberculosis bacteria had reached Eliza's brain. Eliza's physician at the sanatorium was in the sad position of informing her father that they felt in all likelihood she would "go down hill very rapidly," and six days after this letter was written, Eliza died. Before antibiotics, tuberculous meningitis was responsible for about 6 per cent of deaths in the sanatorium, its progress in patients described as "rampant," typically culminating in death within three weeks of the onset of symptoms,[89] which included fever, anorexia, malaise, nausea, vomiting, headache, reduced levels of consciousness, and, at an advanced stage, coma.[90] Stories about experiences such as Eliza's, where disease appeared suddenly and aggressively, heightened anxieties about exposures outside the family home. With tuberculosis widespread in communities, virtually anyone could fall victim to infection and disease.

Differentially Diagnosing Tuberculosis in Childhood

Though a quick and accurate diagnosis might increase the chances of accessing sanatorium care sooner, diagnosing tuberculosis in children was riddled with challenges and difficulties. Comparisons of the results of physical examinations and X-ray findings confirmed that minute physiological changes overlooked by traditional examination methods could often be identified on X-ray images, particularly as the technology improved.[91] Radiology could be powerful in the interpretive hands of skilled physicians but was far from infallible, as pathological changes or small lesions could be masked by shadows created by the diaphragm, the heart, or the bones of the sternum and ribcage, and movements associated with the heartbeat could obscure, in particular, the lung's hilum (an area of particular interest, since the hilar lymph nodes were often involved in primary tuberculosis).[92] Calcified lymph nodes (especially cervical and mesenteric lymph nodes) were relatively easier to identify, provided sufficient calcium had been deposited. The deposition of calcium indicated healing or sequestering of tuberculosis bacteria within granulomas in the lymph nodes.[93] Myers, however, saw little value in chest X-rays in the case of typical primary infection in childhood, arguing that since the tuberculin test could confirm infection and because little could be done in the treatment of primary (not progressive) tuberculosis, "the making of large numbers of films periodically on the chests of children in the future should be looked upon as a waste of time and effort."[94] Where he did see the value in X-rays of children, however, was in determining the extent of primary progressive and reactivation disease. In other words, in children, X-rays were most helpful in tracking changes to pulmonary lesions in active and advancing cases.[95]

Diagnoses based on X-rays were difficult, often requiring the physicians who studied the X-rays to distinguish between tuberculosis and other diseases that could produce similar pathologies. Poor-quality images created difficulties for a sound differential diagnosis, leading to the cautionary reminder to physicians that "radiology can be a good servant, but a bad master."[96] In the case of tuberculosis, a single X-ray could not indicate anything of the status of disease activity, whether patients were experiencing an active and ongoing disease, or if their visible pathologies were old and unchanging, their TB now latent. In this case, a careful monitoring of patients, and attention to the presence of typical symptoms associated with TB, such as fever, night sweats, pallor, and weight loss, along with chronologies of X-rays, could help physicians determine if disease was latent or active and progressing. These symptoms would often come associated with reactivation disease, and, from a clinical standpoint, once these symptoms appeared a clear diagnosis could usually be made "without difficulty."[97]

Though modern doctors may have become more proficient diagnosticians, misdiagnoses were not altogether rare in tuberculosis, and patients had different experiences with this reality. Misdiagnoses leading to admissions to the Toronto sanatorium were certainly not unique. Winnie Gardiner (Gammon), a former child patient at Craig-y-nos in the late 1920s, was thought to have suffered from TB of the stomach. She described the fact that, decades after her discharge, "I was diagnosed with coeliac disease and needed only to be on a gluten free diet."[98] Another former child patient at Craig-y-nos, Edward Ellis Thomas, admitted in 1928 at seven years of age for TB of the hip, was X-rayed years later in the early 1960s because of lower back pain.[99] The X-rays revealed that he had been born with a dislocated hip, the true source of his troubles. As much as tuberculosis was under-diagnosed, particularly in the early stages of the disease, knowledge and awareness of tuberculosis made it a tempting default diagnosis for various symptoms of ill-health. Because tuberculosis was common and could affect many different organs and tissues in the body, it may have been the more often suspected culprit of illness than was actually the case.

Only complicating matters, patients or their families might choose to ignore or downplay a likely tuberculosis diagnosis for various reasons, at least until the disease progressed to its first tell-tale and distressing symptoms. Lillian was only three years old when her father died of tuberculosis.[100] Decades later, she recalled, "My mother knew that I had something wrong with me for years … but she never really admitted that I had anything." Denial was powerful, since accepting that her daughter might have tuberculosis would also mean accepting that she, like her father, might die. The day came, however, when everyone would have to face up to the reality of Lillian's poor health. Lillian remembered it well, the day "my sister and I were having a glass of pop and my sister hit me on the back [because] I got more than she did ... and I brought up some blood." And, just like that, Lillian's tuberculosis could no longer be denied. Shortly after this incident, in 1929, eight-year-old Lillian was admitted to the Toronto sanatorium. In a similar example, in his history of Nova Scotia's Kentville sanatorium, Donald Ripley recounts the events that led to thirteen-year-old Victor Cleyle's unexpected tuberculosis diagnosis and admission, a "hot day in the fall of 1944" that saw Victor and Freddie "heading back to school after lunch, with Freddie perched like an owl on the handlebars of Vic's tired, old two-wheeled bike while the pipecleaner-thin Victor's skinny muscles started the taxing, long peddle to Kentville School. Pushing the weight of Freddie up school hill to the bicycle rack made Victor feel faint; then he coughed and finally he spit up blood. It was a scary time for them both."[101] Of the various symptoms of tuberculosis, haemoptysis (coughing or spitting up blood) was most distressing. A cough was troublesome and concerning, but a cough with bleeding was most worrisome, more than likely encouraging families to seek out their physicians. Haemoptysis strongly suggested that one or both lungs had become cavitary, and this meant that tuberculosis disease was destroying lung tissue.

Among children, there were certainly challenges in distinguishing between latent and active disease, but even the very basics of infection status could be difficult to determine. As part of their illness experience, children would have to weather these periods of indecision, confusion, and repeated testing. When Clark was admitted to the sanatorium in 1943 at ten years of age, tuberculosis was strongly suspected but hard to confirm. Clark had been born on a farm in Ontario, a generally healthy infant who had been breastfed for one month and then weaned onto a cow's milk formula. The family had used unpasteurized milk from the farm's dairy herd, but always boiled the milk used in Clark's formula. When the family's herd was eventually tested in 1937, all of the cattle on the farm were found to be free from tuberculosis. From an early age, Clark had been plagued by lung trouble; a litany of diagnoses had ensued, beginning at three years of age when Clark was diagnosed with bronchitis, followed by a week of asthma, with wheezing and coughing. His troubles with asthma returned periodically, as did his tendency towards bronchitis. In 1940, Clark contracted pneumonia and was confined to bed for two weeks. He was prescribed sulpha drugs and he improved; after three months he was well enough to return to school. Six months later, however, pneumonia returned, followed by another attack of asthma, and Clark remained in bed for six weeks. This time, however, sulpha drugs proved ineffective. Almost a year later, Clark once again contracted pneumonia, followed by bronchitis. Given his ongoing struggles for health, he was referred to a Toronto hospital in July 1941, and there Clark was diagnosed with strep throat and admitted for three weeks. Upon his return home, because of his poor health, Clark was kept out of school for sixteen months, eventually returning to school in September 1942. At this time "he was active ... leading a normal outdoor life without strenuous sports, and resting 1½ hours each afternoon, in bed." In February 1943, however, the whole family, including Clark, was struck down by influenza. His previously dry cough became moist and productive and he developed a high fever. With concerns returning to tuberculosis, Clark was given a series of tuberculin tests in March 1943, all of which yielded results negative for tuberculosis infection. As a result, a firm tuberculosis diagnosis continued to elude poor Clark.

Clark's physicians were more than likely aware that co-infection with other pathogens could compromise TB skin testing results. In 1908, von Pirquet suggested that co-infection (or "intercurrent infection") with viruses (notably, the measles virus) could temporarily suppress skin reactions in tuberculin skin tests.[102] Other disease co-infections would subsequently be considered, including scarlet fever, pertussis, rubella, mononucleosis, and influenza.[103] In 1972, Reed and colleagues published a study involving patients in acute and convalescent stages of influenza virus infection, concluding that typical immune responses could be temporarily impaired by influenza, such that exposure to tuberculin in skin tests would not elicit any diagnostic skin reactivity, even if patients had, in fact, experienced prior tuberculosis infection.[104] In light of these observations of impaired immunity, their study recommended investigating influenza infection as a possible reactivation risk for latent tuberculosis. The possible link between TB and influenza in co-infected individuals has been explored in several recent studies investigating TB morbidity and mortality during, and in the aftermath of the 1918 influenza pandemic (which involved a notably virulent influenza virus strain).[105]

As stymied as they were by Clark's questionable tuberculin testing results, his physicians nonetheless opted to proceed with chest X-rays at a local hospital. Unfortunately, the X-rays were also difficult to interpret, neither confirming nor ruling out a tuberculosis diagnosis. By October 1943, Clark's family physician wrote to the sanatorium wanting him admitted because of concerns that, if tuberculous, Clark might infect his sister. The physician's recommendation for hospitalization met with some resistance, however, from Clark's family, as he suggested Clark's parents were "anything but cooperative." The frustrated physician had "been endeavouring to get a positive sputum for some time" so that he would have the evidence needed to admit Clark to the sanatorium, particularly because the physician believed Clark's "removal to an institution" would be "obligatory under such circumstances." Ultimately, however, the physician was incorrect in this belief and, since admission was not compulsory, the circumstances that led to Clark's eventual admission to the sanatorium a couple of weeks later are not clear. Clark's possible disease and the potential risk to his sister may have been enough to get Clark admitted, even despite the lack of a positive tuberculin test. No greater resolution was achieved at the sanatorium, as Clark continued to produce negative tuberculin test results. Altogether, fourteen sputum and gastric contents specimens returned negative for TB bacteria on both culture and guinea pig inoculation.

Eventually, in March 1944, Clark was transferred to a Toronto hospital where a diagnosis of non-tuberculous bilateral bronchiectasis and chronic maxillary sinusitis was made. Finally, it was understood that Clark was not suffering tuberculosis. All of those negative tuberculin skin tests had not lied. According to one physician's review on the pathogenesis of bronchiectasis, the disease often results from poor pulmonary ventilation, pleural effusion, or the accumulation of mucus in the bronchi.[106] The pressure or blockage caused by the mucus could cause atelectasis, or collapse of the tiny lung alveoli. The atelectasis, in turn, causes pressure to build in the lung, and the bronchi are forced to dilate. That stretching weakens the walls of the bronchi and, over time, leaves them dilated and unable to function properly, even after the atelectasis has resolved. While bronchial pneumonia, often a complication of measles, pertussis, and influenza, was suspected as the most common cause of the stagnant mucosal secretions that led to bronchiectasis, tuberculosis was also considered, though only infrequently, as either a precursor or associated condition. In Clark's case, the mucus may have accumulated because of his ongoing struggles with pneumonia and chronic sinusitis.

Because of shared symptoms such as hemoptysis, sputum production, fever, fatigue, weakness, weight loss, night sweats, and anemia, it is perhaps not surprising that one physician suspected a good "many bronchiectasis patients [were] in sanatoria in whom tubercle bacilli have never been found in the sputum."[107] Reinforcing this belief, like Clark, twelve-year-old Rachel Heatwole, one of Virginia's Blue Ridge sanatorium's first pediatric patients, was misdiagnosed with tuberculosis and admitted in 1921.[108] According to Cynthia Connolly and Mary Gibson, who reviewed Rachel's diary in their study of children and tuberculosis, Rachel spent about a year at Blue Ridge, eating in abundance, sleeping outdoors, and following the regimen of sanatorium life. It was some time later, when she was admitted to another sanatorium, that she was diagnosed with bronchiectasis, not tuberculosis. Since tuberculosis and bronchiectasis shared common treatment strategies, such as "long hours in bed at night and two hours in bed after lunch," heliotherapy in non-febrile patients, assistance with postural drainage of the respiratory passages, expert feeding, temporary phrenic crushes (see chapter 6), and surgical drainage of lung abscesses, it is likely that those patients, like Clark and Rachel, with bronchiectasis (but not tuberculosis) who ended up in TB sanatoria ultimately benefitted nonetheless from the general palliative and specialized regimens of care they received.[109]

Beyond pulmonary tuberculosis, diagnosing extra-pulmonary tuberculosis disease, such as skeletal tuberculosis, could also be challenging. Ira was fourteen years old when he was transferred from a Toronto hospital, suffering from what appeared to be tuberculosis of the left hip. Diagnosing Ira's case had proved difficult, since his physicians knew that conditions other than tuberculosis could be causing the arthritis affecting his hip. There was no history of tuberculosis in Ira's family and no known contacts, though if Ira's affliction proved to be tuberculosis, tuberculous cow's milk was strongly suspected as the culprit. Despite the fact that Ira was admitted in 1947, well past the introduction of routine milk pasteurization in Ontario,[110] contact with raw milk was still possible, since Ira had grown up on a farm with a dairy herd. Ira's recounting of the history of his illness, recorded at the time of his admission to the sanatorium, attests to the difficulties in determining what was ailing him. The illness was mild in its introduction, beginning with a tiredness that Ira noticed in his left thigh towards the end of the school term in December 1946. His daily half-mile walk to and from the school bus soon "aggravated" the condition and was "relieved" only when Ira "took the weight off his left leg by standing on the right." It was around this time that, in the bathtub one evening, Ira "noticed that the left knee seemed nearer his hip than the right," and that "he could not adjust this asymmetry, due to some stiffness." At this point, Ira was taken to the family physician and an X-ray was ordered. Ultimately, Ira's physician believed him to be suffering a broken back, but by early January he advised Ira's parents that he should be taken to hospital to have his hip investigated further. At the hospital, motivated by tuberculosis suspicions, numerous X-ray films were taken and fluid was aspirated from Ira's left hip joint, but the films were inconclusive and the culture for tuberculosis bacteria was negative. At a standstill in his diagnosis, Ira was then transferred to the sanatorium on 28 February for further investigation and observation. Scrutinizing a new set of X-ray films, physicians at the sanatorium believed they were observing some of the early characteristic changes associated with bone and joint tuberculosis, including some generalized osteoporosis and a narrowing of the joint space between Ira's pelvic bone and the head of his femur. Another culture of pus aspirated from his hip joint, however, still did not yield TB bacteria. At this time, Ira's chief complaint was an extreme tiredness of his left hip and leg.

Though his diagnosis was still pending, tuberculosis was strongly suspected, so it was felt that Ira's hip would benefit from a period of traction and immobilization in a hip spica (a plaster cast applied around his hip to immobilize the femur/pelvis joint; see chapter 6). After Ira had spent just over two years in bed in a hip cast, his physicians felt that the disease was sufficiently inactive to allow for a surgical fusion of Ira's hip joint in order to permanently immobilize the affected area (and, hopefully, permanently arrest the suspected tuberculous disease). Ira was transferred to a Toronto hospital for this surgery where an iliofemoral and ischiofemoral extra-articular arthrodesis (surgical fixation of the bones of the pelvis and femur, which would eventually lead to the fusion of these bones, see chapter 6) was performed to stabilize Ira's hip. After some further months of post-operative care and recuperation, Ira was deemed fit for discharge and ready to return to school, his hip then apparently healed and the disease process latent.

Similar to the challenges in diagnosing Ira's tuberculous hip, identifying tuberculosis of the spine could also prove difficult.[111] Evan, fourteen years of age, was admitted to the sanatorium in May 1938, strongly suspected to be suffering from tuberculosis of the spine. In mid-December 1937, Evan had developed a mild abdominal pain. Lacking any other signs or symptoms of disease and working under a tentative diagnosis of appendicitis, Evan's family physician prescribed four days of bedrest and Evan's pain disappeared. A few days after completing his bedrest, Evan went skiing, had a fall, and injured his back. His back pain lasted for a few days and then returned irregularly for some time afterwards. In the meantime, Evan had been excused from his physical education class at school. In the months leading up to his sanatorium admission, Evan, who used to be able to reach down and touch his toes with ease, could barely touch his knees. When asked, he reported that coughing and sneezing did not aggravate the pain he felt, but bending over did, as well as going up or down stairs. His only relief came from lying down.

By mid-April, Evan began to tire easily and the pain in his back had grown worse, now interfering with his ability to do homework at night because he needed to take breaks to rest his back in bed. On the advice of their physician, Evan's parents decided that he would not return to school after the Easter holidays and, in April, he was again examined. Evan's hips were X-rayed, though no abnormalities were revealed. Another set of X-rays was taken further up his spine, and a pathology involving the vertebrae of his lower back was discovered. In between this second set of X-rays, taken at the end of April, and his admission to the sanatorium in the first week of May, Evan had been kept at home in bed with a stiff fracture board placed under his mattress for additional support. He had been allowed up to use the bathroom, but all of his meals were served to him in bed. In his personal history, it was noted that he recalled no contact with tuberculosis and had always consumed pasteurized milk. Until the pain in his back appeared, he had led an active life and walked four miles to school every day. Upon his admission to the sanatorium, Evan was diagnosed with spinal tuberculosis, and he remained in the hospital for just over one year, first immobilized in his bed and then undergoing a spinal fusion (see chapter 6), which arrested the disease. Relatively speaking, this was a fast discharge, particularly for spinal tuberculosis, as most children treated before surgical techniques were refined remained in the sanatorium for years, spending much of that time on bedrest, with casts or traction with weights used to help stabilize their bones and prevent further pathologies and deformities, and with the hope that their tuberculosis disease would not spread to other organs or tissues in the meantime.

Overall, in their attempts to diagnose tuberculosis in children, physicians often relied upon the clustering of symptoms that presented in each case. Unfortunately, the children themselves sometimes overlooked symptoms, unaware that seemingly minor aches and pains could be due to something much more serious. This was the case for Kathryn, who was originally admitted to the sanatorium for the treatment of pulmonary TB in 1931, when she was twelve years of age. The routine physical examination undertaken at the time of her admission revealed a "deformity" in her lower back. She had no sensation or complaints of pain, but upon further questioning it was learned that two years earlier she had experienced some relatively "slight discomfort," which, in retrospect, her examining physician believed probably marked the onset of her spinal trouble.

The "deformity" in Kathryn's back was a moderate kyphosis in the lumbar region of her spine; research suggests that in early stages of kyphosis, deformity results because of muscle spasms, which Kathryn reported she never felt, but in later stages of the disease the deformity is linked to an actual shortening of soft tissue attachments and progressive bone destruction.[112] Apart from the deformity, no other signs or symptoms would have alerted the examining physician to spinal tuberculosis. Kathryn had never experienced pain upon movement. This was not atypical, since Giessler notes that pain is not a constant, some feeling pain upon movement, while others do not, and that the kyphus often becomes visible or palpable before any pain sensations become apparent to the sufferer.[113] One hallmark feature of more advanced spinal tuberculosis, a "psoas abscess" (a tuberculous infection of the psoas muscle) was also not observed in Kathryn's case. Paired psoas muscles attach on either side of the dorsal lumbar vertebrae, run inferiorly on each side of the body down and around the pelvic bones, and attach to the lesser trochanters at the proximal end of the left and right femurs. It is at the site of attachment to infected and pathological lumbar vertebrae that tuberculosis bacteria can spread within the sheath of the psoas muscle, causing infection and abscess. The muscles play a critical role in upright posture, and a psoas abscess is typically associated with restricted and painful movement. Historically, psoas abscesses were so commonly associated with advanced cases of spinal tuberculosis that the presence of a psoas abscess was read as a fairly sure sign of tuberculosis.[114]

An X-ray would reveal what seemed entirely unapparent to Kathryn, a destructive lesion involving the lower half of her twelfth thoracic vertebral body and the upper half of her first lumbar vertebral body, two vertebrae that lay adjacent to each other in the spine. The intervertebral disc between these two vertebrae had been destroyed, eaten away by active tuberculosis disease. In the pathology of spinal tuberculosis, Steinbock targets the first lumbar vertebra as the most common initial site of spinal infection, since tuberculosis bacteria may access this vertebra, in particular, from nearby kidneys and lymph nodes.[115] The intervertebral discs positioned between adjacent vertebra are usually involved early in the disease process, though Aufderheide and Rodriguez-Martin note that complete destruction, as in Kathryn's case, is usually rare.[116] It is likely that because Kathryn's two adjacent vertebra (the twelfth thoracic and the first lumbar) were affected by disease, there was a rapid destruction of the intervertebral disc since, as an avascular structure, it was denied necessary nutrients from both vertebrae (if only one vertebra had been affected, perhaps the disc could have been adequately nourished by the remaining healthy vertebra). The onset of spinal tuberculosis and the destruction of these vertebrae was believed to have developed slowly over a two-year period. Once again, cases like Kathryn's stoked tuberculosis anxieties, with significant bone- or lung-destroying lesions progressing all the while unnoticed by those affected and casting doubts on seemingly well bodies.

Once Kathryn's spinal tuberculosis was identified, she was placed on the "usual regimen." Initially, she had been set up for prolonged recumbency in bed and treated with both heliotherapy and UV light therapy.

She was a "strict bed patient" with no toilet or bathroom privileges. A spinal fusion was considered for Kathryn, as Dobbie explained in a letter to her mother in July 1931, that her tuberculous spine "must either be operated on or else she must lie on her back on a frame perfectly still, for a year or two." Either way, Dobbie suggested, the condition had to be addressed, otherwise Kathryn risked "becoming a chronic invalid with the great probability of her back becoming badly deformed." Since the sanatorium's visiting surgeon, Robert Harris,[117] thought that Kathryn was inclined to be "restless," he felt that surgery would be the better choice for her. The spinal fusion would lead to faster recovery, though she would still be required to "rest quietly on her back" for at least a year afterwards. Dobbie met with Kathryn's mother to review the potential risks and benefits of the surgery, at which time she gave her consent. The fusion was a success and Kathryn left the sanatorium in October 1932. While she was still required to wear a spinal brace for some months, both her pulmonary and spinal disease were felt to be latent.

Bodily Resistance and Susceptibility: Individuals and Populations

For some children admitted to the sanatorium, the road to health could be very long, particularly among those with poor resistance to tuberculosis. Yolanda was a case in point, seven years old when she was admitted in June 1920. Orphaned, her mother had died of TB and her father had deserted the family, Yolanda had been brought to the sanatorium by her grandmother. Because of what appeared to be a very aggressive disease process, her prognosis at that time was not good. In addition to advanced and chronic pulmonary TB and multiple discharging tuberculous abscesses[118] all over her body, Yolanda suffered from spinal tuberculosis, which had severely deformed her spine by both kyphosis (a hump-back curvature) and scoliosis (a lateral curvature). Yolanda's grandmother was far from confident that she could provide the kind of skilled care that Yolanda clearly needed, her condition ever-worsening.

Gradually, Yolanda's condition improved at the sanatorium, but staff had to help her cope with periodic fevers and the discharging abscesses, some of which healed but some of which were much more persistent. The main treatment adopted by the staff, in addition to routine cleaning of the abscesses, was daily UV light treatment. In June 1928, a report on Yolanda's condition was sent by Dobbie to the municipal office that had assumed, increasingly begrudging as the years marched on, her maintenance costs. "While she is in good general condition now and attends school every day," Dobbie advised, "it must not be forgotten that she has had T.B. abscesses on almost every part of her body; that she has had cervical adenitis and T.B. peritonitis; that she has scoliosis and kyphosis of the spine, and the lower ribs flared out on both sides; [and] she still has two small abscesses on the lower part of her back." Dobbie emphasized that, as long as Yolanda benefited by "being treated and kept under good conditions she will probably do well," but that any "lack of these for any length of time would almost certainly result in her going under again" because of her general "poor resistance" to tuberculosis. This report was written just over eight years after Yolanda's admission to the sanatorium summarizing the ravaging effects on her body, from swollen cervical lymph nodes, to tuberculous abscesses, peritonitis, and spinal disease. Despite her exceedingly poor prognosis at admission, Yolanda improved and, in April 1929, almost a year after this note was written, she was discharged and returned to her grandmother's care.

Like Yolanda, many of the children who entered the sanatorium had low resistance to tuberculosis and were hospitalized because they suffered active disease. Yet there was great diversity in the patients sampled, some children experiencing relatively symptom-less primary infection, while others, Yolanda included, suffered more overtly symptomatic and aggressive disease. But what factors could be called upon to account for this great variability in disease expression and vulnerability? Relative resistance or susceptibility to active tuberculosis could be mitigated not only by the strain and virulence of the tuberculosis bacterium involved, but also the size of the bacterial inoculum at infection and the success or failure of individual immune response.

The size of the inoculum relates to the degree and intensity of exposure of children to infectious cases. Research suggests that tuberculosis infection occurring within the family home, particularly the close contacts between parents and children, could be more severe than infection resulting from casual contacts with infectious cases.[119] The duration of exposure needed for transmission to occur varies, depending on the infectiousness of the source case; adults with tuberculous lung cavities (which tend to produce a high concentration of bacteria in sputum), and a high frequency of coughing (which brings both sputum and bacteria up from the lungs and has been found to be positively correlated with the degree of pulmonary involvement) may result in "successful" transmission over lower durations of exposure.[120] Delia was a young schoolgirl when she was admitted to the sanatorium in 1929. While her mother and six brothers and sisters were all alive and well, her father had died of tuberculosis by the time she was hospitalized. Her cot report for 1930 suggested, "It is difficult to trace the source of infection in this case [but] a massive dose it must have been to reduce a young child to poor Delia's state." Delia's father was strongly suspected to have been the source of her infection. Other exposure dynamics relate to factors such as crowding in the home (where a low square footage per person could increase the likelihood of regular contact with an infectious case), and home ventilation, particularly outside (or "fresh") air ventilation, which may help to dilute, redistribute, or remove (with good cross-ventilation provided by windows on opposite walls[121]) tuberculosis bacteria carried in the air and shared by family members.[122] A long period of exposure to airborne bacteria in poorly ventilated homes and buildings was problematic,[123] particularly given Starke's contention that "an adult who would be mildly infectious in an open environment may be highly infectious in a poorly ventilated area."[124]

In a 1920 publication in *Canadian Practitioner*, Dobbie urged greater attention to the age-related risks of infection among children.[125] Children less than three years of age, Dobbie argued, were particularly vulnerable to aggressive tuberculosis disease and high mortality; as a result, he strongly encouraged strict separation of infectious mothers and fathers from their young children. Once past the vulnerable ages under three years, Dobbie reasoned that it would be best for children to experience their first tuberculosis infection (which seemed almost inevitable) outside the home, since smaller dose exposures might gently stimulate (but not overwhelm) immunity. By this time, the family home had been conceptualized as the place of "massive" doses of infection:

> After three years of age ... the child must be carefully introduced to the tubercle bacillus so that he may prepare his defense against it. As the child must soon go out into the world, and there mingle with strangers of all kinds, it is obvious that he will at some time meet with the tubercle bacilli and become infected ... immunity is developed by repeated small doses, and ... disease is produced by massive doses of infection. What we should aim to do then is to protect the child from massive infections such as might be had from tuberculous persons living in the house. These children are not likely to receive massive doses from strangers.[126]

In this sense, Dobbie viewed the family home as a more dangerous site of primary infection than repeated, smaller, perhaps therapeutic exposures and infections occurring via more casual contacts with community and strangers.

In addition to crowding and ventilation, other home characteristics are believed to influence exposure, transmission, and vulnerability. Recent studies have examined the impact of smoking on TB disease, finding that the lungs of TB-infected smokers have a greater tendency to develop more tuberculous cavitary lesions.[127] Since lung cavities are typically associated with higher levels of bacteria released in coughing, speaking, and breathing, children living in smoking homes may have experienced greater exposure to TB bacteria. There is also a possibility that the passive smoking experienced by children in the home may have lowered their disease resistance, resulting in more cases of active tuberculosis disease.[128] Smoking became a more widespread phenomenon in early- to mid-twentieth-century Canada, particularly with the relaxation of gendered smoking norms. In 1920s Canada, women's public smoking gained more acceptability, associated, as it was, with the "strength, passion, sophistication ... independence, and even rebellion" of employed women[129] and with the fashionable "elite feminine smoking culture" as espoused, for example, in the pages of *Vogue* magazine.[130]

It is perhaps ironic that the greater infection risks associated with smoking actually resulted, in part, from anti-tuberculosis measures. In the heyday of endemic TB, public spitting came to be viewed as a highly undesirable and unwanted hazard. Dr Holbrook, of Hamilton's Mountain Sanatorium, targeted improper management of sputum, and careless spitting in particular, as an important source of tuberculosis infection among children. TB bacteria, he argued, could be inhaled "with the dust from city streets due to the polluters of streets by spitting ... undoubtedly, it is a menace to young children who play in the streets, and it is a habit at once so filthy and so easily prevented that it is almost impossible to understand how any persons who give the matter a moment's thought can allow themselves to become offenders."[131] Alongside the mandatory use of cuspidors or spittoons, sputum fears encouraged many municipalities to enact anti-spitting by-laws. Toronto's by-law came into effect on 1 June 1904, when violators could be fined one dollar (plus costs) or given three days in jail if found spitting on sidewalks, in public buildings, or on streetcars.[132] Not only was spitting in these places viewed as "unnecessary" and "disgusting," but also "deadly" in light of the risks of tuberculosis transmission, with bacteria from wet or dried sputum "carried home on people's boots, by ladies' skirts, or wafted around by the wind in the dust" (which begs the question of how much of a direct or indirect influence tuberculosis prevention had on the rising hemlines of women's skirts and dresses in the early twentieth century).[133] As public spitting became a social disgrace, cigarettes offered an alternative to tobacco chewing (which required spitting), and smoking grew more common.[134] Smoking, though strongly discouraged (but not prohibited) by medical and nursing staff, was certainly observed among adult and adolescent patients at the Toronto sanatorium, including nineteen-year-old Garrett, whose tobacco and rolling papers were confiscated after he was found smoking on the post-operative ward following his thoracoplasty (rib removal) surgery in 1936 (see chapter 7).

Resistance or vulnerability to tuberculosis could be shaped by the biological and social realities of life, forces that could either boost or dampen immunity. Generally speaking, good nutrition translates into better immune function and therefore greater individual resistance to a wide variety of pathogens, though not all infectious disease resistance is equally affected by nutritional status. Susceptibility to pneumonia and measles, for example, has been strongly linked to nutritional deficiencies, while nutritional status has no apparent effect on the course of viral encephalitis and tetanus infections.[135] Tuberculosis is an infectious disease with known links to nutritional status as the functioning of cell-mediated immunity (the T_h1 immune pathway) so critical to tuberculosis resistance is particularly vulnerable to the effects of poor nutrition.[136] Since most children admitted to the sanatorium were free patients, their parents or guardians having proven that they were unable to afford the costs of their hospitalization, it would not be surprising if a large proportion of them were either undernourished (not enough food) or malnourished (not enough nutritious food). In 1920, a publication of Toronto's Neighbourhood Workers' Association noted, "There are few starving children in Toronto but there are very many under-nourished children, not receiving food of the right kind, and who are consequently undersized and under weight."[137]

Protein deficiencies have attracted particular attention in relation to tuberculosis-related immunity.[138] Indeed, protein calorie malnutrition (or protein energy malnutrition) has been linked to increased vulnerability to a wide range of pathogens. In their review, Schaible and Kaufmann describe research linking severe protein malnutrition in infants and young children to atrophy of the thymus (an organ of the lymphatic system involved in the production of T-lymphocytes, white blood cells that boost immunity to tuberculosis[139]), ill-developed lymph nodes and spleens, diminished T-cell counts, alterations to protective gut mucosa, reduced abilities of phagocytes (such as macrophages) to engulf and eliminate pathogens, and reduced concentrations of leptin, a hormone produced in adipose tissue that plays a role in activating or regulating diverse immune cells in the body.[140] According to Cegielski and McMurray, studies of protein-deprived tuberculous guinea pigs link protein deficiency with an inability "to regulate the normal recirculation and trafficking of T-lymphocytes," critical to the formation of the granulomas involved in the sequestering of tuberculosis bacteria and the transition to latent disease.[141] The guinea pig studies also suggest that the effects of protein deficiency on immune function are "substantially and rapidly reversible," with positive dietary changes resulting in relatively quick resurgences in immune resistance to tuberculosis.[142]

Along with factors like nutritional status, individual disease histories also play a role in tuberculosis susceptibility. The health of children admitted to the sanatorium was often compromised not by a single disease, tuberculosis, but aggressive synergies resulting from successive diseases or co-infections, often paired with degrees of malnutrition or undernutrition. In early to mid-twentieth-century Canada, a number of diseases, along with tuberculosis, were in common circulation among children. Measles, in particular, was strongly associated with tuberculosis susceptibility. As measles retreated in twentieth-century Canada with ongoing vaccination programs, other diseases that have since emerged in prevalence, such as HIV/AIDS and diabetes, have also been found to increase tuberculosis disease risk. As a result, potential synergies shift as the constitution of population disease environments change. In the sanatorium era, in the case of measles, physicians learned to be on guard for early signs of meningeal tuberculosis in children recovering from measles, particularly "when drowsiness and coma come on more than a week after the measles rash."[143] The metabolic demands of measles infection were understood to lead to nutritional depletion among children in the infection's aftermath and increased their vulnerability to tuberculosis; other common early twentieth-century infections, such as gastrointestinal infections and parasites, have also been linked with malnutrition and tuberculosis vulnerability.[144]

The role of vitamin A has attracted particular attention in these disease linkages with tuberculosis. Vitamin A deficiency not only increases the risks of measles infection, with vitamin A deficient children more likely to die of measles, but the measles infection itself can also deplete the body's vitamin A reserves, setting up a susceptibility to other infections such as tuberculosis.[145] Vitamin A deficiency has been linked more broadly to a number of respiratory and gastrointestinal infections, not only because of immunosuppression, but also because the vitamin plays a key role maintaining the epithelial cells that line these tracts, cells that are important physical barriers to infection.[146] Chandra reports that the epithelial cells of children deficient in vitamin A are more likely to permit epithelial surface adherence, colonization, and mucosal penetration by pathogenic bacteria, rendering them more susceptible to infection and ultimately disease.[147] While naturally occurring vitamin A is found in dairy products, liver, oils, eggs, green leafy vegetables, and orange vegetables and fruit, Kosek and Oberhelman suggest that deficiencies of vitamin A were "extremely common, especially among persons living in poverty," and particularly before the fortification of foods with vitamin A in the 1920s.[148]

Prior to vaccination campaigns, the highly transmissible measles virus caused epidemic outbreaks in Canada regularly every few years.[149] In 1924, measles became a reportable disease and, with a more accurate tracking system in place, the highest Canadian incidence of measles (since 1924) was observed in 1935 with more than 83,000 cases of measles reported in that year alone.[150] Effective measles control evolved in Canada in the mid-1960s with the introduction of the first measles vaccine. By the early 1970s, one-year-old children were routinely vaccinated, and the average annual incidence rate for measles fell dramatically (from 358 per 100,000 in 1949–58 to 30 per 100,000 in 1976–85).[151] For most of the sanatorium era in Canada, therefore, measles was a common disease and, mediated through complex effects such as vitamin A deficiency, may have either facilitated tuberculosis infection or lowered tuberculosis resistance among children. Measles presented a particular tuberculosis vulnerability in the disease ecology of the times, but such ecologies could and did change.

Host resistance, or host immunity, plays a critical role in mediating the interaction between bodies and tuberculosis infection and is the product of both individual- and population-level constructs. Population adaptations to disease environments are grounded in evolution and a genetic perspective on immunity. In the history of human evolution, there are many excellent examples of the interactions between human biology, disease, and the environment; perhaps the classic example involves the evolution of red blood cell hemoglobin variants (sickle cell and the thalassemias) and surviving malaria.[152] Human relationships with *Mycobacterium tuberculosis* have been evolving ever since the pathogen's original associations with human populations deep in antiquity, perhaps 35,000 years ago or so (it was long believed, but now refuted, that the relationship was struck only about 10,000 years ago with the agricultural Neolithic Revolution and cattle domestication).[153] Because of different population histories, trajectories, and subsistence strategies, there were important population differences in ancestral experiences with tuberculosis bacteria. As a case in point, in their research, Larcombe and colleagues explore differences in immune adaptations distinguishing ancestral Old World (e.g., European) and New World (e.g., Indigenous) populations; their research considers differences in immune responses favouring either a T_h1 (T helper 1, linked to cell-mediated immunity and important in tuberculosis) or Th2 (T helper 2, linked to humoral or antibody-mediated immunity) response.[154] Over the course of evolutionary history, as many Old World (e.g., European) populations turned to agricultural subsistence, settled into a sedentary existence, grew in size, and were affected by "crowd infections" such as smallpox, measles, plague, and tuberculosis, they adapted a stronger Th1 immune response (through evolutionary forces such as natural selection and gene flow). Meanwhile, in the New World, Indigenous communities adapted to their environments via different modes of subsistence, some following a more mobile hunting-and-gathering lifestyle with smaller population sizes. Immunity adaptations in the New World may have been less influenced by epidemic or endemic bacterial or viral infections, but more affected by parasitic and fungal diseases.[155] In this case, Larcombe and colleagues argue, selection favoured a stronger Th2 response to protect against these common stressors. Generally, then, Old World populations were more likely to favour the Th1 response, offering protection against tuberculosis, while New World populations adapted a Th2 response towards other important disease protections. While paleomicrobiological studies (involving ancient DNA) have confirmed the presence of *Mycobacterium tuberculosis* in the New World prior to European contact,[156] it has been reasoned by Larcombe and colleagues that the pathogen likely circulated at low frequencies and did not exert a significant selective pressure on immune function among Indigenous populations in Canada. Given these environmentally tailored immunological adaptations, the subsequent importation of more virulent tuberculosis strains to the Americas with European immigration,[157] commingling with the gross inequalities (such as poverty, oppression, and harsh acculturation) that manifested under colonialism, would be devastating for Indigenous peoples in Canada.[158]

Of the 822 children sampled for this study, 736 cases identified the child's ancestry and birthplace. Thirty-nine of the children were of Indigenous ancestry, while 697 were Canadian or immigrant children of other, diverse ancestries. While 15.5 per cent (n = 108) of the non-Indigenous children sampled died at the sanatorium, an overwhelming 51.3 per cent (n = 20) of the Indigenous children sampled died at the sanatorium. A number of factors must be considered to account for this large difference in mortality, including both admission and discharge biases. In comparison to children with primary disease, for example, children admitted with advanced reactivation disease were less likely to benefit from resistance building and survive their disease. Discharge dynamics could also distort interpretations of the numbers. There were many examples evident in the cases sampled of parents who chose to discharge their morbidly ill children from the sanatorium so that they might die at home. There is a discharge bias, however, since this would have been far easier for parents living in the vicinity of Toronto and more difficult for Indigenous parents if they were living remotely or on distant reserves.

The vulnerability of Indigenous children to tuberculosis did not go unnoticed among Indigenous families and communities, understandably raising anxieties and apprehensions over both tuberculosis and hospitalization. As a case in point, Addie, an Indigenous child, was nine years old when she was admitted to the Toronto sanatorium in the winter of 1922. She had lost both of her parents – either to influenza or tuberculosis, the family history was uncertain. When admitted, Addie was described as "very, very ill." Though she "came among strangers" and could not speak English, she was reported to have picked up the language quite easily and to have made many friends at the hospital along the way. In February 1923, Dobbie received a letter from Addie's adoptive mother, clearly expressing her wish, whether Addie was tuberculous or not, to have her daughter returned home: "Please send Addie at this way as soon as you can. I do not want her to die for at that Hospital. You must gave her good medicone [medicine]. The goverment will pay her[159] and her money is over there. It is good for nothing when they go over there[.] the Indains die. If she is sick or not you will send her home ... You must give her some clothes or warm blanket to put over her. This is all. Please send my daughter as soon as you can." It is evident from Addie's mother's letter that there was a general feeling that "Indian" children died in sanatoria and that she did not want to lose Addie in this way. Addie's mother's fear of institutions such as the sanatorium and the prospect of long-term separation from her daughter was far from unwarranted. For generations, since the rise of residential schools in the 1880s,[160] Indigenous children had been removed from their homes and communities as the harsh acculturation agenda of colonialism played out. Since families understood that Indigenous children died at residential schools, it is understandable that faith in the sanatorium, yet another colonial institution, would be questionable. In Canada, the history of such institutions lingers, exerting powerful effects on how tuberculosis and tuberculosis treatment in hospitals is viewed today among some Indigenous peoples.[161] Addie did not die in the sanatorium, but she was also not discharged at the time of her mother's request, spending almost two more years in the hospital before returning home. At the time of her discharge, however, Addie's tuberculosis infection was entirely latent and she returned home to her mother in good health.

A few years later, Walter, a sixteen-year-old Indigenous child from northern Ontario, was admitted to the sanatorium in August 1927. Soon after his arrival, Walter wrote to his mother, expressing his wish to return home. His mother, in turn, wrote to her Indian agent because, like Addie's mother, she was worried that her son would not recover from tuberculosis and wanted him back home with her. The Indian agent wrote to Dobbie for guidance, feeling it relevant to add his personal belief that he did "not think it advisable for his return until he recovers, as they only live the Indian mode of life and camp under tents during 8 or 9 months of the year" (a notable flaw in his argument, since many families bringing home former sanatorium patients set up backyard tents in which to isolate and nurse them in fresh air). In his reply to the Indian agent, Dobbie outlined the seriousness of Walter's condition, "a bilateral case of tuberculosis with involvement of the whole of the left lung and some extensions into the right." Despite the advanced nature of Walter's disease, some improvement had been realized in his case, and this likely inspired a belief that he could benefit from further sanatorium care. Since his admission, Walter had gained fifteen pounds, maintained a normal temperature, and had no cough and very little sputum. Dobbie understood that Walter was terribly homesick but advised that he remain at the sanatorium at least until the spring of 1928, when his condition could be re-evaluated. Despite the initial encouragement of his improvement, however, Walter's disease was advanced, widespread, and unpredictable. His health gradually began to fail, and he died in the sanatorium in September 1928. The inventory of Walter's belongings reveals the careful attention that he had paid to the details of his wardrobe and appearances, from wool and silk socks to the finishing touches of neckties, a set of cufflinks, and a tie pin. At his mother's request and at great expense to her (since municipalities and the federal government would pay only for local burials), Walter's body and belongings were sent home to her via the Canadian Pacific Railway so that he could be laid to rest alongside his father and five siblings.

As evident in Walter's case, Indian agents could exert powerful influence, intervening with their own beliefs and preferences, instead of simply operating as neutral liaisons for communications between Indigenous parents and sanatorium staff. As another case in point, when nine-year-old Samuel was admitted to the sanatorium in January 1925, his prognosis was determined to be very poor. Samuel was diagnosed with advanced pulmonary TB, and tuberculosis of the spine, hip, and knee, a devastating scope of disease effects suggestive of Samuel's low resistance to TB. Samuel spent over eight years in the sanatorium before succumbing to tuberculosis in June 1933. Samuel's chart presents a detailed record of examinations that attest to his prolonged struggle with complicated, fulminating, and advancing tuberculosis. Samuel suffered deep, discharging tuberculous abscesses, and because of them, he could not be considered for any of the surgical treatments for pulmonary or skeletal tuberculosis that were emerging in the 1920s and 1930s, at least not until those abscesses healed (which they did not). As a result, staff were limited in what they could actually do for Samuel, providing him with supportive care, a nutritious diet, and UV therapy to target those discharging abscesses and help build his resistance to the disease; to "brighten the days for this little sufferer," Samuel's cot sponsor was told of the occupational therapy that he was provided with two days a week. Over his eight years of hospitalization, each note to Samuel's cot sponsor emphasized his optimism in the face of such devastating disease; Samuel found "joy" in the occupational therapy, Samuel was "patient and cheerful," Samuel "keeps a cheerful spirit with the help of books which are his greatest delight." Samuel's last cot note was written in December 1932, about six months before he died, and was decidedly more melancholy: "Still another year of bed for poor Samuel and still the same cheerful submission to his fate. The magazines and papers sent to Samuel throughout the year have meant more to him than the donors will ever appreciate. The School Teacher is giving some bedside instruction to Samuel this year but he seems to prefer to live in his own books of adventure – adventures which will always be denied him." Relative to earlier cot notes, this narrative suggests that Samuel had begun to give in to his slow decline by tuberculosis, perhaps realizing that he was getting worse, not better, at the sanatorium.

About three years after Samuel's admission, his mother had travelled a long distance to Toronto to visit both him and his sister at the sanatorium. At the time of her visit, she expressed her wish to take her children back home with her to northern Ontario. Her choice was likely influenced by the fact that, during her visit, she had been informed that, because of his advanced and complicated disease and continuing decline, there was ultimately very little hope for Samuel's recovery. Understanding his fate, Samuel's mother wanted to have her son home if he was going to die. She originally sent her request to her Indian agent, who then forwarded her letter to Dobbie. In his letter, the Indian agent explained to Dobbie that Samuel's mother was living in a very small shack near an out-of-the-way station along the Canadian Pacific Railway tracks. Intervening, the agent explicitly questioned Samuel's mother's abilities to provide her son with the kind of care that he needed. Dobbie responded to the Indian agent, explaining, "I told her that Samuel's condition was practically hopeless; but that he might live for a long time. She was anxious to take him home and let him die there. We tried to discourage her in this, as the boy, owing to the number of abscesses on his body, required skilled nursing care, for the boy's own comfort, and to prevent infection of others ... we agree with you, that Samuel should be left where he is." Sanatorium staff had no real authority or means to prevent the discharge of patients, but Samuel's mother likely did not know that she could have insisted upon the discharge of her son, even if the expectation was that he would die and even if there were infection risks. The inequality is readily apparent, particularly in the authority exercised by the Indian agent who had argued to prevent Samuel's discharge at the time of his mother's request. Much as Dobbie had anticipated, Samuel lingered at the sanatorium in a slow decline for five more years before he died. From both Samuel's and his mother's perspectives, serious questions can be raised about whether it was better for him to have weathered these years in hospital, or to have been returned to his mother's home where he may have lived for only a short time, but died in her care. Samuel's mother's inability to effect her son's discharge furthers the perspective on the trauma of colonialism, as her status, her gender, and her lack of means colluded to prevent her son's return home. In the end, because of her distance from the sanatorium, all that Samuel's mother received was a telegram informing her of her son's death.

The impact of tuberculosis among Indigenous peoples in Canada is linked to histories of marginalization, social and economic repression, and injurious colonial institutions such as residential schools, all of which heightened tuberculosis vulnerability. Potentially low physiological resistance to tuberculosis seated in overwhelming poverty, the stressors of colonization, and deplorable living conditions on reserves led to acute, aggressive, fulminating expressions of tuberculosis, as evident in Samuel's case.[162] But it was also the emotional toll of hospitalization and separation, with many families ultimately permanently separated by death, that lingered in the memories of those most deeply affected by tuberculosis.

Menace, Danger, and Fear: Life with Chronic Infection

Many of the children admitted to the Toronto sanatorium would escape the ravages of tuberculosis and grow up and into adulthood. Although deaths were not uncommon, the majority of children of sampled (83 per cent) were discharged in varying states of health or disease. For those children who were discharged, both their status as ex-sanatorium patients and the enduring presence of latent or active bacteria in their bodies entrenched their lifetime association with tuberculosis. Since the infection could reactivate throughout life, questions might be raised regarding any lingering impacts of diagnosis, hospitalization, and disease in youth. The sanatorium regimen and training ensured that patients knew what this meant and that they would need to lead cautious, measured lives if they were to preserve their health over the long term. A sense of responsibility, sometimes giving rise to an acute self-consciousness, was another by-product of their tuberculosis education, a feeling that they must try to prevent infecting others once they were discharged back to their family homes and communities.

This state of knowing could easily translate into "felt stigma," defined by Graham Scambler and Anthony Hopkins as feelings of shame, self-doubt, or unacceptability, in this case the result of ex-patients' connections with tuberculosis.[163] According to Scambler and Hopkins, "felt stigma" is often fuelled by an underlying fear of "enacted stigma," whereby, in this case, ex-sanatorium patients could be actively discriminated against or stigmatized as a result of their perceived unacceptability, inferiority, or "danger." Scambler and Hopkins believe that felt stigma is often more disruptive to life than enacted stigma, since experiences with enacted stigma are typically less common than the lingering, weighing emotional effects, such as anxiety, unhappiness, and self-doubt, of felt stigma. In reality, ex-sanatorium patients could experience both types of stigma and, for some children, the impact of enacted stigma was immediate. Returning to their communities after discharge with little secrecy about their hospitalization (especially if their municipalities had paid their hospitalization charges), some children were dealt unwelcoming homecomings outside of their families. Such was the case for Lillian, discharged from the sanatorium at ten years of age in 1931. She recalled that the parents of her childhood friend who lived across the street had instructed their daughter that she was no longer allowed to play with Lillian. In fact, she was not even allowed to speak with Lillian, though, as Lillian remembered, "she would sneak over every once in a while and we would play together or talk together." Ultimately, when Lillian returned to school, she experienced the same response, recalling, "People shied away from me."[164] Ostracized by her classmates, "everybody was afraid to talk to you in case they got the disease." Lillian did not enjoy her troubled return to school. Lillian's story, and the stories that follow, highlight a tension in tuberculosis, balanced between individual and community commitments to tuberculosis philanthropy on the one hand, and the fear and even rejection of tuberculosis sufferers on the other.

In one such case, Dobbie received a letter from a family doctor in 1935, concerned because the father of a former patient, Cordelia, had received a note from his school board requesting that he permanently withdraw his daughter from classes. Apparently, the board's "action was taken because of fears expressed by parents of other girls in the class" that Cordelia would infect their daughters with tuberculosis. Cordelia's father was disappointed with the request, since he felt that his daughter had made great improvements since returning home from the sanatorium, eating well, putting on weight, and taking good rest. The doctor asked Dobbie to write to him with his opinion on any potential dangers associated with Cordelia's mingling with her classmates. In his reply, Dobbie judged "that she is not a source of danger to those with whom she may come in contact at school," because her disease had been latent at discharge and because tuberculosis bacteria had never been found in her sputum the whole time that she was at the sanatorium. Dobbie was unequivocal in his opinion that Cordelia was not an infection risk and that she should not be denied the opportunity to attend school. It was easy for others to identify a potential infection risk in Cordelia, since she was obviously an ex-sanatorium patient, but in the era of endemic TB there would be many schoolchildren not hospitalized for TB who were nonetheless both tuberculous and infectious.

Even within family homes, concerns could be raised when a family member returned from the sanatorium. Like Cordelia, children with primary disease, even those discharged against medical advice, typically represented very little "danger." Children with cavitary reactivation disease, on the other hand, could be infectious, but, in reality, just about any children could reactivate in the years following their return home. Jane had been admitted to the Toronto sanatorium at sixteen years of age in April 1936. By June 1938, sanatorium physicians felt that she could be discharged and sent home as long as home conditions were satisfactory, so a letter of inquiry was sent to the medical director in Jane's home town. This doctor seemed to have a good understanding of the family's home conditions and felt that Jane would do well there after her discharge, noting in his letter to the sanatorium that "her people are intelligent," their six-room home was both "clean and well taken care of," they had "an adequate income for necessities," and Jane would have her own separate bedroom. While he did approve of Jane's discharge under these conditions, he had concerns in Jane's potential "menace to the other children in the family," five in total, and ranging in age from early adolescence to young adulthood.

The stigmatizing language of "menace," so casually used even by a physician, alludes to the kind of sentiment that could be directed towards ex-sanatorium patients. Historian Alison Bashford explores this concept, the common language of "danger" and "dangerousness" (in relation to the tuberculosis sufferer's sputum, but also, by extension, the tuberculosis sufferer), and the stigmatizing view of the "infected-as-social threat."[165]

As she argues, voluntary confinement within tuberculosis sanatoria was intended to educate the potentially infectious, thereby allowing their safe discharge back into their communities by instilling a strong sense of "hygienic self-governance"[166] in recognition of "the social responsibilities brought by their own (perpetual) infectiveness."[167] As medical staff at the Toronto sanatorium argued repeatedly, former sanatorium patients were much "safer" than careless, infectious tuberculosis sufferers who had never benefited from a sanatorium education.

Was Jane really a potential threat or danger to her family? In his letter, the medical director noted that all five children in the home had already yielded positive tuberculin tests. This meant that they were already infected with tuberculosis, so, from the perspective of transmission and infection, Jane would have been of little "menace" to her family. Dr McHugh, who responded to the doctor's letter, reassured him that there would be small risk in Jane's return home, particularly since sanatorium assessments suggested that her disease was latent, "completely quiescent," and, as a result, "there [was] no danger to other children in the house." McHugh noted, "She has had no sputum for about a year, and her general condition is excellent." He did, however, advise caution and that, if she began to produce sputum at any point after discharge, it should be examined and that she should be re-evaluated every six months at a chest clinic. Overall, however, he felt "fairly confident … that this girl has sense enough to take care of herself." Jane was subsequently approved for discharge and left the sanatorium in July 1938. Responding to a post-discharge questionnaire eight years after leaving the sanatorium, Jane reported that she had started doing light housekeeping in her parents' home about two months after leaving the sanatorium and attended yearly chest clinics for re-examination. She further reported that her disease had remained latent and that she felt her health was even better than when she had first left the sanatorium.

Stuart, a healthy baby born at the sanatorium in 1950 of a tuberculous mother, was hard to place after he was discharged; the fear of tuberculosis lingered, even at this later time when much more was known about the disease and new antibiotic treatments were emerging. Though Stuart's birth was uncomplicated and his chest X-rays suggested no tuberculosis concerns, when he was placed temporarily with friends of the family he was soon after brought in for examination at a local hospital's chest clinic. According to the hospital's physician's notes, "On physical examination it was noted that he had a palpable spleen. The X-rays showed slight enlargement of Stuart's mediastinal lymph nodes" (located in the mediastinum, or in the central part of the chest between the lungs). Perhaps the greatest reassurance should have been Stuart's repeated negative tuberculin tests, which indicated that he had not been infected. With his family history of tuberculosis and his birth at the sanatorium, however, it was difficult for his foster family to accept that his poor health could be due to anything other than tuberculosis. Even as a unwaveringly uninfected infant, to borrow on the words of Sheila Rothman, Stuart was already living under the shadow of tuberculosis.[168] Over his two-week hospitalization, his lymph nodes and spleen remained enlarged and palpable and the foster family remained wary, so Stuart was instead admitted to a Toronto preventorium.

Since Stuart was an infant, it was others who had doubted his health, but patients themselves could also come to doubt their own tuberculous bodies, tormented by worries over infecting others in their homes once they were discharged from the sanatorium. This was the experience for Ruth, sixteen years old when she entered the sanatorium in 1913. When her mother started inquiring about the possibility of her discharge, Ruth was already over twenty years of age and well-educated about the realities of tuberculosis after so many years in the sanatorium. As Ruth's mother wrote to Dobbie in March 1917, "For some time I have been asking her to come home but she refuses as she is afraid she might endanger my two little children as she says she has a very bad cough." Dobbie supported Ruth's preference to remain at the sanatorium, writing her mother, "I think she is quite right in not wishing to go home to be a source of danger to other children who are in the home." In this case, Ruth was suffering from reactivation disease with lung cavitation and findings of tuberculosis bacteria in her sputum. Cautious and self-conscious about placing her family in "danger," Ruth would remain in the sanatorium for another six months until she was eventually willing to be discharged to the care of her mother in August 1917. Her mother did not share her daughter's reservations and, infectious or not, she wanted Ruth back home.

In addition to anxieties about infecting family and community, ex-patients also suffered lingering concerns over their own health, fearing the possibility that tuberculosis might reactivate at any time. Sidney Hobbs, whose story opened chapter 1, faced such fears. An adolescent patient who was eventually discharged as a young man, Hobbs had personal experience with the symptoms of cavitary (reactivation) tuberculosis. "Our greatest fear was haemorrhaging to death," he recalled, and that "worry of haemorrhaging was to plague me for over forty years."[169] After Sidney was discharged in 1940, he enrolled at a local high school for courses in mathematics and mechanical drafting. Two months later, however, he stopped attending classes, "a bad cold and a positive sputum was recorded and, you guessed it right, [I was] expelled again for active TB."[170] His health returned by the summer of 1941 and he found employment at a local grocery store, delivering groceries with his bicycle. Three weeks into that job, upon meeting with his physician, he was advised that he would have to quit since Ontario's Division of Tuberculosis Control had passed laws forbidding tuberculosis sufferers from handling unsealed food. Sidney subsequently found what was deemed to be a "suitable" position assisting surveyors who worked in the open air for Ontario's Department of Highways.

According to Donald Ripley's history of Nova Scotia's Kentville sanatorium, there had also been lingering fears of tuberculosis for Victor Cleyle, admitted at age thirteen and discharged after a period of treatment. According to Ripley, "Victor's major failing ... was his terrible and almost unrealistic fear of being reinfected with tuberculosis." Fears over the return of disease could lead tuberculosis sufferers to become focused upon their own bodies, particularly sensitive to any perceptible changes in their overall health. For Victor, this meant that "for each cold, chest twitch, sniffle or flu," he sought out his physician, often demanding chest X-rays so that he might be reassured that his infection had not reactivated.[171] Among sufferers, the experience of tuberculosis disease may have been stealthy the first time around, but many educated ex-sanatorium patients were infinitely more attentive to the subtleties of their bodies as a result of those experiences. Some physicians were critical, however, that the "dependence" and "helplessness" associated with prolonged sanatorium care could result in "the overtreated case of mild tuberculosis who becomes a chronic neurotic invalid" even though "signs of activity [would] never again be demonstrated."[172]

Some limitations placed on discharged children had practical implications for the family. When Alex, for example, was discharged from the sanatorium in 1930 at thirteen years of age, Dobbie recommended that he ease back into school slowly, attending only part-time until his health further recovered. Alex's mother wrote to Dobbie shortly after her son's discharge requesting that he write a letter to the Mothers' Allowance Commission's chief investigator to explain why her son was not attending school full-time. The commission had assumed that, because Alex had not returned to full-time studies, he must be working. As a result, they were prepared to deduct five dollars from his mother's allowance. In his letter to the chief investigator, Dobbie explained the situation, reassuring the commission that "later if his physical condition warrants he could go to School full time." With Dobbie's letter of support, Alex's mother's full payment was maintained.

In an earlier case from 1921, four-year-old Jeremy's mother was denied Mothers' Allowance outright, despite the fact that her tuberculous husband had been out of work for some time and eventually hospitalized at the Muskoka sanatorium. Jeremy had seven elder siblings and, in this instance, the commission believed that Jeremy's three eldest siblings should have been able to "keep" their family out of poverty. Jeremy's nineteen-year-old sister, seventeen-year-old sister, and fourteen-year-old brother "had never been able to go to school like other children" because they had all been "forced to eke out a meager living at manual labour" to support the family. Meanwhile, suffering both pulmonary tuberculosis and tuberculosis of the hip, Jeremy spent his time at the Toronto sanatorium in bed and in traction in an attempt to align his diseased hip joint and quiet the active disease. Despite these challenges and likely too young to understand the hardships at home, the cot note written to his patrons in 1922 described him as "the little boy that is always smiling."

Some restrictions on post-sanatorium patients seemed insurmountable. Warren, fourteen years old, was admitted to the Toronto sanatorium in May 1938, and discharged June 1939, for tuberculosis of the spine. He had received surgical treatment, a spinal fusion, which had arrested the disease and he left the sanatorium in good health. Though he had always remained in good health, in a letter he wrote to his surgeon at the sanatorium, he described some of the limitations he had experienced. In 1942, Warren attempted to enlist in the Royal Canadian Air Force, but was refused. In 1943, he was examined in response to a call-up from the army, but was declared medically unfit and "placed in category C-2 because of the liability of recurrence of tuberculosis from the rigors of army life." Despite his apparent health, Warren's treatment in a tuberculosis sanatorium was red-flagged by the army's examining physicians, effectively crushing any hopes he may have held to serve his country overseas. Warren was far from alone in his rejection, however, as the Army had tightened its medical evaluation of potential recruits, in part because of costly lessons learned in the First World War (notably, the number of soldiers decommissioned because of active tuberculosis, and the subsequent long-term responsibilities of government for their disability pensions).[173] As an officer of the Royal Canadian Army Medical Corps explained in 1944, "The recruiting medical boards are like the medical referees of insurance companies. They are employed to see that the country does not lose money by taking into the Army men who will prove bad risks."[174] Warren's C-2 classification was not an outright rejection, but it did mark him as a "bad risk"; only men classified as category E cases were summarily rejected. The C-2 category meant that Warren could only ever be approved for sedentary duties in Canada (not active duty, and not overseas). Recruits falling into category E could be rejected for a host of reasons, including active tuberculosis, asthma, syphilis, diabetes, eye and ear disabilities, hypertension, hernias, and intractable skin diseases.[175]

There were some gender-specific long-term concerns with ex-sanatorium children and adolescents approaching adulthood that reflected gender roles typical of the times. For males, concerns may have been raised about future occupational training, with general recommendations against taking on strenuous or physically demanding jobs. Adolescent female patients may have been aware of the early to mid-twentieth-century conflicted medical perspectives on the advisability of childbearing among women with histories of tuberculosis.[176] In the 1930s, for example, tuberculosis experts felt that the physiological stress of pregnancy, the strains of labour, and the sudden fall of the diaphragm after delivery might fuel a reactivation of latent tuberculosis disease and increase the risk of death among mothers.[177] The first postpartum year was targeted as a time of "rapid hormonal changes, the nutritional strains of lactation, and insufficient sleep," all stressors believed capable of reactivating tuberculosis disease in new mothers.[178] A recent review by Mathad and Gupta suggests that cell-mediated (Th1) immunity is suppressed during pregnancy (to protect the developing fetus); this suppression leaves pregnant women more susceptible to both infection and reactivation of latent, underlying tuberculosis infections and may account for increased risks of developing active tuberculosis disease in the postpartum period.[179] Any pregnancy-related reactivation vulnerabilities would be significant, linking active disease and infectiousness in mothers with the arrival of their newborn and susceptible infants, creating opportunities for the strong intergenerational transmission tendency that characterizes tuberculosis bacteria.[180] Socially and medically, at an extreme, this led some modern era physicians to debate the merits of sterilization to prevent pregnancy among tuberculous women altogether,[181] a daunting and ethically problematic suggestion, had it been seriously considered.

Kathryn, whose story appeared earlier in this chapter, was the twelve-year-old admitted in the early 1930s with spinal tuberculosis, later taken home by her mother following her successful surgical spinal fusion. Despite the gravity of her disease at the time, in a follow-up communication dated to the 1940s, Kathryn reported that she was married, with children, and able to do light housekeeping without fatigue. She did admit that heavy work sometimes resulted in backaches, but that she had never been troubled by coughing or weakness. She contracted pneumonia during one of her pregnancies, and even that combination of stressors did not reactivate her latent TB. In a subsequent follow-up in the 1960s Kathryn reported that she was still in "excellent health," despite the fact that she and her husband had separated, she had taken employment outside of the home, and raised her children as a single mother.

Though patients may have had reservations about their discharge from the sanatorium, much of the correspondence between families and the sanatorium suggests that parents, many times mothers, were unafraid of their children's tuberculosis, often anxious to have their children returned home in order to reclaim their roles as primary caregivers. As one mother hoping to have her son discharged wrote in 1939, "If its only fresh air and sun shine and the right stuff to eat and lots of rest I feel sure I could do that for him." Of course, the staff could not prevent a child from being discharged, but only recommend strenuously against such action, particularly in complicated cases. In some instances, such as when a child's health began to fail after discharge against medical advice, parents sought to have their children readmitted, distressed that they may have been mistaken in discharging their children too soon in the first place. At sixteen years of age, Hugh was admitted to the sanatorium in February 1931. His disease was quite debilitating, another case of spinal tuberculosis. Hugh was placed on a regimen of strict bedrest and then, like Kathryn, treated surgically with a spinal bone graft to fuse the affected area of his spine. Seeming undaunted by the surgery, Hugh's father chose to discharge his son against medical advice in November 1932, though this decision may have been borne out of financial necessity. After his discharge, apparently willing to exert his healing body, Hugh worked hard as a construction camp labourer. By the winter of 1934, however, he noticed that "any over exertion such as walking through deep snow, brought on pain," and, in the summer of 1935, he became troubled with a limp. By February 1936, Hugh needed crutches to walk. From February 1936 until his readmission in July 1936, Hugh lost over twenty-five pounds in weight, a sign of his spiralling health decline. The young man spent almost two more years in the sanatorium, this time for tuberculosis of the hip joint, an indication that Hugh's tuberculosis had reactivated during his time away from the sanatorium. Another surgery, a pelvis/femur fusion, was performed successfully and he was discharged for the second and last time in 1938.

Even if children were discharged by parents against medical advice, that did not mean that sanatorium staff cut all ties with ex-patients and their families. Instead, families sometimes wrote to Dobbie seeking advice on post-discharge care or answers to medical questions. Such was the case relating to eleven-year-old Arthur, admitted in April 1933, and discharged by his parents in July 1934. Arthur had suffered greatly from tuberculous lymph nodes. Surgery was performed while he was in the sanatorium to remove some of the swollen lymph nodes from his underarms and neck. Arthur's mother wrote to Dobbie a number of times because, mere weeks after his release, more swollen lymph nodes began to ooze pus, a problem Myers links to aggressive reactivation disease (as opposed to primary disease, where glands do not tend to rupture, and are more likely to spontaneously heal after a period of inflammation).[182] Arthur's mother's first letter to Dobbie, dated 6 August, 1934, reveals her initial optimism in caring for her son at home, though she may have needed some questions answered and a little reassurance:

> You will … remember that there was one enlarged gland just at the top of the scar where they operated in April. Well that gland looks this morning very much as if it intends to break and discharge now. Arthur seems to have improved very much in every way since coming home … I'm quite sure he has gained both in strength and weight … his appetite is improving and he sleeps well. he is out of doors practically all day long and sleeps in the tent. he goes to bed at 9 P.M. gets up 7 A.M. back to bed at 1 P.M. till 3 P.M. he has breakfast at 7.30 A.M. a glass of milk and sandwich at 10 A.M. dinner at 12 and glass of milk and sandwich at 4 P.M. then supper at 6. Is that what you would think O.K.? he is not bothered as much with that sore feeling across the lower part of his stomach. he has had gas pains a couple of times causing him to vomit, but would be O.K. in a short time again. about that gland just below his ear if it should break and discharge, would you please tell me in what way I should dress it? perhaps I should not ask you this since he is home but I would be very grateful to you if you would be interested enough in Arthur just to tell me this.

Dobbie did not seem to have reservations in guiding Arthur's mother as best he could by correspondence, although typically, and also in this case, he preferred to refer complex questions to family physicians where more practical assistance could be provided. Dobbie confirmed that the routine Arthur's mother had laid out was both "good and proper," and that she should maintain it for as long as possible. As to the gland, Dobbie recommended first and foremost that she let her family doctor see it, particularly if it were to break open. He advised her to keep the gland clean and, should it begin to ooze, to treat it with an antiseptic solution and apply a gauze dressing, using a little sterile Vaseline to keep the gauze from sticking to the skin. He also suggested that "the gland could be exposed to the sun each day for ten or fifteen minutes morning and afternoon taking care to keep the boy's head covered while this is being done." Though discharging glands often took a long time to heal, Dobbie thought that she might have some success with it.

Just over two months later, in October 1933, Arthur's mother wrote to Dobbie once again, worried because "Arthur has not been making the head way lately that he did the first month and half after coming home, he is neither gaining or loosing in weight he is just hold[ing] at 75 lbs." They had taken Arthur to the local doctor, as Dobbie had advised, but she clearly valued Dobbie's opinion. The gland was still troubling, increasing in size and discharging every day. Arthur's mother was dressing the gland in the manner that Dobbie had recommended, but since autumn had arrived, she was finding it more difficult to have the gland exposed to sunlight every day, and she was uncertain if she should go ahead and press the pus out or not. The family was considering moving to southern Ontario because Arthur was "feel[ing] the cold terrible." In his reply, Dobbie reassured Arthur's mother that the breaking down of the gland was not unusual, but to keep dressing it and to avoid squeezing it. Dobbie wrote, "The cold weather is no disadvantage to him, and there would be no gain by moving to another place," since rest, nutritious food, and fresh air (outside, with more layers of clothing as the air grew cooler) were what he needed most of all.

Almost six months passed before Arthur's mother sent another letter. She wrote in response to a letter that she had received from Dobbie, confirming that her son had passed away in January 1935. It had been "rumoured" at the sanatorium that Arthur had died over the winter, motivating Dobbie to write to his mother. As she wrote in her reply,

> We sure do miss him and always will, the poor wee man had suffered so much and was so patient about it all. You ask did he have any more swollen glands, just at the end of the scar from the last operation on his neck a swelling came there running up behind his ear[.] this broke and discharged but in November he started to be very sick at his stomach and vomited quite a lot and he could not eat but very little. Just to speak of food in his hearing would cause

> him to vomit ... he was troubled with gas pains and dioreah [diarrhea], he just gradually got weaker and thinner. On New Years Eve he took very sick with gas pains his stomach was distended. We were told by one of our Drs up here that it was Catarral Inflamation of the Intestines ... On his death certificate it said death was due to Tubercular peritonitis. The Dr told us that while it was in his blood yet it was not in the lung tissue that his main trouble was in the large intestine.

The glandular trouble that afflicted Arthur was part of a more widespread infection, as his final diagnosis, one of "tubercular peritonitis," indicates that tuberculosis bacteria had spread through his body. Such dissemination was reported by Myers to occur in "a fair percentage of cases" of reactivation disease in children and was typically associated with a poor prognosis.[183] Would Arthur have overcome his tuberculosis disease had he remained at the sanatorium rather than returning home? At the very least, his UV therapy could have continued indoors uninterrupted in the winter months with UV lamps, but whether this would have ultimately benefitted him is impossible to know. What is clear is that the commitment of the sanatorium physicians to their patients did not end at discharge. Dobbie's ongoing correspondence with Arthur's mother and the letter that he sent out to her in response to the rumours of Arthur's death are taken as testament to that enduring connection.

Conclusion

Adopting a biosocial perspective, this chapter has attempted to ground the tuberculosis experience in the broader constructs of biology and life, focusing upon the relationship struck between tuberculosis bacteria and children. Considerations of the tuberculosis experience should include the biological perspective, because it influences the manner in which the disease manifests and its type of progress in the body (acute or chronic, active or latent, lungs or other tissues and organs), the symptoms it will produce, and the disabilities it may cause. In the Canadian sanatorium era, in the time of endemic tuberculosis, it was generally understood that many children would be infected with tuberculosis by adolescence. Primary infection and disease was so common in childhood that it was formerly identified by tuberculosis specialists as "childhood tuberculosis." In a time when childhood infections such as measles, chicken pox, and whooping cough were rife, primary tuberculosis disease was often experienced as a minor illness and could easily pass unrecognized by child sufferers and their families before slipping into latency. The latent period was itself an adaptation of tuberculosis bacteria, ensuring each new generation of children would become host to the infection, with reactivation in adolescence or young adulthood making it possible for them, in turn, to pass the infection on to their own children. Reactivation disease, defined by the cardinal signs and symptoms of tuberculosis, was particularly concerning, since lung cavitation could be life threatening. Experiences surrounding both primary and reactivation disease could vary significantly between children.

If tuberculosis infection in childhood was difficult to avoid in the endemic era, then tuberculosis specialists ideally would have liked for exposure to occur in the community, where lower-level exposures to bacterial infection were believed to have a stimulating and resistance-building effect. Infection occurring within the confines of the home was believed to be more dangerous, sites of massive infection, because of the more intensive contact between family members. In reality, in almost half the cases sampled, parents, guardians, or the children themselves had no idea how or when first infection had occurred. In the remaining cases, identifying mothers, fathers, or other family members with reactivation disease as the route to exposure seemed to confirm the prevailing perception that most tuberculosis transmission to children occurred amongst family members within the home.

The challenges involved in diagnosing tuberculosis disease meant that some children without tuberculosis would be admitted to the sanatorium, and other children would be missed, admitted only once the more obvious symptoms of disease emerged. How children experienced both primary and reactivation disease varied according to their own immune resistance, the particular infecting strain of *Mycobacterium tuberculosis*, the route of infection, and children's living conditions and other stressors (such as co-infections and nutritional status). In the end, for those children who were admitted to the sanatorium, the effects of tuberculosis and hospitalization, their own anxieties over the disease and the possibility of reactivation, and the fears or anxieties of family and community members could linger long after discharge. The patient histories highlighted in this chapter capture the variability in the tuberculosis experience engendered by the different ways in which bodies and tuberculosis bacteria interact, from infection through the challenges of diagnosis, treatment, and the nature of their lives following discharge.

CHAPTER 5

Blood and Oxygen: Building Bodies of Resistance

> One who has tuberculosis cannot dodge the fact that an unwelcome visitor has set up housekeeping in his lungs. For the rest of his life he must "put up with" the tubercle bacillus, but in the sanatorium he can learn to keep the villain under his power and thereby enjoy good health.[1]
>
> ~ Canadian Tuberculosis Association

The prescription of bedrest was the most fundamental, pervasive, and enduring form of tuberculosis treatment, both at the Toronto sanatorium and diverse sanatoria across North America. In the absence of fast cures, the tedium of bedrest and resistance building was the reality for most children admitted before antibiotics, but not all children or their families were so patient. A seemingly benign treatment, bedrest could be resisted by patients (or their families), particularly if they saw no practical benefit or improvement. Candice was admitted in January 1927, at twelve years of age in a bad state with advanced tuberculous disease affecting both her lungs. Her father wrote to Dobbie in November 1927, stating his intention "to take her away from there, as she is saying that she can't walk any more, her feets hurt even when she just stands on her bed." Her father was not surprised, writing that it was "no wonder they do, because she's been in bed for all of that time when she's been there," almost eleven months. Since Candice did not "like it" at the sanatorium and wanted "very much to come home," he had decided to discharge his daughter against medical advice, disappointed because he felt "she is a lot weaker [than] when she was taken there." Rather than improvement, Candice's father was convinced that bedrest had created weakness in his daughter and that Candice, with her poor prognosis for surviving tuberculosis, was becoming increasingly miserable at the sanatorium. In his response to Candice's father, Dobbie tried to explain why she was being kept on bedrest, the result of her poor condition and the absence of typical signs of satisfactory progress. Candice lacked an appetite, had not gained weight, and was prone to run fevers. Reviewing Candice's history, Dobbie noted that her temperature was as high as 102.4° to 102.5° each day, occasionally reaching as high as 103°F. She was reported to have a frequent cough with expectoration, and, with her sputum samples continuing to return positive for tuberculosis bacteria, Candice was also infectious. But Dobbie also recognized that Candice's prognosis was ultimately not good, and that if her father wished to take her home and had the ability to look after her, he would not object. Candice, who wanted so much to go home, left the sanatorium just over two weeks later, willing to give bedrest a trial at home, where she might be more content amongst family.

Candice was far from alone in her frustrations with tuberculosis and bedrest. The idea of bedrest conjures the most iconic imagery of tuberculosis patients – long lines of patients resting in beds and lounge chairs on wards, porches, and balconies. Bedrest lay at the core of tuberculosis treatment at many North American sanatoria. But in reality, if not just the bane of sanatorium patients and a worry to their families, what therapeutic benefit did it offer? And how did this aspect of treatment connect with the broader intentions of medical therapeutics? How was the biological effect of bedrest reframed during the transition from the traditional to the modern era of medical practice? This chapter scrutinizes bedrest, focusing on the expanding biological and physiological arguments for its place in the treatment of tuberculosis, and the effects that these new findings would have on the patient experience.

Therapeutic Heroics and Nihilism: Finding Resistance in the Healing Power of Nature

Through the nineteenth century, North American medicine would undergo changes in its therapeutic underpinnings in perceptions of what patients needed to heal and how physicians could play a role in that healing. In the early to mid-nineteenth century, therapies sought to restore the healthy condition of "*natural balance*" and, according to John Warner, this balance was to be regained with the use of depletants in "overexcited" patients and stimulants in the case of "enfeebled and exhausted" patients.[2] The depleting therapies included the use of calomel (a mercury-based compound that, amongst other things, caused sweating and salivation) and emetics (such as tartar and ipecacuanha, to induce vomiting), blistering, leeching, venesection, cupping, and a "low" diet, while stimulating treatments encouraged the patient's system "up to its natural level" with the use of alcohol, iron, cod liver oil, quinine, and a "high" diet.[3]

To treat disease, physicians looked to bodily symptoms to guide the best course of action. In a disease that produced blisters, for example, medical historian Charles Rosenberg notes that physicians attempted to speed healing by intentionally inducing or irritating blisters.[4] Instilled was the idea that through careful attention to the body and its natural responses to disease, physicians might find good models for therapeutic action. Ultimately, inspiration was found with the body itself. The depleting therapies exerted powerful, visible effects on the body (vomiting, diarrhea, blood loss-related exhaustion), evidence that "something was indeed being done" and seemed to affirm the physician's therapeutic power. But in time both physicians and patients alike began to question their use.[5] As Rosenberg has argued, patient likes and dislikes could sway the direction of therapeutics, as "the often draconic treatments of regular physicians – the bleeding, the severe purges and emetics – constituted a real handicap in competing for a limited number of paying patients";[6] if patients avoided the treatments, physicians would not profit. So, in time, treatment regimens were tempered. By the second decade of the nineteenth century, the "heroic depletive therapies" began to fall into decline as physicians themselves embraced a "growing faith in the healing power of nature."[7] The principle was already deeply rooted in medicine, "the Hippocratic heritage" upon which medicine was built "implor[ed] healers to work with nature rather than against it."[8] As physicians "came to doubt their ability to actively cure disease by medical art and transferred their faith to the healing power of nature," they turned to supportive stimulants that "sustain[ed] the patient's vital energy at a natural level while nature's healing powers proceeded."[9]

According to Charles Rosenberg, the shift of attention to the body's "natural defenses" was linked to the therapeutic nihilism that came to define medicine by the middle third of the 1800s.[10] Working within this paradigm, physicians were more willing to recognize their limitations in healing disease and the potentially negative effects of aggressive treatments. At best, those treatments might be "completely ineffective," but then again they might also be downright "harmful."[11] Physicians had always doubted their abilities to treat some diseases; many believed, for example, that the "states of disequilibrium" associated with tuberculosis and cancer "could not be righted."[12] As Rosenberg notes, "The treatment indicated for tuberculosis, as the ancient adage put it, was opium and lies."[13] As physicians began to question the veracity of their healing powers, hopes shifted towards the healing power of the body (or "Nature"). A therapeutic nihilism set in that suggested "the sick had no other hope than the healing power of nature."[14] Explicitly, Christopher Lawrence identifies the affirmation of British physician Alexander Gibson (1875–1950) that "the doctor must recognize that the body had a natural tendency to heal" and that, because of those abilities, patients could and did survive "serious disease" without interventions or remedies.[15] Therapeutic nihilism may have had the benefit of taming overly aggressive nineteenth-century medical therapies, but was also criticized then, as now, for encouraging a therapeutic idleness, as potentially treatable conditions could be resignedly accepted as "inevitable" or simply an "expected part of many illnesses," and thus guide decisions not to treat.[16] Therapeutic nihilism displaced "heroic" cures in favour of more passive treatment agendas. Rosenberg notes, "The physician's duty [was] simply to aid the process of natural recovery through appropriate, and minimally heroic means ... Rest, a strengthening diet, or a mild cathartic were all the aid nature required in most ills."[17] In its earliest years, the Toronto sanatorium would align with this therapeutic restraint, but as treatment strategies changed over time, the move was away from this "noninterventionist position" described by Rosenberg, and towards direct bodily manipulations, a change that became particularly evident in the sanatorium's surgical years.

The tuberculosis sanatorium in Canada arose in the transitional years of this intellectual shift towards nihilism. In tuberculosis, and in the late nineteenth- and early twentieth-century sanatorium era, physicians typically embraced the principles of "conservative treatment,"[18] supporting the body's natural tendency to heal through a specific focus on resistance building. The point of "natural defenses" would be reinforced with tuberculosis once mass tuberculin testing surveys revealed that, despite a wide scope of tuberculosis infection in a given population, only a fraction of those infected actually developed active disease or, more grievously, died of tuberculosis. Among the infected-who-remained-healthy came the affirmation that there existed a "natural resistance" to the disease. Since the body *could* potentially successfully resist tuberculosis, even without treatment, through its natural defences, the tenets of therapeutic nihilism were reinforced in tuberculosis.

From this perspective, physicians began to look more closely at the body and what might constitute natural defences in tuberculosis. If protective mechanisms could be identified, physicians might be in a better position to assist vulnerable tuberculosis sufferers. The clues, physicians believed, would come from the body. As Rosenberg has noted for the nineteenth-century traditional era, the calomel, purgatives, and blistering employed by traditional physicians mirrored "the profuse sweat, diarrhoea, or skin lesions often accompanying fevers" that were "all seem[ingly] stages in a necessary course of natural recovery."[19] As a result, "the remedies he employed, the physician could assure his patients, only acted in imitation of nature."[20] Significantly, it was believed that "medicine could provoke or facilitate, but not alter, the fundamental patterns of recovery inherent in the design of the human organism."[21]

Modern-era tuberculosis specialists did not seek to encourage vomiting or diarrhea in their patients, but they did note other natural processes of the body responding to disease or trauma, and sought to build on those natural responses in their treatment. Here, an older, more traditional orientation of looking to the body to manage disease is seated squarely within the emerging tradition of modern, scientific medicine. The granuloma of tuberculosis became the confirmation and biological symbol par excellence of the body's natural ability to resist tuberculosis. There was real evidence of the "healing power of nature" in the formation of granulomas, observed in the autopsied bodies of seemingly well individuals who had died of other causes yet shown signs of contained tuberculosis infection. Thus, in the same way that Rosenberg has noted that nineteenth-century physicians might encourage blister formation with blistering diseases, twentieth-century tuberculosis specialists noted responses such as granuloma formation and inflammation and aimed to support or encourage those natural body responses in healing. Ultimately, many early twentieth-century approaches to managing tuberculosis were inspired by the nineteenth-century (or earlier) observations, notes, and publications of traditional physicians. Amongst practitioners of scientific medicine, those nineteenth-century insights were revived, recycled, or reinterpreted. In this way, Rosenberg notes a therapeutic continuity, even despite the significant transitions in nineteenth-century medicine: "In the intellectual realm as well as in that of practice, clinicians sought, in a number of ways, to insure the greatest possible degree of continuity with older ideas."[22] Ideas about the body and supporting its natural healing tendency prevailed well into the era of scientific medicine as practised in sanatoria, such as the Toronto sanatorium. Physicians still looked to the body to guide their therapeutic choices in building resistance to tuberculosis.

As a case in point, inflammation and blood supply became focal points of early, modern era therapies in tuberculosis treatment. Here, the early nineteenth century's preoccupation with blood returns under a new guise in the twentieth-century sanatorium; while nineteenth-century physicians sought to achieve a correct balance of blood in the body and used bloodletting to "deplete" and "calm" the "overexcited" body,[23] in the modern, scientific era, blood, through its circulation and delivery of immune cells (later identified as antibodies) would be revered for its association with the healing power of nature. The blood manipulation in diseases like tuberculosis would come to be known as "artificial hyperemia" and was based on the rationale that if the body naturally directed an increased volume of blood to sites of disease and trauma (observed as inflammation), it likely did so for therapeutic benefit. Hyperemia was what nature (or the body) produced, while the "artificial" variant was therapeutically induced by physicians. In this instance, the "artificial" simply plays upon observations of the "natural," and the body ultimately guided perceptions of what was considered "natural."

Arguably, all of the sanatorium era treatments (from bedrest to the tuberculosis surgeries) aimed for the same net effect, to slow the progression of tuberculosis disease and, in doing so, to give the immune system the opportunity to respond more effectively. If tuberculosis bacteria could not be eliminated from the body, they could, at least, be pushed into latency through improved bodily resistance. As one Kamloops, BC, physician argued, "Our aim must *be to so increase the resistance of the tissues* of our patients by every known means that in this way we may overcome the ravages of the bacillus, and so arrest the tubercular process."[24] Clarence Starr, a Toronto physician, referred to "supporting treatment" and the physician aim to "assist the tissues to successfully resist the continuance of the disease."[25] Doctors such as Norman Bethune believed that the natural tendency towards bodily resistance to tuberculosis paired with supportive medical treatments could improve prognoses in tuberculosis. "Pulmonary tuberculosis shows an inherent tendency, a willingness for recovery," he argued, "which when considered beside chronic heart, kidney or liver diseases, which show little or no tendency to cure, makes it unique among the diseases of long duration afflicting man."[26] Bethune felt, "given half a chance, pulmonary tuberculosis will meet the physician half-way towards recovery." Medicine's therapeutic agenda, therefore, was to extend or amplify the body's natural, therapeutic responses in tuberculosis treatment.

Resistance building was a concept that tuberculosis workers promoted widely. Outside the clinical environment of the sanatorium, resistance building intersected more broadly with the principles of healthy living. How one chose to, or could, live was complex, staked in individual preferences and means. Nonetheless, those choices, often filtered through the limitations of inequalities such as poverty, could be used to shift blame for tuberculosis onto the individuals suffering the disease.[27] The point could not be more explicitly made than with Ontario's Division of Industrial Hygiene's 1920s educational film *Her Own Fault*.[28] The film features two women, Eileen and Mamie, both unmarried, working industrial jobs at a footwear factory, and living apart from their families in urban boarding houses, most likely in Toronto. Eileen, "the girl who succeeds," takes care to eat and sleep well, exercises regularly outdoors in the fresh air, and is fastidious in her appearance, her hygiene, and her work. Mamie, on the other hand, "the girl who fails in Life," is caught up in the excitement of city life, she stays out late dancing, appears unkempt, and skips good-quality meals and rest and exercise breaks to go shopping. After setting the scene with these two opposites, we learn that "months later both girls get what was coming to them." Eileen earns a promotion to "forelady" at her factory, while Mamie's supervisor, noting her persistent and worsening cough, her flushed and fevered appearance, and her poor-quality work, advises her to see a doctor. We learn that "Mamie's doctor said 'tuberculosis'" and the film ends with Mamie lying quietly on a bed in a sanatorium. The film suggests that Mamie's tuberculosis was "Her Own Fault," that by her choices and her lifestyle, she had rendered her body vulnerable to tuberculosis, while Eileen's body remained staunchly resistant (all the more remarkable since she had spent many hours each day working alongside Mamie, an openly infectious tuberculosis sufferer). Epidemiological sentiments of "risk" are foreshadowed, linked to a growing sense that individuals must claim responsibility, via their actions, to maintain their health in the presence of endemic tuberculosis. The problem was that many of the "risks" of tuberculosis vulnerability, such as the lack of nutritious diet or overwork, were linked to social inequalities evident in Canadian society and not necessarily individual choice.[29]

It is important to note that for a time, with the rise of antibiotics, attention could focus more directly on ridding the body of tuberculosis bacteria. Though we continue to occupy this era, tuberculosis bacteria have proven their ability to become antibiotic resistant. As a result, the therapeutic pendulum is now swinging back to focus on the body and its resistance to tuberculosis. The most modern emerging treatments for tuberculosis are focusing on immunotherapy, such as providing the body directly with the cytokines (protein signals) that play a role in triggering the intracellular immune responses that are known to be effective against tuberculosis bacteria.[30] Thus, we have returned to the idea of the body's natural abilities to heal, specifically via components of immune function, and the use of supportive therapies to raise that effective immune response. In the sanatorium era, encouraging immunity and resistance was pursued indirectly, through means such as rest and diet, but the approach is now direct, through cytokines. If bacteria can (and do) become resistant to drug treatments, then the body must still be elevated to new levels of immune resistance, a rationale uncannily similar to that of early twentieth-century tuberculosis treatments.

Strengthening the Natural Forces through Diet

Nineteenth-century traditional medicine focused on notions of balance that must be maintained in bodies to ensure health. Most nineteenth-century physicians were familiar with the idea of "vital power" and "the need to support that vitality if the natural healing tendency were to manifest itself."[31] As Rosenberg notes, beginning in the 1850s, physicians increasingly emphasized the importance of diet and regimen to induce a "strengthening and stimulating" effect on the body's "vital power."[32] At the Toronto sanatorium, in the early decades of the twentieth century, patient diet was carefully managed to buffer the body's natural defences to tuberculosis. Aside from rest, the medical management of diet was perhaps one the most ingrained approaches to tuberculosis resistance building. For many patients, weight loss was a key symptom leading to their tuberculosis diagnoses and sanatorium admissions. As a result, overseeing the diet to encourage weight gain, equated with improving health, was an important goal at the sanatorium. In a letter to Toronto's Department of Public Health, Dobbie wrote in October 1924, "Before a discharge a child should at least be free from symptoms and should have attained the normal weight for the height and age," thus weight (and weight gain) served as a guide for timing discharge.

The attention directed towards weight gain are evident in the examples of Iona and Chuck. Iona had been born in 1918 and admitted to the Toronto sanatorium from a shelter run by the Children's Aid Society in December 1927. Her father died of tuberculosis in 1922, followed by her mother's tuberculosis-related death in 1926. About three weeks before the death of her mother, Iona and six of her siblings were sent to the shelter. Given the poor family history for the disease, shelter staff remained vigilant for any symptoms of tuberculosis appearing in the children. The shelter's physician wrote to Dobbie in October 1927, indicating that the children "were almost starved before they came to us" and that Iona, in particular, had been very thin. She had gained some weight over her year at the shelter but was prone to run fevers and coughed a great deal. Clearly a TB suspect because of her family history and symptoms, she was an increasing source of concern for the shelter physician and he wanted her transferred to the sanatorium. Iona was admitted and remained at the sanatorium for just over a year regaining her weight and her health before she was discharged back to the shelter for the Christmas holidays, and then on to a foster home out in the country. Staff understood, however, that children differed in their ability to gain weight. In comparison to Iona, Chuck, "a pale little chap of seven years of age," had struggled to gain weight at the sanatorium. Because Chuck was an active boy, "in perpetual motion," staff were not entirely surprised that his weight gain had been modest and, even despite the small gains, staff felt his condition had improved. In a note to his cot sponsor Chuck was described as "very proud of his personal appearance," though staff were "sure" that he "often wonders if the effort he is required to make is worth the result."

In the early years of the sanatorium era, doctors and nurses alike had subscribed to the practice of "superalimentation," "hyperalimentation," or the "stuffing process,"[33] providing patients with an abundance of protein-, cholesterol-, and calorie-laden foods, including meats, eggs, and milk. Milk, in particular, was favoured for promoting weight gain.[34] Cream, provided only in small quantities "so as not to 'cloy the hungry edge of appetite,'" was believed to be "very strengthening in tubercular cases."[35] Patients were encouraged to eat well beyond their appetites since weight gain was associated with both healing and health, and since many, even in the early stages of active tuberculosis, were often ten to fifteen pounds below the standards expected for height and age.[36] In 1903, J.H. Elliott, the first physician-in-charge of the Muskoka Cottage Sanatorium in Gravenhurst, Ontario, wrote, "The tuberculous patient requires a greater amount of food than the average person, for in addition to that needed to carry on the body functions there must be sufficient to replace the daily waste caused by the disease, and an additional quantity to replace that already lost and to restore the body to the former condition of health and vigor."[37] As a result, new arrivals to the sanatorium and patients with advanced or active disease typically had more food "forc[ed] upon the stomach … than it demands."[38] During her time at Trudeau's Adirondack Cottage Sanatorium at the turn of the twentieth century, Toronto patient Marion Marshall recalled that, in addition to regular meals, she was served "junket [sweetened and flavoured milk curds], poached and soft-boiled eggs (I could not take the raw ones), and about an inch or so of milk in a glass, three times daily."[39] Food was liberal, yet water consumption was carefully controlled (perhaps so that appetites would not be diminished). Marshall remembered receiving "only a pittance of water," and often feeling so "intensely thirsty" that she admitted, "I was tempted to drink from my hot water bottle."[40]

By the early twentieth century, however, attitudes concerning diet were changing. Norton reports that at Tranquille sanatorium in Kamloops, BC, extensive raw egg consumption had been abandoned in 1908, only a year after the sanatorium opened, as the result of unfavourable outcomes. Tranquille's physician-in-chief, Dr Irving, had discovered that "after a few weeks of six to eight eggs a day, patients lost their appetite for all food."[41] In Ontario, in 1912, physicians such as Dr W.B. Kendall, of the Muskoka sanatorium, and Dr Minns, a physician practising in Toronto, were recommending a more relaxed approach to the diet of tuberculosis patients. Minns hoped that the "fad of forced feeding" would never return; in the "worst case" he had treated, the patient had been consuming up to seventeen eggs[42] in a single day.[43] Dobbie knew of instances where patients, desperate in their attempts to overcome tuberculosis, were consuming four to six quarts (sixteen to twenty-four cups) of milk and ten or twelve eggs, in addition to three regular meals, per day.[44] Kendall recounted the case of an adult patient who, before entering the sanatorium, was consuming, in addition to his regular meals, "eight raw eggs a day, sometimes twelve, one pint [two cups] of cream, three pints [six cups] of milk, together with cod liver oil."[45] J.E. Esslemont, an English physician writing in 1911, noted the unsavoury reputation of the sanatorium that arose out of stories of "patients being stuffed with food until they vomited and then having to resume and finish their meals."[46] Of course, improving diet was still considered one of the most significant factors in building up resistance, but not so aggressively and in excess and, as Minns argued, "Emphasis should be given to the necessity of supplying, not luxuries, but milk, butter, eggs, cream, meat, fresh fish, fruits and vegetables" so that good nutrition in managing tuberculosis did not have to cost patients unduly.[47] In the case of patients who had completely lost their desire to eat, insulin was sometimes injected to stimulate appetite, though this practice was not observed among the child patients sampled at the Toronto sanatorium.[48]

The science of the tuberculosis patient's diet came to focus on the particulars of foods consumed. In sufficient quantities, fats and carbohydrates were intended to provide the fuel for the body's everyday metabolic demands, and were meant to spare the proteins provided in the diet. Proteins, Dobbie argued, were "assimilated with difficulty by the body" and were intended to "be used entirely to repair tissue" damaged by tuberculosis disease.[49] J.J. Cassidy, editor of the *Canadian Journal of Medicine and Surgery*, also wrote of the role of protein in "repairing body waste without delay," and recommended meat and eggs.[50] Similar sentiments were echoed by Kendall, who discussed the role of proteins in the "repair [of] tissue waste" and ascribed dietary fats and carbohydrates to the important role of "economizers of protein."[51] With an increasing focus on the quality of the diet, by 1944, diets low in carbohydrates but rich in protein, even if accompanied by some weight loss, were viewed as more desirable by some physicians than diets that simply encouraged weight gain.[52]

In attempts to do what was therapeutically best for tuberculosis sufferers, the anemia of tuberculosis attracted particular attention. The "great white plague" (as tuberculosis was called when it gained epidemic traction in seventeenth-century Europe) often rendered bodies pale and weakened by anemia (hence the "white" descriptor). While a number of symptoms associated with tuberculosis were believed to have therapeutic value, because they were indications of natural defences, anemia was less likely to be perceived as a positive bodily response. This may have been because of the great value placed on blood in healing, and the likelihood that anemia would hinder healthy, therapeutic blood circulation. Since treatments were often grounded in blood's connection with healing, anemia was a problem. While there can be a number of underlying causes of anemia, the anemia of tuberculosis is an "anemia of chronic disease," a by-product of the immune system and its inflammatory reaction to infection and disease.[53]

The case of anemia presents one instance where dietary treatments, furnishing patients with iron-rich diets (particularly all of those egg yolks and red meats), resulted in medical therapeutics theoretically working against the body's natural defences in tuberculosis disease. A cascade of bodily processes are stimulated into action with the immune system's detection of pathogens such as tuberculosis bacteria, a number of which revolve around the body's handling and use of iron. Iron is a key ingredient of red blood cells, part of the hemoglobin molecule responsible for binding and transporting oxygen throughout the body. But iron is also a key ingredient for bacterial growth and replication, so bacteria attempt to liberate iron from the human body in order to fuel their own needs. As a defence against infection, therefore, the body responds by controlling iron, effectively making it unavailable to invading pathogens but also producing the pale and anemic appearance of tuberculosis sufferers.[54] With inflammation, hepcidin, a protein manufactured by the liver, is produced in greater quantity and stimulates less dietary iron absorption from food in the small intestine.[55] Cytokines, the protein signals of the immune system that are called into play with the activation of an immune response in tuberculosis infection, have been found to mediate tuberculosis infection through various pathways, including shortening the life expectancy of red blood cells, and simultaneously reducing any supplemental red blood cell production.[56] Cytokines may also stimulate greater iron storage by macrophages (the same phagocytic cells that also consume tuberculosis bacteria), altering the body's typical recycling pathways in iron metabolism, and this means that less iron is made available for new red blood cell production.[57] Other biologic pathways come into play, but the net effect of all these changes is a strategic "withholding" of iron from tuberculosis bacteria.[58] As a result, the anemia of tuberculosis can be reinterpreted, in this framework, as a protective bodily adaptation to infection, and not just as a symptom or challenge that must be mediated. Despite its protective intention, however, anemia can have detrimental effects on the body, stressing the heart, in particular, because it must work harder to ensure that a smaller number of red blood cells can still be effectively circulated to deliver much-needed oxygen to the organs and tissues of the body.[59] Nevertheless, in instances of bacterial infection, the body can cope reasonably well with low iron availability.[60] While acute infections lead to shorter-lived iron-withholding readjustments, the chronic nature of tuberculosis disease necessarily extends the disequilibrium. As Kent, Weinberg, and Stuart-Macadam note, the fever of diseases like tuberculosis, another by-product of the immune response, is helpful because bacterial iron needs are greater in bodies maintained at higher temperatures.[61] Thus, the body's tendencies toward fever and iron withholding work cooperatively against the needs of tuberculosis bacteria.

Like iron withholding, the fever (pyrexia) response is also triggered by cytokine protein signals of the human immune system and can serve as an adaptive response against pathogens. At the Toronto sanatorium, fever was interpreted as a barometer of disease activity, indicating the immune system was actively fighting bacteria. Though most physicians were wary of the effects of a high and prolonged fever on the body, some considered the possibility that there were important underlying reasons for fever in the tuberculous body. If fever was a natural response of the body, it seemed reasonable to assume that there could be a therapeutic value to this response, and from this perspective the treatment of pyrotherapy evolved. The idea to induce "artificial hyperpyrexia" was not unique to tuberculosis. An intentional, fever-inducing malaria treatment for syphilis sufferers earned Julius Wagner-Jauregg (1857–1940), an Austrian physician, a Nobel Prize in 1927.[62] The initial 104° to 107.6°F cycling fevers of malaria were hypothesized to be adverse to the underlying bacterial infection of syphilis, and once the desired therapeutic effect was reached, it was reasoned that the malaria could be treated with quinine. With tuberculosis, the desire to harness the therapeutic effect of fever through inducing artificial hyperpyrexia was not as promising, for, as Myers noted in the 1930s, it was determined that "the human body cannot tolerate temperatures of such degree as are necessary to destroy the human type of tubercle bacilli."[63] This meant that fever, whether produced naturally or encouraged therapeutically, could not kill tuberculosis bacteria (though it might elevate their iron needs).

With tuberculosis, the typical fever that accompanied active disease was perceived as quite damaging. When fourteen-year-old Elvin was admitted in 1917, a letter from his brother to Dobbie made it clear that he appreciated the dangers of fever. "I understand he has a temperature still," he wrote. "Is it high enough to burn him out in less than a year's time, if not checked?" Elvin's brother wanted to know what sort of treatment was being used, if Elvin had gained in weight, and what Dobbie thought his "chances" were of surviving tuberculosis. The brother's apprehension that Elvin might "burn out" echoed the concerns of some early twentieth-century physicians that fever was "costly," consuming the body's tissues unless energy could be replaced efficiently and effectively through eating. The regular fevers of tuberculosis equalled greater body heat and, to produce that heat, the body's energy reserves were expended. According to Cassidy, "Alimentation during fever being insufficient to supply the 2,500 calories (heat units) required for the existence of an individual of medium weight, the latter is obliged to live on his capital, i.e., his own tissues," and while body stores, such as fats, were consumed, "his energy and vital force decrease."[64] Despite Cassidy's scientific evaluation of diet, the language of "vital force" is a much older concept. According to Charles Rosenberg, in the mid-nineteenth century, "physicians ... spoke habitually of 'vital power' and the need to support that vitality if the natural healing tendency was to manifest itself."[65] Cassidy recommended the therapeutic use of alcohol to offset the fever-consuming effect, even though, in the early twentieth century, there were burgeoning moral concerns with the "evils of the liquor traffic."[66] Socially, alcohol consumption was increasingly frowned upon, but medically, physicians such as Cassidy felt that alcohol still had a place in the physician's therapeutic arsenal, particularly since it was felt that alcohol was easier on the body than other treatments, and more completely "combusted" and absorbed by the body.

Acting on an entirely different cue from the body and its defensive actions against tuberculosis disease, medical attention also focused on calcium. If the body used calcium to consolidate (or solidify) the granulomas (or tubercles) that held tuberculosis bacteria captive, then perhaps medical therapeutics could aid this defence by increasing the supply of calcium to the body. As one physician, Philip Ellman, commented, "A calcified tubercle is less likely to break down and liberate any remaining living tubercle bacilli than a tubercle that is not calcified." On his autopsy of a sixty-four-year-old former sanatorium patient with active tuberculosis gone latent, Ellman reported, "On palpating the lungs carefully ... I [was] able to find a stony hard mass at the right apex, about the size of a large walnut."[67] The "hard mass" of the granuloma was "surrounded by dense calcification," which, upon his attempts to section the granuloma, he had found quite challenging to cut through. In making his case over the potential importance of adequate bodily calcium in positive resolutions of tuberculosis disease, Ellman noted observations of the visiting dentist who treated patients at his hospital. Those patients who had a good prognosis typically also had "good calcification of the jaws and teeth."[68] This the dentist measured by the level of difficulty he encountered upon extracting teeth, where an easy extraction suggested poor calcification. On the other hand, carious teeth were viewed as sentinels of tuberculosis susceptibility, the sign of a more general "decalcification" in the body, which could potentially be reversed with "recalcification" to build resistance to tuberculosis.[69]

It seemed rather straightforward to add calcium to the diet, though the results were less than encouraging: "One knows that nature will utilize calcium in her processes of repair ... but how can we explain the many failures of the past when not only calcium salts have been given by mouth but cow's milk, which contains an abundant supply of that mineral, is equally imbibed with faith and hope?"[70] Cow's milk was a common dietary bastion at most sanatoria, but the milk reputedly delivered calcium to the body in a "non-ionized" form, meaning that the mineral is bound to proteins such as albumin or anions such as phosphorus and, as a result, is not the most therapeutic "biologically active" form of calcium.[71] In the 1920s, as an alternative to dietary calcium consumption, trials were undertaken with hypodermic injections of preparations of calcium.[72] In his late 1930s review of calcium research, Myers reported that patients had been supplemented with calcium "very extensively," and the results, reviewed in both autopsies and X-rays (as physicians looked for calcium deposits in lungs, lymph nodes, and other tissues as indirect evidence for granuloma formation), offered "no proof" that super supplementing patients with calcium "has any definite influence on the healing of tuberculosis."[73] Though perhaps failed in therapeutic effect, the trials with calcium were part of the ongoing attempts to enhance and support the work of the body's natural defences.

It was not only the nature of the diet, but also the manner in which it was delivered that aligned with scientific principles. Clarice was just under two years old when she was admitted to the Davies Cottage at the Toronto sanatorium in 1933. She had been diagnosed with primary tuberculosis affecting her hilar lymph nodes. With her diet and rest carefully scheduled at the sanatorium, Clarice also began to receive regular tuberculin injections in September 1935, in an effort to build her resistance. By January 1937, the sanatorium doctors felt that her disease was latent and that she could go home to her parents, both of whom had also been sanatorium patients. Being separated from her now five-year-old daughter for almost three years, Clarice's mother wrote to Dobbie for direction on how to care for her at home. In his reply, Dobbie outlined the structure of Clarice's daily routine and diet at the sanatorium:

7 a.m.	rise and toilet (washing, teeth and hair brushing, dressing)
8 a.m.	breakfast (porridge, a boiled or poached egg or bacon, toast, cocoa, and a teaspoonful of cod liver oil) and toilet
9 –12	outside play, if possible
10 a.m.	cup of milk or orange
noon	dinner (soup or tomato juice; a small portion of boiled or roast meat or fish; potatoes; vegetable) and dessert (baked apple, or prune whip, or jelly, or rice pudding, or tapioca; a glass of milk) and toilet
1–3 p.m.	rest time and toilet
3 p.m.	cup of milk
3 to 5 p.m.	outdoor play
5 p.m.	supper (soup, or vegetable salad, or poached egg, or plain cooked spaghetti; bread and butter; stewed or raw fruit; sweet biscuit or small piece of cake; a glass of milk)
6 p.m.	warm bath, a visit to the toilet, and then bed for the evening

Overall, Clarice's daily schedule incorporated five hours for play, four hours for eating, bathing, and toilet, and fifteen hours each day for rest and sleep, suggesting the type of resistance-building regimen prescribed for children experiencing primary tuberculosis disease. In Clarice's schedule, we see reflected not only the nature of sanatorium life, but also the hallmarks of Canada's interwar movement into the science of childrearing, which included attention to habit training and feeding.[74] The rising medical specialty of pediatrics had moved beyond a simple focus on the "pathological" to address all aspects of daily life, including feeding and hygiene, that could be monitored or improved to promote overall wellness, prevent illness, and reduce mortality.[75] Infants and children were increasingly routinized and scheduled, much like, as Katharine Arnup has argued, the scheduled nature of workplaces that emerged with industrialization.[76] Not only were eating and sleep times defined in Clarice's daily schedule, but so too were the specific times for "play" and "toilet" activities. Such routines made sense in the order of sanatorium life, but likely influenced perceptions of healthy lives in family homes as well. In dietary practices, it was difficult to find specific proscriptions on feeding the children at the Toronto sanatorium, though it was noted that pork or ham was never served in the children's dining room and that they were not permitted to use pepper to season their meals (perhaps to reduce any transmission risks associated with unwanted sneezing).[77]

"Fashion in Treatment": Bedrest and Gravel Pits

A number of treatment continuities were found across diverse sanatoria, even those established before Koch had identified the bacterial cause of tuberculosis in 1882. The importance of a hearty diet and fresh air met with wide acceptance, but opinions were divided on the amount of bedrest versus exercise that sanatorium patients should experience. In 1960, Edmund Spriggs published on the changing "fashion"[78] of tuberculosis treatment, ranging from a firm commitment to bedrest, to carefully arranged systems of exercise and labour.[79] As Spriggs and others have noted, the earliest (pre-Koch) sanatorium pioneers in Europe generally advocated some form of exercise in their treatment plans. Herman Brehmer, who established the first tuberculosis sanatorium in the German Alps in 1859, and Otto Walther, who established a sanatorium in Nordrach-in-Baden in 1888, both embraced exercise as part of the cure for tuberculosis.[80] According to Spriggs, Walther went so far as to altogether remove the *Liegehalle* (the rest hall) from his sanatorium design, so firm was his conviction that it would not be needed. Exercise advocates might recommend horseback riding, singing, swinging, dancing, and running.

Brehmer had a preference for slow uphill walking, while at Walther's sanatorium, pulmonary tuberculosis patients also walked, their longest travels taking them as far as twenty-four miles (thirty-nine kilometres) in a day.[81] Well into the twentieth century, physicians warned of the dangers of extended bedrest, "the inactive life" believed responsible "for the frail and anaemic condition" of so many patients.[82]

Physicians varied, however, not only in their training and intellectual exposures, but also in their personal experiences with tuberculosis. In the United States, when sanatorium pioneer Edward Trudeau was diagnosed with tuberculosis, his physician recommended he go south, live outdoors, and ride on horseback.[83] Instead, Trudeau retreated to New York State's Adirondack Mountains and pursued a rest-based regimen that saw him slowly return to health. Convinced of the effectiveness of this approach to tuberculosis, he established a sanatorium at Saranac Lake in 1885 and fully committed to the rest cure. So ardent was that commitment that Spriggs notes, Trudeau's sanatorium became known as "the shrine of the rest treatment for tuberculosis."[84]

As Trudeau pioneered the rest cure in North America, his influence permeated international boundaries into Canada. In Ontario, the Board of the National Sanitarium Association followed Trudeau's cottage-style sanatorium design as it selected a peaceful, lakeside location on the shores of Lake Muskoka (just outside of Gravenhurst, Ontario) as the site for Canada's first sanatorium, the Muskoka Cottage Sanatorium, which opened in 1897. The cottage sanatorium's administration building, an informal, wooden clapboard construction with large verandas, was surrounded by smaller treatment cottages that typically housed three or four patients, each with their own private bedroom (Trudeau had followed the cottage plan for its lower construction cost and because he believed that patients would rest better in smaller numbers than if they were congregated in one large building).[85] By the end of the First World War, Rogers argues, "the use of rest ... had apparently won over the majority of physicians in the United States."[86] Likewise, in Canada, the National Sanitarium Association sanatoria in Muskoka and Toronto also followed the rest model of treatment.

As with any treatment, there could be notable variations in how rest was prescribed. Invariably, some physicians and sanatoria carried the principles of Trudeau's rest treatment to extremes. Spriggs notes an information booklet from the New York Tuberculosis and Health Association that explicitly "forbade listening to the radio because it might increase the rate of breathing."[87] In 1979, Dr Alfred Paine, former medical superintendent of the Ninette sanatorium in Manitoba, and Dr Earl Hershfield, director of tuberculosis control with the Sanatorium Board of Manitoba and executive director of the Canadian Lung Association, wrote of the "proven worth of prolonged rest" as "the first effective weapon against tuberculosis."[88] Regimens of absolute rest could be hard on the body, however, producing kidney and bladder stones, blood clots impeding blood flow, obstructions of the coronary artery, nitrogen and calcium imbalances, and increases in resting pulse rate suggestive of reduced cardiovascular fitness.[89] Psychologically, the daily grind of bedrest could conjure boredom and frustration, perhaps even depression. As a result, some sanatoria and physicians were quite averse to the idea of absolute bedrest. Dr Fowler, a consulting sanatorium physician and dean of the Faculty of Medicine at the University of London, England, was convinced that rest was not best: "A patient may lie in the open air till 'all's blue,' including, as I have observed, his cheeks, and be stuffed with food till he is as fat as a Strassburg goose, and yet the disease in his lungs may not be arrested."[90]

Within Canada as well, there were prominent physicians who were opposed to regimes of strict bedrest. John Joseph Cassidy (1843–1914),[91] a University of Toronto medical school graduate who associated with a number of hospitals in Toronto and established his own home practice on Church Street, was a vocal proponent of exercise in tuberculosis treatment and, through his editorship of the *Canadian Journal of Medicine and Surgery*, he encouraged other Canadian physicians in 1900 to adopt "gentle exercise in the open air" in their treatment protocols.[92] Likewise, in England, exercise advocates like Fowler admonished those sanatoria that pursued absolute bedrest.

In the mid- to late nineteenth century, at his sanatorium in Germany, Brehmer had embraced the role of gentle exercise and, through walking, established a "system of training" that aimed to develop "bodily strength."[93] Several decades later, with the opening of the Brompton Hospital Sanatorium in Frimley, England, in 1905, medical superintendent Dr Marcus

Paterson also championed the therapeutic value of activity, but in a much-expanded model of "graduated labour." The system outlined for "the poor classes" admitted to Brompton was intended to ensure that working-class, tuberculous patients were "fit for work" upon their return to life outside of the sanatorium. Fowler outlined the basics of Brompton's labour plan, where patients would exercise and then labour for two 2-hour periods each day. In a ten-step plan, patients would begin with "slow walking exercise, beginning at two miles a day and gradually increasing up to ten miles a day." By step five, they were "carrying a basket of gravel or stones, the weight of which is gradually increased up to 38 pounds." Step ten involved "digging unbroken ground" for six hours each day (an additional two hours over the traditional four-hour day).[94] Fowler noted that the sanatorium was "fortunate in having a public gravel pit on a breezy site close by," since it was there that "any amount of work may be done, and it is found that if a patient at work in the grounds is not making progress he is very likely to do so if sent to dig in the gravel pit."[95] In notable contrast, the Toronto sanatorium, which followed Trudeau's model of rest treatment, despised its neighbouring gravel pit, which, through regular noise and disruption, disturbed the peace and tranquility needed for good bedrest. While such labour-based activities were framed for working-class patients at Brompton, more genteel forms of exercise for middle-class patients included gardening and poultry rearing, in addition to games of golf, croquet, and billiards.[96] Though the Toronto sanatorium did maintain a separate building for paying patients, such distinct class-based treatment differences were less apparent, as the bedrest regimen was followed by all patients.

Wasting and Weakness: Rationales for Rest and Exercise

The different treatment strategies of absolute bedrest or exercise were guided by differing perceptions of what would benefit the body most in building resistance to tuberculosis. To some extent, conceptions of preferred treatment strategies could be influenced by the very symptoms of tuberculosis disease, the weight loss or "wasting" of the body, which met with ideas of rest and "conservation," or the weakness and pallor induced

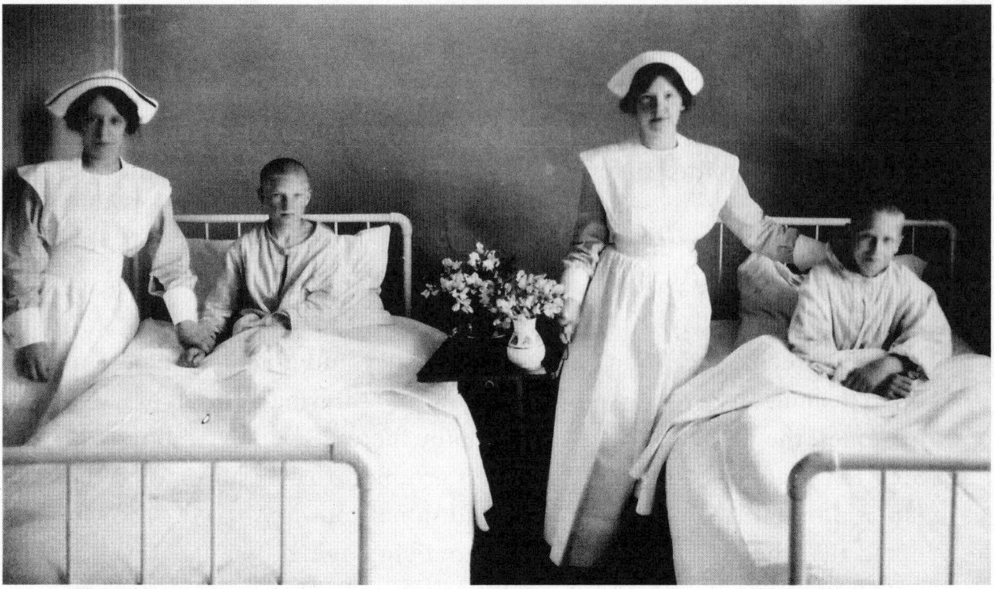

Figure 5.1 Two child patients with a graduate (*left*) and student (*right*) nurse on a ward of the Queen Mary Hospital. Bedrest was an important component of sanatorium treatment.

by poor appetites and anemia, which encouraged activity and strength-building approaches.

In the sanatorium, weight loss was viewed as a sign of disease activity, while weight gain was viewed as a sign of successful resistance building. To offset the wasting or "consumption" of the body by tuberculosis, the rest cure focused on reducing biologically costly fevers and promoting bodily "conservation" of the energies needed to support healing more generally. With the appearance of fever, ambulatory patients would quickly be put back to full-time bedrest. As Trudeau, stalwart proponent of rest, argued, "When any degree of fever is present the course of the disease will be injuriously affected in direct proportion to the amount of active exercise the patient is allowed to take."[97] He reported seeing cases of "apparent quiescent and arrested" disease "fanned into renewed and often uncontrollable activity by one single over-exertion."[98] As a result, he believed "absolute rest, so long as it is taken in the open air, is the best measure at our command to reduce the pyrexia of tuberculosis and to *conserve the patient's energies*, and should be persisted in for some time after the afternoon fever has ceased to be present, moderate exercise again being allowed only with caution"[99] (emphasis added). Over time, physicians developed temperature-related cut-offs for determining when full-time bedrest was appropriate. In 1912, Dr Minns, for example, recommended "under 99°, no restriction; under 100°, considerable rest in a reclining position; over 100°, rest in bed the larger part of the day; over 101°, rest in bed all the time."[100] The passive rest-based cure aimed to overcome disease through supportive care of the body, nourishing it and reducing the work of affected parts, like the lungs, so that the body could instead dedicate itself to healing (figure 5.1). This common sentiment was stressed in an interwar handbook issued by the Canadian Tuberculosis Association:

> Of all the countless remedies advised and tried in the past, rest alone has stood the test of time. Rest is the treatment for tuberculosis whether the disease is in the early or the late stage in whatever part of the body the disease may be. This means rest in the medical sense; not merely a change of scene or work but flat rest, that is, absolute rest in bed. Rest gives the lungs their only chance to heal. A broken leg would never get well if allowed to dangle about. In a splint it has a chance to knit because it is at rest. We cannot put the lung in a splint but we can reduce its work enormously by rest.[101]

In comparison, other physicians focused on the weak and anemic state of the body. In England, for example, it was more common for physicians to engage ideas of "strength building," or building up the body, and the importance of strong blood circulation. This was significant, since blood was believed to play a role in healing. J.J. Cassidy, a Canadian physician who advocated for exercise in tuberculosis, argued that exercise kept the heart healthy, and a healthy heart was "able to maintain a brisk circulation through the somewhat obstructed channels of the pulmonary vessels."[102] Since a "strong heart" was able to support "brisk circulation," the fluid-filled or "dropsical conditions of the lungs," believed to be induced by recumbent bedrest, could be avoided. An active, exercise-based treatment plan aimed to defeat tuberculosis disease through working the body, overcoming TB bacteria through increased lung capacity and an increased supply of blood to the tissues, which would bring along protective "immune cells" carried in the blood. As the body became physically stronger, the rationale went, the more resistant it became to tuberculosis.

So, while some physicians focused on "conserving" the body, other physicians aimed to "strengthen" the body, and that difference encouraged two different treatment philosophies. In 1911, Allbutt and colleagues positioned their discussion of the "defensive forces of the body" somewhere in between.[103] Though they admitted, "What these forces are we do not exactly know," they did believe that blood and other bodily fluids carried "representatives" of the "defensive forces."[104] Fresh air, nourishing food, and careful supervision of rest and exercise were important, they believed, to place the defensive forces "in the best possible condition to fight."[105] While blood could be healing in delivering the "defensive forces," they believed it could also be toxic if carrying large amounts of the "poison" liberated by tuberculosis bacteria. As a result, they argued, critical, individual-level evaluations had to be made about the status of disease activity, to which recommended levels of physical exercise could be tailored. If the disease was active and producing "poison," exercise should be reduced or avoided: "If a man walks several miles, more blood and lymph will go through his lung, and consequently, in the case of a diseased lung, more poison will be swept out than if he lay quietly on a sofa during the same period of time."[106] On the other hand, they believed, if disease was less active, then smaller quantities of liberated poison, if released into the blood, could be therapeutic in stimulating but not swamping the defensive forces of the body. In summary, Allbutt and colleagues stressed the critical role of the sanatorium for its expertise in assessing the needed balance of rest and exercise, based on individual tuberculosis symptoms and disease activity.

The Rest Cure and Apical Vulnerabilities

As prescriptions for bedrest permeated North America in the early 1900s, physicians were exploring possible physiological and anatomical reasons for bedrest's purported therapeutic effect that would carry the rest cure forward in time, even if original ideas concerning "conservation" weakened. The uppermost apical portions of the lungs, located in and around the area of the first rib and collarbone, were of particular concern, long known to be the most typical sites of destructive cavitation among reactivation disease sufferers. Murray notes that Italian physicians Antonio Valsalva (1666–1723) and Giovanni Morgagni (1682–1771), and French physician René Laennec (1781–1826) had all identified the vulnerability of the lung apices to cavitary disease.[107] The challenge, therefore, was to understand why, from a biological perspective, the apices were so vulnerable to tuberculosis. Some physicians believed the apices to be quite rigid and that reduced "functional activity" allowed for an easier lodging of tuberculosis bacteria in this part of the lung; other physicians suggested a "mechanical explanation" whereby the movement of lung apices, "sucked into the thorax during each inspiration and protruded during expiration," allowed for the deposition of tuberculosis bacteria.[108] In reality, the apices were not the usual sites of primary infection, which typically occurred lower in the lung where a larger quantity of inspired air was drawn into the lung; the apices tended to be seeded with tuberculosis bacteria in disease reactivation, as the infection moved hematogenously (via the blood supply) to the apices from those initial sites of infection (the Ghon focus) further down in the lung.[109]

According to Bryan, in 1887, German pathologist Johannes Orth suggested that gravity's influence on the "fluid column of blood" rendered the uppermost lung apices anemic and therefore vulnerable to tuberculosis.[110] August Bier (1861–1949), a German surgeon with interests in homeopathy,[111] championed the therapeutic value of "artificial hyperemia." At the time, some "ranked the hyperemic treatment with Lister's discovery of antisepsis."[112] On the basis of the belief that tuberculosis vulnerability was associated with "anemia of the lungs," Bier advocated for "an increased supply of blood to all tubercular foci."[113] The interest in hyperemia was based on observations that the body naturally produces hyperemia in its efforts to "resist disease or injury," so rather than "opposing its phenomena by rest, elevation, pressure, cold, incisions and drainage," Bier suggested embracing this "wise provision of nature, to be encouraged and increased."[114] "Hyperemia," it was argued, "merely assists the natural inflammatory action when it has not been sufficient."[115]

Artificial hyperemia was based on observations of the body's typical healing response, the premise being that inflammation should not be viewed as injurious and suppressed (often with the use of ice bags), but rather encouraged and enhanced. Into the modern era of medicine, physicians were still manipulating blood, but instead of seeking new states of "equilibrium" through bloodletting, they were now focused on the dynamics of blood flow to sites of disease and trauma. Blood itself was conceived as healing or therapeutic. English physician William Bennett noted that, from Bier's perspective, inflammation was "a protective process designed to fight bacterial invasion," and that the "redness, swelling, and heat" of inflammation must be encouraged, "with a view to increasing the kindly hyperaemia which is necessary in the struggle between the body tissues and the invading bacteria."[116] By increasing the amount of blood circulating to the affected area, Bennett conceptualizes the body's natural inflammatory response as both "helpful" and "kindly." Similar sentiments were raised by Herbert Waterhouse, a London area surgeon, who reported, "I ... look upon inflammation as an attempt on the part of Nature to rid the tissues of the microbic invaders that attack any part of the body. I might almost describe inflammation as having, as its main function, that of excreting microbes."[117] Waterhouse underscores "the antimicrobic action of blood, the value of which Nature abundantly points out to those who study her methods of producing, or attempting to produce, a natural cure in cases of microbic invasion of various tissues of the body."[118] Thus, in this context, artificial hyperemia and encouraging greater blood circulation simply played upon "Nature," furthering the defences that the body naturally elicits. From this perspective, inflammation was not "vicious," but a "protective influence."[119] Bier's method aimed to increase heat, redness, and swelling, through an "increase in the antimicrobic action of the circulating blood" to arrest infection and prevent suppuration, and this was known as active, arterial hyperemia[120]

An alternate measure, known as passive or congestive, venous hyperemia, also attracted attention, aiming to produce "obstructive engorgement" of the target area. Passive hyperemia, often accomplished with the use of elastic bandages or cupping, allowed for arterial blood flow, but was intended to encourage a "sluggish circulation" in venous blood flow.[121] In 1908, William Bennett advised that "the included area should be red or bluish – never white – since anaemia of the parts means starvation and decreased resistance, instead of over-feeding, such as is required in the fight with the bacterial force."[122] Some physicians, such as Herbert Waterhouse, were apprehensive in their attempts to induce passive hyperemia: "To increase the congestion in an already inflamed part appeared to be as unscientific a procedure as was possible to imagine, and it was some time before I could induce myself to try the method. When I did so I used the elastic bandage with fear and trembling, and even telephoned to the medical attendant, asking him to pay the child a visit at midnight for fear lest gangrene of the limb, distal to the bandage applied around the thigh, should threaten."[123] In comparison to the binding restriction of passive hyperemia, active (arterial) hyperemia was often achieved with the use of heat. The wish to encourage inflammation and circulation for healing resulted in a new appreciation for older therapeutic practices involving the use of poultices (soft, warm, and moist dressings of bread, mustard, herbs, or other substances) and fomentations (warm, moist compresses), and newer electro-therapies (such as high-frequency current and galvanism) and heat therapy to relax muscles, to improve vasodilatation, encourage blood circulation to promote healing, and ease pain through analgesic effects.[124] Heat therapy, also known as "baking," and was often used in combination with massage. According to Phelps, there were many different designs for "bakers," though a common model was the "hand-operated, single-bulb type which [could] be moved back and forth over the desired area"; the device was wand-like, with a Bakelite handle into which fitted a narrow glass tube that ended with a flattened glass bulb. When the unit was plugged in, the glass bulb warmed, providing heat and relaxation to the skin and muscle tissue over which it was passed.[125]

Observations of nineteenth-century physicians that heart conditions could influence tuberculosis disease spurred interest in artificial hyperemia and blood flow manipulations in tuberculosis treatment. Depending on the nature of the underlying heart condition, lungs could either be under- or over-supplied with blood. Irish surgeon Atkinson Stoney notes, "Bier himself explains that he got the idea of applying hyperaemia for tuberculosis from the ... observations made by the older physicians. Farre and Travers, in 1815, and Louis, in 1826, called attention to the frequent appearance of pulmonary stenosis in phthisis, explaining it by the pronounced anaemia of the lungs which this form of heart disease produces."[126] Pulmonary valve stenosis is characterized by a narrowing of the pulmonary valve that mediates the flow of blood from the right ventricle of the heart into the pulmonary artery. There is an obstructed flow of deoxygenated blood from the heart's right ventricle into the pulmonary artery, which carries the blood back to the lungs for oxygenation. Whereas a heart defect–related deficiency of blood supply to the lungs appeared to increase tuberculosis vulnerability, as in pulmonary valve stenosis, a heart defect–related excess of blood supply to the lungs was believed to be protective. Significantly, Bier was also aware of the work of Carl von Rokitansky (1804–1878), a Bohemian physician and pathologist, who suggested, in 1838, that those heart diseases "accompanied by fullness of blood in the lungs, offered immunity against tuberculosis."[127] This "fullness" of blood supply in the lungs was viewed among patients with mitral valve stenosis, not an unduly rare condition, because damage to the heart's mitral valve was a common complication of rheumatic fever (an infectious disease caused by streptococcus bacteria). With respect to the lungs, hyperemia occurred naturally among individuals with mitral valve stenosis, because the mitral valve could not open wide enough to allow blood to flow as freely as it should from the left atrium to the left ventricle of the heart. As a result, pressure from the constricted mitral valve causes the left atrium to swell and backs up the free flow of oxygenated blood from the lungs. As blood collects in the lungs, a state of artificial hyperemia is achieved.

Like Bier, many physicians became acquainted with Rokitansky's observations on mitral valve stenosis and its seeming protection against tuberculosis, and new studies were pursued in the modern era with extensive autopsy investigations. In the United States, for example, physician Wilder Tileston analyzed autopsy results for patients at three Boston-area hospitals and published his findings in 1908.[128] Of the 1,900 autopsies from Massachusetts General Hospital scrutinized in Tileston's study, about 18 per cent of those autopsied showed evidence of pulmonary tuberculosis. Of the sixty-six autopsied patients with mitral valve stenosis, however, only 8 per cent showed evidence of pulmonary tuberculosis. Tileston concluded that "passive congestion of the lungs" was beneficial, because the blood supplied a greater concentration of alexins (blood plasma proteins), antibodies, and leucocytes.[129]

On the basis of these observations of the effects of mitral valve stenosis, attention turned to the possibility of inducing hyperemia artificially in the lungs. Tileston had his doubts about the quality of congestion that could be achieved in a reclining posture with feet elevated, though this was popular practice. Instead, he explored a hyperemia-inducing suction mask designed by German surgeon and anesthesiologist Franz Kuhn (1866–1929), a "light apparatus which fits in the nose and mouth, with an arrangement of valves by which inspiration, which is nasal, can be impeded to any desired amount. Expiration, on the contrary, is unobstructed and takes place either through the nose or the mouth."[130] Tileston suggested the net effect of "obstructed respiration" was one of "congestion" and that "the increased amount of blood in the lungs" would be "of the greatest benefit, for it is conceded that it is the relative poor supply of blood or lymph to the apices which predisposes those parts to tuberculosis."[131] Despite the rationale, intentionally obstructing the breathing among those already suffering with tuberculous lungs seems somewhat traumatic. Likewise, for patients with laryngeal tuberculosis, the disease located in the upper part of the trachea in the area of the vocal cords, Howarth, in 1910, recommended "a fairly tight elastic band round the root of the neck," with a buckle so that the band could be tightened, if desired.[132] Patients were to wear the band for twenty-two hours each day, over a period of weeks, in order to encourage hyperemia and blood congestion in the area of the larynx.

As to the question of why the apices had a tendency to destructive tuberculous cavitation in reactivation disease, ideas were centring on the human tendency to spend much of the day with the body oriented in an upright posture and exposed to the effects of gravity. In the upright position, British physician William Ewart argued in 1901, the apices of the lungs would be relatively more "airless" than the bases of the lung. He suggested the therapeutic effects of orienting patients with respiratory diseases such as bronchiectasis on a horizontal plane or, better yet, on an inclined horizontal plane by raising the foot of the bed, to encourage greater air delivery to the apices.[133] A few years later, in 1908, British tuberculosis specialist Alfred Tucker Wise wrote on the benefits of an inclined posture, but rather than extending Ewart's "airless" beliefs, he was concerned with the use gravity to encourage "the drainage of corrupt accumulations in the lung," and, significantly, to modify blood circulation in the lungs. He believed that, because of gravity's effects on circulation, by lying in an inclined position the apices of the lungs would be placed in a more dependent position and therefore receive "a fuller blood-supply."[134]

Tucker Wise emphasized the importance of blood's "bactericidal power" in healing and argued that by inducing "artificial hyperaemia," an intentional increase in blood flow to the apices of the lungs through a correct position in bedrest, some increased resistance to tuberculosis might be gained.[135] He furthered the long-standing belief that the apices were typically quite anemic, and that the "softening" and caseation of lung tissue with tuberculosis resulted because of the "impaired circulation of blood and lymph in this narrow part of the lung."[136] Tucker Wise warned against the popular "semi-supine reclining attitude," propping tuberculous patients up on pillows or the use of reclining chairs, since this relatively upright posture offered none of the therapeutic benefits that could be achieved in a truly horizontal or, better yet, strategically inclined position, to get the apices of the lungs in a more dependent position.[137] Behaviourally, semi-upright reclining may have addressed the prescription to rest, but physiologically, this position was not believed to increase blood flow to the apices, because they were still in a superior position relative to the heart.

It is notable that Tucker Wise had a particular preference for the inclined prone posture (lying, feet elevated, with the face down towards the mattress). According to Ewart's review, "Its advantages are cardiac as well as respiratory. The weight of the heart being completely removed from the diaphragm and from the roots of the lungs[,] the posterior lobes, particularly at the base, are allowed great freedom of expansion, and this in itself eases the circulation through the heart."[138] If these physicians were attempting to modify blood flow in the lungs through manipulations of patient position, then a recent MRI-based study of position and perfusion (blood flow in the lungs) among living people confirms that selected postures can effect such change.[139] Relative to the supine (face-up) position, laying in a prone (face-down) posture results in overall higher

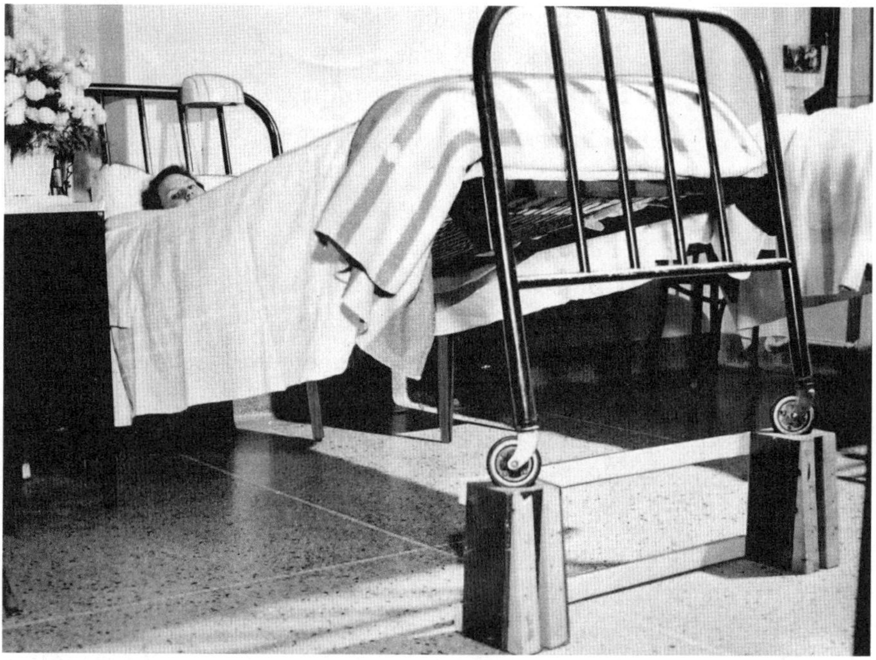

Figure 5.2 The foot of a child's bed raised up on blocks.

perfusion (blood flow) in the lung. The effect is believed to be linked to the relief of lungs from compression that is experienced in the supine position, confirming Ewart's suspicions about the weight of the heart.

Some sanatorium physicians, including those at the Toronto sanatorium, preferred to enhance the effect of bedrest through the use of an inclined horizontal plane, often achieved by raising the foot of the bed (figure 5.2). Ann Peters (Williams), a former child patient at Craig-y-nos sanatorium in Wales, earned the nickname "Ann on blocks" because the foot of her bed had been raised up on twelve-inch blocks in an effort to stop her lung hemorrhages.[140] As patients improved, the foot of the bed was lowered, about four inches at a time, until they eventually lost their incline altogether, in part to ensure no new disease activity emerged as the foot of the bed was gradually lowered, and in part because it was suggested that patients needed time to reorient themselves to the change in position.

Physicians who used tuberculin injections therapeutically to increase resistance to tuberculosis reasoned that they were effective because they produced hyperemia in tuberculous foci and that, by increasing blood supply, they stimulated "more protecting substances to the part which inhibit the growth of bacilli, digest them and the focal products, and carry off the residue."[141] Even vascular surgeons became invested in the idea of encouraging lung hyperemia and explored different techniques that are detailed by John Odell in his review of tuberculosis surgery. Older interests in encouraging lung congestion or lung hyperemia persisted alongside the rise and refinements in tuberculosis-related surgeries. Odell details Sayago's 1921 irritation-stimulating bone graft surgery, which "proposed placement of a bone graft removed from the tibia [the major long bone of the lower leg] and placed in a subpleural position between the first and fourth ribs. The presence of the graft was to excite a reaction in the lung, increasing blood supply and causing growth of fibrous tissue, which would encapsulate the tuberculous lesions."[142] Alternatively, surgeons could also attempt to slow breathing, following along the idea of Kuhn's earlier suction mask. As late as 1929, according to Odell, surgeons were attempting to divert blood flow: "Babcock divided the common carotid artery and jugular vein on the side of the tuberculous lung and anatomosed their proximal ends. His theory was that the diversion of blood would decrease the rate and amplitude of respiratory movements and produce a hyperemia around the tubercles. At 17 days he reported that the respiratory rate in the 28-year-old patient had been reduced such that 11,500 respiratory cycles per day had been saved," and the patient "was discharged with a less productive cough."[143] Even in the rising surgical age, then, interests were still drawn to the possibility of stimulating the body's natural healing forces by manipulating blood supply to tuberculous lungs.

Revisiting the Rationale and Physiology of Bedrest

Bedrest was one of the most enduring and seemingly straightforward aspects of tuberculosis treatment, inside and outside of the sanatorium, and there were two general ideas underlying its use. The first premise was linked to the therapeutic role of blood flow and delivering a greater blood supply to "anemic" apices. The second premise was grounded in the belief that rest was restorative, that only when relieved of excessive work could lungs repair and restore tissue damaged by tuberculous disease. This intuitive explanation was often called upon in reasoning with patients, parents, and guardians for the value and need of seemingly unending and tedious bedrest. While rest for healing was the popular lay explanation for bedrest, the underlying biological rationale, beginning with the anemia/hyperemia perspective, would continue to develop as both experimental data and clinical observations expanded the understanding of lung physiology in health and in diseases such as tuberculosis.

In 1946, physician William Dock[144] of Brooklyn, New York, revived the idea that apical anemia resulted in the apical localization of tuberculosis bacteria, incorporating perspectives on the intertwining influences of posture and gravity. Noting that in the upright posture the lung apices were "well aerated but bloodless," typically for fourteen to eighteen hours each day, Dock suggested that a lack of protective antibodies and phagocytes stemming from limited blood flow was more critical in shaping apical vulnerability to tuberculosis than gas tension or oxygen concentration in the apices.[145] As to the tendency for tuberculosis to reactivate in the lung apices of adolescents and young adults, Dock targeted the social lives of "lively young people who get a minimum of sleep."[146] Specifically, he argued that because young adults tended to spend a higher than average number of hours each day out of bed and in an upright posture, the tuberculosis bacteria already present in their bodies were given "the maximal number of hours of optimal growth conditions and the tissues [of the lung apex] the minimal number of hours when the neutralization and dilution of toxic products, and the supply of antibodies and blood-born phagocytes, are as adequate at the apices as elsewhere in the lungs."[147] What remedial action did Dock suggest? A midday rest, which he believed to be therapeutic in preventing tuberculosis reactivation, because "the highest toxin level occurring each day might therefore be cut in half," such that "in many people where the balance between resistance and susceptibility is so narrow this could easily make the difference between progress and regression of a lesion."[148] Rest may have offered some therapeutic benefit, but it was the recumbent horizontal position that redirected and increased blood flow to the apices and was believed to restore "resistance" to tuberculosis in the upper part of the lungs. Here,

Dock's arguments connect explicitly with the common belief that tuberculosis disease was associated with "overwork," the possibility being that it was not the nature of the work or its physicality, but the number of hours spent upright at work that had the detrimental effect on tuberculosis disease. Likewise, the time spent at recreation, and not rest, was viewed as troubling. In a February 1928 article in the *Globe*, Dr Dobbie, discussing tuberculosis vulnerabilities, lamented the enticements of the urban nightlife: "Today the majority of the young people are wasting their energy in the hue and cry after excitement. Today there is too little sleep, too many late hours, too much excitement, all for what is called pleasure."[149] Once again, Mamie embodied this seemingly careless lifestyle in *Her Own Fault*.

Though Dock addressed, but downplayed, the "aerated" aspect of the apices, and instead focused on the role of blood flow, there was growing attention placed on the possibility that differential oxygen concentrations in regions of the lung had an effect in tuberculosis. Oxygen is important to tuberculosis bacteria, since they are obligate aerobes and require oxygen-rich environments for growth and reproduction. In his history of studies in pulmonary circulation, A.C. Bryan notes that, in 1911, German physician Richard Siebeck published experimental evidence suggesting that the distribution of inspired air in the lung was not uniform.[150] As the understanding of lung physiology grew, so did insights into the complex relationships between oxygen distribution (ventilation) and blood flow (perfusion) in the lungs.[151] According to Bryan, in 1922, Scottish physiologist John Scott Haldane published on the idea of some "proportioning" of regional "air supply" and "blood supply" in the lungs.[152] This relationship would come to be characterized as the ventilation/perfusion ratio.

Examining ventilation and perfusion dynamics in the lung, Robb Glenny notes that both gravity and the closely matched structures of the vascular and airway trees of the lung may influence regional distributions of blood flow and oxygen in the lung.[153] There is an overall tendency to match ventilation and perfusion in the lung, with "airways and pulmonary arteries" that "branch in union with each other"; this close relationship ensures that gas exchange (of oxygen and carbon dioxide) is efficient.[154] Moving from lung apex to base, there are increases in both ventilation (oxygen concentration) and perfusion (blood flow), with the highest measures for both at the base of the lung. However, what does change from apex to base is the degree of "matching" or the ratio between ventilation and perfusion. In an upright posture, the effect of gravity appears to be greater for differential blood flow (or perfusion), as Rhoades notes a "five-fold difference between the top and bottom of the lung" in perfusion, but only a two-fold difference in ventilation (or oxygen supply) from apex to base.[155] Because of this difference, Rhoades argues, the lung apices tend to be over-ventilated (over-oxygenated) in relation to the amount of blood flow they receive (i.e., fewer red blood cells are supplied to pick up the available oxygen for arterial transport). As a result, oxygen-loving (aerobic) tuberculosis bacteria find an ideal niche in the apices, relatively higher in excess oxygen concentration and lower in immune cells and function.[156] According to Bryan, the ability to manipulate combined ventilation/perfusion dynamics (not just blood flow) by changing body position came to be recognized by pulmonary specialists such as Stig Björkman in the 1930s; when the patient lies on one side, the dependent lung receives a greater blood supply and has lower oxygen concentrations, while the non-dependent lung is more deficient in blood supply and higher in oxygen concentration.[157]

Despite the attentions given to blood flow in the lungs and the early hyperemia-based treatments, the potential significance of apical oxygen concentrations, or even just oxygen more generally, was slower to permeate. "The possibility that the lung is more favorably situated for the growth of tubercle bacilli on account of its higher oxygen tension than is any other organ in the body," noted Dr Harry John Corper, of Denver, in 1927, "has been given little, if any, consideration in the past."[158] He considered the lungs to be "especially favorably suited (from the standpoint of available oxygen) for the development of the bacilli." While the long-standing focus on blood dynamics was grounded in concepts of bodily immunity and resistance, the focus on oxygen shifted attention to bacterial needs and why some niches in the body might be more suitable to meet those needs.[159] Reasoning in 1926 that the lung apex was a highly oxygenated environment, Joseph Walsh advocated manipulating blood flow to the apices in order to reduce the high oxygen concentrations that tuberculosis bacteria found so favourable.[160] He believed, however, that the apices were highly oxygenated because of high blood flow, and suggested that to protect the apices, passive hyperemia, or a more sluggish circulation of blood, was needed to discourage tuberculosis bacteria development. In 1936, Burgess Gordon noted that bacterial pneumonia was typically localized in the lung's lower lobes, while tuberculosis had a predilection for the upper lobes and apices. These differences in localization he attributed to the fact that pneumococcus bacteria were aerobic, but optionally anaerobic and could persist in low oxygen environments, while tuberculosis bacteria were strictly aerobic and therefore inflexible when it came to oxygen.[161] Grounded in this perspective, he suggested the possibility that a therapeutic reduction in pulmonary ventilation could inhibit the growth of tuberculosis bacteria.[162]

Given the greater attentions to studies of ventilation and gas tension in the lungs, and the potential importance of oxygen in tuberculosis pathology, Dock would further flesh out his ideas on the therapeutic value of bedrest in a 1954 publication.[163] Presenting a new synthesis of accumulating experimental data, he refocused on apical oxygen concentrations, the effects of which he had recognized but underplayed in his earlier 1946 publication. Dock credited the experimental work of Scott, Hanlon, and Olson for demonstrating that "changes in gas tension created by altered pulmonary flow are of paramount importance in favoring growth of tubercle bacilli."[164] Zones of high oxygen and low carbon dioxide tension would create the most "favorable soil" for tuberculosis bacteria, and this, he argued, was precisely the character of the apices, because of gravity's effects, when humans were in an upright posture.[165] Dock maintained the idea that alterations in blood flow stemming from postural change are important, but because of resulting changes in gas tension in the apices (not because changes in blood flow influence the delivery of antibodies and phagocytes and dilute toxins, as he had argued in 1946). Significantly, he posited that it is not just a general greater quantity of blood to the apices that is beneficial in controlling tuberculosis, but the quantity of deoxygenated blood, in particular, for its effect in picking up and therefore reducing the high concentration of oxygen in the apices. As a result, Dock believed perfusion of the apices with unsaturated or deoxygenated blood held the greatest promise for therapeutically reducing their vulnerability to TB bacteria.

Dock credited the work of Edgar Medlar and colleagues for the idea that posture worked in conjunction with gravity to influence the dynamics of ventilation, perfusion, and sites of lung vulnerability in tuberculosis. Medlar undertook experiments with tuberculosis-infected rabbits, rigging them up in harnesses that artificially held them in the bipedal upright posture of humans. Sure enough, in that position, rabbits developed apical pathologies similar to humans (as quadrupeds, rabbits would typically develop tuberculous lesions along the dorsal non-dependent aspect of their lungs; this was compared to bats, which spent much of their time sleeping in an upside down position and typically developed tuberculous cavities at the base of their lungs). As a result, Dock remained convinced that postural change would have a therapeutic effect for humans, but instead of arguing that lying down and changing blood-delivery dynamics to the apices would influence the provision of antibodies and phagocytes, blood delivery (particularly unsaturated blood) would be important for reducing the high oxygen concentrations that characterized the apices in an upright posture. More unsaturated blood meant more oxygen binding, and the overall reduction in oxygen concentrations would be a detriment to aerobic tuberculosis bacteria. In this model, human anatomy would always render the right lung's apex even more vulnerable to tuberculosis than the left apex, a common observation, because, as Dock described, the more "tortuous course" of the right pulmonary artery means that unsaturated blood will always be delivered less effectively to the right lung in comparison to the left lung.[166] Significantly, Dock also redressed the idea that bedrest was important for "resting" the lung to facilitate its healing, and instead he saw the pure therapeutic effect only in the redirecting of blood flow that stemmed from the horizontal position of bedrest.[167] To Dock, the action of resting was not as important as the position of resting.

A recent study investigating the effects of positional changes and gravity on lung dynamics demonstrates that, in the prone position, there is greater homogeneity in the distribution of oxygen in the lungs and, as a result, there is greater efficiency in oxygenating arterial blood.[168] Glenny and colleagues believe that oxygen concentration may be a more important driver in the effects of positional change on ventilation and perfusion dynamics in the lungs. In particular, oxygen distribution is more greatly affected by changes in gravitational force on the body in the upright versus horizontal position. Changes in gravitational force will stimulate ventilation changes in the lung, and in turn this will effect change in regional perfusion differences in the lung: "Any change in regional ventilation that alters local alveolar O_2 pressures may invoke local changes in perfusion through hypoxic pulmonary vasoconstriction."[169] Overall, from the perspective of the lung's vulnerable apices, by orienting the body in a horizontal, prone position, a more homogenous distribution of oxygen in the lungs combined with higher perfusion to the apices suggests that oxygen could be bound more effectively, reducing some of that excess oxygen in the lung's apices (which would be a disadvantage to tuberculosis bacteria).

Offering these insights on the therapeutic effect of bedrest in 1954, well into the age of antibiotic treatments in tuberculosis, Dock's insights may well have been interpreted as interesting, but no longer as important, since the sanatorium era was slowly drawing to a close. The problem of drug-resistant tuberculosis bacteria was noted early in the use of antibiotics in tuberculosis, however, and, as Dock argued, "strains of bacilli resistant to known and yet-to-be discovered antibiotic combinations may appear, but strains which are insensitive to the tension of gases in venous blood are not known."[170] Further, he believed that the distribution of antibiotics to all areas of the lungs, including the troublesome apices, would be made more effective if combined with the improved blood flow dynamics of bedrest. Dock concluded his article focused on the big picture, indicting the industrial revolution and its supply of "cheap artificial light" for lengthening working hours and the amount of time people spent upright instead of lying down, providing tuberculosis bacteria with a decidedly "vulnerable spot in the armor" of human bodies, their over-oxygenated upright lung apices.[171] Under the direction of sanatorium physicians, tuberculosis patients would spend more time than the average person per day out of the upright posture and lying flat in bed. Overall, Dock was convinced that bedrest, in itself, could offer at least some therapeutic benefit in the control of pulmonary tuberculosis, and was not necessarily just the long-standing bane of sanatorium patients.

Conclusion

From blood to oxygen, it is possible to consider the biological intentions and therapeutic effects of sanatorium treatment. In retrospect, both the hyperemic treatments and the blood and oxygen manipulations of bedrest (from Dock's review) can be considered from the perspective of resistance in tuberculosis. Much of the focus on blood revolved around the belief that, with increased blood flow, would come the delivery of immunity-buffering cells such as antibodies. The role of antibodies in tuberculosis was, however, severely challenged by the emergence of the Th1/ Th2 paradigm, which argues that it is the Th1 pathway that is active in the cell-mediated immunity of intracellular infections (such as tuberculosis), while the Th2 pathway is called into play for extracellular pathogenic infections.[172] The Th1 pathway is linked to a whole cascade of activations, of macrophages, natural killer cells, and CD8+ T cells, whereas the Th2 pathway is linked to antibody secretion in blood and other bodily fluids (and is therefore also known as humoral immunity). It would seem, therefore, that all of the attention given to blood flow dynamics may have been misplaced, since the role of antibodies in tuberculosis came to be conceptualized as minimal with the Th1/ Th2 paradigm. Since the mid-1980s, when the Th1/ Th2 paradigm surfaced, however, researchers have been challenging the notion that these pathways operate independently under "a distinct division of labour," and that, specifically, antibodies of the Th2 pathway may in fact play a role in supplementing the immunity provided by the Th1 pathway in tuberculosis.[173]

How might antibodies play a part in tuberculosis immunity? Glatman-Freedman has argued that even "intracellular pathogens," such as tuberculosis bacteria, "can be found in the extracellular space during their life cycle, either before entering into host cells or after the cell death, and can then be easily reached by antibodies."[174] There are a number of different ways in which antibodies may work cooperatively with the cells of the Th1 system, such as macrophages, one example being the role of antibodies in opsonization.[175] In this scenario, antibodies are opsonins, or intermediaries, which enhance the success of phagocytosis as one part of the antibody binds to antigens that lie on the surface of bacteria, while another part of the antibody binds to receptors on the macrophage. In this way, antibodies may provide a real, physical connection between TB bacteria and macrophages (phagocytes), thus facilitating the macrophage's effective "consumption" (or phagocytosis) of TB bacteria. Alternatively, antibodies are suspected to interfere with the ability of tuberculosis bacteria to adhere to host tissues, a necessary first step in tissue colonization, or antibodies may bind with and neutralize toxins produced by tuberculosis bacteria.[176] It is notable that this was of particular interest to supporters of artificial hyperemia, that is, to increase blood supply to manage the toxic substances produced by tuberculosis bacteria. In this scenario, Abebe and Bjune argue that there may be "a synergy and mutual interdependence" between cell-mediated and humoral immunity, not a discrete polarization of the roles of these two different branches of the immune system.[177] Grounded in this understanding, it is entirely possible that the value sanatorium-era physicians placed in blood flow in better resolutions of lung cavitation and disease could have some biological weight. With this increased blood flow would come a higher quantity of immune cells and a greater chance of stemming the progression of disease.[178] By the 1930s, however, Glatman-Freedman and Casadevall note that there was a deepening intellectual shift away from ideas of antibody-mediated immunity in tuberculosis.[179] Attention was drawn away from the search for protective antibodies (T_h2 immunity) and refocused on the function of cell-mediated immunity (T_h1 immunity) in tuberculosis. Within this shifting paradigm, the focus on blood and antibodies in tuberculosis would lose traction.

Aside from the potential benefits of increased blood flow, the blood flow itself could also affect oxygen concentrations in the lung, particularly the focal area of the lung apices. As Dock argued, it is likely that lowering oxygen tensions in the apices had a therapeutic effect in tuberculosis. What is interesting in this dynamic, however, is that the medical effects in lowering oxygen, albeit unknowingly in the early days of bedrest, once again mirrored aspects of the body's natural defences against tuberculosis bacteria. In this instance the focus is on macrophages. On the basis of mouse studies, Sever and Youmans proposed in 1957 that individual differences in resistance to tuberculosis might be accounted for in part by a "decrease in oxygen tension caused by venous blood perfusing through the lung," but also by "the quality and/or rapidity" of the body's response in directing macrophages to affected lung tissue.[180] They suggested that "a rapid accumulation of macrophages" in affected lung alveoli, with a subsequent "reduction in oxygen tension produced by the macrophages" effectively inhibits tuberculosis bacteria proliferation, giving the body an advantage in healing.[181] Strong, fibrous, calcified granulomas, composed primarily of T cells and macrophages, are created naturally by resistant bodies in tuberculosis;[182] in less resistant bodies, granulomas may fail and become sites of caseous necrosis.[183] Amongst other things, the inner environment of the granuloma is notably hypoxic, low in oxygen tension, and therefore challenging for aerobic tuberculosis bacteria. The bacteria caught within this hypoxic environment are first lulled into lower states of metabolic activity, and then genetically "reprogrammed," to become virtually latent but to "survive for decades in a state characterized by reduced metabolism, nitrate respiration, thickening of the cell wall, and negligible DNA synthesis," all of which can be reversed if the bacteria are at any point "re-exposed to oxygen."[184] According to Nickel and colleagues, the work of the bacteria-containing macrophages situated within the confines of the solid wall of the granulomas is enhanced by the hypoxic environment, stimulating an immune pathway that produces an antimicrobial peptide known as hBD2 which is effective in limiting tuberculosis bacterial multiplication.[185] Thus, both biologically and immunologically, oxygen is significant in tuberculosis. As its best defence, the human immune system creates hypoxic environments within granulomas that are detrimental for tuberculosis bacteria but stimulating for protective macrophages. While positional bedrest and hyperemia may have been intended to redirect blood flow, there were potential underlying effects on oxygen tension that ultimately (but likely unknowingly) mirrored the body's natural mechanisms for reducing oxygen availability to tuberculosis bacteria.

The surgical procedures of compression, explored in the next chapter, may be conceptualized as a natural extension of bedrest, and this was argued from the layperson's explanation, that compression was a form of "aided bedrest," which placed the lung in a type of "air splint." Compression took the intended effects of bedrest, to decrease lung activity, and exerted those effects directly (by putting the lung at rest with collapse).

But compression treatments were being explored well before the more advanced understandings of lung physiology were emerging. Instead, compression was borne out of other insights and brought into the prevailing approach to therapeutic treatment. Like bedrest, the true physiological effects of compression on the lung and its implications for tuberculosis bacteria would come to be understood over the course of the twentieth century, well after the actual introduction of the technique itself.

CHAPTER 6

From Collapse to Cure: The Modern Therapeutics

The day of the sanatorium as a sort of boarding-house is past. The modern sanatorium is a hospital for active treatment. No sanatorium to-day can call itself modern which does not have at least 50 per cent of its patients under some form of collapse therapy.[1]

~ Norman Bethune

By the 1920s and into the 1930s medical therapeutics expanded as surgical treatments for tuberculosis became more common in North American sanatoria. Before the introduction of surgeries, the standard passive sanatorium treatments of diet and bedrest did not cause dramatic bodily changes, just a hopeful, slow tide of steady improvement, as observed in weight gain, returning appetites, and the retreat of fever. Sanatorium patients did not experience the "heroic" cures of nineteenth-century traditional medicine, the calomel, purging, and bleeding, and their "alterative" effects on the body, such as diarrhea and salivation;[2] as a result, resistance building often lacked the tangible reassurance provided by those dramatic bodily reactions to treatment. Without such effects, sanatorium patients and their families had to rely on their convictions of the benefits of supportive treatment and resistance building, even if improvements did not come quickly or predictably. Sanatorium physicians understood that this was why some patients left the sanatorium early in treatment and against medical advice, because either they (or, with child patients, their families) lacked confidence in the somewhat imperceptible nature of sanatorium treatment, or they felt they could manage these treatments just as well at home.

The introduction of surgeries reshaped perceptions of the sanatorium's abilities to influence the course of tuberculosis disease. Belief in the science and expertise of sanatorium therapeutics grew exponentially. Unlike bedrest, surgeries visibly manipulated tuberculous bodies, and though the treatments became more daunting, patients and their families were undoubtedly much more reassured that "something," physically, "was being done,"[3] and seemingly their satisfaction and confidence increased. While greater respect for the abilities and "medical authority" of physicians and their treatments generally characterized the modern era,[4] this effect was enhanced in the sanatorium as it moved into its surgical era. Nobody with a strategically collapsed lung could deny having received the most modern and scientific of tuberculosis treatments. Though the approach to the body changed with surgeries, the intentions remained unchanged; surgeries could not cure the underlying infection, but could, like bedrest and diet, assist the body's natural defences to more effectively control resident tuberculosis bacteria. Canadian physician Norman Bethune, himself an artificial pneumothorax recipient, suggested in 1932, "Rest, either physiological or so-called mechanical, will not by itself cure the disease; it merely induces local conditions favourable for the re-establishing of the body's defensive mechanism, those mysterious and incalculable elements, the sum total of which are called resistance."[5] Decisions to strategically collapse lungs were linked to the underlying ethos of "rest" in tuberculosis, but instead of requiring patients to remain in bed to rest their lungs, the lungs could be artificially placed at rest independent of the body and its actions. With the focus continuing to be placed on lungs at rest, the surgeries introduced at the sanatorium simply extended the rationale of rest treatment already in place.

The use of tuberculosis-related surgeries intensified at the Toronto sanatorium over time. The first official report for the surgical wards at the Toronto sanatorium appeared in the National Sanitarium Association's Annual Report for 1930–31. A couple of years later, in 1933, the Toronto sanatorium introduced a new building to its landscape, the 100-bed Ames surgical building, a modern brick building some four stories high. In addition to pre- and post-operative patient wards, the surgical building featured a solarium on the top floor and balconies on the lower levels intended for supplemental treatments of heliotherapy. The presence of balconies on a sanatorium building constructed in the 1930s may seem somewhat anachronistic, in that balconies and porches were more typical of older, cottage-style sanatoria.[6] On the modern surgical building, balconies emphasized the enduring use of UV light therapy in surgical cases, particularly for bone and joint tuberculosis. Basement space was reserved for a laboratory, diet kitchen, the night nurses' dining room, dishwashing rooms, an employee dining room, storerooms, and thirteen bedrooms for male employees of the surgical building. The operating room complex occupied a separate wing of the surgical building, equipped with an examining room, a surgeons' dressing room, a nurses' dressing room, a scrub room, a sterilizing room, a plaster room (for plaster cast making), and a nurses' utility room. Two observation galleries overlooked the operating room, both equipped with loudspeakers so that surgeons, outfitted with lapel microphones, could lead observers (such as interns and resident physicians) through surgeries. Surgery would remain a priority at the Toronto sanatorium, eventually overlapping with the introduction of antibiotics, and then waning as lungs, bones, and organs were increasingly spared from the ravages of tuberculosis through early and effective antibiotic treatments.

The Origins and Intentions of Artificial Pneumothorax

Surgical treatments for tuberculosis initially entered the Toronto sanatorium with artificial pneumothorax, a procedure intended to strategically collapse (or compress) tuberculous lungs. Conceptions of pneumothorax as a treatment for tuberculosis emerged long before medicine's modern, scientific era. Thomas Daniel credits Italian physician Giorgio Baglivi (1668–1707) for his observation, in 1696, of the seeming improvement of a tuberculous patient who suffered a penetrating sword wound that collapsed one of his lungs (known as a spontaneous pneumothorax).[7] Alex Sakula forwards the chronology, identifying the pneumothorax-related observations of Parisian physician Edmond Claud Bourru (1737–1823) in 1771, and British physician-physiologist James Carson (1772–1843) in 1822. Attempting to duplicate the seemingly therapeutic effects of spontaneous pneumothorax, Carson experimented with inducing lung collapse in rabbits and, later in 1822,[8] enlisted the help of a surgical colleague to induce an artificial pneumothorax in two human tuberculosis patients. Ultimately, however, Carson's procedure failed because of adhesions, a common complication to be explored later in the chapter.[9]

Following Carson's failed attempt,[10] a number of physicians, including Irish physician William Stokes in 1827 and French physician Emile Toussaint in 1880, revived pneumothorax and wrote on their observations that an unplanned, spontaneous pneumothorax (caused by traumas or pathologies) appeared to have beneficial effects in lessening tuberculosis symptoms and disease.[11] Unaware of Carson's work, but having read papers by physicians such as Toussaint, Carlo Forlanini was considering the potential of artificial pneumothorax as treatment as early as 1882 and, in 1888, he attempted to duplicate the effects of spontaneous pneumothorax by inducing an artificial pneumothorax using an apparatus that he had designed with his brother, an engineer.[12] Though Forlanini had already presented his ideas on artificial pneumothorax at earlier medical congresses, it was his 1912 presentation at the International Tuberculosis Congress in Rome, refined through years of work, that Sakula notes, "He was able to present an authoritative report, for which he received a great ovation."[13] Following Forlanini's presentation, artificial pneumothorax gained popularity in North America as a treatment for tuberculosis.[14] Forlanini did not innovate the idea that pneumothorax might be therapeutic, but he did introduce the technology, the pneumothorax apparatus, which, along with the microscope and the X-ray machine, came to be strongly associated with tuberculosis, the sanatorium, and treatment. Accompanying the apparatus, Forlanini also introduced the use of nitrogen gas for inducing lung collapse (he had been dissatisfied with the use of various liquids and found that oxygen was absorbed too rapidly), and a "puncture method," using a pneumothorax needle, to pierce through the outer chest wall and into the pleural cavity.[15] Other physicians would later experiment with an incision method, but it was quickly discovered that "patients responded far more willingly when it was explained that a needle-prick was the extent of the treatment."[16] Using words like *operation* and *cutting* in explaining the incision procedure to patients was "often sufficient to discourage [them] from submitting to treatment."[17] A patient who wrote humorously about his experience with artificial pneumothorax in the Muskoka sanatorium's patient newsletter reveals how relatively minor the puncture method was perceived to be. "There was a slight sting," he wrote, "and I shouted, 'Kill that bee!' but it was all over then. The needle had pierced my side." His first feeling was one of "disappointment," the "soul-searing pain" for which he had "steeled" his "nerveless nerves" was only "about as devastating as a glass of coca-cola to a man who prefers ginger ale."[18] Because of its relatively non-invasive character and reasonable sensibility, Forlanini's puncture method ultimately prevailed.

When the therapy of artificial pneumothorax was introduced at the Toronto sanatorium in the 1910s, it integrated seamlessly with prevailing beliefs in the value and importance of "rest" in tuberculosis. In fact, adoption of artificial pneumothorax greatly extended the rest philosophy in tuberculosis. In 1912, Boston physician Gerardo Balboni reflected on the therapeutic effect of pneumothorax, believing that an "immobilized lung" could take "very little part in the respiratory act," and that "after having obtained immobilization there gradually takes place in the lung the process of repair" and the gradual "evacuation of cavities."[19] Immobilization, or rest, was believed to be important in lung healing, especially if Esmond Long's[20] description of the typical demands of lung activity is taken into account: "Let us form a mental picture, for a moment, of the lung sliding back and forth in its greased box, the pleural cavity, collapsing and expanding, stretching and relaxing, fifteen times, more or less, a minute, nearly a thousand times an hour, twenty thousand times a day."[21] Long likens the possibility of healing in an active lung to that of a cut palm: "Imagine an infected cut across the palm of the hand and ask yourself, What are the chances of ... healing if that hand is opened and shut twenty thousand times a day?"[22] A 1930s handbook issued by the Canadian Tuberculosis Association explicitly connects "rest," healing, and artificial pneumothorax, suggesting that when "lying in bed, even in deep sleep," the lung is still "in constant motion." Artificial pneumothorax, the handbook advises, collapses "the lung so completely that it cannot breathe," giving the lung "extra rest in addition to the rest it gets by lying in bed," and in that state of enhanced and induced "rest the diseased part heals."[23] Just as a broken bone would be hard-pressed to mend properly if not immobilized and placed at rest in a cast, the collapse of artificial pneumothorax was likened to a type of "air splint" for the lung.[24]

In 1911, Boston physicians Samuel Robinson and Cleaveland Floyd explored the idea that the body ("Nature") itself attempted to achieve lung compression in tuberculosis disease: "Nature seeks to reduce the mobility of a phthisical lung by restricting the activity of the thoracic muscles of the infected side, and the chest becomes almost stationary. The ribs approximate [locate closer together] themselves, and the normal convexity of the chest wall is flattened. A partial fixation of the lung thus results spontaneously from the presence of the disease."[25] In addition to the restricted work of the thoracic muscles, the rib approximation, and the partial lung fixation, Robinson and Floyd explored two disease symptoms, pleural effusion and toxemia, as further examples of "Nature's" healing ways in tuberculosis. Pleural effusion occurs when fluid produced by the body's inflammatory response collects in the pleural space between the lung and chest wall (the same space occupied by the nitrogen gas injected with artificial pneumothorax). Robinson and Floyd believed that the fluid helped to compress and immobilize the diseased lung, achieving the same type of compression effect sought in artificial pneumothorax. While physicians had experimented with all sorts of materials to insert into the pleural space to induce an artificial pneumothorax, from nitrogen gas, to oil, wax, and fiberglass, the body and its "pleuritic exudate," they argued, were "Nature's" original attempt at therapeutic collapse.[26] The biological effects of disease are furthered to behavioural changes as Robinson and Floyd suggested that the "general toxemia" caused by tuberculosis disease reduced patient "ambition and activity," bringing about rest in yet another way.[27] On the basis of these bodily changes in tuberculosis disease, Robinson and Floyd further justified modern medicine's commitment to rest in tuberculosis, believing that these "hints" provided by "Nature" of what was best in managing tuberculosis were repeatedly "violated by clinicians," particularly those "who increased the activity of phthisical patients."[28] Since the body itself worked towards lung compression and rest in tuberculosis disease, then according to Robinson and Floyd's perspective, modern medicine was correct in prescribing artificial pneumothorax and rest.

Though compression was advocated as an extension of the principles of bedrest, it actually exerted very different physiological effects, notably in changing ventilation and perfusion dynamics in the collapsed lung. These concepts can be linked back to the bedrest arguments, specifically those suggesting the horizontal orientation of resting bodies (and lungs) reduced bacterial access to oxygen by redirecting more blood flow to the vulnerable apices. Compression treatments such as artificial pneumothorax could achieve the same effect of reduced oxygen availability, but through a different action. As early as 1912, Gerardo Balboni, a Boston physician, suggested that "by strongly compressing the lung," artificial pneumothorax "probably diminishes the arterial circulation" to the collapsed areas.[29] On the basis of understandings reviewed in the previous chapter, and the attention placed on the "healing power of blood," restricting blood circulation by compression could, understandably, be seen as a poor choice for treatment. Compression did, in fact, decrease perfusion in the lung, but it did so as a by-product of oxygen restriction, and here is where the therapeutic connection is made with tuberculosis. With artificial pneumothorax, alveoli in the compressed areas of the lung become "non-ventilated" and hypoxic (deficient in oxygen).[30] Since there is a "tight matching of local ventilation and perfusion in the normal lung," changes in ventilation, or oxygen dynamics, can stimulate the body to make associated changes to blood flow (or perfusion) in the lung.[31] The oxygen-deprived alveoli in compressed lung tissue and the resulting hypoxemia (a deficiency of oxygen in arterial blood) trigger the body's response of hypoxic pulmonary vasoconstriction to redirect blood flow from the hypoxic alveoli to alveoli with higher oxygen tensions.[32] From a biological standpoint this is most efficient, since "the objective of the body is to achieve a normal ventilation-perfusion ratio of 1 in order to optimize blood-gas exchange."[33] Because of the body's efficiency in redirecting blood flow, "a patient affected by a pneumothorax … may barely display a decrease in blood oxygenation," indicating a successful adaptation to this altered state of function.[34]

In its net effect, artificial pneumothorax stimulates less (not more) blood flow to the collapsed tissues and marks a significant departure from the ideas surrounding artificial hyperemia. If oxygen concentrations were ultimately of greater importance in controlling tuberculosis bacteria, however, then artificial pneumothorax followed a more direct route than bedrest in achieving those lower concentrations. In undertaking artificial pneumothorax, by controlling the area and degree of compression, physicians could reduce the risk of extreme hypoxia, even asphyxiation, which can accompany a severe spontaneous pneumothorax.[35] As "the oxygen tension in the collapsed lung parenchyma reaches its lowest possible value, equal to that in mixed venous blood,"[36] there were significant implications for tuberculosis bacteria, which are obligate aerobes in need of oxygenated tissues for growth and reproduction.[37] In effect, then, the artificial pneumothorax created a lung environment less favourable for continued tuberculosis bacteria proliferation.[38] More than just resting the lung for healing, the artificial pneumothorax changed lung dynamics, undermining the potential success of tuberculosis bacteria in the lungs. If compression had beneficial effects because it restricted oxygen availability to tuberculosis bacteria, it is perhaps no coincidence that macrophages, the human immune system's phagocytic cells that consume tuberculosis bacteria, use oxygen deprivation as a key defensive strategy. The hypoxic inner environment of the macrophage is understood to trigger latency in tuberculosis bacteria.[39] Naturally, then, the body uses hypoxia as a defence, while, surgically, hypoxia in affected lung tissue was induced by compression.

Ideally, compression was targeted for the parts of the lung affected by tuberculous cavities, sites typically rife with tuberculosis bacteria. Cavities were "closed" by compression and served with reductions in blood supply and oxygen. While compression could not cure the body of tuberculosis, the altered lung environment did slow the multiplication of tuberculosis bacteria and, in so doing, "shifts the balance in favour of the host's defences."[40] This is a key point, since it meant that the evolving therapeutics of tuberculosis surgeries were still grounded in the sanatorium's original endeavour to assist, support, and encourage the body's natural defences. Ultimately, a "cure" in tuberculosis, more likely a "latency," would come about only through improved bodily resistance, assisted when possible by medical therapeutics such as artificial pneumothorax.

Artificial pneumothorax was one of a number of compression procedures that would evolve to place diseased lungs at rest, with the intention of closing lung cavities and encouraging healing. The "rest" of collapse was accomplished by the insertion of gas, often nitrogen, into the pleural space, or chest cavity. From the patient's perspective, compression therapy had an impressive benefit in the sense that lungs could now be placed at rest (and out of "work") without the need for full-time bedrest. Patients did not have to remain in bed because their diseased lungs could be held immobilized by the compression. As a result, physicians such as Balboni were able to provide patient case reports detailing their successful adaptations to life on artificial pneumothorax, such as a furniture dealer who, despite "having to carry considerable weight up and down flights of stairs," had "not lost a day's work" since his artificial pneumothorax, or the woman with a collapsed right lung who was happily seven months pregnant and doing all of her own housework.[41] Experience suggested that patients who maintained their artificial pneumothorax outside of the sanatorium were neither "crippled" nor "disabled" by the lung compression, instead living their lives, many able to return to employment, "working on gas," as it were.[42] From an infection perspective, pneumothorax was believed to benefit patients and, once discharged from sanatoria, their families, communities, and co-workers by "mechanically isolat[ing]" infection in the patient's body as bacteria became trapped in the collapsed and closed cavities produced by artificial pneumothorax, and cough and sputum production declined.[43] Socially, tuberculosis sufferers with artificial pneumothorax may have been more welcome in their return to life outside the sanatorium, because lung compression typically "limited coughing and spitting, which had hitherto rendered them obnoxious to others."[44]

Artificial Pneumothorax: The Procedure and Experience

To achieve compression, sterile air, most often nitrogen gas, was inserted, via the puncture of the pneumothorax needle, into the pleural cavity in between the pleural membranes lining the outer surface of the lungs and the inner surface of the chest wall (i.e., an "intrapleural" pneumothorax). As gas was inserted, air pressure in the pleural cavity was increased to the point at which it exceeded the pressure inside the lung and caused the lung to collapse. Physicians aimed to control the area and extent of lung collapsed by varying the site and amount of air inserted. Often the artificial pneumothorax would be induced gradually, beginning "with small, frequent injections [of gas], 200–300 cc every few days," and then increasing the amount of gas injected and lengthening the interval between treatments.[45] It is estimated that the pleural cavity is capable of holding a maximum of about 2000 cc of injected gas.

Nurses typically assisted in the procedure, in addition to preparing the pneumothorax equipment, which included the doctor's gown and gloves, towels and a sheet to drape over the patient from which a four-inch square was cut (to define the surgical working space), swabs and gauze, tinctures of iodine, alcohol, and Novocain (the preferred local anesthetic), anesthetizing syringes, and the pneumothorax needle, all sterilized.[46] Patients were placed to lie on the procedure table on the side opposite from the lung that was to be collapsed, positioning a pillow or sandbag under their ribcage and draping their upper arm over their head.[47] Long describes the basics of the procedure:

> The operation is conducted with the usual precautions of asepsis, and is carried out under local anesthesia, a drop of two per cent novocain solution being injected into the skin at a selected spot between the ribs, through which the hypodermic is passed down through the muscles of the chest wall, an occasional drop [of Novocain] being pushed ahead of the point of the needle, until the pleura is reached ... which is well anesthetized with a few drops before the needle is withdrawn. The needle track is next slightly enlarged with a thin bladed knife and the gas needle, protected by a guard from going too far, is inserted and pleura punctured.[48]

Air pressure was then carefully monitored as a selected volume of gas was injected through the pneumothorax needle. Immediately after the treatment, patients, who it was felt experienced "very little discomfort, if any," were encouraged to rest and were provided with a light meal.[49] Air embolism (where air gets into an artery or vein) was a rare complication.[50]

Artificial pneumothorax was naturally reversible, since the air injected into the pleural cavity would slowly dissipate and, as the air pressure fell, the lung would gradually reinflate to its original dimensions. As a result, in order to maintain good lung compression, patients were required to attend regular clinics for "refills" of gas. Refills would likely be required for patients every three to six weeks, often for "a long time, perhaps through life" if a long-term pneumothorax was desired.[51] It was observed that the lungs of patients who were on pneumothorax refills for a number of years sometimes did not re-expand when the pneumothorax was discontinued. In such cases, surgeons could achieve re-expansion by stripping away any fibrous tissue that had grown and restricted the lung.[52] Many patients, some estimate about 50 percent, improved while on pneumothorax.[53] But the return to health could convince some patients that their disease no longer needed such intensive medical management, and as they started feeling better, they might choose to abandon their pneumothorax refills.[54] Here the language of "non-compliance" or "non-adherence"[55] first enters into the realm of tuberculosis treatment. The chronic nature of tuberculosis infection and disease requires a long-term commitment to treatments, be it artificial pneumothorax or antibiotics. The concept of "non-compliance" did not emerge in the era of antibiotics, but was instead borne out of an earlier era. In the pre-antibiotic era, some physicians believed the answer to poor "compliance" with artificial pneumothorax and its necessary repeated refills lay in the selective use of thoracoplasty, a more surgically intensive procedure producing permanent lung collapse that required no patient commitment to long-term maintenance or upkeep.[56]

In order to be considered a good candidate for pneumothorax, patients had to have a least one relatively "good" lung, since it would be relied upon to perform the work of two lungs. With at least one good lung, the body is able to adjust to the lung compression by maintaining adequate levels of blood oxygenation. In the case of a pneumothorax of lesser size, there is "compensatory hyperventilation of the nonaffected lung," which prevents any notable hypoxemia (poor blood oxygenation); hyperventilation also takes place in pneumothoraces of greater size, but the compensatory work of one lung may not be sufficient and patients could experience the effects of poor blood oxygenation.[57] Tuberculous patients already struggling with shortness of breath were not considered good candidates for artificial pneumothorax: "A patient finding difficulty getting enough air into two lungs to satisfy the body needs is not apt to derive much benefit from the physiological removal of one of those."[58] Marked consolidation, where liquid matter such as blood or pus fills previously open air space in the lung, caused by disease activity, often precluded the usefulness of artificial pneumothorax because it would prevent successful collapse, though partial collapse in these cases might offer some therapeutic benefit.[59] For patients with bilateral lung involvement who were not good candidates for pneumothorax, Myers outlines other techniques that were favoured by physicians to achieve at least some compression, including placing weights (bags of shot) on the chest or applying abdominal supports to elevate the diaphragm and reduce lung expansion with each breath drawn into the lungs.[60]

A successful pneumothorax resulted in good compression of the lung in intended and affected areas. If patients suffered other illnesses, such as influenza, then pneumothorax treatments could be suspended in order to allow the lungs to function as fully as possible to clear those infections. Adhesions forming between the pleural surfaces, a by-product of lung inflammation, commonly foiled successful artificial pneumothorax, since the adhesions linking the outer wall of the lung to the inner wall of the chest cavity prevented the lung from falling in and collapsing. There was also a risk of tearing adhesions overlying thin-walled cavities in the lung and, if handled too aggressively, tearing out the wall of the lung and opening a connection between the lung's inner tuberculous cavity and the pleural space.[61] In this instance, the unwanted complication of an empyema, an infection of the pleural space, could result. The problem of adhesions led to a preference for gradually increasing the amounts of gas being injected, allowing for a gentle stretching of adhesions and reducing the possibility that they would abruptly tear. Collapsing well-developed cavities could also be challenging because these cavities typically had hard, thickened walls that resisted collapse.[62] Further, if cavities were located close to the periphery of the lung, then the cavities could rupture with compression, and, if the contents of those cavities were discharged into the pleural cavity, this again could lead to the problem of empyema.[63]

Children with primary tuberculosis (affecting the lymph nodes) did not need artificial pneumothorax (or any other compression-related surgeries), but children with reactivation disease and tuberculous lung cavities could be considered for the procedure. Age was not a restriction, and Myers felt that adolescents with cavitary disease could benefit from artificial pneumothorax, since their lesions were likely to worsen if they were kept on bedrest alone. As he argued, "The logical procedure is to bring about localized rest of the diseased lung at the earliest possible moment, through collapse therapy."[64] In this way, young patients could become ambulatory and return to their lives much earlier in their treatment than if left on bedrest alone, thus avoiding "the hazards of long periods of institutionalization" and becoming "safe associates from the standpoint of [not] spreading tubercle bacilli."[65]

Artificial pneumothorax at the Toronto sanatorium became more common in the 1920s, though trials with patients were undertaken in earlier years, as early as 1914,[66] as staff gained familiarity with the procedure. In 1917, Seth, a fourteen-year-old boy with reactivation disease, was considered for the procedure when he failed to make a "very marked degree" of improvement on bedrest. Though Dobbie recognized that explaining the details of the procedure to Seth's parents would be difficult, he did tell them that "the idea is to give him a better chance for improvement by preventing the poison of the diseased lung being spread throughout his system." By restricting lung cavities with compression, it was generally believed that artificial pneumothorax could prevent further disease dissemination. Seth remained on a regimen of artificial pneumothorax for two years, until his discharge in 1919, when it was advised that his parents ensure their son attend regular clinics for nitrogen gas refills to maintain the compression.

When Alice, thirteen years of age, was admitted in October 1937, it was reported that she had experienced absolutely no symptoms of tuberculosis until the month she was admitted, when a cough developed. She had been examined at the Gage Institute, where a diagnosis of tuberculosis was made. Orphaned since her mother and father had died of tuberculosis when she was an infant, Alice had been living with her grandparents and she did not have any siblings. When the diagnosis of TB was made at the Gage, Alice was taken back home and she remained in bed, on a waiting list, until she was admitted to the Toronto sanatorium in mid-October. Alice's disease was determined to be quite advanced, particularly for her young age. She had a large cavity in the apex (upper third) of her right lung, a classic indication of reactivation disease, and artificial pneumothorax was recommended. Alice's first compression was induced in November 1937, by which time pneumothorax was considered a relatively minor and reliable procedure.

The success of the artificial pneumothorax and its usefulness in arresting disease could vary over time in individual patients. Alice's medical narrative documents her physical progress under pneumothorax. When her collapse was induced on 19 November, a troublesome adhesion sitting at the level of a "thick walled and widely open" cavity in her right lung prevented a good quality collapse of the cavity. In January, her physicians attempted to fully close the cavity by increasing the amount of gas used in the compression, but even with the adhesion "stretching" somewhat, by March it had not yielded enough to collapse the "potent" cavity. In order to achieve a successful artificial pneumothorax, Alice's adhesion would ultimately have to be severed. The procedure, listed as a "closed intrapleural pneumonolysis" in her clinical record, was undertaken in March 1938, as described by Alice's surgeon:

> With the patient lying on her left side, with the upper end of the table slightly elevated, and her right arm held over her head, the right axillary region was prepared with benzene, ether, iodine and alcohol, and draped.
>
> A previously selected spot on the 7th interspace in the posterior axillary line was anaesthetized with 1% novocain. The trochar[67] and cannula[68] were inserted, after the thickness of the chest wall had been duly measured on the anaesthetic needle. The thoracoscope[69] was introduced, and immediately the adhesion came plainly into view, stretching from the upper margin of the well collapsed lung, in an upward and slightly forward direction, to the medial aspect of the second rib.

Once the thoracoscope was in place and Alice's adhesion visualized, it could be assessed for cauterization. Alice had been awake for the procedure, though the use of local anaesthesia (the 1 per cent Novocain that was administered) would have numbed her to it, and with her surgeon working in the area of the posterior axillary line (the midaxillary line runs from the pit of the arm down towards the waist, while the posterior axillary line lies immediately behind the arm), she would not see what was taking place. Tuberculosis-related surgeries, even the rib-removal surgeries of thoracoplasty, were only ever undertaken under local anesthesia because, as Paine and Hershfield explain, there was too great a risk for tuberculosis disease spreading under general anesthesia via the aspiration of tuberculous sputum into unaffected areas of the lung.[70] Returning to Alice's case, upon peering through the tube of the thoracoscope, her surgeon was able to see and describe the "smooth, glistening, and flesh coloured" adhesion, about four centimetres long and half a centimetre wide, that had part of the outer wall of her right lung caught up on a rib and was preventing her successful pneumothorax. He was also able to judge its suitability for cautery. In "galvano cautery," a red hot platinum wire was sent down the cannula and used to slice through the adhesion. Compared to the size of the incision that would have been needed to use a scalpel to do the cutting, galvano cautery was considered a far less invasive procedure.

Alice's trouble with adhesions did not return, and she was kept on a schedule of refills to maintain the artificial pneumothorax. Notations in her chart in the weeks following the pneumonolysis indicate that, after the adhesion was cut, her lung cavity remained well compressed, a "usual good collapse," as noted in April 1938. By June, the report to Alice's grandmother indicated that she was eating and sleeping well and, because her temperature was remaining consistently within normal limits, she had full bathroom privileges (meaning that she could get out of bed to use the toilet and bathing facilities). Overall, she had neither cough nor sputum, and her progress was felt to be quite satisfactory. In December, it was decided that Alice had progressed to the extent that she could be discharged. Alice's grandmother was anxious to have her back home, but had concerns about her abilities to arrange the forty-mile (sixty-four-kilometre) return trip each week for Alice's pneumothorax refills at the nearest clinic. The cost of the treatments was not an issue, since it would be assumed by Alice's municipality. According to the Act that came into effect 1 July 1938, municipalities were "required to provide this treatment and pay the fee to the doctor giving them, which fee is not to exceed $3.00 per treatment."[71] At the end of each year, municipalities submitted patient accounts to the Provincial Department of Health, and the total cost, as paid, was refunded. Alice had her last refill at the sanatorium in December.

When she was discharged to the care of her grandmother, in addition to the weekly refills, moderate restrictions on her exercise and at least twelve to fourteen hours of rest in bed each day were recommended.

Twelve-year-old Evelyn was given an emergency pneumothorax when she entered the Toronto sanatorium in late October 1938. Remarkably, up until only four days prior to her admission, she had been feeling well and attending school. Then, three days prior to her admission, Evelyn expectorated a large quantity of blood, some sixteen ounces (about two cups or 473 mL), and had been admitted to a local hospital. As one physician noted in 1940, "relatively small" hemorrhages experienced by adults were typically under 250 cubic centimetres (or 250 mL) and generally would not cause harm.[72] For a child of her size and age, Evelyn had experienced a significant hemorrhage. A chest X-ray confirmed tuberculosis disease. While in hospital, Evelyn was given morphine in an attempt to control her continued hemorrhaging. Morphine (and its pharmacological relations, codeine and heroin) was an antitussive often used to reduce coughing in cases of hemorrhaging, though some physicians raised concerns that, particularly in large doses, by suppressing coughs it could compromise bronchial drainage and lead to secondary pneumonia complications.[73] Though the overly aggressive coughing in tuberculosis was problematic, cough was still an important "defensive reflex" that functioned to "maintain the health of the lungs."[74] Aside from its antitussive effects, morphine was also intended to serve as an analgesic and sedative; patients, understandably, typically became frightened, anxious, and distressed as a result of hemorrhaging, all emotional states that could raise blood pressure and only worsen an already bad situation.

In addition to the patient experience, hemorrhaging could also be distressing for doctors and nurses. One nurse who worked at the Toronto sanatorium in the late 1910s and early 1920s recalled that many of the young nurses and nursing students, particularly those who had never really been around sickness before, found hemorrhaging events to be "very frightening." As she explained, "A patient would seem to be perfectly all right. You'd been feeding them their dinner maybe and just changing their pillows and making them comfortable for a nap after lunch; you'd go out and leave them and in a few minutes you'd hear that blast; three bells and you'd go on the run and the bed and the wall and everything would be covered with blood."[75] For medical and nursing staff, hemorrhaging was a sure and alarming sign of advanced disease and lung destruction; for patients, it was one of the most distressing symptoms of tuberculosis. According to one physician, the first critical step in effectively managing hemorrhages was to supportively encourage patients into a calm and relaxed state, which it was felt could be influenced by the very presence of the patient's physician, as one physician explained: "The mere presence of the physician with his reassuring smile and hand-clasp will quiet the racing heart and reduce the heightened arterial pressure. As a matter of fact, many bleedings have been known to cease with the coming of the doctor."[76] While this might be read as somewhat arrogant, it could also be understood as an expression of the close doctor–patient relationships and the power of the sympathetic yet medically authoritative consultation defining the modern era of medicine.[77] Once attending physicians arrived, the intent was to "lessen the cough reflex so that coughing is not violent,"[78] so patients were typically given a sedative and encouraged to lie in a position that they found relaxing and caused them to cough less, but still allowed them to raise the blood in order to clear their respiratory passages. Ice was widely used in sanatoria in cases of hemorrhage, with ice-bags placed over the heart and cracked ice given to patients to chew;[79] in this case the goal was to slow blood circulation in this acute event until the hemorrhaging could be brought under control. Ice was so important in this respect that both the Muskoka and Toronto National Sanitarium Association sanatoria included, in their physical plant, ice houses for making and storing ice. By the 1940s, blood coagulants such as fibrogen or thromboplastin had replaced ice and were often recommended for twenty-four to thirty-six hours after a hemorrhage.[80]

Given her hemorrhaging, immediately upon Evelyn's admission to the sanatorium, an artificial pneumothorax (and phreniclasia, to improve the pneumothorax) was induced on her right lung. Though artificial pneumothorax, along with phrenic crushes and blood transfusion, was often induced in long-term hemorrhage management, it could also be undertaken on an emergency basis with the hope of stemming acute hemorrhages (provided adhesions did not complicate the emergency collapse of the affected area).[81] Despite the procedure, however, Evelyn's disease remained active and spread further. A pneumothorax was later induced on her left lung in June 1939, but Evelyn experienced several large hemorrhages after the procedure. According to one report, "Her condition remained only fair until about 48 hours before her death when she complained again of shortness of breath. This was not more severe than on previous occasions but death occurred suddenly with no new symptoms developing." Evelyn died in the sanatorium at the end of August 1939, of advanced bilateral pulmonary tuberculosis. Because Evelyn's disease was so far advanced at the time of her admission, even the assistance of artificial pneumothorax could not slow its progression. As in Alice's case, outlined earlier, the seeming suddenness of Evelyn's onset of symptoms reinforces the insidious character of tuberculosis, a disease where destructive cavitation could eat away at the lungs all the while undetected by sufferers or their families. It was for this reason that tuberculosis workers in the endemic era strongly encouraged routine chest X-rays, even among the seemingly healthy, in order to detect disease at the earliest possible stage when it was theoretically more treatable.

When pneumothorax was successful, it was necessary to determine how long refills would be needed before the disease was considered arrested (or latent) and the lung could be allowed to safely re-expand to its normal dimension. Elizabeth was fifteen years old when she was admitted in March 1935. Soon after her admission, a pneumothorax was induced to collapse the upper lobe of her left lung. Improvement was gauged first by her sputum smears, which began to return negative for tuberculosis bacteria. Positive results were also noted as, over time, the cavity in her left lung closed, her red blood cell sedimentation rate fell to normal levels, and she started to put on weight. Elizabeth was medically approved for discharge and returned home in May 1936, but continued to return to the sanatorium for pneumothorax refills. Overall, her case was progressing favourably. In December 1936, however, Elizabeth caught a cold and, sick in bed, missed her refills. Here is a perfect example of the conflict between the medical ideal of scheduled refills versus the patient reality of unforeseeable complications of life. Unfortunately, according to her clinical notes, when Elizabeth felt better and "did report again" for a refill the "pneumothorax was almost out and widespread pleural adhesions had formed." Because of the adhesions, Elizabeth's pneumothorax had to be abandoned.

Despite her lost pneumothorax, Elizabeth remained well until March 1937, at which time she contracted influenza. Her persistent cough appeared at this point, but she did not begin to produce sputum until after she was re-admitted to the sanatorium in May. At that point, laboratory testing of her sputum smears returned positive for tuberculosis bacteria, confirming that her tuberculosis infection was active once again. A thoracoplasty was considered for Elizabeth, but, because of her general weakness, her physicians opted instead for a less aggressive phrenic nerve crush. A phrenic crush was an alternative to a phrenicotomy, though both procedures aimed for the same result. A phrenicotomy involves sectioning the phrenic nerve and induces paralysis of the diaphragm. The paralyzed diaphragm is pushed upward by the abdominal organs and, through its pressure, compresses a tuberculous lung (the lower lobes in particular). Though phrenicotomies were intended to be permanent, in 25 to 30 per cent of cases the diaphragm did not remain permanently paralyzed unless a "radical phrenicotomy" approach was used.[82] As a result, phrenicectomy, the permanent, surgical removal of a segment of the phrenic nerve, also evolved. A phrenic crush (or phreniclasia), on the other hand, was intended as a temporary measure. The nerve was accessed surgically via an incision about an inch above the clavicle or collarbone. Once exposed, the nerve was injected with Novocain and "crushed thoroughly," the incision then closed. The crush paralyzes the diaphragm for three to six months and, in so doing, typically restricts full lung expansion.[83] Dr Garrett, of the Toronto sanatorium, noted that these procedures involving the phrenic nerve were "used for some years but appeared to be sending a boy to do a man's [or pneumothorax's or thoracoplasty's] work" and could result in an undesirable thinning of the diaphragm.[84] British thoracic surgeon H. Morriston Davies did not believe that phrenic crush had "the slightest value" in the treatment of apical cavities so far up the lung and distant from the diaphragm. Instead, he emphasized the need to spare the diaphragm in the event that a thoracoplasty was required.[85] Similarly, Burgess Gordon advocated for the use of a corset-like medical device to compress the abdomen and elevate the diaphragm, instead of phrenicectomy, since he believed the "propelling force of the diaphragm" should be preserved to ensure future good-quality expectoration.[86]

At the point that a phrenic crush was being considered for Elizabeth, she was suffering from repeated small hemorrhages and had fevers that, on occasion, reached as high as 102°. After the phrenic crush Elizabeth seemed to improve but then, on 11 July, she suffered a "massive hemorrhage" accompanied by a persistent high-grade fever. Seemingly in a desperate race against Elizabeth's advancing disease, other surgical interventions were considered. On 21 July, a plombage involving the upper lobe of Elizabeth's left lung was undertaken. This time, a three-inch incision was made posterior to Elizabeth's left shoulder blade, her third rib resected by about two inches, and the outmost membrane of her thoracic cavity dissected. The apex of her lung was then gently pulled through this opening to allow for the insertion of 300 cc (1 1/5 cups) of paraffin wax. The apex was then tucked back into place and the incision closed in layers. Like artificial pneumothorax, phrenic crush, and thoracoplasty, plombage was intended to compress the lung in areas of tuberculous cavitation. Since the air used in artificial pneumothorax dissipated over time (and could result in difficulties, as evident in Elizabeth's case, to maintain a consistent schedule of refills among discharged patients) and lungs would lose their compression, "it was in the continuing search for substances other than air suitable to fill the space that plombage evolved."[87] In Elizabeth's case, liquid paraffin wax, in use since about 1913, was introduced into her pleural cavity, though other materials, such as gauze, fat, oil, rubber, fiberglass, polythene, and acrylic (Lucite) spheres[88] were also used in the history of the procedure.[89] Dr Garrett, of the Toronto sanatorium, recalled that when liquid paraffin or oil was used, the pull of gravity caused these fluid materials to descend in the pleural cavity and "tended to collapse the lower part of the lung, allowing the upper part, which was usually the diseased part, to expand."[90] Though the use of plombage in the management of tuberculosis was generally abandoned by the 1950s (as a result of the transition towards antibiotic treatments), years later, surgeons were publishing on some of the complications observed in patients due to unwanted migrations of these foreign materials in the body.[91]

In Elizabeth's case, the plombage was performed only as a last resort. It was not an ideal procedure for her, because both of her lungs were also compromised by a pneumonia infection. Procedure after procedure, the sanatorium physicians and surgeons had attempted to collapse the cavities in Elizabeth's left lung. Ultimately, however, the disease proved too aggressive and too far advanced. Forty-eight hours after the plombage, Elizabeth ceased to breathe, apparently in response to the overwhelming pneumonia complications in her right lung.

Thoracoplasty

Unlike the reversible methods of lung compression (such as artificial pneumothorax), thoracoplasty was a permanent method of collapse and sometimes viewed, as a result of its invasive nature, as a last resort in managing pulmonary tuberculosis. As one physician explained in 1943, "The surgeons who advocate radical methods as preferable ... are not the real phthisiologists." Physicians who worked with their patients for years, even decades, knew "the temporary methods are by far more humane and their results more gratifying," particularly if they could "defer the utilization of radical procedures."[92] Often the "less radical methods" were not possible because of complications such as extensive adhesions. On the other hand, adhesions often developed in advanced tuberculosis disease, so the very need for thoracoplasty often suggested delayed diagnoses. In 1932, Bethune argued that "thoracoplasty is usually a sign of neglected or delayed treatment in the past and should be a rare procedure in the future!"[93]

A far more complicated procedure than pneumothorax, thoracoplasty involved the surgical removal of selected ribs, or portions of ribs. Without the structural support of an intact ribcage, the chest wall fell inward, collapsing the lung in the area where ribs were removed. Like artificial pneumothorax, surgeons could control the location and extent of collapse to some extent, though the uppermost apical portion of the lung most troubled by cavitation in reactivation disease still remained the hardest to target for collapse. In Canada, thoracoplasty was first introduced by Professor Edward Archibald, the head of surgery at McGill University in

Montreal.[94] Like other compression treatments, this procedure was reserved for adolescents and adults, because lung cavities and advancing reactivation disease required more aggressive interventions. Adolescents and young adults were believed to fare the best in successfully recovering from the surgery.[95] A study of 231 patients receiving a thoracoplasty at the London Chest Hospital between 1947 and 1949, with only 28 per cent of them receiving a short course of antibiotics, revealed that six to eight years after the surgery, 82 per cent of those with thoracoplasty were living with latent (inactive) tuberculosis, 3 per cent had active disease, 14 per cent had died, and about 1 per cent had been lost to follow-up. The study considered the thoracoplasty results to be "satisfactory," since most had "extensive disease," but few had benefitted from antibiotics.[96]

Perhaps more so than other tuberculosis-related compression surgeries, the irreversible nature of thoracoplasty meant patients had concerns; the physical effects of the surgery would have to be weighed alongside the medical intentions to better manage TB disease. Though the technique had been refined, achieving "a technical perfection which allows us to expect functional restoration of the shoulder and a fairly aesthetic appearance of the chest," one physician, Donato Alarcón, writing in 1943, urged his colleagues to consider "the patient's point of view" and "how dreadful it is for him to face the decision for such a demolishing operation."[97] Recognizing "there is no way to avoid thoracoplasty when it is definitely indicated," Alarcón also noted that it was sometimes "impossible to avoid a deformity and to prevent asymmetry."[98] He felt that, for women, these thoracoplasty sequelae were a matter of particular concern, since "frequently their whole future depends on their physical appearance," while it would be difficult to convince male patients "that with a thoracoplasty he will not be crippled for the rest of his life, morally if not physically."[99] According to the recollections of a former Toronto sanatorium nurse working in the 1930s, thoracoplasty "patients were very ill ... it meant permanent disfigurement with the thoracoplasties ... and they recognized this. I think it was particularly hard for men who saw ... the physical aspects of their living as very important."[100] Bayne notes, "Recovery was slow and painful. Only the most determined person was able to regain a full upright posture, most were left with a hunched gait, and all had, of course, a deformed chest wall."[101] Others, however, have suggested that some patients, when clothed, "appeared to have a normal figure and only physical examination or radiographs would tell otherwise."[102] This variability may have been linked to which ribs and how many were removed.

Spinal curvature, or "thoracoplasty scoliosis," was a post-operative risk experienced, according to one study, in almost all cases.[103] With scoliosis, the spinal column developed a bend towards the side where ribs had been removed, and signs of scoliosis could appear as early as the first post-surgical week.[104] The degree of scoliosis was found to be greater when surgeons resected not only ribs, but also the transverse processes of the vertebrae that articulated with the ribs. Some surgeons felt a complete resection gave better cavity compression, though not all were in agreement on this point.[105] At the Toronto sanatorium, Dr Garrett noted that post-operative physiotherapy was initiated among thoracoplasty patients to help them to retrain the muscles of the thorax and spine, which became decidedly unequal in function, leading to scoliosis in the aftermath of these surgeries.[106] With refinements to thoracoplasty technique, attempts were made to retain the first rib, if possible, to prevent the shoulder from dropping, and to preserve the transverse processes of the vertebrae that articulate with the ribs in order to minimize the appearance of scoliosis.[107]

Regardless, all thoracoplasty recipients would have to learn how to function on less than two lungs for life. There have been recent studies of sanatorium-era thoracoplasty "survivors," a noteworthy descriptor since it implies that tuberculosis patients had to survive not only the disease, but also the surgical treatment of the disease. These studies suggest that while collapse may have inhibited tuberculosis bacteria, there were also negative effects on patient quality of life in the long term, including reduced lung expansion, decreased lung volume, greater work in breathing, hypoxemia (low oxygen levels in the blood), and hypercapnia (excess carbon dioxide in the blood).[108] Working to offset these problematic effects of thoracoplasty was the surgery's perceived success in limiting tuberculosis disease. Paine and Hershfield estimate that about 80 per cent of thoracoplasty recipients at the Ninette sanatorium in Manitoba experienced sputum conversion, signalling a retreat of active disease, in the aftermath of rib removal and lung compression. Unequivocally, they argue, "many patients would have died without [the] surgical aid."[109]

The technique of thoracoplasty would evolve, much to the benefit of patients. Initially, thoracic surgeons had followed the technique developed by thoracoplasty pioneers of the 1910s, such as German surgeons Max Wilms and Ferdinand Sauerbruch, commonly referred to as the "Wilms-Sauerbruch" approach.[110] Both advocated a one-step procedure, where surgeons would typically remove ten or eleven ribs at one time and, irrespective of the underlying TB pathology, all patients would receive the same surgery. In later years, surgeon Noland Carter would argue that there should be "no standard operation ... suitable for all patients," but, instead, "the operation has to be made to fit the needs of the individual patient."[111] The original Wilms-Sauerbruch thoracoplasty was physiologically traumatic for patients, often resulting in high morbidity and demonstrating relatively low success rates for closing tuberculous cavities; Belcher suggests that cavity closure was successful in only about 35 per cent of patients.[112] Typical complications included unwanted rib regeneration, the resistance of fibrous, thick-walled cavities to collapse and closure, and operative and post-operative hemorrhaging due to uncontrolled "bleeders" in resected muscle tissue.[113] Given the number of layers of muscle tissue that thoracic surgeons had to carefully work through in order to expose the ribs for resection, it is perhaps surprising that this was accomplished with patients under only local anesthetic, though, Davies explains, this was accompanied by "heavy doses of hyoscine [also known as scopolamine, used to prevent nausea and vomiting] and morphia" for additional sedative and analgesic effect; patients were insensitive to the pain of the surgery but still conscious.[114] As American surgeon Burr Noland Carter explained, "The safety of having the patient's cough reflexes present and the fact of not being fearful of a long inhalation anesthesia more than outweigh the somewhat greater tediousness of the operation under local anesthesia."[115]

In the evolving world of thoracoplasty surgery, the early Wilms-Sauerbruch approach to performing one big surgery would later be abandoned in favour of smaller, multiple surgeries, often involving three stages with four to eight weeks between each surgery and with fewer ribs removed

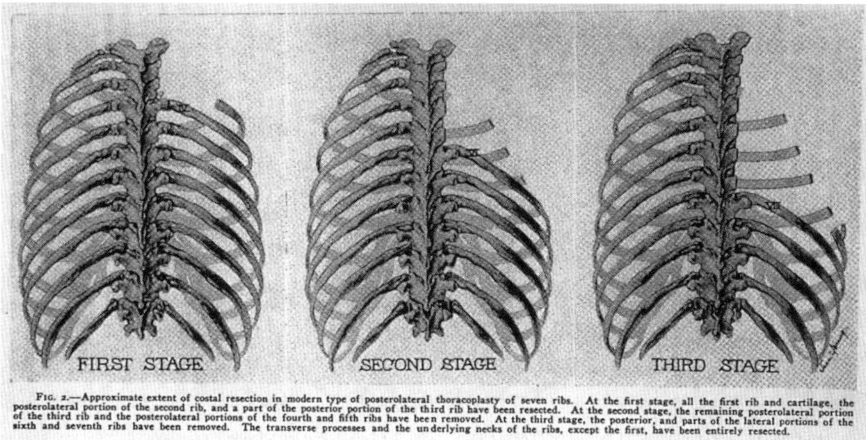

Figure 6.1 American surgeon John Alexander's three-stage thoracoplasty.

at any one stage (see figure 6.1).[116] The staged surgeries were intended to reduce physiological shock and trauma to the body and improve patient survival rates. According to one surgeon, thoracoplasty risk would have to be weighed carefully; the decision was whether it was "better to live with a cavity than die without one."[117] In the 1930s, patients at the Toronto sanatorium typically had three-stage thoracoplasties.[118] Efforts were invested in refining thoracoplasty, since there were few alternatives for patients with cavitary disease, most of whom with unclosed cavities would likely die within five years of cavity formation.[119]

A number of adolescents were admitted to the sanatorium with far advanced and cavitary reactivation disease whose only hope, it was believed, lay in thoracoplasty. When sixteen-year-old Leona was admitted to the sanatorium in 1937, Dobbie already had some familiarity with her case, since he had originally examined her at the Gage Institute in Toronto as a tuberculosis suspect. Dobbie was first questioned about the state of Leona's health in 1934, when the chief attendance officer of the Toronto Board of Education wrote to him in May of that year to obtain a medical certificate to explain why Leona would not be attending school on account of "an illness." In his reply, Dobbie explained that Leona had "an old case of tuberculosis showing some evidence of re-activation and the advice was given that she should be given rest in bed at home." Persistent, by September 1934 the attendance officer was once again writing to Dobbie to determine if she was "now improved and able to attend school," apparently unswayed from insisting upon her return to school even though the school board knew that she was troubled by active tuberculosis. Dobbie responded that "she appears now to be in such a condition of health that she may attend school," so Leona was once again sent back to school. By March 1935, still anxious of her tuberculosis reactivating, Leona's father wrote to Dobbie, concerned that the school was giving his daughter too much homework and that the strain was beginning to harm her health. Dr McHugh responded in March 1935 with a standard letter, which could be shown to each of Leona's teachers to help explain her vulnerable condition, "fair only," and that everyone needed to ensure she took "sufficient rest" to avoid a "recurrence" of active TB. "I think," McHugh wrote, "we should err on the side of giving her a little rather than too much work, because in a case such as this, if she breaks down again, it would take months, if not years, to heal." Despite her delicate condition and the concern that too much homework was a burden, sixteen-year-old Leona left school in December 1936 to begin factory work. It is likely that economic hardships borne out of the Depression years urged Leona's entry into the workforce. Ideally, she should have been resting but, practically, she would help to support her family.

Reinforcing the classical medical perspective on the physical dangers of "overwork," soon after she started at the factory Leona's tuberculosis infection fully reactivated, and shortly thereafter, in February 1937 she was admitted to the Toronto sanatorium. At this time, her prognosis was not good at all, described as advanced, bilateral (the whole of her right lung, and the apex of her left lung) pulmonary tuberculosis with positive sputum. Her physicians acted quickly in their attempts to stop the disease from progressing. Leona's worse right lung was the focus of treatment, first given a trial with artificial pneumothorax and, when this failed, a phrenic crush to paralyze her diaphragm. Showing no marked improvement, a three-stage thoracoplasty for Leona's right lung was initiated in November 1937 and completed in January 1938. Afterward Leona's progress was quite good, her cough and sputum disappearing after her last surgery. Leona was discharged home in February 1939. While she was never heard from again, a note sent to the sanatorium from a friend of the family reported that Leona was still alive and well over two decades after her discharge, having made "a complete recovery from her tuberculosis."

Another thoracoplasty variant was to arise in later years, a technique that came to be known as a Semb thoracoplasty. Norwegian surgeon Carl Semb introduced this new technique at the annual meeting of the British Medical Association in Belfast in 1937.[120] His approach differed from the Wilms-Sauerbruch technique in specifically encouraging collapse (or, as Semb termed it, a "relaxation") of the apex of the lung by resecting ribs and performing an "extrafascial apicolysis," the latter involving the surgical detachment of the parietal pleura, thus freeing up the troublesome apex of the lung to fall downward.[121] By adopting this two-pronged approach, Semb was able to achieve more than just a lateral compression of the lung through standard rib removal.[122] The Semb thoracoplasty procedure gained popularity, precisely because it targeted collapse of the apical region of the lung where reactivation cavitation was more likely to occur. The Semb variant was also favoured because it was less extensive than traditional thoracoplasties. Ribs one through four, closest to the lung apex, were targeted; often the whole of the first rib was removed, six inches of the second rib, five inches of the third rib, and four inches of the fourth rib. Surgeons were also careful not to remove the transverse processes of the vertebrae, an important change in technique that reduced the risk of scoliosis developing in the aftermath of the surgery. For patients, the more moderate Semb approach meant less disfiguration and was a good option if the disease was less advanced or had infiltrated less of the lung tissue. Together with Semb's advances, subsequent modifications in technique by American surgeon John Alexander, who advocated staged surgeries with the removal of no more than two or three ribs at any stage, the conservative removal of ribs, and the preservation of lower ribs (earlier surgeries typically removed the lower ribs first; Alexander began with the removal of upper ribs and left the lower ribs intact, if possible) would lead to a new modern approach to thoracoplasty.[123] Odell reports that Alexander's technique led to lower mortality rates (about 10 per cent) and high levels of sputum conversion (in 75 per cent of thoracoplasty survivors).[124]

In his autobiography, Sidney Hobbs described the two thoracoplasty procedures, or "thoros," as he called them, that he underwent during his time at the Toronto sanatorium. "In October/November, 1935," he recalled, "signs began to appear that my health was deteriorating to the extent [that] operations had to be done. On July 6, 1936, I was operated on for a thoracoplasty, four ribs on the right side."[125] He was "heavily sedated with morphine every four hours" in the days following the surgery and remained in bed for three long months of recovery. In his memoir the small details are remembered, as Hobbs fondly reflects on one of his post-operative ward nurses who "had a real knack of adjusting pillows to ease pain ... done in a certain way to release the pressure on the spine at the stub ends where the ribs were removed."[126] According to Hobbs, "she was always careful and smiling" while going about this work.

In 1937, Sidney's sputum checks continued to return positive for tuberculosis bacteria, indicating that, despite his surgery, he was still experiencing active disease. At this point, he had begun to feel his poor health in earnest, his weight dropping from 125 to only 90 pounds. Sidney recounted that "a series of 12 X-rays taken at weird angles finally located a tiny spot at the apex under my collar bone on my left lung." He was particularly alarmed at this development because he had come to rely on his left lung as his enduringly trustworthy and resilient "good side." Careful monitoring revealed that "as time went on, the spot started to go downward into a crescent shape." Another "thoro" was recommended and, as Hobbs recalled, "September 3, 1939, three days before the War broke out, they took out three ribs and three weeks later they removed another one and a half ribs." In the nine months that he spent in bed post-operatively, the ever-industrious and optimistic Hobbs learned to knit, instructed by both his charge nurse and a fellow patient whom he would come to know and love and later marry.

The Healing Power of the Sun: Treatment and Surgical Adjunct

In addition to a focus on rest, nutrition, and surgeries, the Toronto sanatorium also used heliotherapy (ultraviolet light therapy from the sun) and phototherapy (ultraviolet light therapy from an artificial source) to help build patient resistance.[127] Heliotherapy was undertaken on the flat roofs of the sanatorium buildings and the balconies of the surgical building, while phototherapy was provided by General Electric sun lamps (figure 6.2), a necessary adjunct given Toronto's seasonal climate and low UV

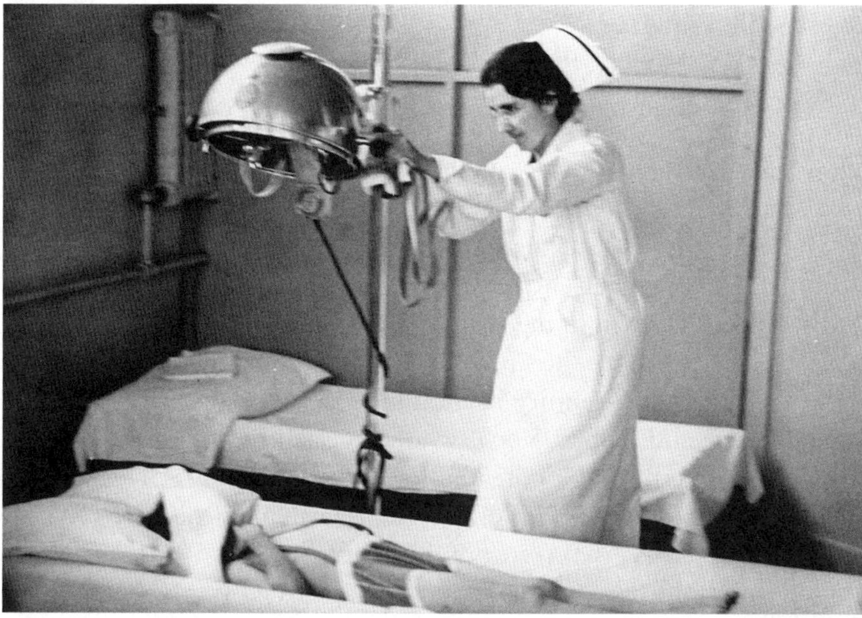

Figure 6.2 A nurse positioning a sun lamp for phototherapy. The child is wearing the type of "sun suit" commonly observed in photographs of children taking heliotherapy and phototherapy.

intensity in the winter months. In the late 1920s, the Queen Mary Hospital added an enclosed rooftop solarium fitted with Via Ray glass, one brand of a new selection of ultraviolet transmitting glasses developed to allow for indoor heliotherapy in hospital solaria.[128] Since UV light therapy was popular in the treatment of tuberculous lymph nodes, this meant that a large number of children admitted to the sanatorium would experience some form of UV therapy (which was also common at children's preventoria). According to a former Toronto sanatorium physician, "sun bathing" was often included in the treatment plans in cases of bone and joint tuberculosis, and was seen as an important adjunct to any surgical management of these cases.[129] During the twentieth century, surgery would become so common in bone and joint tuberculosis, in particular, that this form of tuberculosis came to be known interchangeably as "surgical tuberculosis."[130] Some physicians, including Auguste Rollier, resisted this trend and, throughout the early decades of the twentieth century, argued that patients with extrapulmonary tuberculosis could escape the "mutilations" of surgery through the dedicated and rigorous practice of heliotherapy alone.[131]

Ultraviolet light therapy and a general belief in the sun's therapeutic action have a long history. Roelandts traces the practice of heliotherapy back to 1400 BCE and notes that, with the discovery of ultraviolet (UV) rays in 1801, there was a surge of interest in its use, particularly in the second half of the nineteenth century.[132] Anthrax, rickets, and tuberculosis would all fall within the scope and interests of heliotherapy. In the case of tuberculosis, the therapeutic value of light therapy found its footing in the nineteenth-century bacteriological work of pioneers such as Louis Pasteur and Robert Koch, who suggested that UV light had antibacterial properties, or a potential for killing bacteria.[133] This idea attracted the interests of, among others, the Danish physician Niels Ryberg Finsen, described as "the creator of the light treatment"[134] or the "father of modern phototherapy."[135] Finsen was awarded the Nobel Prize in Medicine in 1903, shortly before his untimely death from Pick's disease at forty-three years of age in 1904, for his work with ultraviolet light and the treatment of tuberculosis of the skin (known as lupus vulgaris).[136] The carbon-arc lamps that he designed specifically for use in his phototherapy work came to be known as "Finsen lamps."

In the first decade of the twentieth century, a number of European physicians, including Oskar Bernhard and Auguste Rollier in Switzerland and Henry Gauvain in England, championed the sun bath method of treatment for bone and joint tuberculosis.[137] Rollier, founder and medical director of the Institutions for Heliotherapy in Leysin, in the Swiss Alps, opened his first UV clinic in 1903.[138] Until this time, Rollier's medical training had focused in surgery, as he studied under and assisted Professor Theodor Kocher, a prominent European surgeon.[139] Despite a promising surgical career, he gave it all up to establish a general medical practice in rural Leysin.[140] In his memorial to Rollier, Billings attributes the physician's change in career path to the diagnosis of Rollier's fiancée with tuberculosis and his belief that the purity of the Swiss Alps air would save her. Apparently, "Madame Rollier recovered her health completely."[141] In his history of sunlight therapy, Hobday also recognizes the influence of Rollier's fiancée's tuberculosis, but adds the tragic case of hip and knee tuberculosis in one of Rollier's close friends, who was treated surgically by Kocher, with Rollier assisting. Ultimately the surgery failed and his friend died, and the experience was traumatic for Rollier, diverting his interests away from surgery.[142] Most practitioners, even Rollier, did acknowledge that some surgical management of TB might be required in selected cases of bone and joint tuberculosis, particularly in aspirating abscesses, manually removing sequestra (dead bone), correcting ankylosis, and possibly even removing tuberculous lesions if patients clearly were not improving with other measures.[143] Surgeons were on staff at the clinics in Leysin, but Rollier's main focus lay in the curative power of the sun.

There were many exceptional cases of tuberculosis disease arrest and cure reported by Rollier in his classic text *Heliotherapy*, published in English in 1923.[144] One case report concerns a thirteen-year-old boy, G.N., who was admitted to the clinics at Leysin with long-standing tuberculosis of the spine. The disease had progressed to such an extent that there was a prominent and advanced spinal kyphosis. There was a history of TB in the child's family, with three of his mother's sisters dying of pulmonary tuberculosis. As Rollier described G.N.'s case history prior to admission, he had been "treated for spinal caries since eighteen months of age" and, since he was three years old, he had been "treated by a well-known orthopaedic surgeon," first with plaster and then canvas corsets. Two years before he was admitted to Leysin, an abscess opened on his thigh and was treated by aspiration. A sinus then formed, but later closed. A year later, another abscess formed and was incised.[145] From Rollier's perspective, the boy was already beginning to experience the "mutilations" of surgery, the incisions and aspirations. When G.N. arrived at Leysin in February 1915, he was described as a "weak, pale child with enormous deformity affecting the greater part of the thoracic and lumbar regions."[146] He also had another discharging sinus, which had formed on the anterior aspect of his thigh. Upon X-ray examination it was revealed that the boy suffered "widespread destruction" of his spinal column from his ninth thoracic down to his first lumbar vertebrae. This meant that five vertebrae were being destroyed by tuberculous disease.

Rollier reported a rapid improvement in the boy's general health at Leysin. Only eight months after his admission, in October 1915, the sinus on his thigh had closed, his temperature had returned to normal, and his hemoglobin counts had greatly improved. The kyphosis had been treated with bedrest, the typical progression of corrective supports used at the clinic (first millet husk, then a sandbag, and finally, a block of wood), and, of course, heliotherapy. Rollier eschewed both surgery and the use of plaster casts, the former because of his personal experiences and beliefs and the latter because of the pronounced muscular atrophy that often resulted after months of fixation.[147] Rollier reported that about two and a half years after he was admitted, G.N. was "clinically and radiographically healed" of spinal tuberculosis, allowed up from bed in December 1917 with support from a celluloid corset,[148] and discharged in July 1918.

"While some of his ideas," Billings wrote in his memorial to Rollier in 1957, "did not gain universal acceptance, there is no doubt that many hundreds of patients who came to Leysin, particularly children with tuberculous adenitis and tuberculosis of bones and joints, made remarkable recoveries under his care."[149] Despite his controversial rejection of surgery, "Rollier's work earned him international recognition and for many years he was head of the faculty of medicine at Lausanne."[150] In his research into Rollier, Hobday also encountered a somewhat uncomfortable acknowledgement of Rollier's work among his medical contemporaries, because his "revolt against the wholesale use of surgery was regarded as extreme." [151] According to Hobday, heliotherapy was perceived as an "unscientific form of treatment" and "slow, careful tanning of the skin" was believed to offer "little prospect of sudden recovery or dramatic cures." Despite the controversies surrounding the effectiveness of heliotherapy, it was a practice that spread widely and the Toronto sanatorium was no exception. The heliotherapy schedule prescribed for one seventeen-year-old patient at the Toronto sanatorium very closely follows Rollier's recommended schedule for sun treatments, slowly acclimatizing patients to the sun through increasing "doses" of UV radiation, beginning with five minutes' exposure of the "feet to ankles" and working up, by the tenth day of heliotherapy, to thirty minutes' exposure of the "feet to neck." All heliotherapy was to be undertaken between 10:30 and 11:00 a.m. The Toronto sanatorium ascribed to Rollier's conservative heliotherapy plan, adamant as he was that heliotherapy was most effective if undertaken with slow and incremental UV exposures. Dr Reyn of Copenhagen, on the other hand, preferred a more aggressive approach, which encouraged erythema, or skin redness, possibly influenced by the ideas underlying the popular hyperemic treatment.[152]

Even while the therapy was practised, there was a vagueness of understanding concerning how or why UV light could promote improvement and healing in tuberculosis. In addressing the "scientific basis of heliotherapy," Dr Rosselet, an assistant physician at Rollier's clinics before becoming a university lecturer, explains the benefits of heliotherapy by virtue of the "bactericidal action of light," the "therapeutic value of vasodilatation" (a widening of the blood vessels to encourage blood flow), and the "increased metabolism of the body."[153] In 1928 Phelps wrote that "the beneficial effects of ultra-violet light that are known are very few ... The effect of ultra-violet light is a *general one* in proportion to the amount of skin exposed and it does not penetrate through the skin more than a millimeter or two" (emphasis added).[154] Indeed, at best, Myers chalks up heliotherapy's benefits to a "tonic effect."[155] In 1923, Reyn writes about "erythema" (redness), "pigmentation," and "a stimulating effect," but again does not pin down the tuberculosis-specific biological benefits of UV exposure.[156] Rollier viewed the skin itself as "an admirable protection against the invasion of micro-organisms," and associated greater pigmentation (the melanin production, or tan, associated with UV exposure) with greater resistance to pathogens, not only in tuberculosis, but also chicken pox and scarlet fever.[157]

Psychologically, the very change of environment associated with heliotherapy was understood to benefit patients tremendously, as even a simple change of scenery from mundane bedroom to porch or sunroom was a welcome diversion during the typically long course of tuberculosis treatment. While sunlight exerted its effect on "the physiologic processes," it also improved "the attitude of the patient," [158] and, with patients feeling that "something of a tangible nature [was] being done," made evident in their tanned skin, they were encouraged to spend more time at the tedium of bedrest.[159] More generally, Rollier wrote of the relationship between "sunshine and happiness," such that "placed on a sunny verandah with a number of other children about the same age, [a child's] fretful, peevish disposition soon gives place to cheerfulness.

Appetite, digestion, and sleep are all improved by the psychical change, and the clinical condition soon follows suit."[160]

Given the remarkable physical and psychological benefits associated with UV therapy, the disadvantages appeared relatively minor. In 1928, Phelps wrote that "the dangers of ultra-violet light are not great."[161] While over-exposure could produce severe and painful burns, Phelps suggested that these "do not seem to be dangerous." However, the eyes were found to be particularly susceptible to UV light, and patients were often photographed with their eyes covered. In comparison to the perceived successes with bone and joint tuberculosis, the possibility of treating patients with pulmonary tuberculosis with light therapy was much more controversial. According to Dr Garrett, when he worked at the Toronto sanatorium, heliotherapy among patients with pulmonary tuberculosis seemed to produce results that were "at least equivocal." Despite the fact that "the amount of skin exposed and the amount of time exposed was carefully regulated," heliotherapy seemed to produce persistent fever and hemoptysis, so it was generally avoided among pulmonary tuberculosis patients.[162] This vulnerability of pulmonary TB patients to heliotherapy was addressed by Rollier in his *Heliotherapy* text, a result that he chalked up to incorrect technique resulting from an "overdose" of sunlight, particularly if, in hot weather, physicians used anything other than the early morning sun.[163] Martin and colleagues suggest that the medical community's promotion of heliotherapy and its result in tanning soon permeated society more broadly and a strong cultural association linking tanning with health emerged. The influential fashionable set began to appear tanned by at least the early 1920s, including Coco Chanel in 1923,[164] and images of tanned bodies in American fashion magazines such as *Vogue* and *Harper's Bazaar* surfaced between 1927 and 1928.[165] Ironically, while the sun's UV rays were lauded for healthful benefits in the treatment of diseases such as tuberculosis, the resulting emerging North American culture of tanning would also correlate with the twentieth-century rise in skin cancer.[166]

It was not until the late 1950s that vitamin D synthesis in UV light–exposed skin would come to be understood as the benefit in treating tuberculosis.[167] Much more has since been learned about vitamin D, a hormone stored in body fat, and immune function. Luong and Nguyen review a number of studies suggesting how the hormonally active form of vitamin D might increase bodily resistance to tuberculosis.[168] These studies suggest an inhibitory effect of vitamin D, reducing the number of viable tuberculosis bacteria in macrophages, possibly because this steroid hormone enhances the fusion of phagosomes (vesicles inside macrophages that have captured TB bacteria) and lysosomes.[169] Such an effect could be beneficial, since lysosomes provide the enzymes needed to destroy the tuberculosis bacteria carried within phagosomes, offsetting the need to simply sequester bacteria in granulomas. Recently Liu and colleagues have demonstrated that macrophages actually carry receptors for vitamin D, as well as producing an enzyme capable of converting vitamin D into an active state, both of which are guided into action upon toll-like receptor activation (which occurs upon encountering pathogen antigens) on the macrophage cell surface.[170] Activation of the vitamin D pathway in human macrophages also signals the CAMP gene, located on chromosome 3, to produce cathelicidin. Cathelicidin[171] is found inside macrophages activated by pathogens or hormonally active vitamin D and is an important antimicrobial peptide effective against tuberculosis bacteria.[172] Ultimately, much more than tanned skin, it was these complex immune pathways that were being activated among patients in sanatoria that followed Rollier's prescription for sun exposure.

Extending the Artificials: Treatments for Bone and Joint Tuberculosis

For all the attention paid to pulmonary tuberculosis and the ways in which the body attempted to naturally resist infection and disease, leading to "Nature"-inspired treatments such as artificial hyperemia and compression surgeries, similar treatments were also sought for bone and joint tuberculosis. As in pulmonary tuberculosis therapeutics, the body served as guide in developing treatments for bone and joint tuberculosis. Adhering to the concept of artificially reproducing "Nature's" effects, physicians observed and took cues from the body's natural attempts to resolve bone and joint tuberculosis. Like lung cavitation, bone tuberculosis is characterized by "degeneration and destruction."[173] The disease process begins at the site of a tubercle and, as bone cells are destroyed, a caseous mass is produced, which in turn incites the production of granulation tissue. If patient resistance is high, the body responds by producing fibrous tissue to encase the pathology, building towards fibrous ankylosis and, finally and most soundly, cartilaginous or bony ankylosis (which, like the granuloma, helps to trap TB bacteria and stop their progression).[174] According to Augustus Wilson, an orthopedic surgeon practising in Philadelphia, it was ankylosis (bony fusion) that was understood to be "Nature's cure" in bone and joint tuberculosis, observed by many an orthopedic surgeon in cases of undiagnosed or unrecognized but resolved tuberculous disease of the hip. While seemingly effective at arresting active disease, the ankylosis of "Nature's Cure" was "objectionable" only because it often resulted in "deformities" that required surgical corrections.[175] So while the body may not have achieved perfection (or perfect form) in bony ankylosis, it did offer a means to resolve active disease. If ankylosis was an effective bodily response, then surgeons would simply follow the example that "Nature" provided, the ultimate objective of ankylosis realized with specialized fusion surgeries for bone and joint tuberculosis; rather than idly wait for the body to produce bony ankylosis, surgeons would intervene by positioning bone grafts to encourage a faster bodily response and fusion of affected bones and joints. These surgeries became more common at the Toronto sanatorium (and elsewhere) in the surgical age of the 1930s.

Non-pulmonary forms of tuberculosis, such as bone and joint tuberculosis, often required specialized courses of treatment. Initially, all child patients with bone and joint tuberculosis were assigned to complete bedrest so that the nature and extent of their pathologies could be evaluated. Plaster casts and other devices (such as traction with weights) were sometimes used to stabilize bones and joints at sites of infection and disease. Augustus Wilson was adamant, however, that successful treatment of skeletal tuberculosis must involve some amount of ambulatory rest. He explicitly draws upon Bier's hyperemic ideas on the healing properties of blood and the dangers of atrophy through confinement to bed: "The excellent results obtained by Bier's hyperaemic treatment require deep thought ... Bier has proven that a large blood supply to a part is almost invariably detrimental to the progress of organisms and increases the resistance to invasion. Weight-bearing is conducive to the benefits obtained by out-door life, and in turn prevent circulatory stasis, thereby securing the benefits obtained by the hyperaemic method of Bier."[176] Rather than absolute bedrest, which some physicians adopted out of fears that tuberculous bones were soft and susceptible to "pathological dislocation," Wilson advocated movement in plaster casts (spicas), particularly when unaided by crutches (to encourage therapeutic weight-bearing), which he believed "conducive to the much-wanted blood supply" to affected bones.[177] Overall, Wilson argued for "vitality," activity, and hyperemia to improve the "resistive powers of the patient," with the best possible resolution of bone and joint tuberculosis observed in solid ankylosis.[178] The alternative to casting was extended bedrest utilizing extensions and traction with weights; the extension, according to Starr, was intended to reduce muscle contractions and the crowding together of inflamed joint surfaces that were brought together by contractions, while the weights provided a type of weight-bearing effect.[179] Spinal tuberculosis, in particular, was comparatively more difficult to manage with casting alone and, according to Moon, "is the most dangerous form of skeletal tuberculosis because of its ability to cause bone destruction, deformity, and paraplegia."[180]

Alongside spicas and traction, bone disorders ranging from fractures and rickets to bone and joint tuberculosis could also be fixated with a variety of splints, including the popular Thomas hip splint.[181] The Thomas splint was typically made of wrought iron and leather and needed to be "sufficiently malleable to admit of being moulded into shape," and yet, "sufficiently unyielding to prevent any modification in shape by movements, voluntary or accidental, on the part of the patient."[182] As patients were seen to improve, their Thomas bed splints could be transformed into walking splints with the aid of crutches and a patten (or a "high shoe") used to elevate the foot on the unaffected side. "No matter how efficient the external fixation," however, a splinted tuberculous joint was rarely found to achieve "spontaneous bony fusion," and a surgical approach came to be understood as the most efficient method to encourage arthrodesis or fusion of the joint.[183]

When four-year-old Walter was transferred from a Toronto hospital in July 1921, he was diagnosed as suffering from tuberculosis of his right hip and both knee joints, and hilar TB (i.e., of the hilar lymph nodes) in his right lung. Walter was described in one of his cot notes as a child who "gets a good deal of joy out of life and radiates sunshine to others." It is not surprising, given the complexity of his disease, that he remained in the sanatorium for almost five years, discharged in May 1926. At the sanatorium, he spent most of his time in bed with splints and traction-supplying weights applied to his legs. While Walter was "strapped to a frame in his little cot," he benefitted from periodic sojourns on the roof for heliotherapy, or the "sun cure," as described in the cot note. In the case of bone and joint tuberculosis, particularly in instances of tuberculosis of the spine, hip, or knee, it was common for patients such as Walter to be placed "on frame" in their beds. There were two common types of frames in use at the time, the Bradford frame and the Whitman frame.[184] The Bradford frame, a rectangular stretcher made up of canvas laced to a gas-pipe metal frame, was innovated in 1890 and intended for fixation (immobilization) of an affected bone or joint; the frame could be used in cases of TB of the hip or knee, diseases of the spine, or for the management of fractures. With patients elevated up off the bed, bedpans could be placed between the frame and the bed so that they could use bedpans without having to move while also reducing the likelihood of soiling dressings or casts. The Whitman frame was a type of curved Bradford frame that had the benefits of the Bradford frame, but, in addition to fixation (immobilization) of bones and joints, it also encouraged hyperextension, particularly of the spine. The degree of hyperextension was decided by doctors in order to achieve the desired corrective position and alignment in each case.

While Bradford and Whitman frames were in common use in the first half of the twentieth century, according to Helen Anderson, a nurse writing in 1948, these frames were "losing favor" in the treatment of spinal tuberculosis.[185] Anderson advised nurses on the use of frames, cautioning that patients often felt "insecure" when they were first placed on a frame, since the frames sat on top of the bed, further elevating patients. As a result, she advised, the frame "should be elevated on sturdy legs and fastened at all four corners by hooks attached to each end of a turnbuckle[,] one hook over the frame, the other on the bed frame."[186] Children could also be given "additional security" by using jacket restraints to hold them onto the frame.

Anderson also addressed issues of comfort and satisfaction. Being "on frame" was restricting, limiting movement and sensory experiences. Many children on frames would typically lie in a supine position (on their backs, face upward), without any elevation of their heads (in order to maintain desired alignment, she notes "most persons with tuberculous spines are not allowed pillows"), so it was difficult for them to see around their rooms or wards. She advised attaching mirrors to the head of the bed, or in any other place that would afford them views of their rooms, doorways, or windows and also to think of occasionally changing the placement of beds to provide patients with new views and interest. As Anderson sympathetically acknowledged, these slight modifications, including the use of mirrors, "help the individual feel more a part of his environment and adjust to living in a horizontal plane."[187] According to Anderson, mirrors could improve mealtimes, allowing supine children some measure of participation in eating by being able to see their food, as well as smell and taste it. Anderson encouraged nurses to use "conversation, stories, good humor, attitudes of plenty of time for eating, and quiet expectation that food will be eaten," not only to improve appetite and digestion, but also because "the child who learns the art of good conversation at mealtime, whether at home or in the hospital, is acquiring a useful social tool."[188] Even among those children restricted on bed frames by skeletal tuberculosis, opportunities for etiquette refinements, apparently, could still find a place in the hospital environment.

When seventeen-year old Chester was admitted to the sanatorium in May 1935, his family physician strongly suspected TB of the left hip and a hilar (lymph node) infection of his lungs. Chester was treated with an immobilizing plaster cast applied to his hip. Known commonly as a "spica," plaster of Paris bandages were used to build casts around affected areas in bone and joint tuberculosis. Casts that immobilized the spine typically extended from head to pelvis, but left the arms free. Particularly in cases of upper vertebral involvement, in the area of the neck, the temporal and occipital bones of the cranium as well as the jaw (or mandible) were also included in the cast to ensure proper alignment and fixation of the head and spine. Casts applied for the immobilization of tuberculous hips typically encased the lower trunk, pelvis, and thighs, and extended down to the lower leg and foot on the side of the affected hip (once again to ensure proper alignment). The Wellcome Library has made the fifteen-minute 1936 documentary "Fillet and Spica Plaster" available for on-line viewing.[189] Set at Abergele Sanatorium, Manchester, England, the documentary illustrates the process of casting for two patients, one with spinal tuberculosis (and involving use of the Bologna suspension apparatus), and the other with tuberculosis of the hip (and involving use of the Stein apparatus). The overall sensations associated with casting are restriction and constriction, particularly for the Abergele child with spinal tuberculosis whose head, neck, and torso are fixed in plaster. The result must have been devastating for the children, trapped, as they were, in their spicas. Unlike a broken bone, which might require some weeks in a cast, it was impossible to predict how long children would have to remain casted for tuberculosis, and that ambiguity in itself must have been disconcerting.

Nurses responsible for the daily care of patients in casts were advised to "consider both the patient in the cast" as well as "the cast itself," particularly as patients adjusted to the "rigid, unyielding plaster."[190] While remaining attentive to any complications, including skin irritation, soreness, burning, or itching, nurses were encouraged to help children and adolescents adapt to new and difficult sensations brought on by casting. Particularly with rigid upper body casts, anxieties could be heightened by the feeling of restricted breathing, often felt as "pressure on the abdomen or pain near the lower margin of the ribs."[191] Edward H. Bradford, of the Boston Children's Hospital and originator of the Bradford frame, noted his difficulties in casting, in which "two children," three and six years of age, "who had worn plaster jackets for two weeks without discomfort, were attacked with dyspnoea [difficulty breathing] so severely that it was necessary to remove the jacket."[192] Nurses were instructed to advise patients "to attempt to lie as relaxed as possible in the cast, to let the cast support him and to localize the sensation of breathing in the upper part of the chest," since patients typically fought the feeling of restriction by pushing their bodies against the cast.[193] Guiding patients in "relaxation, 'feeling small,' and focusing on chest rather than diaphragmatic breathing" were thought to help ease the disturbing sensations.[194] After time in one-piece torso casts, patients would typically transition to "bivalved" casts (split, longitudinally, into two halves; the halves could then be used separately or together), which greatly reduced those feelings of restriction.

Use of plaster jackets in cases of spinal tuberculosis arose, in part, out of the nineteenth-century work of Lewis Sayre. It was Sayre, a New York medical doctor and, later, the first professor of orthopedic surgery in the United States,[195] who, in 1877, published on the use of suspension and plaster of Paris bandages in the treatment of disorders of the spine, including scoliosis and "spinal caries," the latter being an early term for spinal tuberculosis (though the "tuberculous caries" and "spinal caries" terminology would persist well into the twentieth century).[196] Much like dental caries (or cavities), spinal caries was noted for its destructive process on the spine, but its etiology as an infectious disease was not confirmed until after Koch's 1882 discovery of the tuberculosis bacterium. In Sayre's approach, suspension was used to straighten the spine and bring the patient into better alignment before the torso was fixated in plaster (see figure 6.3). He accomplished this with the use of a tripod, where "the individual was literally hung from the device while attached to a specially constructed rope and pulley for head and axillary traction. Only their toes touched the ground, and this was permitted just enough to keep discomfort from becoming too serious. While under this severe traction, a snug-fitting plaster of Paris jacket was applied."[197] Physicians adopting Sayre's technique were candid in their accounts of difficulties in applying jackets correctly, some requiring two or three attempts in order to achieve jackets that were effective, properly positioned, and comfortable for patients.

The patients themselves also had difficulties with Sayre's procedure, one physician relating that, in his experience, "young children were alarmed at being suspended. One young woman fainted. Some, before I could complete my work, became cyanotic. One was seized with a convulsive attack."[198] As a result, gentler methods of extension evolved, such as Stein's horizontal extension[199] and Davy's hammock extension,[200] both of which were argued to offer greater comfort to patients and reduce the risk of fainting. Other physicians, however, such as John Ridlon of Chicago, attempted "forcible straightening" of spines while patients were "profoundly anaesthetized," which was probably for the best, since Ridlon suspended patients by their feet prior to aggressive straightening and casting.[201] With physicians still perfecting the art of anesthesia in the late 1800s, two of the child cases that Ridlon reported on in 1898 "stopped breathing on being turned from the prone [face-down] to the supine

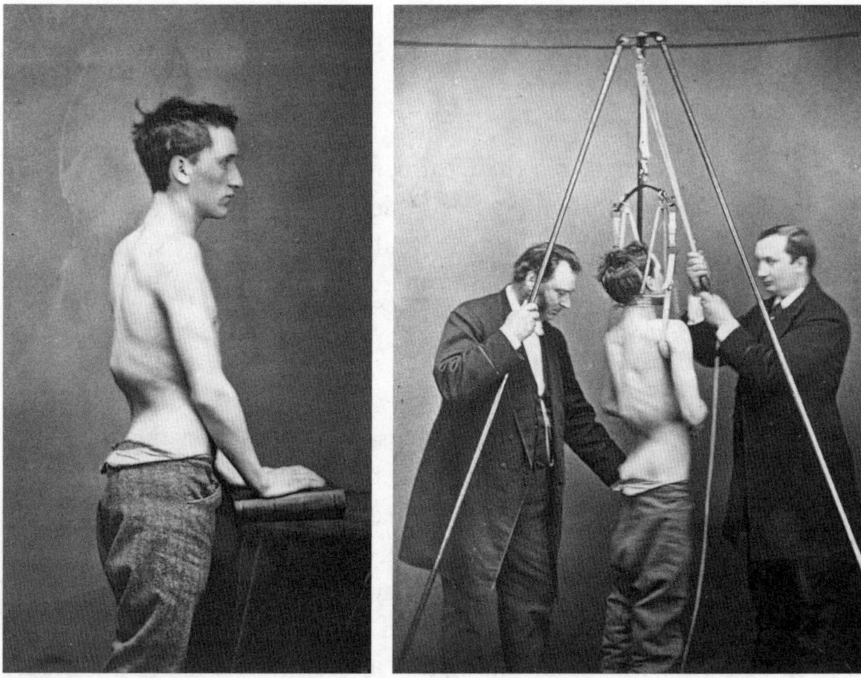

Figure 6.3 Above and opposite Sayre's tripod apparatus for suspension and plaster cast application.

[face-up] posture during chloroform narcosis" though both resumed breathing after a short time.[202] A number of concerns had been raised about the forced straightening of kyphosed spines, particularly those severely kyphosed, including disturbing and further disseminating tuberculous disease, the rupturing of tuberculous abscesses, and the rupture of the aorta if it had twisted around deformed spines. Ridlon noted that in all the cases he treated, the kyphosis had unfortunately relapsed to some extent following the straightening.

Despite overall improvements in technique, there were lingering concerns with the use of suspension and plaster casting in the management of spinal tuberculosis. Dr Grattan, an Irish physician who had learned about this approach during Dr Sayre's visit to Cork in 1877, suggested that some of the "strong prejudice" against Sayre's method resulted because of the misapplication of his techniques.[203] With too much expected

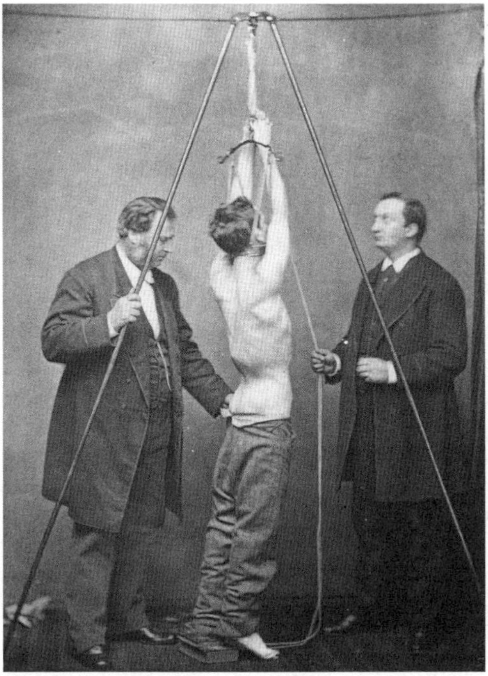

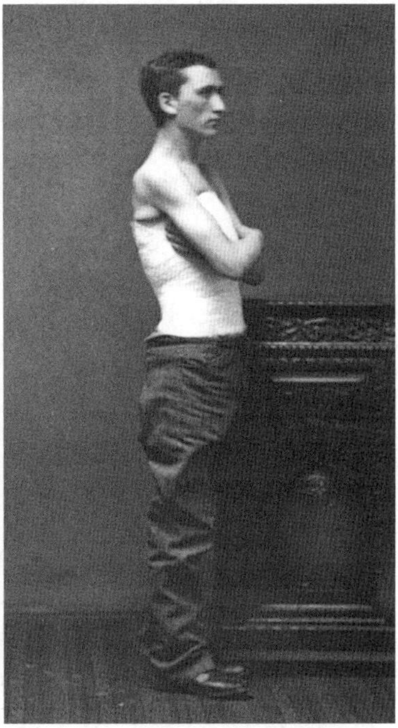

too soon, some physicians attempted severe extension on patients, even among those whose bodies had already attempted to heal via bony ankylosis, instead of, as Grattan quotes from Sayre's 1877 publication, "a very slow extension never beyond a patient's comfort and particularly in cases where bony consolidation had occurred."[204] Bradford had noted Sayre's caution, though he argued that "Dr Sayre's rule that suspension should not be carried beyond the point of relief to the patient is not generally practicable with young children, who are frequently too frightened to relate their sensation."[205] Grattan also noted that many physicians left the plaster casts on for too long, producing "atrophy of the spinal muscles, and consequent weakness, owing to the want of proper exercise" (this also contributed to Rollier's rejection of casting).[206] Plaster casting was definitely not recommended if there was any evidence of active infection, observed in the formation of abscesses and sinuses that worked to drain noxious material from deep in the area of a tuberculous bone or joint.[207]

Ultimately, in Chester's case, it became clear that his hip was not tuberculous, though this took considerable time to determine. Chester's surgeon explained the situation in correspondence with Chester's family physician, that Chester "certainly presented with the usual evidence of tuberculosis of the hip," though his history had been "a bit unusual" because the onset of his disease seemed "very acute." After a "prolonged investigation," in which Chester's tuberculin skin tests continued to return negative for infection, and TB bacteria were never cultured from the pus draining from a sinus on his hip, it was at long last resolved that Chester suffered "suppurative arthritis of the hip joint." After recovering *Staphylococcus aureus* bacteria from Chester's weeping sinus, his surgeon had performed an exploratory procedure on the sinus to investigate further and, in July 1936, discovered, at its focus, a dead bone fragment originating from the head of his femur. Upon removal of this sequestrum, the sinus healed rapidly and Chester's health improved. The determination of the true cause of Chester's hip condition was ultimately critical to his improvement. Though tuberculosis was always suspected, a detailed knowledge of the disease's typical manifestation and the availability of diagnostic tests, laboratory cultures, and exploratory surgeries proved particularly valuable in eliminating Chester's provisional diagnosis of tuberculosis. Rather than lingering in the sanatorium for years, Chester was discharged within a few months of his surgery, in December 1936. Chester did not appear to harbour any ill feelings over his misdiagnosis; instead he was thankful for the resolution to his hip troubles and he maintained a fond correspondence with the sanatorium staff long after his discharge. Just over two years following his discharge he wrote to Dr Coulthard, his surgeon, happily advising him that he was trying to give his bad hip just as much "punishment" as his good hip, for, as his letter attests,

> I might mention that I have taken up dancing again (started about six months ago), square dancing mostly and if you have ever seen any country square dances you will know that as a test that stands by itself as far as getting around fast is concerned.

> I have also done quite a bit of skating this winter but of course I am not another "Chuck" Conacher[208] or Syl Apps[209] on skates yet but that may come with practice. However I think I did fairly good for a "stiff-hipper" as I haven't been on skates since the winter of 1934.
>
> Along with that I have been able to do quite a bit of farm work for instance I put in most of our crop last spring. Did a great deal of haying and am now doing some of the winter chores.

Chester had not been obliged to follow the typical restrictions recommended for a tuberculous post-sanatorium life, instead "punishing" his recovering hip with dancing, skating, and farm work. Chester's lasting gratitude to his surgeon is fully evident when, in 1949, he again wrote to Coulthard sentimentally acknowledging that, with his help, "thirteen years ago this month it was possible for me to walk out of the San." The card included a newspaper clipping of the birth announcement for his first child, "another milestone" he felt he had reached because of his "new lease on life."

Raymond, a nine-year-old Indigenous child, was admitted to the sanatorium in 1923. With moderately advanced pulmonary tuberculosis and tuberculosis of the spine complicated by multiple abscesses, Raymond's prognosis was even poorer than Chester's had been. As his disease progressed and his condition worsened, Raymond died in September 1929, after over six years at the sanatorium. Tuberculosis had ravaged his spine, causing a marked kyphosis. Since there is a natural curve that defines the alignment of thoracic vertebrae, which were affected in Raymond's case, the kyphosis tends to progress more rapidly in this part of the spine.[210] Between the time of his admission in 1923 and his death in 1929, Raymond's spine had been continually stabilized by a series of splints and braces in order to reduce any further progression of the kyphosis. Immobilization in plaster was not an option for Raymond, because he suffered persistent discharging sinuses, another indication of active disease.

The results of regular physical examinations attest to the tenacity of Raymond's disease and the frustrations that he suffered, as reflected in a lengthy medical narrative of treatment. The ebbs and flows of tuberculous disease are evident in Raymond's experience, and while he sometimes benefitted from slight improvements, his overall decline is painfully evident. Though the clinical record aims ultimately to document physical findings, nonetheless some qualitative statements concerning Raymond's condition were noted: "improved some" on 24 September 1924, "general condition is fairly good" on 15 September 1925, "not doing well" on 14 January 1928, and "condition fair only, not improving" on 30 May 1928. These humanistic impressions provide insights into Raymond's changing prognosis, the kind of notations that would increasingly disappear from clinical charts over time because they were felt to be "imprecise and 'unscientific' expressions" of a patient's condition.[211]

Raymond's persistent discharging sinuses were a concerning sign of disease activity, reinforced by other observations: the need to begin using a sputum box in September 1927, the X-ray confirming that Raymond's hilar lymph node infection had moved beyond this focus to his lung tissue (parenchyma) in November 1928, and his loss of appetite that became apparent in July 1929. Because of Raymond's poor condition and the degree of disability that he experienced as a result of the spinal kyphosis and discharging sinuses, he had been kept in bed for most of his time in the sanatorium. Despite his poor condition, Raymond was able to take breaks from bedrest to go up to the roof for heliotherapy, to play on the ward (particularly around Christmas), and to play out on the grounds one day (but one day only) in 1924. Sanatorium staff were aware of the importance of balancing a good (but measured) quality of life with the demands of managing persistent, chronic spinal tuberculosis. The longest period of time that Raymond spent continuously in his bed (with bathroom privileges) was between May 1927 and May 1929, marking two full years of bedrest. Despite his long stay in the sanatorium, Raymond had only a modest collection of possessions, mostly clothing and crafting tools, which he left behind at the time of his death, including two embroidery rolls, an embroidery hoop, a pair of scissors, a box of paints, a box of beads, and a ruler. Though staff had held out hope for Raymond's recovery, his experience in the pre-antibiotic era depicts the long drawn-out struggle between failing bodily resistance and aggressive bacteria. Raymond's story is one of persistent and chronic disease, marked only by a few brief periods of improvement within a much longer narrative of slow decline so characteristic of tuberculosis.

Surgeons were cautious in deciding when it was safe to proceed with surgeries for bone and joint tuberculosis, and it was the need for some preoperative stability that most likely precluded sufferers such as Raymond from surgery. Even when surgeries were carefully timed, however, they did not come without risks. Frank was seventeen years old when he was admitted to the sanatorium in June 1934, suffering from a tuberculous hip. His hip had begun to trouble him in August 1933, causing pain when he moved his left leg. Frank "continued on his feet" until May 1934, when an increase in pain and difficulty in movement forced him to bed. Growing concerned with this pain, Frank was seen by his family physician and, with a tuberculosis diagnosis, sent to the sanatorium shortly afterwards. On examination, the physicians at the sanatorium noted Frank's limited range of movement and the extensive bone destruction at the head and neck of his left femur. The articular cartilage between the head of the femur and the socket of his pelvis was nearly destroyed, causing pain when the bones rubbed together and limiting Frank's movement. While surgery was being considered, Frank's hip was treated with prolonged fixation in a plaster cast.

By November 1934 Frank was more robust and his disease stationary enough that his planned surgery, an arthrodesis for his left hip, could proceed. The arthrodesis, or surgical fusion (by means of bone grafting) of the hip, was delayed by disease activity, since surgeons preferred that the limits of bone destruction be more or less established before attempting the surgery (since the graft could fracture or be eaten away as a result of continuing disease activity).[212] Frank was to have an iliofemoral graft, a stabilization and fusion of the hip joint accomplished through the fixation of the ilium (part of the pelvis) to the femur. The iliofemoral approach adopted in Frank's case was one of a number of evolving techniques in arthrodesis (see figure 6.4). Writing in 1948, just as streptomycin was emerging, Nissen reviewed these procedures, noting that the earliest graft procedure, the Hibbs procedure, had all but "gone out of fashion" because the developing hip in early adolescence could not reliably support this type of graft.[213] The type of iliofemoral arthrodesis that Frank was to receive, illustrated in figure 6.4b, gained prominence in the interwar years, but was usually performed only on children at least ten years of age or older. The arthrodesis, or graft surgery, involved cutting out "an oblong of full-thickness iliac bone" and wedging the graft "into slots cut

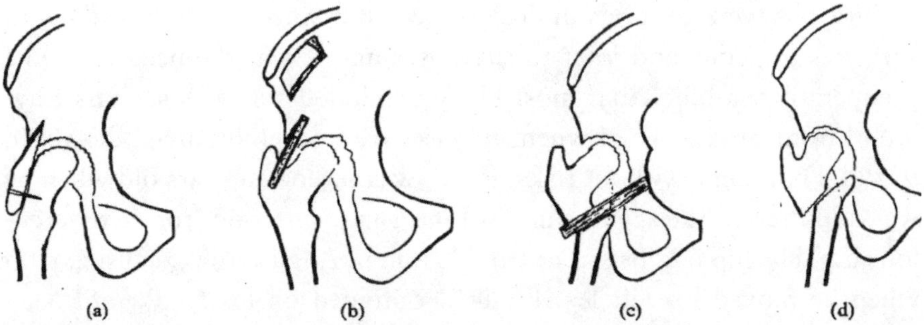

Figure 6.4 The evolution of surgical procedures for the arthrodesis of the tuberculous hip: (a) Hibbs procedure, (b) Seddon procedure (iliofemoral graft), (c) Brittain procedure (ishiofemoral graft), and (d) Wilkinson procedure.

in the greater trochanter [at the proximal end of the femur] and in the ilium [of the pelvis] just above the joint."[214] Nissen reported a success rate of about 70 per cent with this procedure, with failures due largely to graft fractures; other complications included unintended damage to the sciatic nerve and the resulting sciatica that could leave patients with long-lasting pain and restricted mobility.[215] Fixation in a cast was used post-operatively to keep the site stable so that the body could respond to the surgical trauma by laying down new bone and solidly fusing the graft. That fusion and bony ankylosis would then help to quiet the tuberculous disease process.

Since parent or guardian consent was required for any surgeries involving patients younger than twenty-one years of age, Dobbie wrote to Frank's mother, explaining that the surgery "will ensure Frank against a recurrence of disease in this joint, but will leave him with a stiff hip." A "stiff hip" was considered a reasonable compromise if Frank's destructive tuberculous disease could otherwise be arrested, and Frank's mother provided her consent. The surgery had two stages, the first required the surgeon to pop the head of the Frank's femur out of the socket of his pelvis so that pathological granulation tissue could be removed from both surfaces, exposing a clean femoral head and a clean socket receptacle in the pelvic bone. The head of the femur was then placed back into the socket. According to Frank's surgeon's notes, "a very excellent exposure" of the hip joint was achieved "without a great deal of haemorrhage." In the second stage of the surgery, two bone grafts were prepared; these grafts were intended to hold the femoral head and pelvis together in a fixed position, one end of each graft attached to the femoral neck and the other ends secured to the wing of the ilium. Small bone fragments were then packed into the pelvis's socket. Both the grafts and the "screws" used to secure the grafts were fashioned out of Frank's own bone, all cut from the wing of his pelvis's ilium. Ideally, over time, the grafts and bone fragments would encourage a solid, bony fusion of Frank's femoral head and pelvis. Following the procedure, in his notes, Frank's surgeon expressed his satisfaction with the outcome of the surgery, "the best operation for arthrodesis of the hip that I have yet performed." After the incision was closed and sutured, a plaster spica was applied around Frank's pelvis and, before he was taken out of the operating room, he had received 500 cc's of blood and 500 cc's of saline (about two cups of each). Despite the apparent success of the arthrodesis and all of the precautions taken, Frank died about eighteen hours after his surgery, the result of an unforeseen embolism.

While the risks of surgeries weighed heavily in deciding the best course of treatment for patients, when successful, these surgeries could put an end to the long, chronic suffering of bone and joint tuberculosis. George, fourteen years old, entered the sanatorium in May 1938 with tuberculosis of the spine. For the first six months he was in the hospital, George was kept immobilized on a Whitman frame. When he had made satisfactory progress and built up his strength, George was then given a spinal bone graft. Six months after this surgery (and twelve months after he was admitted), George was allowed to get up out of bed. An examination revealed that George's bone grafts were fusing satisfactorily to the spinous processes, and that the vertebral bodies of the twelfth thoracic and first lumbar vertebrae would soon be fused. George was then fitted for a supportive steel brace and discharged thirteen months after he was originally admitted. He was in excellent health at this time, though his range of movement was restricted to about 25 per cent of what it normally would have been. George was cautioned about over-exercising his spine as he slowly became ambulatory after his surgery. In June 1961, about twenty-two years later, the physicians at the sanatorium received a note from a colleague in Toronto who thought, out of professional courtesy, that they might like to know that George had "remained well ever since [his surgery] and has been doing active heavy work and has grown up into a fine, strapping man with no evidence of his old troubles." In this case, the surgical fusion had achieved the intended results and entirely resolved George's spinal tuberculosis, even in the era before antibiotics.

A New Therapeutic Regimen: Drug Treatments and *Mycobacterium tuberculosis*

By the 1940s, drug treatments were slowly making their way into use at the sanatorium. Finding effective drug treatments for tuberculosis was a long-standing challenge, partly due to the bacterium's behaviour in the body. As one tuberculosis specialist explained in the 1930s, "Because the tubercle bacillus is so soon walled-off after it enters the body, it seems highly improbable that we shall ever be able to disinfect the body by the use of any drug, as we are able to do in the case of organisms which remain free in the blood stream."[216] Mercury, copper, arsenic, gold, and iodine had all been tried, "but none has been found which penetrates the tubercles in such concentration as to have a germicidal effect."[217]

Emerging drug therapies for tuberculosis were evaluated in clinical environments, sanatoria and hospitals, to establish effective dosages and durations of treatment. The new drugs were used in combination with bedrest and, in some cases, surgical management, particularly important because, especially in the early days of streptomycin use, patients could revert to active disease even after completing treatment.[218] As drug-based treatments gained success, however, there were notable changes in the medical procedures undertaken. In 1955, a time when multi-drug treatments had become established at the Toronto sanatorium, both bedrest and surgical resections of tuberculous lungs (actually removing tuberculous lung tissue from the body) were still fundamental to treatment regimens, but all of the collapse therapies (artificial pneumothorax, phreniclasia, plombage, and thoracoplasty) had become virtually defunct.[219] No new artificial pneumothorax procedures, for example, had been undertaken at the Toronto sanatorium beyond 1952. With the aid of effective antibiotics and improvements in thoracic surgery, resectional surgeries of lungs had become more refined with less tissue removed; pneumonectomies (lung removals) and lobectomies (lung lobe removals) increasingly gave way to segmental and wedge resections where only a smaller portion of affected tissue was removed from the lungs, often with significantly less bodily trauma.[220]

In some instances, the rise of antibiotics extended surgical possibilities that, in weighing the benefits and risks to patients, surgeons had previously avoided because of the high risk of complications. Spinal tuberculosis was notable in this respect. According to Johnson and colleagues, as far back as the eighteenth century, English surgeon Percivall Pott was advocating the drainage of vertebral abscesses in spinal caries (spinal tuberculosis), a practice that they state he credited as far back as Hippocrates.[221] This approach was contentious, however, and by the early twentieth century, surgeons became increasingly apprehensive of disturbing tuberculous abscesses around the spine, concerned with the very real risks of further disease dissemination, secondary bacterial infections, and pulmonary reactivations of tuberculosis. The advent of streptomycin would allay some of these concerns and generally increase physician confidence in direct manipulations of tuberculous pathologies. In the early 1950s, for example, Johnson and colleagues performed direct vertebral biopsies (which greatly improved the difficult differential diagnosis of spinal tuberculosis) and even evacuated abscesses around the spine in a much more confident surgical climate, aided, as they were, by streptomycin. Encouraged by positive patient outcomes, they advocated doing away with the typical "conservative" approaches characterized by long periods of immobilization and non-interference with persistent abscesses (such as those suffered by Raymond) that effected "extensive destruction of tissue and alteration of blood supply," for which very little could be done in the aftermath.[222]

In the chronology of emerging twentieth-century drug treatments, some more or less useful in tuberculosis, sulphonamide (sulpha) drugs came first and became available at the Toronto sanatorium in 1938.[223] The history of sulpha drugs emerges in the work of German scientist Paul Ehrlich, who had brought dyes from the manufacturing and textile industries into the laboratory to stain tissue samples and microbes, improving the contrast needed for Ehrlich's specialty in thin sectioning samples for microscopy.[224] Dyes worked differentially and, according to Frank Ryan, Ehrlich realized that "this must mean that the surface membranes of the cells, or micro-organisms, had different affinities for different dyes."[225] In the first decade of the twentieth century, he reasoned "it must surely be possible to construct dyes, or chemicals, that would kill bacteria while not killing the human being infected by the bacteria."[226] Erhlich's revelation would be realized in 1931, when continued research into his pioneering work led German researcher Gerhard Domagk to isolate a dye effective against aggressive β-hemolytic streptococcal bacteria responsible for much human suffering.[227] The red dye, with its chemical "sulphonamide" side group, came to be known as *Prontosil rubrum*. It was the first synthetic antibacterial drug that had minimal side effects in humans. A few years earlier, in 1928, Alexander Fleming unknowingly observed evidence of antibacterial activity in culture dishes contaminated with the common environmental mould *Penicillium notatum* that had entered his "stiflingly stuffy" laboratory through the windows he had opened.[228] It would be some years before Fleming came to realize what he had observed in those culture dishes, the dawning insight inspired by a 1935 presentation by Domagk in London. In 1939, Fleming travelled to New York for a microbiology conference and met with Selman Waksman. Waksman was, in turn, inspired by Fleming's insights into the effects of naturally occurring airborne mould, and he and his colleagues renewed their interest in the potential antibacterial properties of microorganisms found naturally in soil. In 1943, Albert Schatz, a graduate student in Waksman's laboratory, found what they were looking for in the soil bacterium *Actinomyces griseus*, later renamed *Streptomyces griseus*, and from which the antibiotic streptomycin, the earliest effective agent against tuberculosis bacteria, would be subsequently refined.[229]

The Toronto sanatorium was not isolated from these monumental discoveries in science and medicine, in some instances actively participating in clinical trials of potential anti-tuberculosis treatments. Anthony, a fifteen-year-old schoolboy, was admitted in May 1942, identified with a positive skin test and regularly producing tuberculosis bacteria in his sputum samples. He was treated first with artificial pneumothorax, followed by a pneumonolysis (to sever adhesions) and thoracentesis (to drain fluid that had accumulated in his pleural cavity), and finally a thoracoplasty. The aggressive approach to his case was indicated by his diagnosis of active and far advanced pulmonary tuberculosis. While in the sanatorium, Anthony was put on "various forms of sulpha drugs," the most "effective" found to be Dagenan, which he was given both intravenously and by mouth in the amount of six grams per day. At this time, Dagenan, a sulfapyridine, was well known for its successful treatment of pneumonia, meningitis, and gonorrhea, though the impact of this sulpha drug on tuberculosis bacteria did not seem as clear or promising.[230] Physicians quickly came to appreciate some of the side effects associated with Dagenan. In 1941, two case reports from the Toronto sanatorium documented anuria (an inability to pass urine from the kidneys into the bladder) due to blockages caused by crystal formation in the ureters.[231] It was soon determined that abundant fluids would have to be administered with Dagenan.

Papers published in the late 1930s and early 1940s reported discrepant results with sulpha drugs, "those claiming a definite degree of protection" and "those that failed to demonstrate such an effect" in tuberculosis.[232] William Feldman and Corwin Hinshaw, two physicians at the Mayo Clinic in Rochester, Minnesota, were testing a new variant, Promin, on tuberculosis bacteria. Though some scientists were certain that "in one of the sulfones is to be found the first chemotherapeutic agent against tuberculosis," repeated trials revealed that, at best, sulpha drugs were only mildly bacteriostatic (inhibiting bacterial growth or reproduction, but not killing bacteria outright).[233] Other disadvantages were noted, key among them the fact that sulphonamides had to be administered immediately upon infection: "when the treatment was delayed until seventeen to twenty-four days after inoculation the drug failed to alter the macroscopic appearance of the tuberculous lesions."[234] Even worse, the sulpha drugs being tested required initial doses be administered even *before* infection took place.[235] As a result, these drugs were poor candidates for practical, clinical use. Despite the seeming failure of sulpha drugs, it is notable that Feldman and Hinshaw had refined a "reliable research technique" through their work with these drugs, so that when the time came to test streptomycin's anti-tuberculosis capabilities, these two scientists were entrusted with the research.[236]

At the Toronto sanatorium, Anthony progressed well following his thoracoplasty, maintaining consistently negative sputum samples until he was discharged in April 1944. His discharge was recommended "with the idea of being treated by penicillin when available." Penicillin did come into use at the Toronto sanatorium later in 1944,[237] though it proved to be of limited use in the treatment of tuberculosis as in vitro laboratory testing suggested "inhibitory" results, at absolute best.[238] Its impact was important but nonetheless indirect, as penicillin was found to be effective in controlling secondary or opportunistic bacterial infections in tuberculosis patients.[239]

Streptomycin, the first drug found to be effective against tuberculosis bacteria, was first used at the Toronto sanatorium in January 1946. At this time, supplies of streptomycin in Canada were very limited and only a small quantity could be obtained from the United States in an effort to treat sanatorium staff physician John F. Mulligan, thirty-five years of age, who had become critically ill with tuberculous meningitis.[240] The quantity was so limited, however, and the disease so aggressive, that he died on 5 January 1946.[241] Medical journals, such as the *Canadian Medical Association Journal*, dating to the late 1940s are rife with studies and case reports of the new era of tuberculosis patients receiving streptomycin treatment. Detailed with side effects (for example, among children, tinnitus, deafness, vomiting, neck rigidity, "cerebral irritation," deepening unconsciousness;[242] side effects typically appeared ten to fourteen days after the beginning of streptomycin therapy, to be endured for a long forty- to sixty-day course of treatment[243]) and patient progress (or non-progress) on the new drug, these articles all share some similar findings or conclusions. First, that recommended dosages and the duration of treatment needed to be refined. By the 1950s, the recommendation was for one gram of streptomycin twice weekly, in combination with other drugs.[244] By 1969, one report indicated that streptomycin was given at one gram intramuscularly each day for the first month, followed by twice weekly for up to three months; other dosing schedules were established for para-aminosalicylic acid (PAS) and isoniazid.[245] In its initial use, streptomycin had been given more frequently, every three to four hours, modelled after the dosing schedule that had been established for penicillin. Experiments by Feldman and Hinshaw revealed, however, that streptomycin was not cleared by the body as rapidly as penicillin, meaning that wider dosing schedules could still achieve the same "cumulative effect in the body."[246] Feldman and Hinshaw recommended two intramuscular injections of streptomycin per day, approximately twelve hours apart.[247]

As physicians may have debated, from a clinical perspective, the most effective dosage and length of treatment on streptomycin, for those who did not qualify for free streptomycin, the duration of treatment could be influenced by the weight of the "patient's purse."[248] The number of patients wanting streptomycin easily swamped the quantity that cities and provinces could provide for free. When Vancouver's Division of Tuberculosis Control was first issued streptomycin in 1947, for example, the city could only afford nine grams of streptomycin per day, and since the recommended dosage at that time was three grams per patient per day, the city could fund the treatment for only three patients.[249] In 1949, the Mountain Sanatorium in Hamilton was prescribing streptomycin in sixty-day courses, up from forty-two days when the drug was first put into use.[250] By 1955, a time when the Toronto sanatorium had adopted multi-drug treatments, patients could expect to be on streptomycin anywhere from twelve to twenty-four months.[251] The fear of tuberculosis struck deep and, as Aronovitch and Lewin noted, "in spite of its high price and the fear of complications it was increasingly evident that the general public was waiting eagerly for wider use of the drug in tuberculosis."[252]

Another significant observation shared by many of these early publications was that streptomycin was, at best, bacteriostatic (bacteria are not able to reproduce, but they are not destroyed), not bacteriolytic (destroys bacteria), and that the rise of bacterial resistance was proving to be a monumental problem. In the early days of streptomycin monotherapy, critiques were raised concerning whether or not "the purpose of chemotherapy" could actually be achieved given the short period of the drug's effectiveness; the American College of Chest Physicians reported that 75 per cent of patients had streptomycin-resistant tuberculosis bacteria after only three to four months of treatment, a notably short period of effectiveness for chronic, slow-reproducing tuberculosis bacteria.[253] As a result, in 1949, though the efficacy of streptomycin was "no longer open to doubt," reports of its use were "tinged with caution," sometimes "hint[ing] at disappointment."[254] While physicians understood that streptomycin was beneficial in the treatment of TB, the possibility that this drug alone could cure the disease was a matter of debate.[255] Streptomycin's limitations would come to be remedied with the introduction of multi-drug therapies. This was a significant innovation, since emerging bacterial resistance to streptomycin meant that once patients went off the drug, they could not be put back on streptomycin (since it would be ineffective), even if their disease symptoms returned.[256]

From the patient's perspective, streptomycin held obvious appeal, despite the side effects, because many would quickly experience remarkable improvements in their symptoms: "Within very few days there is a rapid subsidence in the toxic effects of the disease. The temperature comes down, the pulse slackens, the patient experiences a sense of well being, eats better, sleeps better, and starts to gain weight."[257] Physicians, however, remained more guarded in their perceptions of the drug's impact since, among some patients, the effects were "illusory, as the pulmonary lesion may spread in spite of the feeling of well being."[258] Aronovitch and Lewin recommended that physicians remain "cautious in stating the prognosis is improved," at least until multiple serial X-rays could be taken to assess whether or not tuberculous lesions and cavities were actually responding to treatment.[259] Physicians, they argued, could testify to "improvement" only if symptoms were resolving *and* there were "signs of radiological clearing in serial X-rays or conversion of sputum to negative."[260] Sputum conversion was the most definitive sign of improvement, irrespective of the patient's feelings on symptoms, but, that said, Aronovitch and Lewin qualify "improvement" further, to include cases that benefited from streptomycin to the extent that they were brought "to a stage where other procedures," such as collapse therapy, "could be tried."[261] It is clear that in this early stage of drug therapy, streptomycin, even though not reliably effective in controlling tuberculosis bacteria in patients (because of emerging resistance issues), was seen as an invaluable ally to traditional sanatorium therapies. Not only could streptomycin help to ready patients for collapse therapies, it could also improve on incomplete results arising from collapse therapy, such as patients who had received thoracoplasties but remained sputum positive. "These patients," Aronovitch and Lewin note, "are a problem since they feel well, have little sputum and are … ready to leave the sanatorium," but cannot be readily discharged "for fear" that they would infect others.[262] Aronovitch and Lewin used streptomycin in seven of these difficult cases and noted that, in four cases, patients' sputum became negative for tuberculosis bacteria. Overall, however, physicians remained guarded about streptomycin's potential. Even Hinshaw and Feldman, working with streptomycin in the laboratory, cautioned against the drug's growing reputation, given concerns that patients would choose to forego traditional therapies, including collapse therapy, if they overestimated streptomycin's capabilities.[263]

In May 1948, sixteen-year-old Annie was admitted to the Toronto sanatorium as a stretcher case from a local city hospital. The history of Annie's case suggested that she was likely infected in 1943, "when she was in contact with a family of tuberculous children." Annie's mother explained that while on vacation at a cottage, Annie had played with the children who, she understood, had subsequently died of tuberculosis. Annie had been monitored with regular chest X-rays, about every six months, for a few years afterwards. In February 1948, Annie experienced "bilateral pleuritic pain" with a high fever of 103° and "was treated with sulphathiazole" (a sulpha drug formerly used in the treatment of pneumococcus and staphylococcus infections until toxicity concerns limited its use). The drug treatment was not effective, and Annie suffered "three subsequent attacks of pleuritic pain," which "became localized in [her] lower chest" but produced neither cough nor sputum. It was this enduring respiratory pain that had precipitated Annie's hospital admission in February 1948; at this time, her pain was ascribed to an "acute pleurisy." Further examination revealed hilar cavitation in Annie's left lung, findings suggestive of tuberculosis. Artificial pneumothorax was induced at the hospital in April 1948, but complications arising from widespread adhesions caused some concern and Annie was transferred to the sanatorium in May 1948. In June, Annie would undergo a bronchscopic examination of her respiratory passages. At this time, a rigid bronchoscope would have been used, the long tube of the bronchoscope passed down Annie's throat into the bronchus and allowing the physician to see inside her lungs. At this time, bronchoscopy offered yet another option in the evaluation of the lungs, alongside the traditional examination measures, and the technologies of planograms[264] and X-rays. Along with the visualization of Annie's lungs, the bronchoscopy was also used to target sputum samples for testing, and samples collected from her left bronchus and pleural fluid tested positive for tuberculosis bacteria. Annie's gastric samplings also tested positive for tuberculosis bacteria. On the basis of these positive samples, there was no question that Annie's tuberculosis was active. Annie's gastric samples continued to test positive for tuberculosis bacteria until 15 November 1948. After this date, seven consecutive gastric specimens all returned negative for tuberculosis bacteria, a result her physicians chalked up to Annie's treatment with streptomycin. Annie was begun on streptomycin on 14 October and remained on the antibiotic for sixty-five days, at one gram per day. Early planograms continued to show signs of cavitation in her left lung, but the pathology became less obvious with each new planogram series. On discussing her case at a sanatorium medical conference, it was agreed that, prior to Annie's discharge, she also be given a phreniclasia (phrenic nerve crush). The drug therapy and the surgical intervention together were believed to give her the best possible chances for recovery. The left phreniclasia was carried out in January 1950, and she was discharged in February 1950. Two years later, Annie was still alive and well, with her tuberculosis remaining latent and her sputum continuing to test negative for tuberculosis bacteria.

In addition to streptomycin, in 1948, the Toronto sanatorium became involved in early clinical trials with PAS.[265] Given the frustrating reality that tuberculosis bacteria were quick to acquire resistance to streptomycin, the drug was paired with PAS to increase effectiveness of treatment. Gale notes that while PAS "was, in itself, a very weak drug, [it] had the remarkable effect of preventing (or at least delayed for a long time), the onset of … resistance to Streptomycin."[266] When seventeen-year-old Winona was admitted in February, 1948, she was diagnosed with far advanced pulmonary tuberculosis, defined by a large tuberculous cavity in her right lung. Winona was prescribed half a gram of streptomycin twice a day and ten grams of PAS daily for eight weeks beginning in May. Following Feldman and Hinshaw's recommendation, streptomycin was typically injected intramuscularly, or as one former patient expressed it, "two shots in the rump each day, one in the morning, the other around supper time."[267] As new anti-tuberculosis drugs were developed, new multi-drug treatments, typically utilizing three drugs administered in combination, became the norm, with new drugs, such as isoniazid (1952) and rifampin (1970) and ethambutol (circa early 1970s), introduced at the sanatorium over time.[268] Not all physicians embraced the three-drug approach, such as the streptomycin, PAS, isoniazid combination that emerged in the early 1950s, because they believed it was dangerous not to have additional drugs "in reserve" should antibiotic resistance emerge.[269] It is still standard practice today to hold some drugs in reserve and use them only when all of the standard drugs have proven ineffective.

As described earlier, the rise of more effective drug treatments did not result in an immediate abandonment of surgical procedures. Many patients placed on early drug treatments, such as Winona, were also considered for supplementary surgeries. In Winona's case, while drug therapy combined with pneumothorax was considered, the latter was not undertaken because it was thought that the lower lobe of her right lung might already be partially collapsed (atelectatic). On a drug treatment regime alone, Winona's X-rays did suggest improvements, but in June 1949 it was noted that a moderate-sized density in the base of her right lung still lingered. This was the only persistent problem, however, since both the large cavity and widespread disease originally affecting her right lung had essentially resolved. In order to target the base of her lung, an artificial pneumoperitoneum (injection of air into the abdominal, or peritoneal, cavity) was induced in order to collapse Winona's lower lobe in October 1949, with the hope that this might prevent a recurrence of her disease. Weekly refills in the amount of about 900 cc of gas were recommended for at least three years. Winona was discharged in February 1950, agreeing to return to the sanatorium each week for her refills.

Despite demand, when prescribed use of streptomycin was introduced for use in tuberculosis in the late 1940s, it was strictly controlled by governing bodies and, in the infancy of its use, the drug was not routinely administered in all cases. Some cautiousness was to be expected, since researchers and physicians were only just learning about dosages and effectiveness. At three years of age, Sally was admitted to the Toronto sanatorium in September 1948. She was identified as a contact of her father, who had already been admitted to the Toronto sanatorium suffering from far advanced pulmonary tuberculosis. Sally's X-rays were suggestive of tuberculosis and her tuberculin skin tests returned positive on two separate occasions. As a result of her contact with her father, who was probably highly infectious in his advanced disease state, and the fact that another young member of her household had recently developed miliary tuberculosis, a serious and life-threatening course of infection, Sally was considered for streptomycin therapy. The drug did not materialize, however, since her admitting physician noted that, in Sally's case, "streptomycin therapy did not fall within the scope of the criteria set down by the Ontario Streptomycin Board at that time, and Streptomycin was decided against for the present time." Sally was suffering from primary disease, and use of streptomycin had not yet been approved for patients with primary disease. Nevertheless, with regular sanatorium care, Sally was discharged in September 1949 with her disease then latent. Though she remained vulnerable to reactivation disease, her primary disease had not progressed. A couple of decades later, when a potential employer required that Sally undergo a physical examination in the early 1970s, her prior history with tuberculosis and the fact that she had never received any antibiotic treatment led to the recommendation that she start prophylactic isonicotinylhydrazine (INH), or isoniazid, treatment. She spent six months on the treatment and, at her next exam two years later, it was suggested that she be removed from active follow-up, since her original lesion had been unchanged for years. Sally was left with the choice to continue yearly chest X-rays, just for her own reassurance that the infection remained latent.

Sally's case had brought to light an important issue in the rise of streptomycin treatment as to whether or not the drug should be used to treat primary tuberculosis disease in children, or reserved only for cases of reactivation disease, especially in light of streptomycin's toxic side effects.[270] When drug treatments began with streptomycin alone, the feeling was that the drug had "outstanding value … in the virulent cases that do not respond to ordinary treatment such as miliary, meningeal and rapidly advancing exudative lesions," but that primary tuberculosis foci were largely "unaffected" by the drug.[271] By 1955, however, with the rise of multi-drug treatments of streptomycin, PAS, and isoniazid, physicians noted that primary tuberculosis of the lymph nodes also yielded well to treatment.[272] The question, at least in the early days of streptomycin when the expensive drug was in such limited supply, was whether or not streptomycin was actually critical to successful recovery, given that the majority of children survived primary infection (though they would be left with viable, latent TB bacteria in their bodies). In the early days of streptomycin, attention focused on progressive and aggressive disease where there was little hope of recovery, and as a supporting "adjuvant" to surgical cases.[273]

Despite the hopes offered by streptomycin in the new era of tuberculosis treatment, it was a sad reality that even this promising new antibiotic could not save everyone. Jane, a critically ill two-year-old, was transferred to the sanatorium in March 1949 from a city hospital. "The baby ... [was] carried in by [her] parents evincing a marked toxic pallor associated with listlessness, irritability, marked weakness, and in a semi-comatose state." Tests of Jane's cerebrospinal fluid returned positive for tuberculosis bacteria, indicating she suffered tuberculous meningitis, the most fatal form of tuberculosis for children, and her prognosis was extremely poor. Streptomycin had been administered to Jane prior to her transfer to the sanatorium, but only after failed penicillin and sulpha drug treatments. At the sanatorium, dihydrostreptomycin[274] was administered at a dosage of 0.5 gram intramuscularly daily, and 50 milligrams of streptomycin was given via a lumbar puncture (intrathecally) to introduce the drug directly into the fluid-filled space surrounding her spinal cord. This was undertaken three times a week from 15 to 31 March 1949. and Jane received a total of 8.5 grams of streptomycin intramuscularly and 400 milligrams of streptomycin intrathecally. Despite the streptomycin, Jane remained feverish. Her temperature averaged 101°F in her first week at the sanatorium, 102° in her second week, and fluctuated in the third week, reaching a high of 108° prior to her death, which occurred eighteen days after her transfer to the sanatorium. An autopsy confirmed tuberculous meningitis as the principal cause of death; an examination of the child's lungs also revealed the existence of a "small peripheral primary complex [in her] left lung." In attempting to determine Jane's exposure to tuberculosis, her parents could only think of her grandfather who had died of tuberculosis in 1947, though he had never lived in their home.

Conclusion

For much of the sanatorium era, the essence of tuberculosis treatment hinged on observations of how the body naturally responded to trauma and disease, attempting to manipulate those responses to encourage the body and its immune system to work more effectively against tuberculosis infection. From artificial hyperemia (increased blood supply), to artificial hyperpyrexia (inducing fever), artificial pneumothorax (selective lung collapse), and even artificial arthrodesis (surgical fusions), all of these "artificial" treatments were attempting to induce changes that might increase bodily resistance, shifting the balance of success to the immune system and trading active TB disease for latent infection. As scientific medicine impelled its therapeutic objectives forward, there was a shift from the more passive objective to support the immune system to build resistance, to surgical intentions to manipulate lungs, bones, or other tissues directly to increase bodily resistance by creating environments less hospitable to tuberculosis bacteria. With streptomycin, however, physicians were able to engage tuberculosis bacteria directly, their focus less exclusively occupied by the underlying state of the immune system. The story of treatments at the sanatorium, as presented here, ends abruptly with the introduction of streptomycin. A whole new chapter would unfold in the wake of antibiotic treatments – the rising therapeutic confidence that led to the demise of Canadian tuberculosis sanatoria, the need for new multi-drug treatments and directly observed therapy, and the North American epidemiological shift away from endemic tuberculosis. As antibiotic treatments become increasingly compromised by adaptive tuberculosis bacteria, however, attention has necessarily returned to the body and the complexities of immune function.

CHAPTER 7

Children and the Sanatorium: Conduct Sheets and Report Cards

Mind and body are inseparable in the experiences of sickness, suffering, and healing.[1]
~ Nancy Scheper-Hughes and Margaret Lock

Tuberculosis specialists of the sanatorium era understood that mind and body were inseparable in this chronic infectious disease. All of the demands of resistance building, and particularly all of the hours committed to quiet bedrest, would require a mind willing to cede to the limitations imposed by tuberculosis. The sanatorium was meant to be a disciplined environment, where rules aligned with the goals of hospitalization and treatment. The challenge of tuberculosis was typically no acute, short-lived experience, and it held great power in influencing how those infected, with or without active disease, might structure their lives and how they treated their bodies. Within the sanatorium, as physicians and nurses aimed to build biological resistance to tuberculosis, they could do so only with patients' acceptance of (or resignation to) the treatments and limitations that aimed to guide them back towards health. As Alison Bashford has argued, physicians believed "discipline and struggle produced stronger bodies with a greater capacity to resist and contain the effects of the disease."[2] As a result, the role of the sanatorium extended well beyond building physiological resistance, towards strengthening the underlying mental resistance of patients to the chronic infection of tuberculosis. Bashford notes that "for most experts and patients, enhancing 'resisting power' meant working on character and attitude as much as bodies."[3] From the staff's perspective, the minds of patients had to yield to sanatorium expectations so that their bodies could persevere and heal. The hope was that, as child patients aged, they would apply what they had learned at the sanatorium, ensuring an adequate diet, taking care to rest, breathe fresh air, and avoid taxing their bodies through overwork.

Surviving tuberculosis would require both effort and cooperation. Paine and Hershfield reflected on the temperaments and attitudes of the "miracle patients" of the sanatorium era, those who "showed moral strength, courage and perseverance in fighting their disease ... Scarcely anyone recovered without being a better person, more mature, better adjusted and educated, and with a higher potential for giving and receiving than ever before."[4] They note that with the rise of antibiotics, attention shifted "from the miracle patients to miracle drugs." Antibiotics meant that cure became "easy" and, as a result, "removed some of the moral fiber, the striving urge to recover, so characteristic of the old time patients." To achieve cooperation and encourage patients to take an active role in controlling their tuberculosis, sanatorium staff had to build positive relationships and ensure a good experience at the sanatorium; for their part, medical and nursing staff respected those patients who fought through or stoically endured incurable and potentially deadly tuberculosis. But for patients, especially children, facing TB and hospitalization, behaviour was also the key to resistance, both misbehaviour and complaints serving as important behavioural expressions of resistance to the sanatorium and the frustrating limitations imposed by illness and disease.

Views into patient expression, albeit in this chapter stemming mostly from incidents of misconduct and complaints about the sanatorium, help to flesh out not only the inner workings of the sanatorium, but also its social context, apart from and in connection with its medical function. It is through the narratives of misconduct, for example, that we learn of the fluidity connecting the sanatorium to the larger community of Weston and the abilities of children to resist strict institutional isolation. In many ways, these stories provide some of the richest perspectives on life inside the sanatorium that would not exist if all children had behaved accordingly, or if there had not been such a commitment to documentation among sanatorium staff. Indeed, lacking this material, a very different perspective on life in the sanatorium may have emerged, one that did not recognize the degree to which children could and did exercise their agency and wilfulness.[5] It is also those children who resisted (some more brazenly than others) the expectation of an ordered life in the sanatorium who provide some of the more compelling insights into the diversity in patient character as they interacted with and influenced the sanatorium environment through their misbehaviour. The stories of misbehaviour animate the sanatorium's child patients in ways that no other source could.

Sanatorium staff were ultimately responsible not only for the physical but also the social well-being of the children who were admitted. Being admitted into a medical institution could be stressful for children, many away from home and apart from their families for the first time in their lives and under difficult circumstances. Given the family and household context of tuberculosis, a large number of the children admitted would have already experienced terrible hardship, often disease and death within the family home, sometimes at young ages, and they brought those emotional traumas with them to the sanatorium. While some children may have found reprieve or comfort in the sanatorium, others would struggle, less receptive to the staff, the other children, the treatment protocols, and the rules. According to Dobbie, bedrest, a central feature of treatment, shaped a "passive, automatic, almost vegetative existence," particularly among those most unwell.[6] Patients who were not as incapacitated by tuberculosis, including children with uncomplicated primary disease, would be more likely to struggle with the limitations on their freedoms. At Craig-y-nos sanatorium in Wales, children who would not stay in their beds for bedrest could be tied down in their beds with "restrainers," but this practice was not reported for the Toronto sanatorium (which is not to say they were not used, but just not documented). Ultimately, according to Linda Bryder, sanatoria aimed for "passive and submissive states of compliance" to achieve a level of cooperation that did not require such restrictive practices.[7] But in considering how demoralizing the sanatorium rules could be for adults in American sanatoria, Sheila Rothman has argued that wilful and knowing disobedience could serve functional purposes, perhaps relieving boredom and loneliness, or as a way that patients could remember and assert their individuality.[8] Disobedience marked a lack of cooperation, a mindful rejection of the limitations of disease and hospitalization.

Among adults, this type of resistance could result in their early discharges from the sanatorium, whether medically advised or not. To some extent, misbehaviour among the child patients played a similar role, reflecting their resistance to disease and hospitalization, but for other children, their misbehaviour was simply a by-product of their youth. Whether children were admitted to the sanatorium from family homes or other institutions, they were likely already accustomed to being held accountable to rules and authority. There is a good indication that sanatorium staff were fairly tolerant of misbehaviour among child patients, even in cases of repeated misbehaviour. Susan Haugh has also argued that staff at Waipiata sanatorium in New Zealand were generally tolerant of minor infringements of the rules, allowing for "relatively harmless rule breaking," such as reading during rest hours, "in order to alleviate the more dangerous aspects of frustration with treatment."[9] More contented perhaps by these allowances, patients may have felt less motivated to actually leave the sanatorium. The strictness of rules that typically characterized adult sanatoria was difficult to impose in the children's sanatorium. The discipline of the children's hospital had as much to do with socializing and educating the children about acceptable conduct, as it did with instructing them on the dangers and limitations of tuberculosis. As will be evident in this chapter, child patients were usually considered for early discharge only if they were prone to what was viewed as excessive or particularly grievous misbehaviour.

Amidst the rules, the illness, and the loss at the sanatorium, there were emotionally important reprieves. Children, if sufficiently healthy, could attend the sanatorium's Board-certified school, receive instruction in arts and crafts, and enjoy playtimes, both indoors and out, in addition to the toys, dolls, puzzles, books, and magazines provided to offset the boredom of hospitalization (figure 7.1). At the Queen Alexandra Solarium for children on Vancouver Island, Lenora Marcellus notes that "many of the children participated in social events that their families would usually not have had access to because of low family economic and social status, including motor-boat rides, car rides, circus shows, moving pictures, and visits from royalty."[10] Great emphasis was also placed on celebrating happy occasions, such as birthdays and holidays, often arranged by the nurses and particularly important to child patients. In his first year at the sanatorium, fourteen-year-old Howard wrote two letters in August 1919, one addressed to Dobbie (see figure 7.2) and another to Dobbie and Dickson, wanting to remind them of his upcoming birthday, and endear-

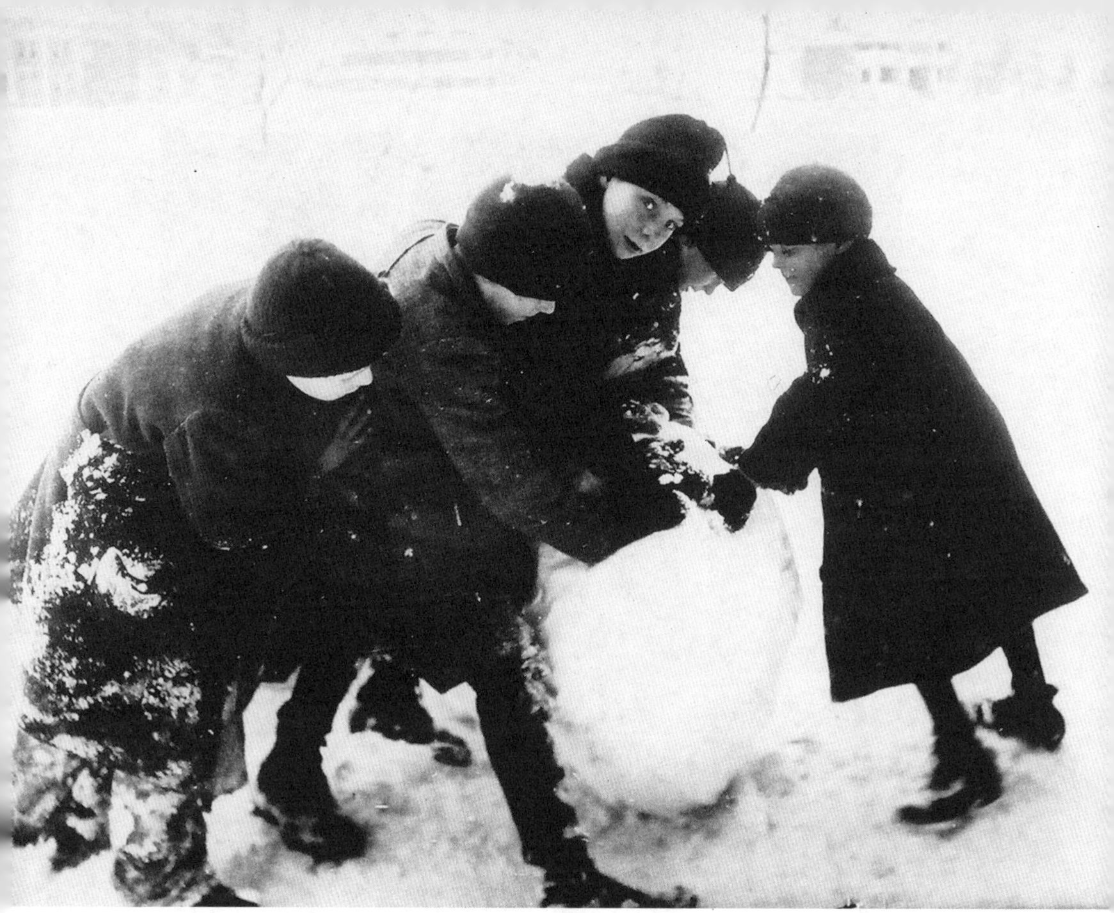

Figure 7.1 Children building a snowman at the Queen Mary Hospital.

ingly specifying exactly how he wished to celebrate this milestone. "Dear Miss Dickson and Dr Dobbie," he wrote. "I would like to ask you would do me a favor, that is to give me a birthday party." He wanted the celebration to take place during supper, and to have "nice" sandwiches, cake, fruit, and lemonade served. He wanted to share in his celebration with the boys who usually sat at his table in the dining room. "I will thank you very much if you will let me have it," his letter concluded. There is no documentation of Howard's birthday party but, reading between the lines, it seems Howard had been satisfied, as he wrote a thank-you note to Dickson in the days that followed. "Dear Miss Dickson," it began, "I thought I would write you a few lines to thanke you for the cake what you have sent me for my birthday." Howard noted that everyone who had a piece of cake seemed to like it. Somewhat surprisingly, the letter continues, "I did not have a very good time but I had lots of birthday

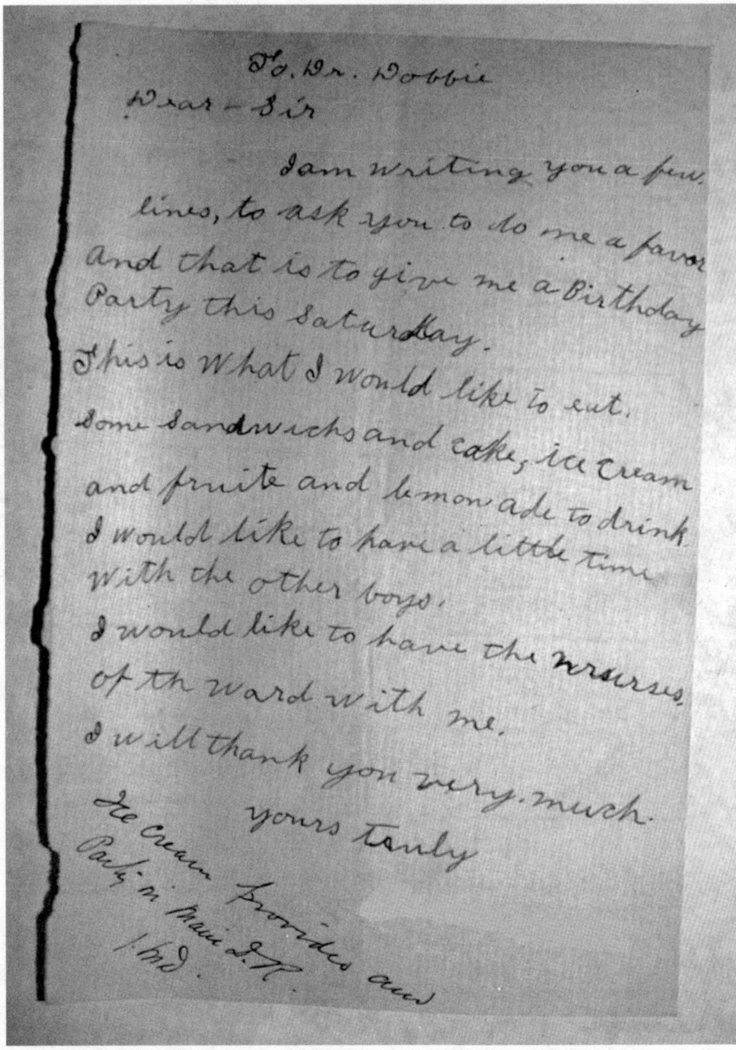

To. Dr. Dobbie
Dear-Sir
I am writing you a few lines, to ask you to do me a favor And that is to give me a Birthday Party this Saturday.
This is What I would like to eat.
Some sandwichs and cake, ice cream and fruite and lemonade to drink.
I would like to have a little time with the other boys.
I would like to have the nurses of th ward with me.
I will thank you very. much.
Yours truly

Ice Cream provided and Party in Main D.R.
[illegible]

Figure 7.2
To Dr Dobbie
Dear Sir
I am writing you a few lines, to ask you to do me a favor and that is to give me a Birthday Party this Saturday. This is what I would like to eat. Some sandwichs and cake, ice cream and fruite and lemonade to drink. I would like to have a little time with the other boys. I would like to have the nurses of the ward with me. I will thank you very much.
Yours truly
Dickson's note in the bottom left corner: Ice cream provided and party in Main D.R. [dining room].

prazents." Though Howard did not account for his disappointment in any greater detail, he did clearly appreciate the celebration. "I did not think I had so many friends as I did," he wrote, while also expressing his thanks for "the flowers on the table," the many "nice things," the "candie fruite," and the money that was given to him. Howard need not have worried that his birthday would be overlooked, because it was typical that such occasions were celebrated with decorations, cake, ice cream, and presents, the happy occasions that staff embraced with the children to offset all of the other challenges of hospitalization, treatment, and tuberculosis.

With the support and contributions of philanthropic groups (see chapter 8), the sanatorium staff tried to make holidays, in particular, special for the children who were away from their homes and families. On Christmas Day in the 1930s, children were seated at their decorated tables in the dining room to enjoy a special dinner of cream of celery soup, creamed chicken, mashed potatoes, peas, pink junket,[11] bread and butter, and fruit drink. A former child patient recalled that at Christmastime a limousine was hired, and each night staff took a different group of children out to see the Christmas lights and decorations in the neighbourhood.[12] When eight-year-old Amalie was admitted from northern Ontario in 1929, she had never heard of Santa Claus until, in December of that year, "her bed was brought out into the corridor to hear him speak over the radio." Quickly grasping the idea of Saint Nick, Amalie happily set about selecting her (imaginary) gifts for everybody she knew from a department store catalogue, her list then "sent to Santa" so that he could see to delivering the gifts. In the Christmas update sent to her cot patrons, staff noted proudly that modest Amalie had asked for nothing for herself, already content with her favourite doll that she had brought with her to the sanatorium.

It is easy to understand that child patients could perceive hospitals as "foreign, sometimes hostile, places."[13] Vulnerable at admission and meeting nurses "at times of crisis in their lives," Fleitas notes that children often found a particular "protective intimacy" in caring nursing staff, developing new relationships to help "buffer their fears" over hospitalization.[14] Those relationships could become so powerful that some children came to view the sanatorium as home, and staff as family. Eight-year-old Lillian, for example, was admitted to the Toronto sanatorium in the summer of 1929 and was quite ill for the first six or seven months of her hospitalization. Reflecting back to that time, Lillian recounted that because her mother was widowed, with four children at home and without a car, "in those days cars were quite a luxury," she had very little contact with her mother between 1929 and her eventual discharge in April 1931. She remembers, "I saw her twice, the first Christmas I was in when I was very, very ill and they didn't expect me to live, they called her, and then I saw her once after that."[15] Her brothers and sister also visited her a handful of times, "but other than that," she was essentially left alone at the sanatorium and came to feel "the hospital was more my home." When the day of her discharge grew closer and the nurses asked if she was looking forward to going home, she remembered that she had told them, "I am home," and when she did return home, she remembered feeling "quite strange among all these other people."[16] This sentiment of sanatorium-as-home was a common finding for children who had been long-term sanatorium patients, spending their formative years in the hospital and acclimatizing to such an extent that deep connections endured long after discharge.

While ward nurses were most directly involved with the children and often developed the closest relationships with them, all staff members would ultimately play some role in their care and supervision. If any problems came to light, the nurses were supposed to apprise both Dr McHugh (in charge of the Queen Mary) and Dr Dobbie. It was not uncommon for correspondence to pass between the nurses, Dobbie, and McHugh until consensus was reached over the proper resolution to a particular situation. Miss Dickson or Miss Wilkinson, lady superintendents, could also intervene in discipline-related matters. In addition to the administrative, medical, and nursing staff, the general staff, including maintenance and kitchen workers, also assisted in watching over the children. The night watchman noted any unapproved comings-and-goings, sometimes even returning errant children to the sanatorium, while teachers at the Queen Mary school monitored progress in education and conduct.

Misbehaviour: Resisting the Sanatorium

Most problem behaviour noted on the conduct sheets was pretty standard fare for children who could be found saucy, noisy, disobedient, refusing to go to bed, or using bad language. When older children or adolescents were involved, staying up after hours, sneaking out of their rooms, getting into fights, and leaving the sanatorium grounds were common problems. Serious misconduct was a rarity, and most of the children sampled did not even have conduct sheets in their files. Some children such as twelve-year-old Hazel, however, outdid themselves, as she upset staff with her ongoing threats to murder her roommate at the sanatorium. Other children had quite lengthy conduct sheets, which suggest that staff were somewhat patient in their dealings with the children, often building long trails of documentation before any decisions on discharge were made. Most often this meant that the privileges that children attained due to improving health status could be temporarily withdrawn, such that children who had been given school, play, or dining room privileges could be sent back to bed for "extra rest." This tactic could be problematic since measures such as bedrest, framed as treatment, could then be confused with punishment.

Responsible for the whole of the sanatorium, including both the adult and child hospitals, it was Dobbie who ultimately decided on appropriate disciplinary actions, determining if early discharges or other measures were warranted. On a few occasions, Dobbie had to caution staff members against taking matters of discipline into their own hands. One such occasion involved a dining room employee and the boys he served at his tables, one of whom was "getting beyond" him. Fifteen-year-old Jackson was found fighting at the table one day and was late for a meal the next. The dining room employee wrote to Dobbie in 1917, explaining, "I put him on bread and milk as I do the other boys when they are late." Jackson, however, had his own ideas and "refused to do as he was told and went on and ate a regular meal." Dobbie had not been particularly happy with the staff member's choice of discipline, interfering as it did with a fundamental of sanatorium treatment to provide good, nourishing, and plentiful food and encourage weight gain. In future, Dobbie advised the staff member to document any cases of misbehaviour in the dining room, which he could then present to Dobbie at the end of each week, leaving the administrative staff to "set the punishment required."

In researching the history of the sanatorium, Gale noted a ledger-style "discipline book," the rows and columns of which listed patient, complaint, and punishment; in serious cases, fighting, swearing, lying, and the destruction of hospital property could each earn a patient two straps.[17] Though discipline does not really find a place in an average hospital, the sanatorium was different because of its characteristic long-term hospitalizations. Given the time period, parents may have subscribed to this discipline regimen, especially since a number of parents sent their children to the sanatorium precisely because they felt their children would not respect the discipline needed to pursue the rest cure at home, a treatment fundamental to overcoming tuberculosis. In this respect, the sanatorium, like schools, became an extension of home discipline. Disciplining even for minor infractions such as swearing may have been important, since any loss on the footholds of basic discipline might jeopardize the medically important commitment to the more tedious rules of the sanatorium, such as quiet rest in bed. In more grievous cases, often after recurrent misbehaviour, the ultimate recourse was to discharge the child, even if, from a medical perspective, a longer stay may have been beneficial. Parents were often dismayed to learn that, because of disobedience, their children were being returned home early. Ultimately, in such cases, it was felt that children were only undermining their own opportunities to become well.

In a hospital full of children, not all of the children would get along together all of the time. Children occupying beds on wards or in rooms with other children could try to relieve the monotony of hospitalization and bedrest by irritating, sometimes "tormenting," one another. On a Sunday night in May 1922, for example, five adolescent boys sharing a room in the unsupervised pavilions amused themselves with a food fight. The nurse who came on duty the following morning found their room in a "disgraceful condition," egg and pineapple from their supper trays littering the floor and beds. Behaviour problems noted in the case of five-year-old Maureen, a long-term resident of the Davies Cottage for infants, led staff to the conclusion that it was time to transfer her into the company of older children at the Queen Mary Hospital. Maureen had a tendency towards what was described as "juvenile sadism," as she was caught on two occasions biting and scratching younger children. The transfer was finally undertaken after she was discovered holding another child's arm against a hot water radiator long enough that it burned. Despite these incidents, staff noted, "she is not bad tempered or unpleasant otherwise."

Fourteen-year-old Heather became very unhappy during her stay at the sanatorium in 1933 and was discharged within only three months of her arrival. Heather had experienced tensions with other girls on her ward, the situation culminating the evening one girl pulled away Heather's bedcovers, while another girl slapped Heather's face and called her a "charity brat." Inconsolable, Heather ran away the next day, returning to her home in Toronto, but her parents promptly returned her to the sanatorium the same day. Though Dobbie recommended that the girls "should all start over again and try to get along amicably," Heather was determined to leave, so her parents packed up her belongings and took her home. With many of the children at the sanatorium from homes in Toronto, there were other children who, like Heather, found their way home from the sanatorium only to be brought back by parents or other guardians. Personal conflicts, homesickness, and boredom were all strong motivators to venture home, particularly if children were feeling well enough.

Some children who entered the sanatorium became persistent and determined runaways, those who obstinately could not or would not settle into life at the sanatorium. Eldon was one such child. He was admitted in October 1914 at twelve years of age, orphaned by the tuberculosis-related deaths of his parents. Of Eldon's two brothers, one was alive but suffering from TB, and the other had died of TB. Of his five sisters, three were alive and well, but two had also died of TB. Before his admission to the sanatorium, Eldon had been living with an adult sister in her Toronto home. According to an April 1915 chart note concerning Eldon, he simply could not come to terms with the idea of remaining at the sanatorium and on a Wednesday afternoon "ran away and went to the residence of his sister." The next day, she returned her brother to the sanatorium, "reporting that she had no place in which to keep him, and that he must stay" at the sanatorium. If Eldon returned to her home, she was prepared to get the police involved. Eldon was readmitted, but within minutes he had once again "disappeared." On Friday morning, Eldon was seen on the sanatorium grounds, and a staff member was sent out to retrieve him. Seeing the man coming for him, Eldon ran, wading into the Humber River "until such time as the current threw him off his feet, and it was necessary for the man to plunge in, in order to prevent him being drowned." Brought back to the hospital, Eldon was given a hot bath and put to bed, but by noon he had once again disappeared. Eldon's story is one of rejection, his sister so adamant that he could not return to her house that she was willing to report him to the police if he reappeared. While she argued that she did not have space for him, it is questionable whether her concerns could have had more to do with a fear of Eldon's tuberculosis, particularly if she had children and because she had already witnessed the deaths of her parents and three siblings. Regardless, this was the last that anyone heard of Eldon. He never returned to the sanatorium and his discharge was formalized on 10 April 1915, for reasons of "French Leave" (i.e., he had run away).

Few children were motivated to go so far as to run away from the sanatorium, but a good number did treat themselves to unsupervised sojourns, sometimes alone and other times in the company of fellow patients. Recalling the two years that she had spent at the Queen Mary Hospital, eventually discharged at ten years of age in 1931, Lillian recounted the children's secret evening ritual of "lights out." Once the Queen Mary was quiet, some of the boys from the upstairs ward would sneak down the back stairs and "come through our ward," she remembered, "and we would open up the window and we would sneak out and go down to the play yard ... we used to go down there and we would climb the fence and ... cross over this rickety old bridge."[18] Their destination was a little convenience store on the other side of the Humber River, where they would treat themselves to bubble gum. According to Lillian, "We were not allowed gum to begin with, but it was fun." Interestingly, children at Craig-y-nos sanatorium in Wales were also not allowed to have gum. According to Pat Davies (Cornell), "We were told that it was very bad for us. After one visiting day, a little girl on the balcony died and we were told it was because she'd eaten chewing gum."[19] In Weston, in addition to the convenience store, there were other local attractions that the children found difficult to resist. In 1935, twelve-year-old Perry was apprehended by the watchman leaving the sanatorium grounds, on his way to get an order of fish and chips from a popular local restaurant. He wrote a letter of apology to Dr Dobbie, reassuring him, "Dr Dobbie I will promise that I will stay with in the hopitel grounds [and] obay all the reuls in feucher" and, with that, the matter was resolved.

In another instance, on an evening in 1919, a night nurse went in search of a commotion she had heard coming from a ward in the Queen Mary. Upon finding two boys awake and out of their beds, the nurse brought them into her office so that the other children on their ward could sleep. In the office, the boys had apparently laughed at the nurse and made fun of her, so she gave them each a slap on the back of the head. The boys ran away later that night, but were brought back the next afternoon by one of the boy's mothers. Upon inquiry, the nurse admitted that she had slapped the boys, but insisted in her defence that she had not been severe and the boy's mother was satisfied. Dobbie reprimanded and warned the boys, one of them later offering Dobbie five promises, in writing:

> I promise on my word of honor to take my rest.
> To go to bed at the right time.
> To do as the nurse tell's me.
> Not to make to much noise so as to disturb the men.
> To come and tell you if we fail to do any of these things.

This last point is endearing, the boy promising that if he found himself breaking his other promises, he would report himself directly to Dobbie. This case reflects the sanatorium's preferred approach to discipline, looking to the children to recognize and take responsibility for their misdeeds, and ultimately accepting the apologies that children offered (thankfully in writing, otherwise these exchanges would be lost to history).

With her father dying from tuberculosis in 1926 and her mother suffering from active tuberculosis disease (and later becoming a patient in the Muskoka sanatorium in the early 1930s), Aileen was considered to be at high risk for developing the disease. She was admitted to the IODE

Preventorium in Toronto and remained there for eighteen months. She was removed from the preventorium in 1934 and placed in the care of her grandmother in Toronto. She attended school in the city until June 1935, when, upon X-ray examination of her lungs, a city order was placed for her admission to the Queen Mary. Aileen was eleven years of age at this time and now showing signs of active disease. During her treatment in the sanatorium, she suffered complications, including bronchiectasis[20] and a spontaneous partial collapse of her left lung. Despite these problems, she gradually improved and was discharged as a latent case in December 1939.

Aileen first attracted the attention of the medical and nursing staff in January 1939 when she and another patient sneaked out of the sanatorium sometime after 11 p.m. on a Sunday, arriving at the nearby Mount Dennis Theatre for the midnight show. As Aileen and Nancy made their way into the theatre, they unknowingly took seats in the vicinity of three of the sanatorium's nurses. One of the nurses used the telephone at the theatre to call the sanatorium, but interference on the line meant that the nurse receiving the call could not make out the specifics of the message, and was uncertain which of the patients had been seen at the theatre. The rooms were searched, but all appeared to be in order. It was not until the next day, when the nurses at the theatre came back on duty, that the identities of the patients were revealed and, when questioned, the girls readily admitted that they had gone to the show. In a note to Dobbie, Aileen wrote, "We didn't have any special reason" for going, "we just wanted to have some fun." When Aileen's mother came to the sanatorium a day later to take her daughter to the dentist she was told of the incident; apparently annoyed with her daughter, she had stern words for Aileen. A few months later, Aileen disappeared once again, this time on a Saturday night, with another girl. Both were unaccounted for between 7:30 and 9:30. When they reappeared, they said that they had been playing in the basement, hiding in the cleaner's cupboard. Dobbie seriously doubted their story, however, since the next day, Aileen sought treatment for blisters on her feet and a ward maid reported that she had found Aileen's shoes wet. To reprimand the girls, Aileen was put back to full bedrest. Because staff were involved in most aspects of the patients' lives, soiled clothing, wet shoes, and skipped meals did not go unnoticed. When a group of five young boys were conspicuously absent at lunchtime, it did not take staff long to realize, upon scrutiny of their "very wet and muddy condition," that they had been playing in the Humber River. In this case, the boys were given hot baths and put to bed for extra rest.

Some patients were admitted to the sanatorium as children, but stayed for such an extended time that they matured into adolescence or even young adulthood. Accordingly, childhood preoccupations could evolve into more serious adult interests. Described by Rothman as "cousining," boredom-relieving personal relationships in sanatoria were fairly commonplace.[21] For those with love interests outside of the sanatorium, visiting days could bring their own excitement. On an internship in the 1940s at Grace Dart Hospital (a tuberculosis sanatorium in Montreal), Dr Bayne recalled the spectacle of visiting day on the women's wards with "2 rows of young women, dressed in frilly nighties, their hair stylish, their cheeks flushed with fever and touched up with make-up and lipstick."[22] They were anticipating the arrival of "boyfriends and young husbands whose interest in them had to be maintained despite this illness and the long separation it caused." It is clear that a tuberculosis diagnosis did not mean the loss of romantic interests, probably in part because the disease was so common, it could simply be accepted as part of the person. Such interests were certainly observed among adolescents at the Toronto sanatorium. In January 1931, the night supervisor reported that four adolescent girls who shared a room were visited by a boy. It was believed that sometime between 7:30 and 8:15 p.m. the stealthy visitor had entered the girls' room through a window. The night nurses searched in vain for the "intruder," but the girls were strategically unwilling to admit that they knew the boy, so nobody was reprimanded in the incident.

Rosemary was admitted to the Queen Mary in 1931 when she was fourteen years of age. Her father had died an accidental death, and pulmonary TB had claimed her mother at just thirty-nine years of age. The death of her parents left Rosemary and her sisters orphans in Toronto. In 1935, now eighteen years old, Rosemary had finished with her education at the Queen Mary School and spent most of her time resting in bed, sitting outside when the weather permitted, and either reading or sewing a little. Rosemary and other girls were found missing from their rooms without permission one summer evening. It was soon learned that they had left the sanatorium grounds and made their way to Weston's local dance hall, the details provided by Rosemary in the letter of apology she wrote to Dobbie a day after the incident. Rosemary explained that, along with fellow patients Naomi, Shirley, and Gwen, they had arrived at the dance hall at 7 p.m. While Naomi left the group over the course of the evening, Rosemary and the others "started talking to some fellows who had been around there for quite a while," the men "persuading" them to "go for a car ride." Soon realizing that the men "wanted the night kind of company," Rosemary, Shirley, and Gwen requested that the men drop them off near the dance hall at 11:30 p.m. so that they could make their way back to the sanatorium, following the trail of the Humber River. "But," she noted, "the fellows thought it wasn't safe for us as it was all in darkness so we went back to the car where two more younger boys joined us. From there we went back to the hospital and got out of the car in the side lane." Though Rosemary did "not like to promise to keep away from dance pavilion," in case she should break that promise, she did resolve that she would "try and keep away from it." Rosemary remained at the sanatorium for almost five years and was nineteen when she was discharged with minimal and latent pulmonary TB.

The local dance hall, known as Hunter's Dance Pavilion, was located alongside the Humber River, somewhat problematically within walking distance of the sanatorium. It was a temptation that many patients found difficult to resist, and the lure of the dance hall kept the sanatorium's night watchman on his toes. Over the years, a number of the sanatorium's adolescent patients frequented the dance hall, though Rosemary admitted that it was a "pretty 'low' place," perhaps because of the company or maybe because of the "port and other liquors" that were sold. Naomi had been out with Rosemary and the other girls from her ward, but had parted with them just after 9 p.m. at the dance hall. In her letter to Dobbie, Naomi explained that she had gone for walk with a man, whom Dobbie characterized as a "useless ex-employee." Like Rosemary, Naomi also resolved "to try and do my utmost not to go down to the dance pavilion on the Humber any more," as she had "come to the conclusion that it is not the place for decent people to go." She did ask Dobbie, however, if he had any objections to her seeing the young man she had been out with, because she had clearly developed an interest in him.

Despite the regular forgiving of minor incidents, there were some more serious conduct-related matters that staff could neither overlook nor correct with letters of apology or extra bedrest. Clarence was admitted to the sanatorium at fifteen years of age in 1931 and remained for just over two years before Dobbie discharged him rather dishonourably. Clarence had been given a bed in the pavilions, sharing a room with two other patients, Andrew and Jason. Over the course of a single evening, the three had left the sanatorium and shared two bottles of wine, intending to see a movie at the Mount Dennis Theatre. For Dobbie, the most disturbing aspect of the evening was the fact that they had brought along with them a young female patient, Patricia. By the time they reached the theatre, "the girl was very much under the influence of the drink and was vomiting." Being refused admission, the four then returned to the pavilions. Deeply intoxicated, Patricia "was very noisy and restless and had to be taken into the Main Building and given a sedative to quieten her down." Dr Garrett sought out Dr Dobbie, and when the two "had the girl's assurance that she had not been molested" they "allowed the matter to stand over till the next morning." The following morning, the now-sober Patricia recounted to Dobbie what she remembered: "She told me she had taken four glasses of wine at the request of the men named. She said she felt certain that she was not molested; she admits that she was much nauseated and for a while had only an indistinct memory of what was going on around her." Dobbie then interviewed Clarence, Andrew, and Jason, "who said that they got the two bottles of wine lying in a parcel at the back of the dance hall at the Humber. They all admitted drinking and having given drink (wine) to the girl." Determining "I cannot have such men as these in the hospital," Dobbie summarily ordered immediate discharges for Andrew and Jason, informing them that they might be called upon by the police for breaching the Liquor Control Act and in supplying alcohol to minors (both Patricia and Clarence were underage). Clarence was also to be discharged but, lacking in funds, Dobbie instructed him to "write to his people for enough money to take him home," allowing him to remain at the sanatorium in the meantime. Despite the concession granted to him, Clarence chose to leave after the incident. Staff later learned that he had been taken in by the Salvation Army in Toronto until he could gather the funds for his train fare back home.

Children at the sanatorium could find amusement and distraction in many forms, including petty thievery. One nine-year-old girl, Olive, a patient at the Toronto sanatorium between 1919 and 1921, was caught stealing from a number of different children over the period of a few weeks. Although one of the ward nurses had spoken with Olive "sternly" about her stealing on a number of occasions, the child could not seem to help herself, and her conduct notes documented the diverse and growing inventory of stolen goods found in her possession: oranges, a pair of socks, biscuits, doll's clothes, chocolates, handkerchiefs, black shoe polish, seventy-five cents, a box of snapshots, a bag with fancy work, two dollars, a bank, perfume, soap, writing paper, twenty-five cents, and toothpaste. Tommy, a six-year-old who spent about eight months in the Toronto sanatorium in the late 1930s, was also described by staff as "light fingered." In his conduct notes, it was recorded, "He is cute enough to realize that there is only one nurse around at night and watches for every opportunity to sneak into the office and take things from drawers, cupboards and off the desks." Tommy knew this was wrong, but kept it up, "often remark[ing], 'well, if you lock it up I can't get it.'" Tommy was discovered in his bed eating what remained of a box of chocolates late one night. He was brought into the nurses' office and, when asked about it, apparently "spoke a number of lies" and was told he would not be allowed to go back to bed until the truth came out. According to his conduct sheet, he sat quietly on a chair in the office for five minutes, and then had a temper tantrum, jumping up and down, for another five. Eventually, "he owned up that he knew he should not have taken them but he just wanted to take something." Rather than feeling remorseful, even when he was told that the chocolates were intended as a gift from one of the child patients to her mother, "he seemed to think it was a great joke." Tommy's amusement did not end there, however, and, over the course of the next two months, he was apprehended taking "a box of powder which he had opened and spilled part on himself and part on the floor," the greater part of a basket of fruit, of which a half-eaten apple was found on his nightstand (the rest of the fruit handed out to the boys in his room and stashed at the bottom of their lockers), more food, a rag puppy doll, a crucifix, nail polish, thread, red and blue ink, a pen knife, and a pen. These items were all taken from patients while they slept. Perhaps this tendency towards thievery can be better understood by Rothman's conclusion that in the "closed world of the patients, privacy and even private ownership practically disappeared. Clothing, radios, and love letters became communal property."[23] At the Craig-y-nos sanatorium, this whole problem was avoided altogether with a rule of communal property; anything that came into the wards immediately became the property of all.[24]

According to his conduct sheet, Tommy's problem behaviour did not end with stealing. About a month and a half prior to his discharge in 1939, it was reported that Tommy had gotten into the habit of pulling up the skirts of the nurses and ward maids when their hands were otherwise occupied. One nurse noted, "To-day when I was busy bathing another patient he had crawled out of bed and along the floor so that when I turned around I found him lying on the floor and trying to look up under my uniform." Furthermore, she noted, "I have frequently walked into the room and found him exposing his buttocks and parts of his body in a most disgusting way to the other boys in the room. On one occasion he threatened to urinate on my uniform." Apparently, when questioned about looking up the nurse's skirts, Tommy cried and said he was sorry, but then, according to his conduct notes, upon returning to his ward, he was overheard laughing and telling the other boys, "Hee ha that is over with." The matter did not end there, as the nurses quickly learned that urinals could not be left with Tommy unattended because he liked to empty their contents on the floor or in his bed and did the same with urinals belonging to the other boys on his ward. Growing increasingly concerned about Tommy's well-being, a psychiatrist was called in to meet with him. Following the evaluation, Tommy was pronounced "normal," and since the staff at the sanatorium felt that everyone, patients and staff included, had grown tired of what was taken to be his boredom-relieving antics, he was transferred to another sanatorium for a "fresh start."

Fourteen-year-old Kenneth was admitted on 2 September 1935, but also needed a "fresh start" just over a year later. Although Kenneth was a young patient, his health was sufficiently good that he had been placed in an outlying pavilion (with other adolescent and adult male patients). Dobbie documented Kenneth's staunch resistance to the sanatorium, frustration mounting since staff had "tried everything to induce this boy to take the cure," from "persuasion" to "coaxing and mild threats," all "without much success." A fellow patient, a schoolteacher in her life outside the sanatorium, had agreed to give Kenneth daily lessons "in an attempt to make him content," but after several lessons, she discovered five dollars missing from her dresser. "While she is not sure he took it," Dobbie wrote, "she will not give him any more lessons." On another occasion, when contemplating running away from the sanatorium, Kenneth had taken a watch and pair of binoculars belonging to other patients; in that instance, the items were recovered and returned to their owners. In the two months leading up to his discharge, more troubles came to light: going down to the Humber River to bathe, offering cigarette butts and matches to younger children, being absent from his bed in the pavilions in the late evening and early morning hours, striking the face of an adult male patient ("which was returned"), and the theft of money from other patients in the pavilions (fourteen dollars and counting). Dobbie felt that Kenneth would need at least another three to six months of care under supervision, but made arrangements for his transfer to another sanatorium. Dobbie felt the other patients had grown to "distrust him" and that "it would be better in his own interest that he should be taken away from here as soon as possible, so that he may have a fresh start in a new environment."

In one other case sampled, a child's conduct seemed so incomprehensible to sanatorium staff that, like Tommy, upon the child's discharge, a psychiatric evaluation was advised. Hazel was twelve years old when she was admitted to the Queen Mary in November 1936. There was no history of TB in her family, and Hazel was the only member of her household who skin tested positive for tuberculosis infection; she was admitted to the sanatorium with a diagnosis of minimal pulmonary tuberculosis. For the rest of 1936 and all of 1937, Hazel's hospitalization was seemingly uneventful. In 1938, however, a series of incidents arose, all meticulously documented with supporting materials in her conduct sheet. Hazel's first attempt to run away was noted in April 1938. According to a ward nurse's report, "Last night at the Queen Mary at 7.30 Hazel got dressed and went out. The maid went after her. Found her at the fence behind the Davies Cottage and brought her back." In June 1938, Hazel again tried to run away from the hospital. And once again she was brought back. When asked why she wanted to run away, she wrote, "I have a reason for running away; I couldn't bear to say it in words. Here is the reason. Love. But please don't tell my mother because she had a stroke once and if you tell my mother I hate to think what might happen." Hazel claimed she had received a couple of letters from a boy encouraging her to run away, but that she had torn up those letters and thrown them away. After what was at least her second attempt at running away, McHugh wrote to Hazel's mother advising her that after speaking with Hazel "at considerable length," they had decided to move her to an upstairs room and "to start her on light needlework and knitting" in an effort to "occupy her mind with something interesting and instructive." Hazel had been placed in a smaller room off the wards, which she shared with a "quiet girl" named Elaine. This room had a chain on the door that, if necessary, could be secured at night to prevent Hazel from sneaking out.

Hazel, however, was even less content in her new room and wrote notes to the ward nurses asking to be returned to the main ward downstairs. Given her history and propensity to run away, Hazel's request was not entertained. Dissatisfied, Hazel turned her attention to her roommate, Elaine. Sometime in August, Hazel began threatening Elaine, outlining her intention to "murder" her. An undated note, preserved in Hazel's chart, was passed between the girls, each girl's response written onto the single piece of paper:

> HAZEL: I think that I'm going to run away to-night. And also murder. If you get what I mean. You see I told Ramona something. Now I'm sorry I told her. Because she might tell and then I'd get in lots and lots of trouble. Answer the truth.
>
> ELAINE: And may I ask: What might your mum do.
>
> HAZEL: Say do you think I can read my mom's mind.
>
> ELAINE: Well if your going to start that again [threaten murder] I might just as well tell my mom to-day[.] are you going to start that again or not[,] yes or no.
>
> HAZEL: That's not the point. First I'm not starting anything again. I said I might run away. The reason you know and I mentioned something about murder. Answer.

ELAINE: Yes but if you start any thing about murder again I'm going to tell mom to-day.

And, in a subsequent note also passed between the girls:

HAZEL: Tell me what you will tell the nurse. Don't say you don't know because you do. Tell me what you'll tell the nurse. Then we will decide what our play will be about.
ELAINE: Well heres the answer[.] I'm not having a play if you start that again and I just tell the nurse if you start that again.
HAZEL: Yes. But … Would you say: Hazel tried to murder me. Yes or No. The Truth. P.S. What nurse would you tell. Are you going to tell your mother … Ans. Yes or The Truth.
ELAINE: ~~I don't know what I'd say~~. Yes I'd say Hazel tried to. I don't know what nurse I'd tell and I'll tell my mom if you start that again.

According to a note passed to Elaine on 1 September, then confiscated by the staff for Hazel's file and never answered by Elaine, Hazel wrote, "You think that I'm scared to attempt to murder you. At least that's what I think. Are you going to tell the nurse; just because I'm writing you a note. Take a guess at why I want to murder you. Answer. P.S. Have this answered and ready for me when I come from Prayers." Apparently Elaine had not kept Hazel's note a secret because it ended up in the hands of a ward nurse. The next day, Hazel wrote to the nurse, explaining, "I'd … be scared to run away; let alone murder Elaine. I think murder is a horrible thing … I'd be scared to murder anybody. I want to get well and go home. But I can't get better if I try to do anything so horrible." Hazel begged the nurse for "one more chance," feeling "terrible when I think that nobody trusts me." She reassured the nurse, "I have nothing against Elaine – I think she's a swell girl. On my word of honour – I won't run away or even think of murder. Elaine and I get along fine. We have a few quarrels. I guess everybody has quarrels." On the same day that Hazel wrote this letter, she had been moved to a room of her own, staff cautiously separating her from Elaine. McHugh felt obliged to write another letter to Hazel's mother, concerned that Hazel's "mental condition has become much worse." He admitted to feeling "very much disturbed" by her letter "threatening to murder Elaine, the little girl in the room with her." He encouraged Hazel's mother to come to the sanatorium to see Hazel, feeling "we cannot take responsibility for her much longer in her present condition." Responding promptly to the sanatorium's concerns, Hazel was discharged and taken home by her mother five days later.

On the day of her discharge, McHugh wrote a letter to the medical officer of health in Hazel's home town. In it, he outlined the three main reasons why Hazel was being sent home: because she was not infectious, because she was not resting well at the sanatorium and had wanted to go home for several months, and because he felt that her mother could probably handle her and convince her to take the required rest. He also suggested that Hazel be evaluated by a psychiatrist for her behaviour, the details of which he outlined in the letter, and a psychiatrist was sent to Hazel's home within two weeks of her discharge. According to what he determined, Hazel was "very much attached to her mother so that it was quite a mental shock to the girl when she had to leave home for treatment at the Sanatorium." He believed that she was a "highly imaginative type of child," fond of school, reading, and writing letters. He concluded, "A good deal of her behaviour was deliberately staged in order to encourage discharge home" and that this "home-sick girl who was highly imaginative ... chose this way to bring about her return to her family." He did not believe that Hazel ever posed any real threat to Elaine. In the end, Hazel had manipulated her way home, going to such lengths as threatening to murder poor Elaine, which sanatorium staff could not ignore.

Like Hazel, other children in the sanatorium tried various means to achieve their discharges. Some were successful. Often preying on the frustrated sympathies and lingering guilt likely experienced by families when children were hospitalized, children could write home with the words they thought would bring about their discharge. Erin, admitted in 1928 at fourteen years of age, had been orphaned, losing her mother to tuberculosis and her father to accidental causes. Erin kept up a regular correspondence with her elder married sister, and it was this sister who wrote to Dobbie in 1929, concerned about Erin's situation. "I received a letter from my sister Erin," she wrote, suggesting "she has a hearth [heart] trouble" and had to stay in bed. "If she has a hearth trouble," the sister believed, "she need a kind good nurse to look after her." Erin had written unkind words about her nurse in her letter to her sister and, on that account, the sister worried that with the nurse that Erin had, "she never will come home alive but in a coffin." In her letter, she begged Dobbie, "Please give her a good nurse," not a "mad" nurse, otherwise, in her worried state, she felt she would soon be his next patient. In his reply, Dobbie expressed his disappointment that Erin had not been truthful with her sister. Apparently, "she had not been diagnosed as a heart case, she has not been confined to bed ... she is going to school every day, and her general condition is good." Dobbie was also "sorry too that she should be so unfair" to the nurse "to whom a great deal of credit for her progress is due." The nurse had "been very good to her in every way, in spite of the fact that Erin is not always as polite and obedient as she should be." Dobbie was certain that her nurse "would not bother to be 'mad' at her about anything, though, of course, it is necessary for all of the Nurses to see that these children do as they are supposed to do." Dobbie felt that Erin was telling her sister these stories because she wanted to go home and he wrote that, provided home conditions were good, Erin could be discharged from the sanatorium. Less than two months later, Erin had been discharged into her sister's care. Like Hazel, Erin had achieved her goal of discharge.

Parents often supported the sanatorium discipline, even going so far as to elaborate on their children's behavioural challenges. When nine-year-old Maureen's mother was admitted to the Toronto sanatorium in the early 1930s, her daughter was sent to Toronto's IODE preventorium, where she spent ten months. She was then transferred to a boarding house for a further six months. While in the boarding house, she caught a cold that developed into pneumonia and was subsequently admitted into a Toronto hospital where tuberculosis suspicions were raised. Maureen was then transferred to the Toronto sanatorium in July 1933, her mother still a patient at the sanatorium. By August 1934 Maureen began to attract attention as a conduct problem, often found walking around the hospital in the evenings, perhaps because she was feeling better. On one evening in particular, Maureen "persisted in going into the kitchen" at the Queen Mary Hospital, and three times in the space of five minutes, a nurse "sent her out." After the third rejection, Maureen flew into "a violent temper and said she was going home.” Instead, she ran to her mother’s room, crying to her mother and father that the nurse “had slapped her on the face.” Maureen’s father returned his daughter to the Queen Mary and, on inquiry, the nurse dismissed the accusation, reporting that “she only touched her in getting her out of the kitchen” and “never slapped her on any occasion.” Despite Maureen’s insistence that she wanted to return home with her father, he left her at the sanatorium and Maureen “screamed loudly all the way upstairs to her room and continued in a bad temper all evening,” though the staff managed to convince Maureen to return to her bed just after 9 p.m. In this matter, the staff had the full support of Maureen’s parents, her father describing his daughter’s “very stubborn temper” and her mother agreeing that “she was a difficult child to handle.”

Maureen remained agitated for much of August, causing minor troubles for the Queen Mary staff. By the third week of August, Miss Dickson provided Dobbie with a note explaining why Maureen was spending her days sitting on a chair in the hall outside the main office. First, Maureen had been found “riding on the dumb waiter,” apparently entirely oblivious to “the danger she was in.” Second, Maureen had followed the night watchman to the basement one evening and was discovered alone in the Queen Mary kitchen, “vandalizing” it with oatmeal and beans. Finally, Maureen had gotten into a medicine cupboard and taken iodine, a nurse arriving just in time to discover her pouring it on some sugar. Maureen had overheard Dr McHugh telling a patient that iodine was a good treatment for goitre, so she wanted “to see what it was like.” Frustrated, Dickson resolved that Maureen was to “sit outside our Office in a Camp Chair,” going to the Queen Mary for meals and sleeping, until her father’s next visit. Dickson explained, “I told her that when her Father comes I would tell him to take her home or punish her here, as we did not punish children who had parents to do it.” Maureen would ultimately remain at the sanatorium, but a few months later, at her parents’ request, she was discharged and returned with her family to the “Old Country.”[5]

Though staff exercised patience, children could sometimes be discharged for recurring bad behaviour. Such was the case for David, admitted when he was nine years old, in 1919. By 1922, three years older and growing bolder, David had regained both his strength and his health. On 2 February, upon Dobbie's request, one of the nurses compiled an expanding list of David's misdeeds:

> Insolent to the Nurses.
>
> If sent back to wash himself in the morning would refuse to come to Breakfast.
>
> When in the Dining Room would throw Bread at the different tables; whistle and shout.
>
> If sent from the Dining Room would dance and make faces outside the glass doors.
>
> When taking a Bath would fill his mouth with water and squirt the newly painted walls.
>
> Stole Fruit from the other Boys' commodes [their dressers].
>
> Went down the Hill [to the Humber River] without permission.
>
> Disorderly in Church, talking most of the time and refusing to walk in line to and from Church with the other children.

David's improved health and his growing list of misconduct, behaviours suggesting a burgeoning resistance to the sanatorium, led Dobbie to conclude that it was time he be discharged. Accordingly, David left the sanatorium on 9 February, seven days later.

Along with the observations of ward staff, the Queen Mary School teachers sometimes reported problems among the students in the classroom. Randall was ten years old when he was admitted in 1921 and remained at the Queen Mary for just over two and a half years. Teachers who worked at the sanatorium appreciated the fact that some of the children under their charge might have behaviour or learning problems as a result of their illness, but they still expected the discipline of any regular school. One teacher felt obliged to report Randall's misconduct in the classroom to Dobbie, seeking "punishment" for his "refusal to obey." In general, the teacher felt that "his work has been careless, when he has done it," and that, when he was not watched, "a good deal of his time has been spent in idleness." She believed that Randall had not even shown up on several occasions when he was expected to be at school. The teacher reached the end of her patience when Randall "was asked to copy sentences from the Speller on Page 85 Section 5. Instead of this he did Page 90 Section 15." Even then, she discovered several spelling mistakes and expected him to make the corrections. Instead, she noted, "He sat without working at all for sometime, and I asked him whether he was going to correct his work, and he said he was not." The teacher then sent Randall out, and the matter was forwarded to Randall's ward staff. A nurse spoke with Randall about his disobedience in the classroom. He reassured the nurse that he wanted to go back to school, was ready to apologize to the teacher, and would do the work he should have done the previous day, with an added promise to respect the teacher in future. The question of any reprimand was left unanswered, since all seemed satisfied with Randall's genuinely apologetic response to the incident.

From time to time, more notably disruptive children distinguished themselves at the sanatorium, including three brothers who were admitted together in the late 1920s. Marvin, the youngest, spent six years in the sanatorium. When he was about eight, he and his brother, Keith, who was one year older, grew restless and the troubles began. Marvin let the air out of two tires on a visitor's car, while Keith pulled the wires out of the loudspeaker connected to the sanatorium's radio system and moved the assembly hall piano (which was on casters). One evening, Keith attempted an unsavoury deception, a nurse at the Queen Mary noting, "Keith urinated in a tin drinking cup and tried to get Sally, Warren and some of the other children to drink it. He told them it was orangeade."[25] When Keith complained of an earache, a nurse provided him with a hot water bottle, which he then punctured with a needle. The eldest of the three, Nathan had a milder temperament than his brothers. The only complaint in his chart concerned his resistance to heliotherapy; on three consecutive mornings he had just "folded his arms and absolutely refused to take his clothes off." This problem appears to have been resolved by sitting down with him and explaining the importance of sun treatment.

All of the brothers were discharged to the care of the Children's Aid Society, their mother having died at the Muskoka sanatorium of advanced pulmonary tuberculosis and, though their father was alive and well, they were not returned to him. Between the time of youngest brother Marvin's discharge in February 1934 and his readmission to the sanatorium in

September 1935, he had been shuffled between three different boarding houses on account of behaviour problems. Marvin's readmission was felt to be warranted by the results of a chest clinic examination in August 1935, which suggested some extension in his old primary disease. His readmission note summarized his growing list of conduct issues while in foster care: "He is very untruthful, is given to stealing, constantly in mischief such as setting fire to buildings, in trouble at school, and indecent in his personal habits. It has been necessary to keep him separated from small girls living in the same house." Marvin, however, was subsequently discharged only a month after his readmission to the sanatorium. Medical staff determined that he was not experiencing any active disease, the primary disease affecting his hilar lymph nodes remained latent, his admission likely motivated by behavioural troubles and not tuberculosis. Marvin's discharge was guided by the administration's explicit belief that the sanatorium should never serve as a refuge for the "hard-to-place," but always maintain a strict medical function in the treatment of tuberculosis.

Like Marvin, other children attracted attention over persistent behavioural issues. Garrett was admitted to the sanatorium when he was fourteen and spent over ten years in the sanatorium. Suffering from advanced and cavitary pulmonary TB, he was placed on an adult ward and would eventually undergo thoracoplasty surgery in an attempt to better control his disease. Like many of the children who entered the sanatorium, Garrett had suffered great trauma at the hands of tuberculosis, losing both of his parents to the disease prior to his own hospitalization, and this likely factored into his defiant behaviour at the sanatorium. Garrett's conduct sheet was among the most lengthy of all the child patients sampled, with many documented incidents spanning the years between 1931 and 1939. Eight of Garrett's incidents involved staying up or out late, after 10:30 p.m., particularly after his transfer to the pavilions in 1932. Sometimes the late nights were uneventful, perhaps sitting on chair outside the pavilions or out for a walk. On other nights there were dramas, such as the evening a curious Garrett put a light bulb on a hot radiator long enough for the light bulb to explode. That evening, Dr McHugh, in charge of Garrett's ward, had had enough, resolving "the trouble in the ... ward ... at night has reached a point where it must be stopped." Making a "thorough investigation," McHugh identified Garrett as "the worst" of the four boys causing troubles. "He shouts, whistles, argues and quarrels almost constantly," McHugh noted. Further resisting sanatorium rules, Garrett had been "known to throw his legs up in the air and jump out of bed as in the most rigorous gymnastic exercise" and, if staff spoke to him about this, "he will sulk or slam doors." Two of Garrett's incidents concerned fights with other patients. Regarding the first fight, in 1931, Garrett explained that he had entered a men's ward on a Sunday when a patient approached him and "got hold" of his housecoat and tore it. "I caught a hold of his hand and pulled it away," Garrett reported. "When I done this he threw me on the bed and kicked me on the chest." The two then "struggled" and "rolled on the floor," Garrett's buttons torn from his housecoat. "He then told me that if I went in their again he would do worse," Garrett concluded, "but he lets other patients in not saying a word to them because they are bigger and stronger." Staff investigated the incident, suspecting that Garrett had provoked the altercation, but also acknowledging that the adult patient was known to many as a "rough customer." The second fight took place between Garrett and his two roommates in the pavilions in 1933. McHugh's investigation the morning after the incident revealed that they had made a game of "putting porridge in the beds of the others," but, upon finding the porridge in his own bed, one "flew into a rage and threw the porridge and clothes all over the place." When the cleaner arrived in the morning and protested the state of their room, the still irritated patient "attacked" him. When McHugh then approached him, the patient "again flew into a rage using filthy expression," threatening to strike the doctor. This patient was ultimately discharged. Two of Garrett's reprimands, in 1938 and 1939, concerned visiting the women's wards, though he had been "spoken to before about this." He had excuses: he had gone to "see a book" or to show a visitor to the ward, but staff suspected other motivations. Garrett's final reprimand stemmed from the post-operative ward, where he was recuperating after having ribs removed in his thoracoplasty surgery and where he was also found smoking. "He states he has only smoked one a day, but knows that he should not have done so," his conduct sheet noted. "The materials he had for making cigarettes" were taken away and he was "advised that no more be brought in."

Garrett was discharged in the early 1940s, by then a young man. For the most part, as the staff themselves had commented, Garrett's misbehaviour had only ever amounted to "minor infractions of the rules."

Frustration mounted, however, because his misbehaviour was believed to be defeating the good intentions behind his treatment; in 1931, it was noted that all the benefit achieved through a few hours of rest during the day was undone by his "fiendish actions at night" and, in 1933, that he was just "wasting time" at the sanatorium, not pursuing his fight against tuberculosis in earnest and with discipline. Staff were as frustrated by Garrett's behaviour and resistance to the rules as they were in their belief that he was only undermining his best opportunity to get better. In part, Garrett's conduct sheet was lengthy because he had spent more than a decade in the sanatorium, not because he was bad natured, but with all of the warnings and cautions, its lengthiness is also testament to the staff's enduring patience with his continuing misconduct.

Like Garrett, Dwight's behaviour was also perennially troublesome. And, like Garrett, he was also given many chances, though the nature of his troubles suggested that he was feeling well and likely ready for discharge (he had been admitted with minimal and seemingly relatively inactive disease). Overall, thirteen-year-old Dwight would spend just over two years in the sanatorium before he was discharged in 1938. Shortly after his admission, Dwight had gotten into the habit of leaving his bed at night, being noisy, and creating mischief with two fellow patients, Gary and Elliott. After cautioning the boys on a number of occasions, it was felt that Dwight would be best transferred to the pavilions, splitting up the trio. Medically, this seemed acceptable, given that Dwight only occasionally ran a 99° temperature. It was in the less-monitored pavilions, however, that most of Dwight's conduct incidents (staying out late after bedtime, cutting down trees behind the occupational therapy buildings) played out. Most grievous, perhaps, was the incident in August 1936, when Dwight was found "in the wash room floating a toy boat in one of the basins. He had gasoline in it and had set fire to it." Another patient had brought a small bottle of gasoline into the pavilions to remove stains from his clothing, but Dwight had found it and filled his toy boat. The patients were warned "of the extreme danger of gasoline, or fluids in which gasoline is an important constituent being taken to the [wood frame] pavilions."[26] When Dwight was reported to have been seen out walking on Weston Road in May 1938, staff finally resolved that he would likely be best transferred back to the Main Medical Building, since they did not believe he had the maturity to handle the freedoms of the pavilions. Despite the transfer, almost a month after this last incident Dwight was discharged from the sanatorium because he just could not settle and his health was much improved.

Not all behaviour noted in the conduct sheets related to misconduct, as some of the children were actually praised for their good behaviour in their conduct sheets. Theresa was admitted to the sanatorium in 1928 suffering from primary tuberculosis of her hilar lymph nodes. She remained in bed for her first full year at the sanatorium, her temperature periodically spiking to 102°F. While her continued fevers meant that Theresa was never permitted much activity, her condition did improve over time. She took an active interest in the domestic science class taught at the Queen Mary School and occupied much of her time in bed reading and sewing. By the time she was eighteen, she had completed the school program and was assisting the hospital seamstress for a few paid hours of work each morning. Theresa's skill with needle and thread won her numerous prizes in the annual sewing competitions at the Canadian National Exhibition in Toronto. The sanatorium staff held Theresa in very high regard, writing, "She is almost as much credit to the hospital physically, as she is to the church school morally." Theresa spent eight years in the sanatorium before she was discharged into the care of her mother.

Cot notes provide other insights into the endearing aspects of the children's behaviour, as observed by staff. Fiona, seven years of age, and Vivian, six years of age, were sisters admitted together in 1935, and placed in beds on the same ward to keep each other company. Ward nurses noted that Fiona "loves having something pretty to wear – and to 'dress up,'" playing "in a little world of her own imagery." Fiona liked to sing with her sister, the nurses amused that "on a piece of paper they have laboriously presented their repertoire, from which we must make a selection." Vivian was described as a "very neat and orderly" girl who, despite her own young age, loved to "'mother' the smaller children." The sisters were discharged home together in 1936.

Grumbles, Complaints, and Report Cards

As much as patients were expected to cede to the sanatorium rhythm and routine, they were also invited to comment on their satisfaction (or dissatisfaction) with the institution. The invitation was open and standardized as, each morning, patients who were old enough were provided with a Patient's Daily Report Card on their breakfast trays. Patients could use the report card to comment on any and all aspects of the sanatorium, including the quality of the day's meals, the services of the sanatorium staff, and any other matter. These report cards were reviewed by staff, but it was typically Dobbie who responded directly to each patient (with the original report card, a copy of his response, and any other supporting material filed in the brown envelope of the patient's chart). These report cards provided the opportunity for all patients, irrespective of whether they were free or paying patients, young or old, to comment on the sanatorium and the care they received. The care taken in providing feedback, in addressing and responding to concerns, and sometimes, as a result, in modifying circumstances or protocols clearly suggests that the concerns of patients, even younger patients, received timely and respectful consideration. There were good reasons for the medical institution to solicit patient feedback and to be accountable through change. First, because philanthropy was an important source of ongoing funding for the sanatorium, administrators were accountable for evidence that good-quality care was being provided at the institution with high levels of patient satisfaction. Second, since patients could leave of their own free will from this voluntary institution, it was important to ensure their voices were heard in the regular operations of the institution so that any chronic deficiencies or complaints could be resolved to everybody's satisfaction and prevent future patients from simply deciding to leave.

Some of the returned report cards suggest that the food at the sanatorium was a source of disappointment. Complaints about institutional food were, however, far from unique to the Toronto sanatorium. In British sanatoria, for example, Linda Bryder has noted that patients raised complaints, but that "tuberculous patients were reputed to be particularly finicky about their food and therefore complaints in that direction were not taken seriously."[27] Since tuberculosis itself interfered with appetites, food complaints could be explained away for medical reasons and not given serious attention. In 1910, the editor of the *Canadian Journal of Medicine and Surgery* suggested that because tuberculous disease hampered the ability to effectively oxygenate the body's blood supply, patients "will not take enough oxygen into the blood to carry on in a proper manner the ordinary purposes of life, much less to dispose of a large and very nutritious diet. They have no craving for food; the appetite is poor, and forced feeding is not relished."[28] In effect, he was arguing, tuberculosis patients did not have adequate oxygen in their bodies to carry on with normal functioning, let alone maintain a healthy appetite. So, of course, the rationale went, they would struggle with food and eating.

It is likely that, in some cases, dissatisfaction with food or mealtimes was symptomatic of deeper sources of discontentment. What and how we eat is, after all, one of our most profound connections to home, family, culture, and religion. The foreignness of different foods prepared in unfamiliar ways might have just reinforced yearnings for home and comfort. According to Connolly and Gibson, when twelve-year-old Rachel Heatwole wrote home to her parents from Virginia's Blue Ridge sanatorium, she noted, "The cooks made good chicken but they didn't clean the feathers off very well."[29] As one woman hospitalized at four years of age in the 1940s in Australia recalled, "I can remember how desperate I was to have my mother's food."[30] Like everyone else, children took note of the foods they were obliged to eat, even remembering the food in particular many decades after they were discharged.

If food concerns were raised by child patients in their report cards, Dobbie or Dickson coordinated investigations. From time to time, for example, Dolores used her Daily Report Card to comment on the quality of the food she received. On 3 August 1918, she indicated that breakfast, dinner, her room, the nursing, and overall general aspects were all "OK." She did comment, however, that "not enough" food was served at tea. Dobbie duly reviewed the menu for this meal – cabbage salad, bread, butter, canned pears, tea, and milk – and noted that food was served "in abundance." In light of his findings, Dolores's complaint was considered "unjustifiable and unreasonable." Dolores was a long-term patient, and her next objection about the food was filed years later in July 1930. Once again, she noted that the tea meal was problematic and, specifically, that the potatoes had been served burnt and slathered in butter. Dobbie referred this complaint to the lady superintendent and, after conferring with the sanatorium's dietician, he wrote to Dolores to explain the adjustments that he had made, ensuring Ward F was to be served instead with scalloped potatoes. Dobbie himself had "tasted the jellied Veal," but would check on it again as it was served with supper. The chef had been further instructed to "provide more variety in the way of supper dishes." Dobbie hoped that these adjustments would "prove more satisfactory." A successful resolution for Dolores, perhaps, but sometimes it was not so easy to effect change. In August 1919, for example, Shirley lodged a complaint that she had been served meals on dirty dishes. Dobbie responded, "Sorry this is the case," but drew her attention to the fact that "because of war conditions we have been unable to procure competent help for this work." The sanatorium experienced acute staffing shortages during both of the world wars, as staff left the sanatorium to pursue more lucrative industry-related employment. Dobbie wrote Shirley, "While every effort is being made, I cannot promise that this condition will not prevail from time to time." He suggested further, "Perhaps you could lend a hand yourself and persuade some others to assist you." It was felt that patients, if well enough, could contribute to the proper functioning of the sanatorium in such times of crisis.

While adult patients may have been better equipped to voice their concerns, children also bettered their sanatorium experience. Grady, a fifteen-year-old Indigenous schoolboy admitted in 1929, suffered advanced pulmonary tuberculosis. He had made specific food requests, and according to staff, this was not uncommon for gravely ill children, many struggling to regain their lost appetites. In support, staff typically obliged these requests, preparing special meals in the Queen Mary's diet kitchen, a small kitchen located just off the wards (figure 7.3). Not all children understood this allowance, however, seeing only that some of their ward-mates were receiving special privileges. It was precisely this misunderstanding that had created friction in Grady's ward, Ward C, at the Queen Mary. In a note to Dobbie, the sanatorium dietician explained that on Ward C, "the majority" of child patients actually "resented" the fact that "one or two of the sick ones [were] getting extras." As a result, when a new head nurse was appointed to this ward earlier in 1930, she had decided to dis-

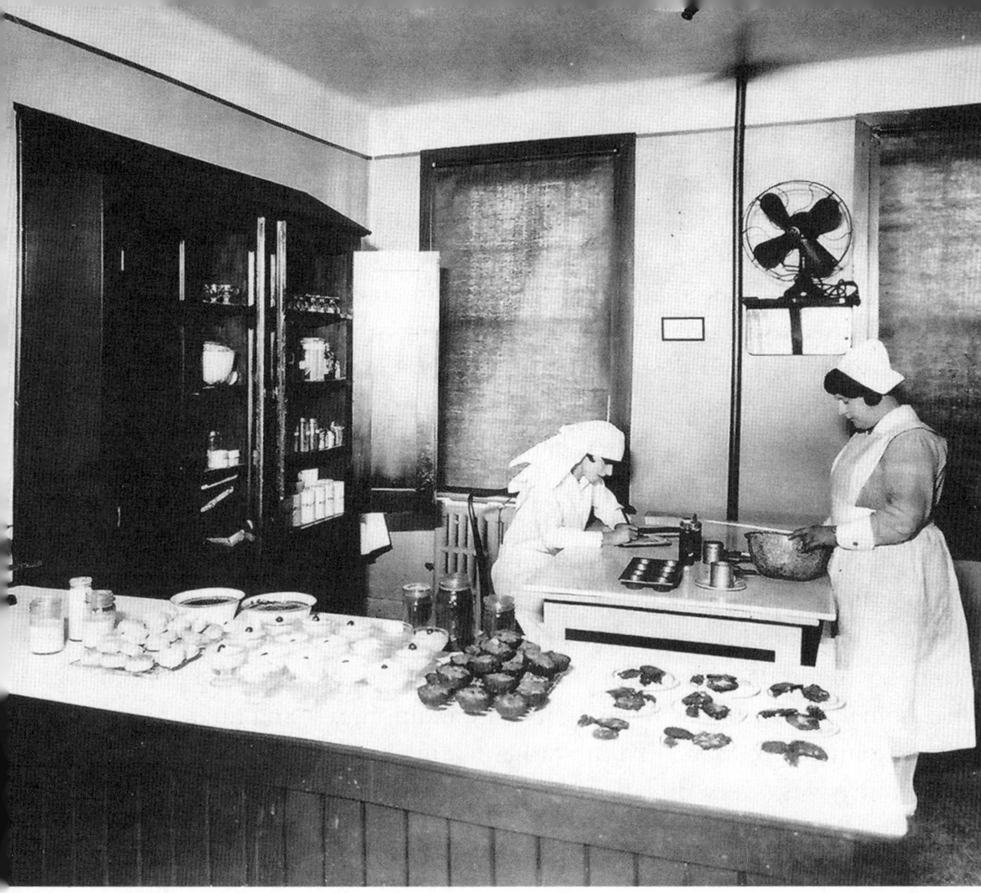

Figure 7.3 A ward diet kitchen, circa 1930, where tea meals and special meals were prepared. Note the slanted top on the cupboard, designed to minimize dust collection.

continue the privilege of special diets, a decision that was subsequently reversed by Dobbie. Accordingly, Grady and other acutely ill children on his ward were to be provided with the foods that they desired most, in order to encourage their appetites. In November 1930, Grady requested lamb chops and roasted chicken for lunch (chicken was typically restricted to Sunday lunch only), and fried eggs and fried meats for supper. The diet kitchen was instructed that Grady should be provided with baked potatoes every night with his supper, as per his request. The children on the ward would just have to be made to understand that this was not special privileges, but an important aspect of treatment in the sanatorium.

While children were able to effect change, families could also be vocal on their children's well-being at the sanatorium, either in person during visits or by correspondence if family members could not be present. In some cases, the complaints seemed more likely to be borne out of frustration and powerlessness in the face of tuberculosis and hospitalization than actual failings of the sanatorium. When Faith entered the sanatorium in 1937 at fifteen years of age, she was suffering advanced pulmonary tuberculosis, with active disease in her entire left lung and the upper half of her right lung, and signs of small cavities developing throughout. Her prognosis, even from the outset, had not been good. Though an artificial pneumothorax had been considered for Faith, because she feared the procedure and was a poor candidate for it anyway (because both her lungs were diseased), it was not attempted. Faith's father wrote to Dobbie in January 1938, nearly eight months after his daughter was admitted, outlining his intention to discharge her, understanding "that the chances of recovery of our daughter Faith are very slight, so we have decided to bring her home." Acknowledging that "in her condition, rest and nourishment are absolutely necessary," Faith's father felt justified in the decision, since the family was "very dissatisfied with the catering at the Queen Mary Hospital." The first line of Faith's father's letter is most telling of why he wanted to discharge his daughter, though he seemed to add value to the decision with the distractions of catering complaints. In his response to Faith's father, Dobbie expressed his disappointment at not being able to do more to better her prognosis, but noted that the severity of her disease had made this impossible. Few formalities would come associated with Faith's discharge, since the family was quite wealthy.

Although Faith would soon be leaving, Dobbie promptly referred the catering complaint to Miss Wilkinson, who, within three days of the letter from Faith's father, looked into the matter and wrote up a memorandum. Wilkinson noted that, prior to the letter from Faith's father, neither her parents nor Faith herself had ever complained about the food service, though there had been minor criticism about bologna. On the contrary, staff had tried hard to keep Faith satisfied, as Wilkinson explained to Dobbie:

> If Faith stated that she does not fancy any particular article served, she has been asked the reason and if there was something she would wish substituted. Her appetite has been noticeably failing, and [a nurse] states that she has stayed with her when she had

> tried to eat. She has never been refused anything that she particularly asked for. [Faith's mother] has brought fruit, chicken, special meat and special soup in for her which has been cooked or served as the mother requested. It is understood that Dr McHugh was approached regarding the food sometime ago. This was not reported to me at the time. Criticism at that time was concerning some bologna which was served with cold meat for supper. I feel that the nurses have tried in every way to make this patient comfortable in hospital. Special privileges have been allowed in that the patient's own silver and dishes were brought from home, which necessitated extra care and supervision.

Only once had Faith's personal silverware found itself on the wrong patient's tray. The real problem, according to Wilkinson, was Faith's failing appetite in the face of advancing tuberculosis disease, and not the quality of food. In the end, this upset likely had less to do with bologna or the mismanagement of Faith's silverware and much more to do with her parents' anxieties that they would ultimately lose her to tuberculosis. Finding a reason to justify the discharge of their daughter in their own minds, Faith was taken home by her parents a few days later.

The complaints of Toronto sanatorium child patients (or their families) about food paled in comparison to the grievances of former child patients of Craig-y-nos sanatorium. Winnie Gardiner (Gammon) unequivocally described the food as "horrible," remembering that the sanatorium always "smelled like lamb stew."[31] Despite the fact that children may have disliked particular foods, they were told to eat them anyway. Douglas Herbert "couldn't stand" cabbage, but he remembered being "force-fed cold cabbage," so very unappetizing to him that it made him vomit.[32] Other former child patients recalled finding undesirables in their meals, often slugs that had been unintentionally served with vegetables.[33] When Ann Shaw discovered a "plump brown" slug in her salad, her nurse had suggested, "If you didn't go looking for these things then you wouldn't find them."[34] Betty Thomas (Dowdle), admitted in 1941 when the sanatorium was experiencing wartime food shortages and rationing, remembered being advised that she should eat her porridge and "put the maggots" that she found within it "alongside."[35]

Local parents tried to take an active role in their children's care at the Toronto sanatorium, and, like Faith's mother, brought in extra home-cooked or store-bought food. For parents and children alike, food was a tangible expression of love and nurturance. At times, however, staff felt this was unwarranted, and possibly even an interference with the treatment regimen. Diet and nutrition were the cornerstone of sanatorium treatment, and dieticians were hired to ensure that patients were not only eating, but eating well-balanced meals high in protein. Fourteen-year-old Gregory was a model child patient, who, staff noted, had endured a year of bedrest admirably. Overall, he seldom complained and was characterized as "a very co-operative patient," content to fully absorb himself in building model airplanes. The problems the staff had with Gregory had more to do with his family's behaviour. As one nurse noted to Dobbie in 1934, "He is visited by some of his people every day, and they bring him rich pastry from the store, meats, and preserved fruits, etc, knowing it is against the rules of the hospital." The problem was, according to the nurse, "They continually force him to eat it, and send back the hospital food." Six-year-old Sylvia's mother also liked to bring her daughter food. Described in a cot note as a little girl with "a pale little face and deep set eyes," Sylvia enjoyed her paper dolls and assured her nurses that "she will sing and dance for them" once she was no longer a full-time bed patient. Sylvia's disease status always remained in question, and even at the time of her discharge she remained only a suspect for primary disease of her hilar lymph nodes. The staff felt that the girl had "progressed favourably but was retarded by frequent visits from her mother who not only disturbed her by her frequent visiting but each time [also] brought her unsuitable food to eat."

Some children struggled to find contentment, apart from their families and thrust into a strange new social environment of hospital life; not only did the children have to adapt to diet, they also had to negotiate interpersonal relationships with other patients. Iris was ten years old when she entered the sanatorium in 1935. Iris's father was alive and well, but her mother had been readmitted to the Toronto sanatorium not long after her daughter's admission. It was reported that Iris had been feeling well until about two weeks prior to her admission, when she caught a cold from a boarder who had stayed in the family home for about a week.

Iris's family history showed that in addition to her mother's active disease, the most likely source of Iris's infection, her maternal grandfather, had died of TB.

Having been readmitted to the Toronto sanatorium, Iris's mother was well aware of the nature of life in the institution and was not likely surprised when, within weeks of her admission, she received a note from Iris, unhappy because she had to stay in bed in a room by herself and because she did not like some of the children she was meeting at the sanatorium. Iris wanted to go home. In her gently worded reply, Iris's mother tried to reassure her daughter that things would get better, that she would soon be moved to a downstairs ward with other girls, and that once she started going to school things would be different:

> Dear Iris –
> Mamma got your letter and I am sorry dear you don't like it over there. You told me on Sunday you liked it over there. You be a good girl the rest of this week and see if you don't like it down stairs away from all those bad kids. You worry Mamma terrible for I don't know where I could take you … Just be a good girl the rest of the week. You will be going to school and won't have to stay in bed like you are now. I will write to Dr Dobbie and tell him how the kids carry on and fight with you. He will stop them. Let daddy know after you get down stairs and go to school if you don't like it any better and if not I will try to get you out and get some one to look after you. I think — might take you. Cheer up and don't cry for you make mamma cry too. Write Mamma again. Love Mamma.

Iris's mother then explained to Dobbie what she believed to be at the heart of her daughter's discontentment:

> I do not like to make any complaints to you in regard to this institution for it is my second time here and I always got treated fine. Through the kindness of you my daughter Iris has been admitted here in the Queen Mary and she is very discontented as we expected she would be for awhile. She is associating with rough young boys, they are always quarrelling with the little girls, going in their rooms

> and taking their things and always exposing themselves indecently. I do not feel my child is better than other children but she has never been in the habit of playing with boys. I wonder if she could be moved with other girls, she is lonely and crying all the time being in a room by herself. If she keeps on fretting I will have to do something for I feel under that strain I can't take the cure as I should. Would it be possible for me to go to the Queen Mary?

The "rough young boys" were a source of Iris's unhappiness at the sanatorium. As Iris's mother explained, her daughter was not used to playing with boys. One, coincidentally, was Marvin, whose problem behaviour at the sanatorium and in foster care was detailed earlier in this chapter. Iris and Marvin were at the Queen Mary at the same time in 1935, though Marvin had been readmitted only for a month before his final discharge in October of that year. Meanwhile, on the back of the letter, Iris replied to her mother (see figure 7.4):

> Mama
>
> I am down stairs now and I do not like it here ~~I was going to run away to night~~ Mama I do not like it down stairs please take me home please please please and I get up for one meal please let me go home ~~to morrow~~ go home tomorrow today.

Following her mother's suggestion, Iris gave her new bed in the downstairs ward a chance, to see if she might come to like it as her mother suggested. As evident in Iris's reply, however, she was no happier with the sanatorium and firm in her desire to go home (either tomorrow or today, she seemed undecided), even suggesting she might run away (though she had crossed out that thought in her letter). A nurse discussed the note with Iris's mother, explaining that she was not actually up for one meal. If that were the case, and Iris was considered physically well enough to be an up patient, perhaps she would have had a stronger case for returning home. As it was, Iris remained at the sanatorium until the end of June 1936. Iris's experience highlights the importance of interpersonal dynamics at the sanatorium, where one child's disobedience could

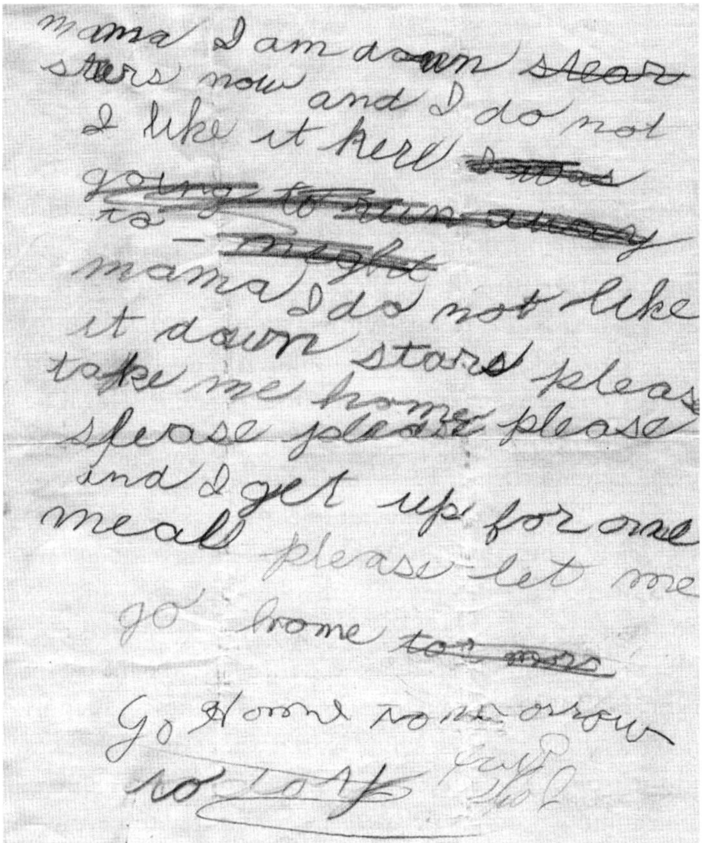
mama I am down stairs now and I do not like it here
mama I do not like it down stars take me home pleas please please please and I get up for one meall please let me go home
Go Home tomorrow
no today

Figure 7.4 Ten-year-old Iris's original (1935) letter to her mother (who was also a patient at the Toronto sanatorium) indicating that she did not like her move to a "downstairs" ward and wanted to go home "tomorrow" (if not "today"). In the end, she remained at the Queen Mary Hospital for another nine months.

easily lead to another child's discontentment. At times, interpersonal relations between child patients could lead to significant dissatisfaction. To some extent, it was expected that children would have to work out positive social relationships on their wards, or at least to do their best not to irritate each other.

Conclusion

Non-medical aspects of the sanatorium's patient charts help to provide fresh insights into the sanatorium and its operations, shattering misconceptions of the patient experience inside the sanatorium. There were rules and regimen, but, particularly for child patients, there was also forgiveness. Children developed their own routines and rhythms of life at the sanatorium, incorporating all the pleasures and celebrations of childhood – birthday parties, Santa Claus, school, the playground, and whatever else they could think to get up to. The children's stories also help to better appreciate the connections of the sanatorium with the local neighbourhood in Weston. At this sanatorium, tuberculosis patients were not locked away, isolated, and restricted. To do so would be to ignore the large number of infectious yet undiagnosed tuberculous persons out and about in the disease's endemic years. Instead, the children's stories emphasize the many connections of the sanatorium: with the local fish and chips restaurant, the convenience store across the river that sold forbidden bubble gum, the tempting but seemingly scandalous dance hall, the movie theatre and its midnight shows. On an even finer level, these notes and reports also reveal something about children's lives on the wards, including their friendships and their disputes. These insights can be pieced together, but only because the administration so vigorously committed to keeping anything and everything pertaining to patients, even bits and scraps of paper, notes passed between the children, at least those confiscated by staff and tucked away in their charts. These non-medical stories breathe a sense of life into the sanatorium, help to define it as a lively place where against a sobering milieu of illness, suffering, and death, there were also friendships, fights, and adventures. The (mis)adventures are revealing, because they reframe the children as agency-possessing, decision-making, life-embracing, animated persons, even as they lived apart from their homes, in a hospital, and under the "shadow of tuberculosis." While they may have been learning how to live with tuberculosis, they were also discovering and negotiating their way through the world around them and, for many of the children, that world had been hard on them.

Rules and regimen formed the cornerstone of sanatorium treatment, though both adult and child patients sometimes resisted the construct out of boredom, homesickness, and frustration. In some cases, the perceived usefulness of sanatorium treatments were questioned, particularly in advanced and declining cases where futility and hopelessness permeated any of the good that the sanatorium had to offer tuberculosis sufferers. All patients, including child patients, had a voice, either loosely heard or formalized through the patient's report card. As a result, patients could effect change in the sanatorium and their experience. Patients and their families could resist or uphold sanatorium regimens, but may have been less accepting of features like the idleness of long-term bedrest, particularly in child patients who were improved or failing in health. Ultimately, as an open institution, patients or their families could secure discharges, and this was often the recourse among those most discontented with hospitalization. Sanatorium staff had to negotiate a challenging position – they had to be firm in the rules of treatment and sanatorium life, but also sensitive to patient satisfaction. As a voluntary institution supported largely by philanthropy, it was critical that the sanatorium functioned as successfully as possible. As a result, staff had to try to maintain patient satisfaction, even as the limitations of treatment regimens such as bedrest tended to inspire discontentment.

CHAPTER 8

Tuberculosis Support and Philanthropy

We shall not need to say to any victim of Tuberculosis, struggling in the icy waters of sickness and poverty, "We cannot help you."[1]
~ The Samaritan Club

Like physicians and nurses at the sanatorium, families and communities also acted collectively to help children build resistance against tuberculosis, assisting them both materially and emotionally. Generally speaking, the ongoing or acute crisis of infectious disease, endemic or epidemic in its manifestation, may bring out the best or the worst in humanity. While much has been explored on the negativities engendered by anxiety, fear, stigma, and scapegoating in disease, it is also important to emphasize the acts of kindness and caring within and between families, and among neighbours and community members. Families may have been at the core of support for tuberculous children, but families were often weakened or traumatized by the illness and losses of tuberculosis. The children's stories provide some insights into how people worked together, offering support and assistance, in the years of endemic tuberculosis. Both George Jasper Wherrett and Katherine McCuaig have detailed aspects of organized philanthropy relating to tuberculosis, including the massively successful Christmas Seals campaign that was introduced in 1927.[2] This chapter considers more localized forms of philanthropy that connected directly with the children of the Toronto sanatorium.

In the first half of the twentieth century, Canadian families had to cope with not only the emotional toll of children's hospitalization, but also the entangled reality of financial costs. As noted in the Queen Mary Hospital's first annual report for 1913–14, most of the child patients admitted were, according to the Consumptives Act, considered "indigent" and in need of financial and material support. Ninety-five of the children came from families who could pay little or nothing towards the maintenance of their children, leaving only four child patients classified as "paying" patients.[3] Nonetheless, families did what they could to support their hospitalized children, even if municipalities[4] were responsible for actual hospitalization costs. This chapter will consider some of the complications associated with this model of funding, including disputes over responsibility and the erosion of family privacy. Other than municipal councils, there were other sources of "practical" (financial and material) support, including Children's Aid and Mothers' Allowance, that affected the lives of hospitalized children and their families. This chapter explores the particulars of formal and informal networks of support provided by families, municipalities, institutions, and philanthropic groups in attempts to improve and enrich the lives of children affected by tuberculosis and hospitalization. In the sanatorium era, the social context of tuberculosis received particular attention, while the medical aspect of the disease claimed greater scrutiny in the wake of the Second World War with the rise of streptomycin and multi-drug treatments.[5] It was at this turning point, according to sociologist Paul Draus, that "the ability to consistently cure TB in individuals made ingestion of drugs the single most important measure in controlling TB, more important than housing, nutrition, or income."[6] Recent resurgences of tuberculosis, the longstanding persistence of tuberculosis in vulnerable communities, and a rising tide of antibiotic-resistant tuberculosis bacteria have brought social concerns back to the forefront, once again embedding tuberculosis in its social context and targeting the insidious effects of social inequalities and poverty in shaping disease vulnerabilities.[7]

Family and Friends: Informal Networks of Support

Parents typically expressed loneliness, sadness, and regret upon the hospitalization of their children, fearing for their happiness, their potentially long struggles with tuberculosis, and their possible death away from home. Many families tried to provide extra comforts for their children in the sanatorium, even as they struggled to provide for their other children who remained at home. If they could not care for their hospitalized children in their illness, then every pair of shoes, shirt, or toy sent to them in the sanatorium took on special significance, tangible expressions of their love and caring, however distant. In 1919, for example, one mother was determined to keep her ten-year-old daughter Charlotte suitably clothed during her time at the sanatorium, feeling that this was her maternal responsibility. In her letter to Miss Dickson, the sanatorium's lady superintendent, she indicated that she tried to get to the sanatorium every two or three weeks to visit her daughter, always bringing her "clean changes of underwear, and any possible comforts and necessities" that she could afford. Charlotte's mother made a point of noting that she had spent over six dollars on the underwear, which was double the amount she had spent on her two other children at home, in addition to the "goods for that dress she is wearing, and warm cotton eiderdown for a kimono [a housecoat], some shoes $3.50, stockings, hair ribbons, soap, etc." She worried, however, as the season was easing towards winter, that her daughter was "not sufficiently protected against inclement weather" and wanted to know if the sanatorium or the city provided anything "in the way of rubbers, mitts, etc. for the severe weather." She wanted to ensure that her daughter received at least rubber boots and "overstockings." She had already borrowed money from "a sympathetic person" to purchase Charlotte the warm mitts she needed, and had "begged a pair of old boots for her to wear." But she wanted to know if Miss Dickson could provide her with the "address of any kind Christian" to whom she could write for warm stockings, and either rubbers or, even better, overshoes. As she wrote, she "would lose no time in appealing" to that person.

In her reply, Dickson assured Charlotte's mother that her daughter would be provided with anything needed to keep her adequately clothed and comfortable, taking the time to detail the sanatorium protocols in this respect. Children who were provided with clothes by their families and caregivers could wear those clothes. If those clothes were not sufficient, then the sanatorium would provide extra clothing, as needed. If nothing else, Dickson noted, families and caregivers often provided boots and shoes. The sanatorium avoided "woolen underwear" because of its "prohibitive price," the insufficient quantities available, and, most importantly, because woollens could not be "boiled in washing." For children whose families or caregivers could not provide any clothing support, the sanatorium's seasonal "outfit" was provided to them. For the winter of 1919, Dickson noted, "the complete winter outfit consists of long sleeved vest, ankle length underwear, corset waist, underskirt, blue serge skirt, light blue middy, tan stockings for girls and black for boys, overcoat, mitts, and woolen caps." The specifics of the colour and style of clothing provided to children varied by season and by time. Over one summer, for example, light cotton polka-dotted dresses for the girls had been favoured. Though undoubtedly practical, the colour-coded, standardized clothing provided to indigent children who needed support was perhaps reminiscent of the identifiable and potentially stigmatizing uniforms provided to poor orphaned children in charity schools.[8] The children at Craig-y-nos sanatorium in Wales also had standardized clothing and appearances. One ex-patient recalled "brown tunic tops and shorts," with the girls' hair "cut almost above our ears in a basin crop."[9] As Craig-y-nos's assistant medical officer explained to one mother whose daughter's long curls had been cut away, hair had to be kept short, otherwise "all the strength's going in the hair and not in the body."[10] It is likely that longer hair would require more maintenance and that children would be tempted to fuss with it, and in this way expend precious energies on their hair. As a case in point, girls at the Welsh sanatorium were not permitted to use curlers, since this would have required them to lift their hands up to their heads, making too great a demand upon their resting bodies. Short hair was likely sensible since ex-Craig-y-nos patients remembered that their hair often went unwashed for long periods.[11] At the Toronto sanatorium, children's hair was washed once a week.

Even modest expressions of caring were captured in the charts. In 1938, Bert's father sent Miss Wilkinson, lady superintendent, a dollar to spend on whatever his twelve-year-old son needed most. For her part, Wilkinson purchased Bert "three pairs of good woollen socks." The socks would keep Bert warm through the winter, she assured his father, and, in respect for the dollar spent, they were "marked with his own name" and would be "kept mended for him." While Bert also needed trousers, Wilkinson thought it best to ask Santa to provide them, Santa's gifts provided by the women of the Weston Sanitarium Club. Wanting to be helpful to Bert's father, Wilkinson suggested, "If you wish to send him a little parcel at Christmas, I would suggest that you buy him a shirt which need not cost more than .75¢ or $1.00, or if you would like me to buy it for you, I would be glad to do so, and would see that it is nicely parcelled with your name on it."

It was not rare to find cases where members of the extended family also stepped in to provide care, especially for orphaned children, either during their hospitalization or when they were discharged. Often, though not always, the children's aunts played a prominent role. When thirteen-year-old Alvin entered the sanatorium in December 1923, he had recently lost both of his parents, his father known to have died from tuberculosis. He was placed in a sponsored cot; according to the note written to his sponsors, "on admission," Alvin "looked very tired and hungry." First arriving at the sanatorium close to 7 p.m., Alvin had been provided with pyjamas and settled into his new bed for the night. The nurse assisting him asked him if he would like to eat anything before going to sleep, but the woman who had brought Alvin in interjected, stating, on his behalf, that this was unlikely because his appetite was so poor. Upon considering the nurse's suggestion, however, Alvin had looked up at her and said, "I could eat sumthin if it was sort a tasty." Cooking up some bacon and a fresh egg in the nearby diet kitchen, the nurse brought Alvin's light supper in on a tray and, she noted, "In a few minutes he had eaten up all his supper and by way of appreciation he said, 'thanks that's the best dinner I ever tasted, and gee, its fine to have such a good bed to sleep in.'" Alvin improved at the sanatorium, gaining over sixteen pounds, and regularly attending classes at the sanatorium school. Responsibility for the care of Alvin and his younger siblings had fallen willingly to his aunts. When Alvin and a sister who had also been at the sanatorium were discharged, an aunt living on a farm in western Canada took them in, while another aunt in Ontario welcomed Alvin's other siblings.

In another case, nine-year-old Pearl was taken in by her aunt and uncle following her discharge from the sanatorium. Being "very fond" of Pearl and without children of their own, Pearl's aunt had "persuaded" Pearl's father to send her to live with them. After Pearl's mother died, her father had remarried, bringing a new wife and two younger children into the "small flat" the family occupied. Fearing "Pearl would not have the care and nourishment ... which would be absolutely necessary to her" and to protect the health of those younger children in the household, Pearl's aunt had stepped in, both she and her husband wanting to do everything they could "to keep her well and strong." At their home, Pearl had been provided with "a large, bright, airy room to herself" and would always have "the best of nourishment and comfortable clothing," but Pearl's aunt and uncle did "not want to make any avoidable blunder," so they wrote to Dobbie for advice on her post-sanatorium care. In his reply, Dobbie advised that what she needed, more than anything else, was "a good home where she will be given the proper amount of rest." He recommended that Pearl be put to bed no later than 7:30 p.m. and that she should also have a two-hour midday rest, as was customary at the Queen Mary. He advised them that she did not need special medicines and that she should be provided with an ordinary, nutritious diet.

Where families fell short in their abilities to provide for children, unexpected sources of support sometimes materialized. In the years between the death of Alma's mother from tuberculosis in 1915 and Alma's entry into the sanatorium at thirteen years of age in 1925, her father had remarried. She was in rather poor condition when examined by her family physician, and he grew concerned that if the family did not have her admitted she would likely continue to fail in health. Financial difficulties were preventing her from entering the sanatorium, and, in this case, the sympathetic family doctor was willing to contribute personally to her hospitalization costs. In his letter, he described Alma as a "poor kiddie" who "never had a chance." He clearly did not like Alma's father, "ignorant and careless," and stepmother, "who takes no interest in her." According to the physician, both had "neglected" and "underfed" Alma, leaving her "to run wild." Fortunately, Alma's maternal grandparents had taken her in, caregivers who he felt were "very kind and decent," but were ultimately living on limited means and unable to contribute to the costs of her hospitalization. Medically, upon examination, the physician had noted "very marked signs of involvement" in the upper lobe of Alma's left lung. While he felt it "possible that she may recover," he did not believe she would do so under the conditions at her grandparent's house. As a result, he was willing to contribute $2.50 per week to the costs of Alma's hospitalization, at least for a few months, "to secure her some chance in this world." He felt her grandfather might possibly be able to manage the other $2.50 per week needed. Alma was admitted in early July, but soon after discharged in September to board a train and return to her father's house. Her father had heard she was "losing ground" and wanted her back home if there were no prospects for her recovery, even despite the family doctor's indictment of his parenting and Dobbie's strong urging that she was best left where she was.

Other family physicians also stepped in to help support children when hard-working families had fallen on hard times. When thirteen-year-old Frederick was admitted to the sanatorium in 1936, his father was not in the best of circumstances. Fred's mother had died of TB at the Toronto sanatorium six years earlier. When Miss Wilkinson wrote to Fred's father informing him that his son would need about $3.50 to provide him with the clothing that he needed, it was the family's physician who wrote back, enclosing the amount requested. "The father is most poor," he explained, "but a very good father" to both Fred and his ten- and eleven-year-old daughters. Frederick's father had been on relief "for a very long time" and was "not very healthy." The physician had "operated on him" about a year earlier for a double inguinal hernia, progressing well, but yet still "poorly" in other respects. "I am glad to help him," the physician wrote, "because of his devotion" to his children. Wilkinson accounted for the money that the family doctor had sent along, used to purchase Fred two suits of underwear ($1.96), a pair of trousers (.57¢), and a sweater (.79¢), leaving a balance of eighteen cents. At Miss Wilkinson's suggestion, the doctor agreed that the remainder of the money could be used to purchase Fred a little toy for Christmas. The hospital, in turn, would provide him with a pair of shoes.

Marie, a French-Canadian girl living in northern Ontario, was fourteen years old when her tuberculosis was discovered in early 1936. By March, she had been admitted to the Queen Mary. Her case was one of minimal pulmonary TB, but she also suffered an unrelated bone infection that required treatment. Marie's mother first wrote to Dobbie in March, while her daughter was in transit to the hospital: "Will you please write as soon as Marie my little daughter gets their at the hospitell is she very lonsome please be real good to her and God will help you with all your undertakers" [a rather unfortunate misspelling which was meant to read "undertakings"]. Since Marie could not write, she relied on other patients to assist with letters home to her mother and, not hearing from her daughter regularly, Marie's mother grew anxious, so she wrote to Dobbie in July. She asked after her daughter's arm, which, in her last letter home, Marie had said she had hurt while playing. "Did she break it or not?," Marie's mother asked Dobbie. "I have asked her severall times about it as I am worried about her." In her letter she also asked about "the slippers and stockings I sent her in June ... she has not told me if got them." Her mother felt it was "two bad she cant write her selfe," explaining "she was not very strong and she had five miles to walk to school so it was impossible for us to send her to school that far." Marie's mother felt "very lonsome for her," so much so that she felt she was "failing in healthe my selfe." According to a note sent to Marie's cot patrons in December 1936, she had come along very well at the sanatorium. The staff related the fact that she had arrived a very thin little girl, "apprehensive of everything and everybody" when she travelled alone from northern Ontario. By December, she was in better health, putting on weight and her confidence growing as her English language skills improved. According to the Christmas-time note, "She is one of the happiest and most appreciative children we have, and is always saying 'I am so glad I came to this hospital.'"

At the sanatorium, Marie's physicians quickly realized that something was wrong with her vision and that she would need glasses, so Dobbie wrote to Marie's parents in January 1937. From her mother's prompt reply, it was clear that her parents knew of Marie's difficulties, but could not afford the cost of the necessary glasses: "I knew she had a very weak eye sieght but it was impossible to have her fited with glass as we were on Reliefe and still are." Marie's father was out of work, and the family of ten was only just surviving on relief. Over the winter, the Relief Board had provided the family with $25 a month. Understandably, food was Marie's mother's main concern, emphasizing in her letter the difficulty in ensuring the family had sufficient "potatoes and vegitables and meat." With her parents already hard-pressed to provide even food for their large family, and not wanting to leave Marie without the glasses she needed, Dobbie discretely paid for them himself, making the notation in her paperwork, and ending all correspondence on the matter.

Orphanages and Foster Care

Outside of family homes, a number of children admitted to the sanatorium were connected with custodial institutions such as orphanages or foster care placements, often arranged through local chapters of the Children's Aid Society. In many instances, diseases such as tuberculosis were responsible for the death or disability of one or both parents, which then led to the children's attachments to these support networks. Generally speaking, children leaving the sanatorium presented special challenges for the shelter and foster care systems. Dobbie advised full disclosure, that anyone thinking to foster or adopt children discharged from the sanatorium should be made fully aware of the children's medical and family history of tuberculosis. Some shelters were wary of admitting former sanatorium patients, even though their disease would have typically been latent or patients otherwise non-infectious prior to their discharge from the sanatorium. Despite reassurances, fears normally surfaced that a shelter full of potentially susceptible children were vulnerable to infection by confirmed tuberculous children.

Placement difficulties also ensued if the children being discharged required special provisions, often extra bedrest, hearty diets, and additional supervision. Some discharged children were recommended for regular follow-up examinations at tuberculosis clinics, which could be problematic for foster families if travelling clinics reached their areas only irregularly, perhaps once a year or so. It was generally easier to place "working" children, those who could help around the house or in farm labour, for example. Many post-sanatorium children could not be asked to perform this kind of work, since extra rest and, at best, only light work were often recommended. Ideally, Dobbie felt that discharged children should be placed in homes without other children, more for the focused care they would receive and not usually over concerns of infectiousness (though there were exceptions). Despite these challenges, child welfare groups worked hard to find appropriate homes. Ten-year-old Gordon, for example, was to be given an "exceptional opportunity," placed by Children's Aid in a "very refined" country home with unmarried, childless, adult siblings. As explained in a letter to Dobbie, "the Lady has just lost her only Sister. They lived together in the Old Homestead. Her

Brother is a Principle of a School and away from home a lot and she is so lonely." The Children's Aid worker believed "she would have plenty of love to give Gordon" on a farm without other children and much opportunity for good quality "individual care." Despite his placement in a foster home, Gordon was not a true orphan. While Gordon's mother had passed away, his father was alive but suffering a worrisome, unidentified "chronic cough," and unable to provide a suitable home for Gordon at the time of his discharge.

Municipal Responsibilities

While sanatorium treatment was not truly "free," the families of most child patients admitted to the Toronto sanatorium were not responsible for the costs of hospitalization. Instead, where it could be demonstrated that children came from "indigent" (poor or destitute) families, the costs of hospitalization were typically shared by the province and municipalities. Provincial support included contributions towards the cost of sanatorium construction (in 1908, the province would grant one-fifth of the cost of sanatoria established by municipalities or other recognized associations, but would not exceed a maximum $4,000 grant), as well as contributions towards the maintenance of indigent patients (in 1908, for example, municipalities were responsible for $1.50 per week per patient, and the province would provide an additional $1.50 per week per patient).[12] Provincial support, for both hospitalization costs and aftercare, was particularly important for patients admitted from northern Ontario's unorganized territories, where there was little municipal infrastructure.

By the time the sanatorium era was under way in the twentieth century, Ontario's municipalities were already accustomed to their responsibilities for their residents, funding basic services and education, and paying part of the cost for residents admitted to hospitals, children's homes, and orphanages. Many municipalities struggled under the weight of these responsibilities, since the capital raised by land taxes was often quickly exhausted.[13] As a result, "indigent" children admitted to the sanatorium could place significant burdens on municipal coffers, particularly given the long average length of hospitalization. A review of the sampled cases revealed numerous instances of contended municipal claims, which, upon meticulous review by municipal clerks, generated substantial correspondence. According to Dr Holbrook, of Hamilton's Mountain Sanatorium, the process of municipal review could be "so humiliating" that some families chose to keep tuberculosis sufferers at home and take their chances rather than be reviewed for municipal support.[14] Families who went through this process undoubtedly placed their children's health above the inevitable scrutiny and possible family shame.

Given the financial costs placed on municipalities, the process of determining a sanatorium patient's municipality of origin could be contentious. In an attempt to clarify, paragraph 23 of Bill No. 176, 1926, "An Act to Amend the Hospitals and Charitable Institutions Act," outlined not only the obligations of municipalities to their citizens, sharing the financial costs of hospitalization with the province and covering the maximum $15 charge for local burials in the case of death, but also how municipal residence was to be determined. The critical question of municipal responsibility was to be determined by assessing a patient's residence in the five months preceding hospitalization; the municipality in which the patient resided for three of those months was determined to be the municipality of residence. If, however, a patient had travelled from one municipality to another "for the purpose of seeking medical advice or treatment or seeking admission to any hospital," that could not be considered in the three-month count. Clerks of municipalities receiving "statutory notice" of an indigent patient's hospitalization had thirty days in which to contest that notice by registered letter, otherwise, by default, that patient would be determined a legitimate, indigent resident of the municipality. "Statutory notice" was a form letter sent by the sanatorium to municipal clerks, notifying clerks that a resident of their municipality had been admitted and presenting the particulars (name, age, length of residence in the municipality, and so forth) of the patient. Valid reasons for contesting the notice included errors based on incorrect residence allocations or the belief that patients (or, more specifically, their families) were not truly indigent. Indigence was typically claimed by the majority of children hospitalized. For example, of all patients admitted to the Toronto Free Hospital and Queen Mary Hospital in 1919–20 the overwhelming majority, some 85 per cent (of 280 patients), were indigent and received municipal support.[15]

Given the financial implications, municipal clerks reviewed these notices thoroughly. Sometimes, when admitting children, information was supplied by whoever accompanied the child or, at times, by the children themselves. And sometimes that information was not complete or entirely accurate. When two-year-old Ernest was admitted in 1915, for example, and his municipality was served with the statutory notice, Dobbie received a prompt response from the town clerk staunchly refusing to accept any financial responsibility for his case, claiming that the child had not lived in the municipality for over two years. "We earnestly protest from being made the dumping ground for all the indigents of the County," the clerk wrote, "and we want you to investigate this case before making any demand upon us, as we absolutely refuse to pay for his keep." Dobbie replied diplomatically, explaining that there was no wish to charge the municipality "unfairly," but that an incorrect address had been supplied by the child's guardian when he was admitted. The correct municipality was subsequently contacted and assumed responsibility for Ernest's hospitalization. By February 1916, however, that municipal council believed it was no longer responsible for Ernest because his father had died and his mother had since moved and was no longer a resident of the municipality. Dobbie's reply made it clear that maintenance payments could not be discontinued for this reason, because "according to the Act relating to Hospitals and Charitable Institutions, Section 23, Sub-section 1," it was the place of residence of a child at the time of admission that determined municipal responsibilities, not the whereabouts of family members if they chose to move during the course of a child's hospitalization (which, given the length of time some children were hospitalized, was not unheard of).

Orphanages created problems for municipalities if their charges were admitted to the sanatorium. Municipalities complained that only those "poor children properly belonging to them" should be their responsibility, and not the myriad children sent to local orphanages "from all over the Dominion." Such children were viewed by municipalities as "outsiders" who had the potential to significantly and artificially increase the responsibility placed on local taxpayers. Disagreements and controversies over support for orphanage children often caused acute difficulties for the orphanages, particularly if a sick child could not be effectively segregated from the larger population at these institutions while awaiting an order for admission. This was the experience for one matron of an Ontario orphanage that was home to sixty-five children. Twelve-year-old Peggy was already a two-year resident of the orphanage when her tuberculosis disease became active. She had arrived with three siblings "practically homeless and destitute," her mother dying of unknown causes and her father unable to provide for them. The matron's frustration grew evident as the municipality from which Peggy had been sent and the municipality in which the orphanage was located debated over their responsibilities for her sanatorium costs. To some extent, the sanatorium held power in this negotiation, since a child could be admitted with the default always being to simply charge the maintenance to the municipality in which the child was last living prior to admission, leaving the municipalities to debate and correct the issue, if required. With the introduction of the Sanatoria for Consumptives Act, 1931, the situation had been addressed, stating that "for the purpose of this Act, no patient shall be deemed to be a resident in a municipality, (d) by reason of having been a patient or inmate of a hospital, sanatorium, house of refuge, orphanage, children's shelter or child welfare institution, etc."

Sometimes families or even referring physicians did not thoroughly understand this process for receiving municipal support. Selma, eleven years of age, was admitted to the Toronto sanatorium in 1925 with moderately advanced tuberculosis disease affecting both of her lungs. Within a week of the girl's admission, the rector of her church wrote to Dobbie on her father's behalf informing the physician-in-chief that, because of an inability to pay, Selma would have to be removed from the sanatorium, explaining that Selma's father, "a poor man" who was "unable to contribute very much towards the cost of his daughter's maintenance" had been under the impression "that this sanatorium was 'Free,' or he would not have taken the child to Weston." The rector was adamant that Selma should "not be returned" home, "for the sake" of her seven young siblings living there. One child had already been buried earlier in the year, and two more a short time before that. Letters from members of the clergy familiar with the financial and living conditions of families connected with their churches were often provided as testimonials in determining potential municipal responsibilities. Dobbie replied to the rector's letter, informing him that if Selma's father could not pay the maintenance charges of $10.50 per week (the daily charge being $1.50), then the amount would be charged to his municipality. On the basis of the rector's letter, a statutory notice was sent to Selma's municipality. Within thirty days, however, the clerk had written back to Dobbie, informing him that the council did not believe this child to be indigent and that, therefore, maintenance costs would not be paid by the municipality. In the end, Selma's family somehow bore the costs of her care, and she remained in the sanatorium for thirteen months.

All indigent cases considered by municipal councils were carefully scrutinized by all means that councils had at their disposal, including tax rolls and property registrations. Ownership of land, homes, or automobiles seriously undermined indigent claims. When one eight-year-old boy was admitted to the sanatorium in 1926, a clerk for the city of Toronto determined that the boy's father owned property and had been a long-term city company employee. The clerk was even able to determine the amount of money, deemed "considerable," that the father held in a Dominion Bank account. On the basis of these findings, the clerk felt that the boy could not be considered "indigent" as defined in the Hospitals and Charitable Institutions Act and, as a result, the family was obliged to assume responsibility for his sanatorium costs.

Ultimately, however, many different factors had to be taken into account, including the number of people in the household supported by the principal breadwinner. Douglas was admitted to the sanatorium with advanced pulmonary tuberculosis and, after only forty days of hospitalization, died in July 1932. Dobbie wrote to the city clerk for Toronto requesting $60.00 in arrears for his treatment, which was billed at the standard rate of $1.50 per day. The clerk returned the application, the city refusing any responsibility for these charges. Douglas's father had died and, at the time of his admission, Douglas was living with his mother. On examining her situation, the council found that she owned a property in Toronto, which she valued at $4,600. The clerk's office undertook an independent valuation and their estimation weighed in at $4,875, adding, furthermore, that the property was owned free and clear of all encumbrances. In light of his mother's property holdings, the city council refused to consider Douglas's family indigent.

Though established municipalities had their own difficulties negotiating which cases they felt they were or were not responsible for, the matter of sanatorium charges for patients coming from Ontario's unorganized districts presented other challenges. In 1930, disputing liability for $109.50 in hospitalization charges for four local patients, one industrious clerk of a northern township cited recent case law, "a Judgement handed down by Judge Middleton in a case of the National Sanatorium Association v. Town of Bracebridge." That judge had determined that unorganized districts were "not legally liable for the maintenance of indigent patients in Sanatoria for Consumptives." Exceptions made for unorganized districts were not without reason, principally because, without solid foundations, some of these municipalities simply did not generate the revenue or have the resources to support patients in the sanatorium. Even in smaller municipalities, one clerk argued, it would take but one long-term surgical case to drain any available financial reserves. Another clerk wrote to Dobbie in 1935 expressing the frustrations of a municipal council that had determined it "almost impossible" to cover the expenses of a child patient, Horace, who had been admitted to the Toronto sanatorium. He explained, "This Township only raises about $1000.00 every year for roads and running expenses." In addition to the $550.00 per year that it would cost to keep Horace at the sanatorium, the township's local hospital was also demanding $264.25 to cover the costs of Horace's hospitalization earlier in the year. In this instance, for this municipality, the costs of even one patient's hospitalization seemed both overwhelming and impossible. Even more daunting, the municipality now had another sick resident, "the same" as Horace and "just as poor." In effect, given the mismatch between revenue and demand, the clerk was arguing to Dobbie that the sparsely populated municipality itself should be considered "indigent" in comparison to larger, often urban, and more financially stable municipalities. In reality, these inequalities at the municipal level led to notable regional variation in the rates of sanatorium hospitalization and undermined the whole notion of accessible "free care" for any in need.[16]

Given the chronic nature of tuberculosis, municipalities could easily be entering into long-term support commitments for children at the sanatorium. As a case in point, Bruce was six years old when he entered the sanatorium in June 1913. He was classified as an indigent patient, and his municipality accepted responsibility for his care. In April 1914, however, the town clerk wrote to the sanatorium to find out when the boy would be discharged, anxious because Bruce had been there almost a year. Although this was, by far, a modest length of hospitalization, given the early date of this case in the rise of sanatoria in the province, the municipality may simply not have had a good sense of the kind of commitment that it was entering into. Bruce's prognosis was not good, as Dobbie makes clear in his reply: "I do not think that we are going to be able to bring about a sufficient degree of improvement to make his recovery anything like a permanent nature." Bruce's tuberculosis disease was both active and far advanced, and Dobbie acknowledged that "he may continue in his present condition for a considerable time," but "that ultimately there will be only one end." Of course, Dobbie was unable to estimate the possible date of Bruce's discharge or death.

Not all municipalities were patient. Some municipalities attempted to pressure parents to remove their children from the sanatorium, intimating that they intended to cancel maintenance payments, particularly in cases where it seemed (to the municipality) that children had been hospitalized for unduly long periods of time. Ultimately, pecuniary concerns led to differing municipal and medical opinions on the necessary lengths of hospitalization. Impatience with long treatment regimes, however, was regularly encountered with tuberculosis, given the chronic, slow nature of the disease. Margie was admitted to the Queen Mary in April 1919, at five years of age. She remained in the sanatorium until July 1923, just over four years later. By early summer, discussions with Margie's mother were underway about her potential discharge. The public health nurse from Toronto's Department of Health who had visited the home to assess Margie's living conditions upon discharge was confronted with a mother who was not prepared to have her child home. In early July, Dobbie received a letter from the city stating that Margie's mother "seemed to be of the opinion that Margie could stay in the hospital indefinitely and was not willing to discuss any other plan." The Department of Health was sympathetic to the difficulties that Margie's mother, a single mother, faced in making arrangements for her daughter's discharge, but, in order to motivate her in that direction, she was sent a letter stating that since her daughter no longer required hospital care, the city order for her daughter's maintenance would be cancelled. In defence of precedent, Dobbie dismissed the actions, writing to the Department of Health that it did "not actually [have the] power to cancel the order in this way while the child remains in residence in accordance with the terms of the Act relating to Hospitals and Sanatoria for Consumptives." As the sanatorium administrator and as a physician, Dobbie would not "turn the child out until some other provision is made for her." As a result, he was insistent that "her maintenance charges must continue to be met by the City of Toronto until she is placed elsewhere." As it turns out, perhaps in response to the letter that she received from the Department of Health, Margie's mother arrived at the sanatorium and discharged her daughter against medical advice within the space of a few days. Margie, however, suffered a resurgence of her symptoms and was later readmitted, once again at cost to the city, on two further occasions.

Despite vested interests, not all municipalities pushed to have children returned home as quickly as possible, and the experience of Calvin's family is a case in point. Calvin was six months old when he and his sister were admitted to the sanatorium in July 1932, their mother having already been admitted to another sanatorium. Once Calvin's mother had become well enough to return home in the spring of 1933, she and her husband wrote to Dobbie, now ready and wanting to have their children back home with them. Dobbie wrote to the town clerk of the municipality that had been maintaining the children in the sanatorium, informing him of the parents' desire to have them discharged. As the town clerk explained to Dobbie, however, the town council wanted the children to remain in the sanatorium because of their mother's physical condition and the fact that the family was living on relief with no employment prospects for their father on the horizon. "While we appreciate the parents' desire to have their children with them," he wrote, "the parents should have the best interests of the children in mind." The council urged the parents to consider leaving the children at the sanatorium, particularly since they were "being well cared for" and since they would "require the best of food," which their parents would be unable to provide on their limited means. The clerk asked Dobbie to write to Calvin's parents to explain that the council was not "unfriendly," but only had "the best interests of the children in mind." Though the council was financially responsible for Calvin and his sister, it ultimately lacked any power to either order or prevent their discharge. Less than a month after this matter came up for discussion, despite the fervent wish of the town council, the children were removed from the sanatorium by their parents.

Adding to the debates of municipal responsibilities were broader, national issues concerning the matter of residence and the problems that mobility, in particular, caused for the funding of tuberculosis treatment. Charles Hodgetts, Ontario's former chief medical officer of health, was arguing as early as 1912 that tuberculosis and responsibilities for its control and treatment needed to be considered a federal, rather than a municipal, or even provincial, phenomenon. According to Hodgetts, as a result of the chronic or "prolonged character of the disease, the sufferer often moves from place to place in the search of health, and for a time moves about without becoming a burden on any particular community." At the moment, however, "when he fails both financially and physically, and some person or place must care for him," it was often "not the place of his citizenship, and frequently not his home province."[17] Attention focused on the tide of health seekers drawn to the much-lauded healthful climates of western Canada who then fell ill and became charges "in districts which can ill afford and have not the accommodation" for their care.[18]

Problems with municipal funding led to the introduction of a new Act in July 1938. With the passing of this Act, the province assumed complete responsibility for maintaining indigent tuberculosis sufferers in hospitals and sanatoria, thereby relieving municipalities of this responsibility; however, municipalities were still required to fund half the cost of hospitalization for conditions other than tuberculosis and were not altogether relieved of tuberculosis-related responsibilities. Instead, rather than funding sanatorium hospitalization charges, as of 1938, municipalities became responsible for funding the aftercare of patients discharged from sanatoria. The provincial legislature had approved this measure to ensure more efficient admissions of newly diagnosed cases into sanatoria by circumventing disagreements over which municipalities were responsible for which patients.[19] Indeed, it has been reported that in 1938, some 80 per cent of Ontarians were admitted to sanatoria within one month of their diagnoses.[20] In Ontario, Katherine McCuaig notes that this move towards provincial responsibility for maintenance was intended to address the inequalities in municipal tuberculosis mortality rates and rates of hospitalization that resulted, since "the municipality was an inadequate financial base for an efficient, comprehensive anti-TB program."[21]

At the Toronto sanatorium, concerns were raised over two distinct repercussions stemming from this new approach to funding patients.[22] First, it was suspected that, relieved of financial responsibilities, municipalities would no longer have vested interests in prevention-related activities, such as home supervision and contact tracing, and that the valuable role that municipalities played in this respect would be lost. Second, concerns were raised that sanatorium beds would quickly fill with "maximum benefit" cases (i.e., those patients who had benefited from sanatorium care, but for whom no additional period of hospitalization would be beneficial), since the provision of adequate aftercare (boarding and lodging ex-patients, for example), now the complete responsibility of municipalities, might be more troublesome to arrange. As a result, patients might be more efficiently admitted but more difficult to discharge, even when medically approved. As McCuaig notes, however, the government ensured that municipalities complied with their aftercare responsibilities "by insisting that any municipality failing to arrange for former patients' care within thirty days of notification of their discharge was liable for the patients' maintenance charges in the sanatorium until they were provided for."[23] McCuaig argues that since hospitalization was more costly than aftercare, municipalities were likely motivated to meet their responsibilities.

The Samaritan Club

Like other early twentieth-century health movements in Canada, voluntary charitable organizations played a critical role in supporting tuberculosis work and the sanatorium. In Toronto, and in association with the National Sanitarium Association, tuberculosis philanthropy was linked with two women's groups, the Samaritan Club and the Weston Hospital Sewing Club (later renamed the Weston Sanitarium Club). The co-existence of these two clubs suggests that philanthropy itself could be divided along class lines, the Samaritan Club reflecting a middle-class ethos, while the Sewing Club's membership included women from affluent Toronto homes. Late nineteenth-century and early twentieth-century women's groups have been viewed critically as vehicles by which society could spread middle-class, white, patriarchal ideals,[24] often motivated by religious sentiment.[25] However, in the years before support systems became institutionalized through policy and government, these grassroots and voluntary charitable organizations played a key role in supporting families in times of crisis and through chronic diseases such as tuberculosis. While government supports such as Mothers' Allowance were introduced in the early twentieth century and were intended to offset some of the hardships of family life, these schemes could be so exclusionary that they only ever supported a small fraction of households needing assistance.[26]

The stimulus for the formation of the Samaritan Club came from the work of Julia Stewart, a registered nurse and the National Sanitarium Association's first visiting nurse. Working out of the offices of the National Sanitarium Association's Gage Institute in Toronto, Stewart was responsible for following up on Toronto patients discharged from the NSA's Muskoka and Toronto sanatoria, attempting to visit discharged patients in their own homes at least once, as well as visiting other families connected with the Gage Institute clinic. Visiting nurses, Barbara Bates has argued, brought the "concepts of science" into the home, such that the home could be made into a safe and effective place for the ongoing care of those suffering tuberculosis.[27] Through her work, Stewart gained an insider's perspective on Toronto homes and quickly realized that much needed to be done in the support of families affected by tuberculosis. In collaboration with William Gage, she called together a group of women one afternoon in 1912.[28] It was reportedly Gage who suggested the organization be named "The Samaritan Club of Toronto."[29] At the time of her retirement in 1929, Stewart was lauded by the women of the Samaritan Club as a woman of "lofty vision and penetrating judgement."[30] As the activities of the Samaritan Club expanded, the women became masters at fundraising and supported Stewart's health visiting, providing her with a motor car in 1913 and an assistant in 1914, both of which enabled Stewart to increase the number of home visits undertaken (1,670 visits in 1913–14, representing 670 more visits than the previous year) (figure 8.1).[31]

Though tuberculosis was her main focus, Stewart's general nursing background guided her belief that health had to be grounded in a more comprehensive understanding of society and disease. For families living in Toronto, the Gage Institute's visiting nurses worked in collaboration with the institute's Samaritan Club to provide medical care, advice, food, shelter, and sundries, and partnered with physicians in health-related matters. Prior to his admission to the Toronto sanatorium in 1940, four-year-old Donald had been under the care of a visiting nurse. Donald's family had been tuberculin skin tested and while Donald's father tested negative, Donald, his mother, and his three siblings (two of whom were under two years of age) all tested positive for tuberculosis infection. The only suspected point of contact for the family had been Donald's grandfather, who had "always had a bad cough" and who had died ten years earlier, some years before Donald or his siblings were even born. Donald's grandfather likely passed on his tuberculosis infection to Donald's mother and she, in turn, was the most likely source of her children's infection. Donald was examined in October 1939, but his chest X-ray was negative for signs of disease. At this point, Donald's parents were advised that he should receive extra rest throughout the day. In an effort to improve his nutrition and build up his resistance, the Samaritan Club provided the family with extra orange juice and cod liver oil. The nurse who visited the family home quickly determined that since the entire family lived in two small rooms, it was proving difficult to ensure that Donald was getting his extra rest. In February 1940, another chest X-ray was taken, this time showing enlarged hilar lymph nodes in his lungs, physical evidence that he was not improving at home, and Donald was recommended for sanatorium treatment.

Sophie was a fifteen-year-old schoolgirl living in Toronto with her family when she was admitted to the Toronto sanatorium in January 1924. Her father had died of TB when she was only three months old; her mother had subsequently remarried and had two more babies. Sophie was referred to Dobbie at the Gage Institute Clinic and he confirmed, via chest X-ray, tuberculous lesions in both of her lungs, the left lung in particular affected by "extensive tuberculous infection." Sophie, however, was re-

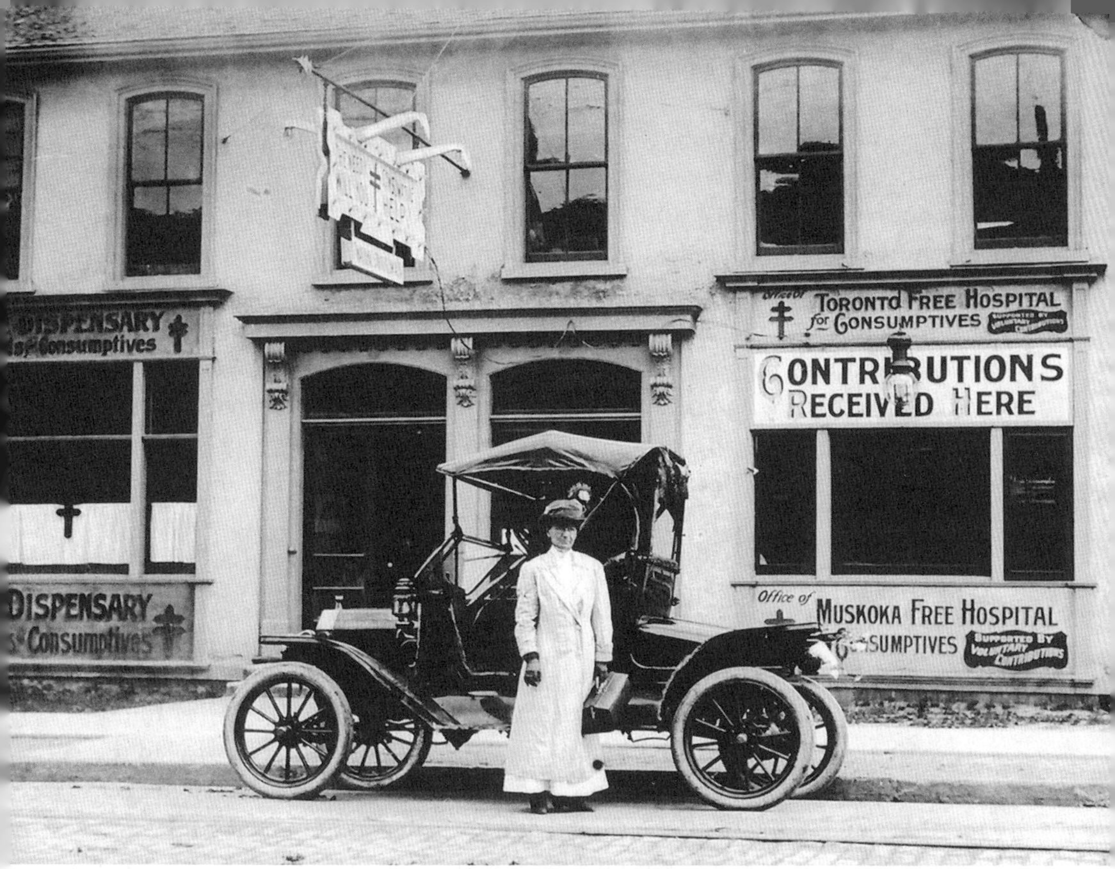

Figure 8.1 Julia Stewart is pictured in 1914 with the motor car secured for her use by the women of the Samaritan Club to facilitate her home visits. Behind her are the original National Sanitarium Association headquarters and free dispensary located at 345 King Street West, Toronto. In 1915, the Gage Institute (including a clinic, X-ray department, free dispensary, and space for the Samaritan Club) would open in a newly built headquarters at 223–5 College Street.

sistant to entering the sanatorium, and because she could not be forced to go, a Gage Institute public health nurse was assigned to visit the family periodically, providing support as best she could. Potentially infectious for some time, Sophie was perceived as a danger to her younger siblings; her two-year-old brother Earl, "pale and thin," had already been infected, though her four-year-old sister Martha appeared healthy, for the time being. While Sophie's parents respected her wishes to remain at home, as the visiting nurse notes, both her parents and the family's physician were "anxious" that she be admitted to the sanatorium. Upon her visit on 5 September 1923, the Gage nurse characterized Sophie as "difficult to manage," noting that she did "not want to rest." She spoke with Sophie about her "condition" and "the harm that she might cause by remaining at home." The public health nurse returned five days later to discover that Sophie, determined to remain with her family, wanted to take a seven-month trial at home, so the nurse advised Sophie's mother as best she could and planned return visits every two weeks or so as they adjusted to this arrangement. By 24 September, Sophie was perhaps "a little better" and "carrying out instructions," but the family physician was "still anxious that she be admitted" because it was felt her mother had "no control over this child." On 10 October, the nurse noted that Sophie had a cold with an elevated temperature and a rapid pulse. Nonetheless, Sophie "refuses to go to Hospital." The notation of 8 November finds Sophie "very ill" and "confined to bed," though her room was "neat and clean" and she was receiving "every necessary attention given by mother." Despite her resistance, Sophie's continuing decline led to her eventual admission to the sanatorium at the end of January 1924. In the space of three short months, however, Sophie's condition declined further, quickly and dramatically. Feeling that her death was imminent, and wanting to be back at home with her family, she was discharged by her stepfather in April.

Twelve-year-old Kate was admitted to the sanatorium in October 1923, but only after her family had been visited numerous times by a Gage visiting nurse between 1921 and 1923. Attention turned to the family because Kate's father had been diagnosed with tuberculosis and admitted to the Toronto sanatorium. Kate, her mother, and her six siblings remained in the family home, all considered tuberculosis suspects because of their long-term exposure to Kate's father. The visiting nurse's report accompanied Kate upon her admission to the Toronto sanatorium and, from that report, some of the inner workings and challenges that she and her family faced can be surmised. During August 1921, when the nurse began to visit, concerns were focused on Kate's tonsils, significant because diseased tonsils were believed to predispose children to tuberculosis.[32] While her mother had thought of having Kate's tonsils removed, she changed her mind on the advice of the nurse. While concerns in the fall of 1921 revolved around Kate's tonsils, the nurse's reports for the fall of 1922 were defined by whooping cough, slowly making its way through the children in the home. The reports also document two occasions when

Kate's father was given leave of absence from the sanatorium. On both occasions, the visits correlated with the family moving from one home to another. When breadwinners such as Kate's father were hospitalized, it was often difficult for families to maintain their standard of living, and some found it necessary to move to lodgings with lower rents. In the wake of each move, the visiting nurse lost track of the family's whereabouts. While home visiting could be perceived as invasive, and perhaps this was why Kate's family did not seem conscientious about providing the visiting nurse with their new address each time they moved, it also worked to facilitate support. The visiting nurse's attention had likely connected Kate's family with the women of the Samaritan Club, who in turn covered the costs of trips to the dentist and a summer camp holiday for Kate's mother and her siblings in the summer of 1922. Kate was eventually admitted to the Toronto sanatorium in October 1923, with a diagnosis of minimal hilar tuberculosis. She remained until October 1926, three long years, when her disease was determined to have become latent.

The Samaritan Club called its first general meeting to order on 6 May 1912, at the Dispensary of the National Sanitarium Association, then located at 345 King Street West in Toronto. In 1915, the Dispensary was renamed the Gage Institute and relocated to a new brick building at 223–5 College Street (known today as the "Gage Building" and part of the University of Toronto's St George campus); in recognition of the importance of the club's work, William Gage ensured the women were given working space and meeting rooms in the new institute building. Nineteen women were present at the inaugural meeting and Mrs R.N. Burns was appointed the club's first president. Its central mission was to assist the work of the National Sanitarium Association by providing support to "families and individuals crippled by the disease and by poverty."[33] The club realized that the families of Toronto patients sent to the Toronto and Muskoka sanatoria needed "sympathetic supervision" and "material assistance" if those remaining at home were to be spared from tuberculosis and poverty.[34] The Samaritan Club focused on assisting the "tired, over-worked wife" and the "under-fed anaemic children" to increase their resistance to tuberculosis and reduce the possibility that they too would someday require sanatorium treatment. They believed that their support meant that adult patients admitted to the National Sanitarium

Association sanatoria, particularly breadwinners, were "relieved from anxiety" about the fate of their families and could therefore focus more fully on making "more rapid strides towards recovery."[35] In Toronto, the emotional welfare of family members, as well as their clothing, shelter, fuel, and food needs all concerned the women of the club. From the original nineteen women who had met on that first afternoon in 1912, the club had over four thousand names on its membership roll by 1914. While not all of these women took an active part in the club's activities, they were noted for showing their sympathy for the tuberculous by entering into a "liberal subscription" with the club and therefore at least supporting the club's activities on a much-needed financial level. In its first year, the club began to supply food and clothing to families in need, at least as much as it could muster on the $477.93 that members raised in the first year.[36]

Revenue would increase substantially as the club's membership grew. In the 1914–15 operating year, for example, the club amassed $2,159.78.[37] Then, in 1918, the Samaritan Club became a member of the Federation for Community Service, an organization founded in the same year by the Rotary Club of Toronto to raise and distribute funds to charitable member organizations in the form of stipends.[38] There was some resistance among Samaritan Club members, those who feared that members would lose interest if the club was simply provided money through the federation; however, other club members believed that, freed from the massive undertaking of fundraising, members could instead devote their time to assisting families and in the work of tuberculosis education.[39] By 1921–2, with the federation's support, the Samaritan Club managed a sizable annual budget of $18,235.00.[40]

In order to improve overall efficiency, the club partitioned its work into task-oriented committees. The Clothing Committee purchased bolts of fabric, which were sewn up to meet clothing needs. The Christmas Cheer Committee "saw that gladness was brought into many homes ... by distributing practical gifts where there was no money to spare for this purpose."[41] The Relief Committee, which supplied milk, eggs, meat, and sundries, was reported to have "frequently helped the anxious mother to solve the problem of how the rent was to be met, how the coal bill was to be paid, and where the medicine was to come from that had been ordered for the ailing one."[42] The Relief Committee typically consumed a large portion of any year's operating budget; for 1915–16, for example, groceries, meat, and milk cost the club $2,658.45, or 51 per cent of the $5,250.11 budget for that year.[43] While food and milk supplies were intended to benefit families generally, the health of children was a particular concern, especially given the understanding that proper nutrition was critical to building tuberculosis resistance. For 1921–22, Julia Stewart, at this time the director of nurses for the Gage Institute, describes two such cases supported by the women of the Samaritan Club, one of a boy being raised by his grandparents, both over age seventy, having lost his parents to TB. The grandfather earned some $12 per week, viewed as "inadequate to give the child the care he should have," so they were supplied with milk and an allowance for food and clothing.[44] The second case was that of a twelve-year-old girl, described as "several pounds under weight, but with no definite T.B. diagnosis." Her father, a TB suspect, had been unable to work, so her mother went out to work to support the family. Stewart reports, "It was found by one of our nurses that the child was caring for the home, doing practically all the work," and, as a result, she did not attend school. Her situation was reported to the Board of Education, and she was recommended for the Orde Street Open Air School.[45] While this was being arranged, she was being supplied with milk. The club particularly espoused this type of "case work," believing that focusing attention intensively on a smaller number of families was better than scattering meagre attention across a large number of families. On the downside, families becoming subjects of such case work sometimes attracted unexpected attentions. The case of the twelve-year-old girl detailed by Stewart resulted in a report to the Board of Education's attendance officer, to the benefit of the girl so that someone with authority could advocate for her education, though her mother and father, focused on their own dire situation, may have had a different perspective on the importance of her education at the time.

A notable expense for the 1915–16 operating year was Restholme Cottage, which drew $821.46, or almost 16 per cent of the Club's budget. Restholme, "The Haven of Working Mothers and Their Children," was the centrepiece of the Club's "Fresh Air Work," and despite the fact that some club members thought it a costly endeavour, it proved too popular among other members to abandon the work. Fresh air camps were enduringly popular in other Canadian cities as well. For Montrealers, Poutanen and colleagues note an expansion of camp work in the 1930s and 1940s, with an increase in the number of campers and the length of their "therapeutic stay" at camps increasing to six to eight weeks.[46] The Samaritan Club's Restholme Cottage, which William Gage had donated for the club's use, was originally located in Muskoka.[47] Julia Stewart had raised the idea of a retreat for Toronto's mothers and children in 1913, wanting to create a refuge where she could send "her tired mothers and their delicate children for a holiday."[48] Though club members realized that they could never change the daily lives of Toronto's poor and struggling households, they did see benefit to a short reprieve for health and morale building. The cottage's second summer saw eighty-six mothers and children arriving in Muskoka, each family given a two-week holiday.[49] Because it was far from Toronto, the cottage proved costly, so by 1917 the club had been forced to abandon the cottage loaned to them by Gage.[50] By this time, however, the club had many "generous friends,"[51] and Mrs E.L. Bonnick donated $1,500 towards establishing Valdai Rest Home, located about forty-eight kilometres (thirty miles) outside of Toronto in Cheltenham, in memory of her daughter. Not only was the cottage much more accessible to the city but, in its rural location, fresh fruit and vegetables could be "procured in abundance" in the summer.[52] Increasing demands for space occasioned by a growing number of women and children using the camp led to a final relocation, and Valdai Rest Home was reopened on the Glen Sibbald property at Jackson's Point on Lake Simcoe in 1923 (figure 8.2).

The idea of the rest home was enduringly popular, that vacationing women and children, tired, overworked, and perhaps poorly nourished, would benefit from their time away from home and city to rest, relax, and, most importantly, build up their resistance to tuberculosis. None of the women and children themselves had ever suffered active tuberculosis, but since their "homes [had] been invaded by the dread disease," their risk was believed to be high.[53] It is clear that many club members believed very strongly in the benefits of the rest home and that the Fresh Air Work was the single most important contribution that they made to Toronto's mothers and their children. This belief is highlighted in one annual report,

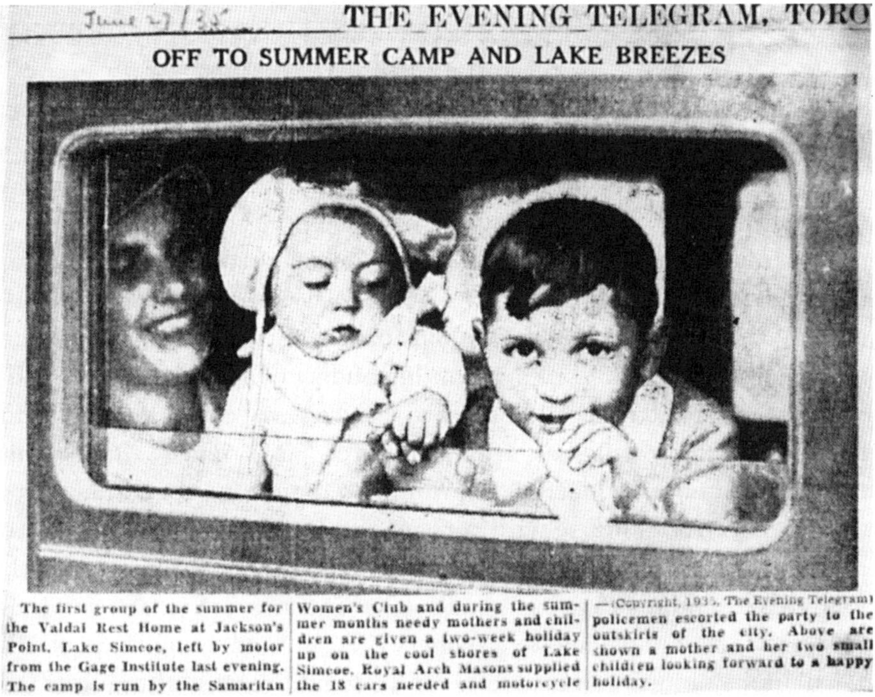

June 27/35 THE EVENING TELEGRAM, TORO

OFF TO SUMMER CAMP AND LAKE BREEZES

The first group of the summer for the Valdai Rest Home at Jackson's Point, Lake Simcoe, left by motor from the Gage Institute last evening. The camp is run by the Samaritan Women's Club and during the summer months needy mothers and children are given a two-week holiday up on the cool shores of Lake Simcoe. Royal Arch Masons supplied the 18 cars needed and motorcycle policemen escorted the party to the outskirts of the city. Above are shown a mother and her two small children looking forward to a happy holiday.

—(Copyright, 1935, The Evening Telegram)

Figure 8.2 A mother and her two children on their way to the Samaritan Club's Valdai Rest Home at Jackson's Point, Lake Simcoe, June 1935. All mothers and children had examinations at the Gage Institute clinic prior to their vacation to ensure that they did not have active tuberculosis disease.

perhaps in response to persistent criticisms over the great expense incurred by the club in this one endeavour, when one mother was asked how she was enjoying her holiday at camp. "Oh it is just like Heaven," she had responded. "I've never slept out of my own home, not once in all the nineteen years I've been married until I came up here."[54] Her response, and similar sentiments from hundreds of other women, conjured the understanding that "'Nature's charms may be free alike to all,' [but that] all may not have the opportunity of enjoying them," reinforcing the Samaritan Club's belief that their "exploit of faith in the purchase of such a home … has been fully justified."[55] The rest home and the club's Fresh Air Work continued to run well into the 1940s, by this time generously supported by the *Toronto Star*'s Fresh Air Fund.[56] Valdai was eventually sold in 1948 and, after this time, Toronto families were connected with other camps run by various community and volunteer associations.[57]

One of the greatest struggles that the Samaritan Club found affecting families was an inability to establish any savings to buffer their homes when breadwinners were unexpectedly hospitalized. The inability was linked, quite simply, to the high cost of living in the city. Carefully scrutinizing the budgets of some of the club's families, Stewart concluded that the prospects for struggling families of the early 1920s to "live decently," even in "respectable" neighbourhoods on the outskirts of the city, were nearly impossible. She used the monthly budget of a family consisting of father, mother, and two children, six and eight years, as an example, with the breadwinner earning an average of $100 per month.[58] Almost half the family's budget, some $48.40, would go to housing costs alone ($35 to rent a six-room house with furnace, $8 for fuel, $3 for gas, $1.40 for light, and $1 for water). Additional monthly expenses would include food ($30), clothing ($10), insurance ($4.50), carfare ($3), and sundries such as soap, stamps, and newspapers ($2.75). According to Stewart's calculations, a meagre balance of $1.35 would remain after all of the necessary expenses had been deducted. As Stewart argued, "It does not require much play of the imagination to realize what happens when tuberculosis occurs in such a family," since any alteration in income would easily leave the family without sufficient funds to get by.[59]

In 1971, well after the advent of antibiotic treatments for tuberculosis, the Samaritan Club surrendered its Charter and disbanded. The women felt that their work had been done, confident that Toronto's struggles with tuberculosis were behind them: "Many of our projects have been assumed by the Government. The hospital sojourn has been curtailed since the introduction of the 'Wonder Drugs,' which are also controlling the disease. Thus we can resign with pride at having fulfilled our Mission and with the hope that Tuberculosis is in the capable hands of the Scientists."[60] There is a certain irony here since, only decades later, it would become apparent that "wonder drugs" and science alone could not cure societies of tuberculosis, and it is precisely the type of community-focused, supportive work undertaken by groups such as the Samaritan Club that would be critical to successful tuberculosis control programs.

The Weston Sanitarium Club

In addition to the women of the Samaritan Club working with the National Sanitarium Association's Gage Institute and Toronto families, another group of women aligned with the National Sanitarium Association to support patients at the Toronto sanatorium. Originally known as the Weston Hospital Sewing Club upon its creation in 1912, by 1915 the charitable organization had come to be known as the Weston Sanitarium Club.[61] The women of the Sanitarium Club were residents of Toronto's wealthy High Park neighbourhood (to the west of Toronto's downtown core). The co-existence of these two clubs, the Samaritan Club and the Sanitarium Club, and the differences in their intentions and charitable work, suggests that tuberculosis philanthropy itself could operate along class lines. While members of the Samaritan Club worked at the grassroots level, meeting with women and families, teaching them valued skills (in sewing, for example), entering their homes, and interacting directly, the women of the Sanitarium Club were more removed, making important contributions to the support of sanatorium patients, but from a distance.

In September 1912, ten women inaugurated the Sewing Club with "the purpose of helping the hospital to clothe its needy patients and to give such other assistance as might be feasible."[62] The Sewing Club quickly grew to some fifty members and met regularly on the first Tuesday of every month,[63] enjoying the "hospitality of the largest homes in the High Park district."[64] At its height, the club had a membership of about one hundred women. Contrary to the club's name, no sewing actually took place at meetings. Instead, a subcommittee of women worked in between meetings to cut out garments that were handed out to members at meetings, each woman taking a garment home and sewing it up in time for the next meeting. At the end of the club's second year, it had cut over one thousand yards of flannelette, fashioning garments for Toronto sanatorium patients most in need of support.[65] While the club was initially focused on patients "so unfortunate as to contract tuberculosis during their declining years," a growing membership meant that attention could be expanded to include all adult and child patients.[66]

It is notable that both the Samaritan Club and the Weston Hospital Sewing Club shared an interest in sewing. Daughters forming the Junior Samaritan Club, an offshoot of the Samaritan Club, taught sewing to poor women, helping them to develop skills in thriftiness to stretch their modest, perhaps near non-existent, household budgets. The "sewing" aspect of the Weston Hospital Sewing Club also reflected class-based and gendered notions of women's work, where women of high social standing would have been schooled in the art of needlework, alongside the languages, literature, music, and gardening. Though these women were wealthy and could likely have more easily supplied the funds for store-bought clothing for sanatorium patients, sewing staked a more personal involvement in their philanthropic work and also gave evidence of more admirable social and economical values, such as frugality; simply handing over money would have been a vulgarity and would have undermined the belief that charity should come with work. As with many other charitable organizations in Ontario of the time, the work of the Sewing Club was guided by Christian spiritual underpinnings, perhaps most evident in the Weston Hospital Sewing Club's lofty guiding motto, which directly referenced the Gospel of Matthew: "Inasmuch as ye have done it unto one of the least of these, my brethren, ye have done it unto me."[67] In comparison, the more utilitarian and middle-class Samaritan Club's motto was, quite simply, "Prevention is *better* than cure."[68]

In addition to their philanthropic focus, the regular meetings of the Sewing Club were also intended to be social occasions. The club often arranged for talks by notable people who worked "among and for consumptives,"[69] including Miss Dickson and Dr Dobbie of the Toronto sanatorium, Mr W.P. Gundy, chairman of the executive committee of the National Sanitarium Association, Miss Gordon, of the Nursing-at-Home Mission, Miss Edith Brindon, deaconess of Little Trinity Parish, Dr Helen MacMurchy, government inspector of hospitals and public charities, Mrs A.M. Huestis,[70] president of the Local Council of Women, and Miss Julia Stewart, representing the Samaritan Club.[71] In the Sewing Club's early years, Miss Dickson served as its link to the sanatorium, keeping the women informed of the patients' needs. In addition to regular Christmastime visits to the sanatorium, club members enjoyed special tours; reflecting on their sanatorium tour in June 1915, it was reported,

"Amidst beautiful surroundings we come face to face with the afflicted ones we are endeavoring to assist, and a fresh impetus is given us to keep on doing our part to make them more comfortable, and help along with their recovery."[72] In 1924, the women of the club were invited to the sanatorium to meet with Dr Pepperdene for a demonstration of the sanatorium's X-ray machine.[73]

The social nature of the Sanitarium Club was also reflected in its fundraising activities which, over the years, included garden parties, teas, socials, and invited speakers who presented on diverse topics, such as the "Sandwich Islands," "Women's Work," "Serbian Relief," "Patriotism," and "Greece." Bridge and euchre parties were the club's most enduring fundraisers. In a single day, special events such as rummage sales or lawn parties held on the grounds of High Park mansions could raise hundreds of dollars to support the club's sanatorium work;[74] in December 1919, a successful sale of "home-made cooking and fancy articles" and a "musicale" raised over $2000.[75] Club members were also given Self Denial Mite Boxes to fill during the summer months. Mite boxes (also known as "alms boxes" or "poor boxes") were a common feature for charitable collections at churches, again reinforcing the Christian model of philanthropy that guided these women. For those of great wealth, the alms boxes reminded them that it was important to remember those who were struggling by experiencing the act of self-denial.

While always remaining true to its underlying sewing mandate, the club's efforts expanded as the women sought to brighten the lives and increase the comfort of sanatorium patients. Each year of the club's annual report provides a detailed accounting of their work and accomplishments. In 1924, for example, "768 yards of flannelette, 190 yards Eiderdown and 2 lbs wool were purchased."[76] A total of 776 articles were sewn or purchased and donated to the hospital in this year, including 156 white nightgowns, 158 coloured nightgowns, fifty-four pairs of cloth slippers, 175 napkins, eight boys' nightshirts, two pairs of panties, two pairs of hand knit socks, two pairs of gloves, one pair of spats, as well as one pair of brown shoes for a child. Every year, they also organized a "Christmas Treat"; in 1927, for example, in addition to the regular Christmas tree they provided for the children of the Queen Mary, the women purchased fifteen pounds of candy, twelve boxes of crayons, and twelve pounds of peanuts to fill eighty-four Christmas stockings for the children (which also included a "new nickel," an increase over the "new penny" that had been provided in previous years). Other Christmas contributions for that year included sixty-six bed jackets, fifty-three boxes of notepaper, sixty writing pads, thirteen pairs of hand-knitted slippers, seven pairs of children's bed slippers, twenty-three pairs of mitts, one child's toque, two baby jackets, one pullover, one toy, one parcel of unfinished fancy work, thirty jars of jam and other preserves, four baskets of books and magazines, and $8 to provide a cut flower, often a rose, on every patient's Christmas breakfast tray.[77]

Aside from Christmas, throughout the year the club also organized "showers," such as "showers of fruit," "showers of stationery," and "showers of books." Over the years, surplus funds or special fundraising drives resulted in donations of hammocks, reclining chairs, rocking chairs, wheelchairs, a regularly maintained "boot and shoe fund" for the ever-growing children of the Queen Mary, $500 towards the construction of a chapel and recreation hall, $25 to purchase movies for the sanatorium's Pathescope movie projector, and, in 1939, the club donated a piano for the use and enjoyment of the children of the Queen Mary.

Conclusion

In the endemic years of tuberculosis, control of this disease and care for its sufferers was perceived as a community responsibility. The cause was embraced philanthropically with the construction and support of sanatoria such as the Toronto sanatorium. The province of Ontario and local municipalities had explicit fiscal responsibilities to support tuberculosis sufferers, particularly those who were determined to be "indigent." Case investigations could be unsettling, exposing families to scrutiny and criticism in the midst of the intrusions into the typically private family dynamic. In addition to formal networks of support, the extended family, friends, sympathetic strangers, and orphanages also helped to support families struggling with tuberculosis.

As the solid infrastructure of tuberculosis support materialized in the form of the Gage Institute clinic and the Toronto sanatorium, clusters of women's organizations sprang up to support these institutions and the patients and families that they served. Philanthropy itself could be marked by class dynamics as the largely middle-class Samaritan Club and affluent Weston Sanitarium Club organized with their independent yet complementary mandates. If resistance to tuberculosis was to be built, it would require far-ranging supports, from family, to community, to government.

CHAPTER 9

Conclusion

Although auto traffic was blocked, one could walk up the driveway under the now-tall trees to the sloping plateau that looks over the Lehigh River. Weeds were now high, but many of the old buildings were still standing. In the silence, it was easy to hear the ghostly voices.[1]

~ Barbara Bates

In the conclusion to her social history of tuberculosis in the United States, Barbara Bates describes what remained of Pennsylvania's decommissioned White Haven Sanatorium in the mid-1980s. In Canada and the United States, these abandoned institutions, both monuments and artifacts of TB's endemic years, conjure the memories of the thousands of sufferers who struggled to survive tuberculosis. This qualitative case study has explored the stories and experiences of tuberculous children who were hospitalized for resistance building at the Toronto sanatorium in the years before the rise of antibiotic treatments. Several findings of this study are not surprising, nor unanticipated. Parents and children might try to evade or deny the reality of a tuberculosis diagnosis, and they might be hesitant about hospitalization, at least until symptoms such as hemoptysis or discharging abscesses could no longer be ignored. Parents missed their children, and children who were obliged to leave their homes and families were often sad and frustrated. Parents sought the "truth" of their children's prognosis, wanting to know if they would survive the disease, while children at the sanatorium observed the "truth" first-hand – this was a disease that could torment and shorten lives. Everyone was afraid of dying of tuberculosis, but sufferers and their families could sensibly prepare for that possibility with the help and guidance of physicians and nurses. Many of these findings are intuitive, and could not be expected to be otherwise, but they are richly detailed in the particulars of the individual life stories that have been revealed in the charts. Important subtleties of experience also emerged, helping to expand our understanding: the sister who was too afraid to leave the sanatorium over fears that she might infect her younger siblings at home, the children growing up in Ontario, virtually surrounded by tuberculosis, the hopes that patients nurtured in medicine and the sanatorium, the confidence that physicians and nurses placed in the healing power of the body, and the individual variability in commitments to resistance building.

The study has explored the different effects of tuberculosis on the body – from the slow torment of tuberculous lungs and spines, to the urgency of tuberculous meningitis and miliary tuberculosis. Tuberculosis was itself a complex disease, sometimes difficult to diagnose because symptoms such as swollen lymph nodes were non-specific, and misdiagnoses were ultimately made with the result that children without tuberculosis were admitted to the sanatorium. In both primary and reactivation disease, children were admitted to strengthen their bodies against tuberculosis through the long process of resistance building. Some children were not diagnosed until their disease was well-advanced, when supportive treatments were provided a little too late perhaps to have been effective. Tuberculosis could be a stealthy disease, seemingly unapparent to sufferers until the more distinctive symptoms emerged, often the disconcerting appearance of a sudden hemorrhage in pulmonary tuberculosis.

While the case study focuses on hospitalized children, the "site" or "context" of their hospitalization – the Toronto sanatorium – is also illuminated. Along the same lines as the studies by Susan Haugh, Lynda Bryder, Greta Jones, and Barbara Bates, the findings of this case study also contribute to a fairer-minded perspective on the sanatorium and hospitalization, dispelling the perception that it was generally an unkind or uncaring institution, Rothman's "waiting room for death." While some children did reject the sanatorium and hospitalization, other children seemed to make the best of their situation, even thriving at the sanatorium. Children adapted in various ways, from Sidney's general industriousness and his make-the-best-of-it attitude, to those children discharged within days of their admission, or those so convinced they did not want to be there that they took matters into their own hands and ran away. For most children and their families, the sanatorium represented hope and prognosis, the best evaluations of their improvements and declines and ultimately their potential to survive tuberculosis. For those children who adapted, they joined a community and created their own lives at the sanatorium, many making friends, securing an education, and learning from their physicians and nurses how best to live with tuberculosis.

The children in this case study shared in the experience of hospitalization and treatment, but that experience would change as new approaches to tuberculosis were adopted. While strict bedrest could be tedious and even depressing, examining the underlying biological rationale for rest helps to dispel the notion that medicine was just controlling and "mean-spirited." In the end, it appears that all of the Toronto sanatorium approaches to treatment, from bedrest to artificial pneumothorax and thoracoplasty, mirrored, in one way or another, the body's (or "Nature's") underlying strategies for dealing with tuberculosis infection and disease. Hospitalization and treatments ultimately aimed to build the resistance of tuberculosis sufferers, especially the very youngest. For the patients, the sanatorium was both hospital and community, a prominent and vibrant institution, visible, vigorously funded, well-supported, and staffed with recent graduates of modern medical and nursing training; promising new trainees would nurture their chosen professions at the sanatorium. The children were thus admitted into a vital and hopeful institution, not tucked away and forgotten in a remote sanatorium.

The biosocial grounding of this case study has emphasized both the biological and social aspects of the tuberculosis experience, highlighting the amazing adaptability of the body and many of the mechanisms that come into play in its natural attempts to heal tuberculosis infection and disease. Building resistance to tuberculosis would ultimately be driven by the body; but bodies could be either nurtured or harmed by the social, economic, political, and physical environments that they inhabited. In a detailed case study such as this, the biosocial grounding was paramount, emphasizing the important exchanges between body, bacterium, nutrition, living and working conditions, and stressors such as measles that crafted the particular environments and niches in which tuberculosis flourished.

In the attempt to distil key points that run through this case study, four themes emerge: adaptability, tuberculosis genealogies, resistance building, and responsibility. Despite the decades that have passed since the closing of the Toronto sanatorium, there is a timelessness to these key themes, as relevant as they were to the children at the Toronto sanatorium as they are to children experiencing tuberculosis infection and disease today.

Adaptability

The remarkable adaptability of tuberculosis bacteria and their tenacious persistence is best captured by Christian Lienhardt and colleagues' aphorism: "Tuberculosis is an ancient disease, but not a disease of the past."[2] This case study is but one small story in a very large, globally and historically entrenched narrative. The global persistence of tuberculosis, rooted in national and international social, economic, and political inequalities, the resurgence of tuberculosis in new syndemic contexts involving diseases such HIV/AIDS and diabetes, the vulnerabilities in developing countries with burgeoning populations and massive, sometimes unplanned urban growth, and the alarming rise of variants of multi-drug-resistant (MDR), extensively drug-resistant (XDR), and totally drug-resistant tuberculosis (TDR-TB) bacteria emphasizes the understanding that tuberculosis and its control is anything but historical. Recent estimates suggest that one-third of the world's population is currently infected with tuberculosis bacteria, testament to the bacterium's exceptional transmission capabilities.[3] According to John Grange and colleagues, should existing drug therapies become ineffective, "we will very soon be at a very real risk of massive epidemics of tuberculosis that will be exceedingly difficult to control."[4] In his foreword to the World Health Organization's *Antimicrobial Resistance: Global Report on Surveillance* (2014), Keiji Fukuda, assistant director-general of health security, warned, "A post-antibiotic era – in which common infections and minor injuries can kill – far from being an apocalyptic fantasy, is instead a very real possibility for the 21st century."[5]

Most studies of past tuberculosis sanatoria conclude with the next, antibiotic phase that emerged in the history of the disease. It is a dramatic point of departure, since antibiotics revolutionized the tuberculosis experience, both for sufferers who could now be cured of their tuberculosis infections, and for the institutions themselves that began to close in neat succession in countries like Canada in the 1960s and 1970s. The Toronto sanatorium was no exception, an institution that began its slow and steady redefinition, its own adaptation, as a long-term-care facility in the late 1960s. Across Canada, tuberculosis sanatoria either found a new medical niche or were permanently closed and abandoned. But the rise of effective antibiotics was, it appears, its own time-limited adaptation to tuberculosis, golden decades where a cautious but robust confidence in cure rose to new heights. If we are indeed entering a twenty-first-century "post-antibiotic era," then the next chapter of this continuing journey with tuberculosis remains to be written, but the scope of infection success and the massive status of global infection does not bode well as a starting point in this new, emerging phase of TB bacterium/human co-adaptations, all grounded in very old and tenacious evolutionary relationships.

Tuberculosis Genealogies

The idea of "genealogies" furthers the more biological intergenerational construct, recognizing the long-term interconnectedness of humans and their experiences and understandings of tuberculosis, the children of this study representing but one or two generations in the past and future of the disease. Understanding the strong longitudinal grip of tuberculosis on humankind, the children in this study are, however, unique generations: they were amongst those who became patients at a sanatorium (a specific type of hospital that existed in Canada for only the first six or seven decades of the twentieth century), they were hospitalized at a time when tuberculosis was understood to be a bacterial, infectious disease (not a hereditary disease), they would see the rise of effective antibiotics such as streptomycin in their lifetime (if they survived TB), and they experienced tuberculosis in a time when it was endemic, so common that tuberculosis infection was reckoned as a rite of passage to adulthood. Children who were not admitted to sanatoria, or those who experienced the disease when it was believed to be hereditary, or those who developed tuberculosis when it was epidemic in appearance would all have different experiences with infection and disease.

In its endemic era, tuberculosis wielded a powerful influence over family life in Canada. Children grew up in a time when, in addition to baby weighings, vaccinations, and dental examinations, most children could expect to be subjects of both tuberculin testing and chest X-rays. School field trips transported busloads of students to chest X-ray clinics so that maturing lungs could be visualized and evaluated; the sooner that tuberculosis disease was diagnosed, the better. For many children and adults, these public health measures kept the disease front and centre in their consciousness, unnecessary for many, however, since there were seemingly few children who would pass through childhood without grim reminders of the disease's presence – the illness or deaths of mothers or fathers, grandparents, siblings, aunts, uncles, friends, and neighbours.

Ultimately, this case study is built on the stories of 822 Ontario children who were admitted to the Toronto sanatorium for resistance building. But their stories are connected to a much larger and longer narrative of tuberculosis, the first half of the twentieth century just one brief moment compared to the much longer history of tuberculosis in human populations around the globe. And yet the children in this study were invariably connected with these deeper histories of tuberculosis, such as Villemin's successful rabbit infection, Koch's twenty-ninth birthday present from his wife, Trudeau's search for health in New York State's Adirondack Mountains, and Forlanini's trials to perfect artificial pneumothorax. The children were likely unaware of these early physicians and scientists and their role in shaping ideas of infection, tuberculosis bacteria, bedrest, and lung compression, but these ideas would nonetheless affect their lives with tuberculosis at the twentieth-century sanatorium. And their experiences at the sanatorium would, in turn, influence future antibiotic treatments and tuberculosis experiences. This is the reality of tuberculosis – it has persisted, resisting all measures to control infection and disease. Tuberculosis bacteria rely on generational connections, exploiting them by adapting a tendency to reactivate in adolescence and young adulthood with routes of transmission finding their way to the bodies of young, uninfected infants and children. Biology plays an important role in defining the enduring success of tuberculosis across time, particularly the ability of tuberculosis bacteria to fall into latency, only to reawaken, conveniently, in early adulthood when new generations of vulnerable children are born.

The genealogy theme can also be extended to the physicians and nurses who attended to the children at the sanatorium – they were a product of their modern, scientific education, knowledgeable about the bacterium and issues of transmission, the difficult and changing prognosis of tuberculosis, and the sometimes unpredictable deaths, but they were also positioned in a conflicted time when they could treat but not cure the thousands of tuberculosis sufferers, including all of the infants and children who came under their care. Temporally, the sanatorium staff can be framed by what they did and did not know about tuberculosis in the first half of the twentieth century. They were, for example, well aware that tuberculosis was a bacterial, not hereditary, disease, that protein-rich diets were important for resistance building, and that handwashing was one of the most fundamental protections against tuberculosis infection. What they did not know, however, is that tuberculosis bacteria can become airborne and, not knowing this, they placed little importance on the regular use of masks, and this heightened occupational risks of infection. As scientific knowledge advanced, this generation of physicians and nurses would learn new ways of treating tuberculosis, experiencing the introduction of artificial pneumothorax, thoracoplasty, and the tuberculosis surgeries and manipulations that would appear, eventually eclipsed by the arrival of streptomycin. As a result, in addition to respecting the demands of palliative care for patients on bedrest, these physicians and nurses would also experience the first inroads into active, manipulative treatments of the body and the knowledge that they would, in turn, pass on to the next generations of physicians and nurses.

This study has presented a focused and localized case study of children admitted to one modest Ontario sanatorium. But tuberculosis is of course far from localized in Ontario or Canada, presenting one of the global population's largest and ongoing challenges. As a result, global connectedness extends the genealogy to the global population. Since the more locally focused sanatorium era, a number of widespread, global control schemes have emerged, massive efforts coordinated by the World Health Organization, including directly observed treatment, short-course (DOTS), the Global TB Programme, the Stop TB Strategy, and the End TB Strategy.

In the End TB Strategy, WHO Director-General Margaret Chan calls for "intensified global solidarity and action to ensure the success of this transformative" program with goals to reduce cases of TB, reduce TB deaths, and reduce poverty amongst TB-affected families.[6] These large-scale, sophisticated, coordinated efforts are targeted against a simple bacterium that, through its very flexibility and adaptability, has persisted in association with humans for tens of thousands of years. Humanity experienced a brief golden era, the early antibiotic era, when confidence in controlling this pathogen rose to new heights. In Canada, as sanatoria were closing in the 1970s, George Jasper Wherrett wrote *The Miracle of the Empty Beds*.

Genealogies are often characterized by linkages and connections through time. There were few facets of life that tuberculosis did not affect in its endemic age in Canada. From massively successful philanthropic fundraising campaigns, tuberculosis was also a driving force behind the rising culture of tanning (which then fell as skin cancer rates increased), the shortening of women's dresses and skirts (to prevent dragging TB bacteria off the streets and into homes), the rise of pervasive cigarette smoking (which also then fell as lung cancer and other pulmonary complications emerged), the innovation of unembellished Modernist design, and the health culture visible in ubiquitous paper tissues, vacuum cleaners, and pasteurized milk.[7] Even as a child, I remember that my mother had an aversion to cluttering our home with knick-knacks, or "dust collectors," as she called them. I realize now that this was probably a perspective and terminology that she had inherited from her own mother, who managed to raise ten healthy children in the thick of Ontario's endemic tuberculosis era. The enduring genealogies of tuberculosis extend through the reality of changing cultures – from behavioural changes, to new technologies and even esthetics.

Building Resistance

In keeping with general treatment objectives in the sanatorium era, children were admitted in order to build up their resistance to the chronic infection and disease risk of tuberculosis. Some parents were reluctant to hospitalize their children, confident that with a little knowledge and assistance they could provide adequate home care, particularly if children suffered only from familiar symptoms such as fever or swollen lymph nodes. Children, too, could be resistant to the idea of hospitalization and, once at the sanatorium, become bored, frustrated, and overwhelmingly homesick. Parents may have struggled with hospitalization, sympathizing with their children and wanting them back home, but many also understood that their children's best chances for recovery might be realized at the sanatorium. Few families had the abilities or resources to improve the home, or provide the routine, discipline, and diet for resistance building. As long as the sanatorium continued to offer hope or comfort through its treatments, even if it could not promise cure, it remained an appealing institution.

The concept of "building resistance" has been a key theme in this case study, an idea that is all about nurturing the body and immune system to help prevent underlying tuberculosis infection from developing into active disease or to coax active disease into latency. Through mass tuberculin testing surveys it was generally understood that high levels of infection prevailed in the sanatorium era, but that only a fraction of those infected would actually fall victim to active tuberculosis disease. This observation contributed to the understanding that, in infectious diseases, infection did not equal disease and that the well-maintained body could, all by itself, potentially control tuberculosis by trapping bacteria within the granulomas that would see them fall latent, perhaps for life. The premise was important for medical understandings and treatments – if the body had the potential for its own ingrained protections, then perhaps those most vulnerable to disease just needed some support to encourage their natural resistance. In the early years of the Toronto sanatorium, resistance building was essentially palliative, and patients were provided with abundant, nutritious meals, encouraged to follow a strict schedule of bedrest, to breathe fresh air and expose their bodies to UV light, and to take only carefully planned, medically advised exercise. In the sanatorium's later years, various surgeries and procedures would supplement the approach, many of these surgeries in the case of pulmonary tuberculosis meant to rest the lungs without the need to physically lie in bed, though even a strategic, midday nap was reasoned to have significant effects in reducing bacterial access to oxygen in the lung apices. From lung compression, to the bony fusions for skeletal tuberculosis, surgeons were following procedures that yielded results comparable to what the body might achieve if left to its own devices.

The sanatorium offered support, but ultimately, before antibiotics, it was up to the body to push an active tuberculosis infection into latency. There were two competing realities in resistance building, however: the body (or "Nature") and its adaptations to infection and disease, and the resistance adapted by tuberculosis bacteria. Ultimately, bacteria had their own survival strategies, able to weather the hypoxic environment of granulomas, holding out for a lull in immune defences, which would allow for their resurgence into active infection. Just as remarkable is the adaptation of tuberculosis bacteria to increasingly survive antibiotic exposures. Strong, healthy bodies are best equipped to overcome the challenges of tuberculosis infection. Resistance building was really a biosocial construct, the biology within the domain of medicine, while social aspects fell within the purview of public health and communities in general. As the assuredness of antibiotics continues to wane, we are best to remember the value in resistance building, placing a strong emphasis in building healthy bodies, homes, and communities. Tuberculosis bacteria are known to thrive in the great potential offered by social inequalities, where some bodies are better nurtured and built or seasoned for resistance than others. As physician-anthropologist Paul Farmer notes, inequalities and infection often act together to "wither bodies slowly."[8] Sociologist Paul Draus acknowledges that the rise of antibiotic treatments shifted attention to the simple act of swallowing pills, where patients could easily be divorced from the realities of their daily lives; invariably, however, the ability to access the pills to be swallowed is compromised by social inequalities.[9] Like the sanatorium-era physicians and nurses, it is imperative to once again become invested in tuberculosis sufferers – not only the particulars of their disease and bodily effects, but also their overall well-being – their family relationships, their homes, their economic well-being, and the quality of their lives. In Canada, such inequalities are not just historical; even today, Indigenous communities continue to carry the burden of alarmingly high tuberculosis rates, which are influenced by social, economic, and political issues evident in poor access to medical care, poor nutrition, lack of potable water, and extreme housing crises.[10]

Responsibility

If we acknowledge the significance of both biological and social factors influencing tuberculosis, then issues of support can be framed by personal, communal, governmental, and structural responsibilities, a concept widely embraced in the resistance-building era. Improvements to individual, community, and population health do not come easily. In Canada, population health began to improve in the late nineteenth century, even in the face of epidemic infectious diseases, by virtue of large-scale attention and improvement to sanitation and water and food supplies. Into the twentieth century, further improvements in living and working conditions, widespread lessons on how to live healthily, and the rise of sanatoria were believed to hold the promise of improving overall population resistance to tuberculosis.[11] As Katherine McCuaig has emphasized, "To cure TB, one had to cure society," and particularly support the poor and working-class, whose struggles for health and well-being had become abundantly obvious and inspired the philanthropy evident in the National Sanitarium Association and the building of the Muskoka and Toronto sanatoria.[12] Feelings of responsibility fuelled both fundraising and philanthropy, visible in endowed beds and donations to the sanatorium. In Toronto, for the women of the Weston Sanitarium Club, this meant sewing and donating spirit-lifting gifts and clothing for patients at the sanatorium, while women of the Samaritan Club ensured that children in poor homes were provided with milk, that mothers could afford the fuel needed to heat their homes in winter, and that mothers and children of TB-stricken homes could be sent to camp for fresh air therapy and a reprieve from their lives and the city. Providing the means to build stronger bodies became a community responsibility. Because of disease and death, families and family responsibilities could be quite fluid in the sanatorium era. In the sanatorium narratives, parents often relied upon orphanages or other informal sources of support, sometimes placing their children with family members, friends of the family, or even "sympathetic strangers" when needed. As was so evident in the stories of Ontario children, building resistance cannot be achieved in isolation – people need the support of family, friends, communities, governments, and practical philanthropy to build resistance and control tuberculosis. In the midst of endemic tuberculosis, everyone had responsibilities: physicians to diagnose and treat, public health to educate, parents to support children and children to support parents, sufferers to be disciplined and careful, municipalities to cover the costs of hospitalization or aftercare, and communities and individuals to be philanthropic. Arguably, tuberculosis was one of the first health challenges to encourage collective community support and action, including large fundraising campaigns that, by the next century, would be directed at heart disease and cancer research.

Much of this was to change with the introduction of antibiotics. "Antibiotic therapy," sociologist Paul Draus argues, is "remarkably effective at curing disease," but it "often does so while leaving the patient in exactly the same position as before."[13] With the advent of effective drug therapies, broader concerns over patients' housing, lifestyle, and nutrition waned, and those community-level supports were slowly lost. Further complexities would reveal themselves: if antibiotics were supplied at a cost to patients, were they actually affordable; would patients follow the whole, often long-term antibiotic treatment program; once DOTS strategies evolved, could patients afford, for example, to take time off work in order to take their regularly scheduled dosages of antibiotics at hospitals or clinics? "Much more than chemotherapy is needed," Charlotte Roberts and Jane Buikstra argue, "to control tuberculosis."[14] The failure to consider social contexts is one of the biggest limitations in attempts to control tuberculosis today, a limitation rooted in recent history when the seeming magic bullet of streptomycin was introduced in the 1940s. Gone were the days when, in addition to treating the body, tuberculosis control also meant ensuring adequate housing, nutrition, and living conditions.[15] As medicine comes to terms with the failing surefire success of antibiotics, however, new approaches to tuberculosis control have emphasized older paradigms focused on the importance and mediation of social contexts.[16]

Notes

CHAPTER ONE

1 Risse, *Mending Bodies, Saving Souls*, 9.

2 Hobbs, "Before the Sanatorium."

3 With respect to the use of *sanatorium* or *sanitarium*, according to Elliott, "The word *sanatorium* has its origin in the Latin verb *sanare*, to heal, to cure, and is properly restricted to an institution where treatment is undertaken. The word *sanitarium* is from the substantive *sanitas*, health, and should be used in speaking of any healthy district, or of a resort for convalescent patients, for example the Adirondacks, Colorado, or the foothills of our Canadian Rockies" (Elliott, "The Sanatorium," 113–14).

4 Ibid.

5 Where both biological and social aspects are considered; anthropologists also engage "biocultural" approaches. In this case study, I felt that I was more often considering social dimensions than cultural dimensions, so the "biosocial" descriptor was applied. Arguably, the project is also biocultural in a broader sense, since TB was experienced within the context of the culture of biomedicine, at the sanatorium.

6 On case studies and "how" and "why" questions, see Yin, *Case Study Research*.

7 Merriam, *Qualitative Research and Case Study Applications in Education*, 41.

8 Ruddin, "You Can Generalize Stupid!," 808.

9 Merriam, *Qualitative Research and Case Study Applications in Education*, 29–30.
10 Baron, "Introduction to Medical Phenomenology," 609.
11 Stake, *Art of Case Study Research*, 65.
12 Creswell, *Qualitative Inquiry and Research Design*; Stake, *Art of Case Study Research*.
13 Stake, *Art of Case Study Research*, 63.
14 Klaver, "Illness Memoir"; Haugh, "Hill of Health."
15 Haugh, "Hill of Health," 2.
16 Ibid., 2.
17 Rothman, *Living in the Shadow of Death*. See chapter 15, "The Sanatorium Narrative," 227–8, 238.
18 Bryder, *Below the Magic Mountain*; Jones, *"Captain of All These Men of Death."*
19 Bates, *Bargaining for Life*, 321.
20 Haugh, "Hill of Health," 3.
21 Ibid., 10.
22 Ibid., 17.
23 Ibid.
24 Ibid.
25 Ibid.
26 Klaver, "Illness Memoir," 309.
27 Ibid., 310.
28 Haugh, "Hill of Health," 16.
29 Stake, *Art of Case Study Research*, xi.
30 Yin, *Case Study Research*, 12.
31 Rubaie, "Rehabilitation of the Case-Study Method," 32.
32 Klaver, "Illness Memoir," 310.
33 Firestone, "Meaning in Method," 16.
34 Ibid.
35 Creswell, *Qualitative Inquiry and Research Design*, 39.
36 Ibid., 57.
37 Starks and Trinidad, "Choose Your Method," 1376.
38 Stake, *Art of Case Study Research*, 65.
39 Baron, *Introduction to Medical Phenomenology*, 609.
40 For a review on the biosocial and syndemic perspective, see Singer and Clair, "Syndemics and Public Health."

41 Ibid., 429.
42 Farmer, "Anthropology of Structural Violence."
43 Singer and Clair, "Syndemics and Public Health," 429.
44 Starke, "Tuberculosis: An Old Disease."
45 Jacobs and Eisenach, "Childhood Tuberculosis," 24.
46 This response was not unique to tuberculosis, as Esyllt Jones has detailed a similar impact on Winnipeg families affected by the 1918–19 influenza epidemic. Jones, *Influenza 1918*.
47 Poutanen et al., "Tuberculosis in Town," 83.
48 Bloom and Murray, "Tuberculosis," 1057.
49 Gaikwad and Sinha, "Determinants of Natural Immunity," 415.
50 Kochi, "Global Tuberculosis Situation."
51 Grange et al., "Biosocial Dynamics of Tuberculosis."
52 Stone et al., "Tuberculosis and Leprosy in Perspective."
53 See McCuaig, *The Weariness, the Fever, and the Fret*.
54 Gagneux, "Host-Pathogen Coevolution in Human Tuberculosis," 855.
55 It appears that TDR tuberculosis bacteria possess some novel biological characteristics and adaptations, such as a greater tendency towards a round shape and a thicker cell wall, both of which may influence infection dynamics and antibiotic effectiveness. See Velayati, Farnia, and Masjedi, "Totally Drug Resistant Tuberculosis (TDR-TB)."
56 Young, "'Little Sufferers'" 131.
57 Stuart, "Ideology and Experience."
58 Young, "'Little Sufferers,'" 131.
59 Jardine, "Urban Middle-Class Calling," 179.
60 Neff, "Government Approaches to Child Neglect and Mistreatment," 179–80.
61 Ibid., 183.
62 Neff, "Role of the Toronto Girls' Home"; Neff, "Government Approaches to Child Neglect and Mistreatment"; Neff, "Education of Destitute Homeless Children."
63 Neff, "Education of Destitute Homeless Children," 7.
64 Ibid., 8.
65 Neff, "Role of the Toronto Girls' Home"; Neff, "Role of Protestant Children's Homes in Nineteenth-Century Ontario."
66 Neff, "Education of Destitute Homeless Children," 8.
67 Struthers, "'In the Interests of the Children.'"

68 Jones, *Influenza 1918*.
69 Marcellus, "Tiny Cripples and the Sunshine of Life."
70 Young, "Divine Mission," 72.
71 Ibid.
72 Young, "'Little Sufferers,'" 132.
73 According to Young, Robertson became interested in the work of the HSC following the death of his daughter from scarlet fever. Young, "Divine Mission," 81.
74 Young, "'Little Sufferers,'" 138.
75 Ibid., 139.
76 Marcellus, "Tiny Cripples and the Sunshine of Life," 411–12.
77 Stuart, "Ideology and Experience," 114.
78 Brown, "Infant and Child Welfare Work."
79 Stuart, "Ideology and Experience."
80 Rooke and Schnell, "Child Welfare in English Canada."
81 Ibid., 499.
82 Dodd, "Advice to Parents," 207.
83 Ibid., 208.
84 Rooke and Schnell, "Child Welfare in English Canada," 499.
85 Shorter, *Bedside Manners*, 131.
86 Duffin, *History of Medicine*, 325, 327–9.
87 Meryn Stuart notes that in 1920, Ontario's Board of Health sent public health nursing representatives to remote northern and rural areas of Ontario to promote the work of health education. While these communities may have been interested in securing public health nurses, the reality was that many municipalities, already challenged with funding other necessities and improvements, did not want to raise the taxes of labouring people further in order to secure the capital needed. Stuart, "Ideology and Experience."
88 Dodd, "Advice to Parents," 211.
89 Ibid., 204.
90 Ibid., 221.
91 Ibid., 223.
92 Ibid.
93 Arnup, "Raising the Dionne Quintuplets."
94 Ibid.

95 Struthers, "'In the Interests of the Children.'"
96 This would not be the first Mothers' Allowance plan in Canada, however, since the province of Manitoba first offered Mothers' Allowance in 1916.
97 Struthers, "'In the Interests of the Children,'" 70.
98 Little, "'Manhunts and Bingo Blabs,'" 220.
99 Struthers, "'In the Interests of the Children,'" 70.
100 Gale, *Changing Years*.
101 Ibid.
102 Warren, "Evolution of the Sanatorium."
103 Daniel, "History of Tuberculosis," 1864.
104 Ibid.
105 Jeanes, "Tuberculosis"; Daniel, "History of Tuberculosis," 1864.
106 Warren, "Evolution of the Sanatorium."
107 Sakula, "Robert Koch: The Story."
108 Sakula, "Robert Koch: Centenary of the Discovery of the Tubercle Bacillus."
109 Ibid., 246.
110 Koch, "Die Aetiologie der Tuberculose"; Kaufmann and Schaible, "100th Anniversary of Robert Koch's Nobel Prize."
111 According to Sakula, the discovery of the importance of heat had been somewhat fortuitous: "It was by accident that Ehrlich learned of the benefit of heating the slide. In his laboratory there was a small iron stove in which the fire had been out for some hours that evening. Before returning home, he placed the stained preparations to dry on the top of the cold stove. The next morning he was annoyed to find that the stove had been lit, but when he examined the slides he was astonished to find the bacilli in clumps showing up even more clearly." Sakula, "Robert Koch: The Story," 6.
112 Ibid.
113 Warren, "Evolution of the Sanatorium."
114 Ibid.
115 Cassidy, "Bacteriological Diagnosis of Diphtheria," 129.
116 Ibid., 130.
117 Shorter, *Bedside Manners*.
118 Trudeau, "Adirondack Cottage Sanitarium," 373.

119 Proctor, "Pulmonary Tuberculosis," 154.
120 Levine, "Good Doctor," 245.
121 Warren, "Evolution of the Sanatorium."
122 See, for example, Crichton-Browne, "Address on the Treatment of Tuberculosis"; Morland, "Essay and Plans for the Erection of a Sanatorium"; Williams, "Oration on the Sanatorium Treatment"; Fowler, "Therapeutic Value of Sanatorium Treatment."
123 Warren, "Evolution of the Sanatorium," 471.
124 Also known by his Roman name, Aesculapius. See Stanton, "Aesculapius."
125 Warren, "Evolution of the Sanatorium," 475.
126 DasGupta, "Between Stillness and Story," e1385.
127 Elliott, *Present Status of Antituberculosis Work in Canada – 1908.*
128 Tremblay, "Historical Statistics Support a Hypothesis."
129 Dobbie, "Provincial Program," 494; Editorial Comment, "Trends in Tuberculosis," 626.
130 Elliott, *Present Status of Antituberculosis Work in Canada – 1908*, 4.
131 Dobbie, "Provincial Program," 494.
132 Elliott, "Treatment of Pulmonary Tuberculosis," 381.
133 Canadian Tuberculosis Committee, "Housing Conditions That Serve as Risk Factors"; Lux, *Medicine That Walks*; Waldram, Herring, and Young, *Aboriginal Health in Canada.*
134 Smith and Nickel, "From Home to Hospital."
135 Corish, *Health Knowledge.*
136 Ibid., 506.
137 Ibid., 508–9.
138 Ibid., 509.
139 Ibid.
140 Ibid., 553.
141 Minns, "Practical Management of Pulmonary Tuberculosis," 168.
142 Dobbie, "Hygienic, Dietetic and Medicinal Treatment of Tuberculosis," 158.
143 Poutanen et al., "Tuberculosis in Town."
144 Ibid., 94.
145 Marshall, "My Personal Experience of Tuberculosis."
146 Ibid., 491–2.
147 Ibid.
148 Hodgetts, "National and Provincial Responsibility," 217.

149 The aversion to, or even disdain for, cod liver oil as a tuberculosis treatment may seem antithetical to our contemporary focus on the important immune-boosting properties of Vitamin D (which is present in cod liver oil). However, the science of vitamins (and their discoveries) was in its infancy in the early twentieth century. Concerns over rickets and osteomalacia led to animal-based laboratory and human field studies in the 1920s and 1930s and the subsequent identification of Vitamin D, its presence in cod liver oil, and, later, in UV-irradiated food and skin. See Wolf, "Discovery of Vitamin D"; and Rajakumar, "Vitamin D, Cod-Liver Oil, Sunlight, and Rickets."

150 Though not specified, this would have most likely been wood creosote, as opposed to the more toxic coal tar creosote.

151 Proctor, "Pulmonary Tuberculosis," 157.

152 A salt compound of guaiacol and carbonic acid taken by mouth. Since the stomachs of tuberculosis sufferers were believed to contain "an abnormally large quantity of saprophytic and parasitic bacteria, the compound is split up and a large amount of guaiacol set free by the fermentative processes. This arrests the development of the bacteria, and finally entirely frees the stomach from its unwelcome guests." The drug was believed to ease symptoms, improve appetites, and augment "the general resistance of the organism to diseases." Harper, "Guaiacol Carbonate in Phthisis."

153 Used as an antiseptic.

154 Proctor, "Pulmonary Tuberculosis," 157.

155 Ibid.

156 Porter, "Choice of a Climate," 346.

157 Dobbie, "Hygienic, Dietetic and Medicinal Treatment of Tuberculosis"; Minns, "Practical Management of Pulmonary Tuberculosis"; Lyman et al., *Practical Home Physician*, 158–9.

158 Price-Brown, "Treatment of Laryngeal Tuberculosis," 76.

159 Porter, "Choice of a Climate."

160 Proctor, "Pulmonary Tuberculosis," 155.

161 Dobbie, "Hygienic, Dietetic and Medicinal Treatment of Tuberculosis," 155.

162 For home, Minns recommended the use of paper or small individual handkerchiefs of any material that could be held in front of the mouth while coughing or to wipe the lips; these disposable handkerchiefs could

be collected in a paper bag pinned to the side of the bed and then burned (never washed). See Minns, "Practical Management of Pulmonary Tuberculosis," 167.

163 Marshall, "My Personal Experience of Tuberculosis."

164 Ripley, *Thine Own Keeper*, 62.

165 Fleming, "Responsibilities and Opportunities of the Private Practitioner."

166 Shorter, *Bedside Manners*.

167 Bates, *Bargaining for Life*, 263.

168 Marshall, "My Personal Experience of Tuberculosis."

169 Porter, "Tuberculosis Association," 513.

170 See, for example, Uhlin et al., "Adjunct Immunotherapies for Tuberculosis."

171 Holbrook, "Present Need of the Tuberculosis Campaign," 469–70.

172 Myers et al., *Tuberculosis among Children and Young Adults*.

173 Dobbie, "Provincial Program," 499.

174 Ibid., 498.

175 Ontario Provincial Department of Health, "Development of Public Health," 110.

176 Minns, "Practical Management of Pulmonary Tuberculosis," 166.

177 Editorial Comment, "Trends in Tuberculosis."

178 Ibid., 626.

179 van der Geest and Finkler, "Hospital Ethnography," 1995.

180 David S. Crawford, emeritus librarian, McGill University, has compiled an extensive bibliography of studies on the histories of Canadian hospitals and nursing schools, see http://internatlibs.mcgill.ca/hospitals/hospital-histories.htm.

181 Young, "Divine Mission," 72.

182 van der Geest and Finkler, "Hospital Ethnography," 1996.

183 Starr, *Social Transformation of American Medicine*.

184 Adams, *Medicine by Design*, 109–11.

185 National Sanitarium Association (hereafter NSA), *First Annual Report of the Toronto Free Hospital for Consumptives*, 1904–5, 19.

186 Gale, *Changing Years*, 19.

187 Burke notes that in in his invited lecture "On Bacteriological Research," August 1890, Koch identified "guinea-pigs, which are known to be particularly susceptible to tuberculosis." Burke, "Of Postulates and Peccadilloes," 796.

188 Bates, *Bargaining for Life*, 98.

189 Ibid.

190 Ibid., 103.

191 Ibid., 107–8.

192 Gale, *Changing Years*, 19.

193 Adams and Burke, "'Not a Shack in the Woods.'"

194 Shorter, *Bedside Manners*.

195 NSA, *Annual Report* (hereafter *ARNSA*) 1916–17. The photographs are featured opposite pages 20, 21, 24, and 25.

196 Adams, Schwartzman, and Theodore, "Collapse and Expand," 915.

197 Shumsky, Bohland, and Knox, "Separating Doctors' Homes and Doctors' Offices"; Adams and Burke, "Doctor in the House."

198 van der Geest and Finkler, "Hospital Ethnography," 1996.

199 See, for example, Lux, *Separate Beds*.

200 Risse and Warner, "Reconstructing Clinical Activities," 184.

201 Ibid., 186.

202 Ibid., 190.

203 Warner, "Uses of Patient Records by Historians," 103, 108.

204 Risse and Warner, "Reconstructing Clinical Activities," 189.

205 Ibid., 200.

206 Noll, "Patient Records as Historical Stories," 413.

207 Gillis, "History of the Patient History since 1850," 491.

208 Shorter, *Bedside Manners*.

209 Ludwig, "Emotional Factors in Tuberculosis," 887.

210 Noll, "Patient Records as Historical Stories," 415.

211 See Condrau, "Patient's View Meets the Clinical Gaze."

212 Noll, "Patient Records as Historical Stories," 419.

213 Shaw and Reeves, *Children of Craig-y-nos*, 7.

214 Ibid.

215 Gale, *Changing Years*.

216 Davies, "Night Soil, Cesspools, and Smelly Hogs."

217 See, for example, Barton, *Driven by a Dream*; Baston, *Curing Tuberculosis in Muskoka*; Flanagan and Raina, *Clara's Rib*; Mierau, *Memoir of a Living Disease*; Norton, *"A Whole Little City by Itself"*; Ripley, *Thine Own Keeper*; Sims, *Life Consumed*.

218 For a summary of West Park Healthcare Centre's history, see www.westpark.org/en/AboutUs/History.

219 Vassar and Holzmann, "Retrospective Chart Review."
220 Creswell, *Qualitative Inquiry and Research Design*, 75.
221 Flyvbjerg, "Five Misunderstandings about Case-Study Research," 229.
222 Stake, *Art of Case Study Research*, 56.
223 Levy, "Case Studies," 8.
224 See http://www.babycenter.com/babyNameYears.htm.
225 Warner, "Uses of Patient Records by Historians," 110.
226 See Marais et al., "Natural History of Childhood Intra-Thoracic Tuberculosis," 393; Schaaf et al., "Adult-to-Child Transmission of Tuberculosis."
227 See, for example, Drees, *Healing Histories*; Grygier, *Long Way from Home*; Kelm, *Colonizing Bodies*; Lux, *Separate Beds*; Lux, *Medicine That Walks*; Waldram, Herring, and Young, *Aboriginal Health in Canada*.
228 Moffatt, Mayan, and Long, "Sanitoriums and the Canadian Colonial Legacy," 1597.
229 Ibid., 1594.
230 "Little sufferers" was a common reference for child patients, at the sanatorium and in hospitals more generally. See, for example, Young, "'Little Sufferers.'"

CHAPTER TWO

1 Esslemont, "Sanatoriums from Within," 1641.
2 Pulver Ungar and Bach, "Gage, Sir William James"; Parker, "Distributors, Agents, and Publishers," 43.
3 Hart Massey was born in Haldimand Township, Upper Canada, 29 April 1823, and died in Toronto, 20 February 1896. The Massey Manufacturing Company specialized in agricultural equipment, particularly tractors and binders, which subsequently merged in 1891 to form the Massey-Harris Company Limited (and later merged in the 1950s into Massey-Harris-Ferguson, but shortened to Massey-Ferguson). See Roberts, "Massey, Hart Almerrin."
4 Massey memorialized Fred Victor with the opening of Toronto's Fred Victor Mission in 1894.
5 Filey, *Mount Pleasant Cemetery*, 154.
6 In his memory, Massey had funded the building of Massey Music Hall, which opened in June 1894.
7 Pulver Ungar and Bach, "Gage, Sir William James"; Parker, "Distributors, Agents, and Publishers," 43.

8 NSA, *First Report of the Muskoka Cottage Sanatorium for Consumptives*, 1898, 13.

9 *ARNSA*, 1901–02, 9.

10 Site selection proved difficult. Originally, a site had been selected in High Park, then in Wychwood Park, but "Health authorities" in the city of Toronto did not approve either of these locations for a tuberculosis sanatorium, likely as the result of fears over transmission. In retrospect, the Weston site seemed ideal, overlooking the Humber River and unlikely to be surrounded by other buildings. Dobbie, *History of the Toronto Hospital for Consumptives*.

11 According to Garrett's history, at its height, the Toronto Hospital had 667 patients.

12 Southam, "Secretary's Report," 7.

13 Gale, undated research notes.

14 *ARNSA*, 1901–02, 9.

15 Gale, *Changing Years*.

16 The fire began around midnight and, according to Dobbie, "all the patients were removed without injury or loss of life." Dobbie, *History of the Toronto Hospital for Consumptives*, 3.

17 Porter, "Tuberculosis Association," 512.

18 Gale, undated research notes.

19 Holbrook, "Present Need of the Tuberculosis Campaign," 464.

20 The Woodstock tuberculosis beds were provided at the site of the expanded Ontario Hospital, Woodstock, originally opened in 1906 to care for patients with epilepsy.

21 The hospital in Moose Factory provided beds for Indigenous patients. The hospital opened in September 1950 and was constructed in the shape of the Cross of Lorraine, symbolism associated with tuberculosis and lung disease. The hospital is now known as the Weeneebayko General Hospital. See Grygier, *Long Way from Home*.

22 Gale, undated research notes.

23 Grzybowski and Allen, "Tuberculosis: 2. History of the Disease in Canada."

24 Foster-Carter, "Sanatoria," 509.

25 Committee for Survey of Hospital Needs, *Tuberculosis Care*, 12.

26 Ibid.

27 Canadian Tuberculosis Association, *Handbook for Tuberculosis Patients*.

28 Currently the site of West Park Healthcare Centre.

29 *ARNSA*, 1905–06, 6. Tuberculosis was also known as the "white plague," because of the pallor that tuberculosis sufferers exhibited as a result of anemia.

30 Gooderham, "What the Daughters of the Empire Are Doing toward the Prevention of Tuberculosis," 190.

31 Gale, *Changing Years*, 23.

32 See 1911 Census of Canada, Library and Archives Canada: data2.collectionscanada.gc.ca/1911/jpg/e002038626.jpg.

33 Dr Finnerty.

34 Nurses Bolwell, Bas, McMahon, Wells, Sharpe, Alway, Surrler, Bryden, Jones, Jones (Daisy), Donnelly, Fisher, and Lovett.

35 Gale, *Changing Years*, 25.

36 "News," *Canadian Medical Association Journal* 3, no. 6 (1913): 530.

37 "Report of the Secretary and Treasurer, R. Dunbar," *ARNSA*, 1913–14, 6.

38 Adams, Schwartzman, and Theodore, "Collapse and Expand," 909.

39 Gale, *Changing Years*, 24–5.

40 Dobbie, *History of the Toronto Hospital for Consumptives*.

41 Adams, *Medicine by Design*, 58.

42 "Report of the Physician-in-Chief, W.J. Dobbie," *ARNSA*, 1918–19, 20.

43 There was also a Queen Mary Pavilion that provided an additional twelve beds. By 1926, however, the pavilion was turned over for use by adult patients; see *ARNSA*, 1926–27, 9.

44 Bliss, "Davies, William."

45 Ibid.

46 Adams and Burke, "Not a Shack in the Woods," 435.

47 For biographical details on Dr MacMurchy, see McConnachie, "Methodology in the Study of Women in History."

48 According to George Reid, the NSA's business manager and secretary-treasurer, "The past year, financially, has been one of the hardest in the history of our Association. Commodities have been scarce, and high in price; physicians and nurses have been difficult to secure; satisfactory help almost impossible to find. All this has increased the operating expense of our Free Hospitals, until now the cost per patient per week averages $19.13, which is nearly $7.00 per week in excess of the statutory maintenance allowance received from the Government, from municipali-

ties or from patients themselves." "Report of the Business Manager and Secretary-Treasurer, G. Reid," *ARNSA*, 1919–20, 3.

49 "Extract from Report of Dr Helen MacMurchy," *ARNSA*, 1916–17, 27.

50 *ARNSA*, 1913–14, 37.

51 Shaw and Reeves, *Children of Craig-y-nos*.

52 "Annual Report of the Physician-in-Chief, W.J. Dobbie," *ARNSA*, 1914–15, 40.

53 "Annual Report of the Physician-in-Chief, W.J. Dobbie," *ARNSA*, 1920–21, 21.

54 *ARNSA*, 1913–14, 37.

55 Ibid., 37.

56 *ARNSA*, 1915–16, 18.

57 "Report of the School," *ARNSA*, 1928–29, 11.

58 "Report of the School," *ARNSA*, 1929–30, 9.

59 "Annual Report of the Physician-in-Chief, W.J. Dobbie," *ARNSA*, 1925–26, 27.

60 Davies, "Night Soil, Cesspools, and Smelly Hogs on the Streets," 12–13.

61 Gale, *Changing Years*.

62 Jackson and McLeod, "Tuberculosis in Infants, Children, and Adolescents," 419; Starke, "Childhood Tuberculosis in the 1990s," 552; Kline and Lorin, "Childhood Tuberculosis," 147.

63 Adams, *Medicine by Design*, 9–14, 10.

64 Trudeau, "Adirondack Cottage Sanitarium," 371.

65 Adams, *Medicine by Design*, 14.

66 Shaw and Reeves, *Children of Craig-y-nos*, 84.

67 van der Horst and van der Veer, "Changing Attitudes towards the Care of Children in Hospital"; Lindsay, "Comments on the Article 'Changing Attitudes towards the Care of Children in Hospital'"; Robertson and McGilly, "Comments on 'Changing Attitudes towards the Care of Children in Hospital.'"

68 Wood, "Bowlby's Children," 122.

69 Marcellus, "Tiny Cripples and the Sunshine of Life," 417.

70 Committee for Survey of Hospital Needs, *Tuberculosis Care*, 6; Gale, "Oral Histories – Grant."

71 van der Horst and van der Veer, "Changing Attitudes towards the Care of Children in Hospital," 124.

72 Jackson and McLeod, "Tuberculosis in Infants, Children, and Adolescents," 419.
73 Kirby and Madsen, "Institutionalised Isolation."
74 Street, "Affective Infrastructure."
75 Kendig Jr and Inselman, "Tuberculosis in Children," 241.
76 Gale, *Changing Years.*
77 Dobbie, "Hygienic, Dietetic and Medicinal Treatment of Tuberculosis."
78 Myers et al., *Tuberculosis among Children and Young Adults*, 202.
79 McCuaig, *The Weariness, the Fever, and the Fret*, 13.
80 "Annual Report of the Physician-in-Chief, W.J. Dobbie," *ARNSA*, 1915–16, 18.
81 Canadian Tuberculosis Association, *Handbook for Tuberculosis Patients*, 28.
82 Myers, *Tuberculosis among Children and Young Adults*, 202.
83 Bates, *Bargaining for Life*, 277.
84 McCuaig, *The Weariness, the Fever, and the Fret*, 161.
85 Myers, *Tuberculosis among Children and Young Adults*, 292.
86 Goffman, *Asylums.*
87 In 1918, an "up-to-date steam laundry" was installed to service the hospital. Rather than sending out laundry, the on-site facilities proved more cost effective, saving the hospital more than $2,000 in the first six months of operation. "Annual Report of the Physician-in-Chief, W.J. Dobbie," *ARNSA*, 1918–19), 20.
88 The Toronto Free Hospital for Consumptives, the King Edward Sanatorium, and the Queen Mary Hospital for Consumptive Children.
89 Dobbie, *History of the Toronto Hospital for Consumptives*, 5–6.
90 The sanatorium cultivated some twelve acres of land on the hospital grounds for growing a variety of vegetables. This small-scale farming operation kept the patients supplied with vegetables for a few months out of each year while providing light exercise for some of the healthier patients.
91 The hospital ran its own hennery, capable of housing about one thousand birds; the hennery supplied patients with some 77,891 eggs in 1916–17, for example, while some of the fowl was also reserved for "table use." "Annual Report of the Physician-in-Chief, W.J. Dobbie," *ARNSA*, 1916–17, 20.

92 The piggery provided a convenient means for recycling the large quantity of food waste produced by the dining rooms and kitchens. Pigs raised on sanatorium "leftovers" were subsequently sold at market and the money was, in turn, used to support the sanatorium. Given TB transmission concerns, all tray and table waste was "boiled by live steam" before being fed to the pigs. See "Annual Report of the Physician-in-Chief, W.J. Dobbie," *ARNSA*, 1923–24, 28. Over time, the piggery grew in order to accommodate the growing volume of food waste produced by an increasing number of patients occupying an ever-expanding number of beds. As Dobbie explained, the piggery was the most economical means of food waste disposal: "As has been explained before it is difficult to dispose of this material in an institution of this kind. It cannot be sold, as is similar material from hotels and clubs; it is difficult and costly to either burn it or bury it. By feeding it to pigs it becomes a source of revenue." See "Annual Report of the Physician-in-Chief, W.J. Dobbie," *ARNSA*, 1930–31, 23. The money earned through the sale of pigs was not colossal, only 0.7 per cent (or $427.85) of the standard revenue for 1924–25, for example, but it did bring in some money while offsetting disposal costs.

93 Shortt, "Canadian Hospital in the Nineteenth Century," 5.

94 Ibid., 5.

95 Ibid., 6.

96 Ibid., 9.

97 Heron, "Baillie, Sir Frank Wilton."

98 Ibid.

99 Boye, "Finding Amy Sternberg."

100 Heron, "Baillie, Sir Frank Wilton."

101 Taylor, "In the Limelight," 3.

102 Hopkins, *Canadian Annual Review of Public Affairs*, 43.

103 Iles, *Ask the Grey Sisters*, 52.

104 Bergey, "Martin, Jesse Bauman (1897–1974)"; Erb Street Church Cemetery, "Jesse B 'JB' Martin and Naomi Collier Martin," erbstchurch.ca/who-we-are/cemetery/.

105 The Hospital for Sick Children did, however, retain a role in tuberculosis work. On 24 September 1928 the first patients were transported to a new convalescent hospital known as the Country Branch of the Hospital for Sick Children, located in Thistletown, Ontario (now known as

Rexdale, on the outskirts of Toronto's city centre). When it opened, the convalescent hospital had a capacity for 120 patients, but plans were in the works to expand to 300 beds. The hospital was "particularly equipped for the sun treatment of tuberculosis, arrangements having been made so that all patients can be moved directly out of their wards into the sunshine." "News Notes," *Journal of Bone and Joint Surgery* 11, no. 1 (1929): 168.

106 Archives of Ontario, series MS 935, reel 14.

107 Obituary, "Dr William James Dobbie," *Canadian Medical Association Journal* 46, no. 6 (1942): 625.

108 University of Toronto Yearbook entry, "Dr William James Dobbie," University of Toronto Archives, file A73-0026/85 (38).

109 Ibid.

110 "Bury Dr W.J. Dobbie, Long Hospital Chief," *Star*, 22 April 1942, scrapbook article from "Dr William James Dobbie," University of Toronto Archives, file A73-0026/85 (38).

111 Shorter, *Bedside Manners*, 78.

112 Ibid., 130.

113 Ibid., 51.

114 Ibid., 128–30.

115 Ibid.

116 Gale, *Changing Years*, 13; according to Dobbie, *The History of the Toronto Hospital for Consumptives*, Adams had served as physician-in-chief when the Toronto sanatorium opened in 1904, a position he had accepted after working as an associate physician at the National Sanitarium Association's Muskoka Free Hospital for Consumptives in Gravenhurst, Ontario.

117 Gale, *Changing Years*, 13.

118 Obituary, "Dr William James Dobbie"; "Noted Fighter against T.B. Dr W.J. Dobbie Stricken," *Telegram*, 20 April 1942, scrapbook article from "Dr William James Dobbie."

119 Gale, "Oral Histories – Robinson."

120 Paine and Hershfield, "Tuberculosis: Past, Present and Future," 57.

121 Williams, Healey, and Gow, "Death Throes of Tradition," 553.

122 Hobbs, "Before the Sanatorium."

123 Gale, "Oral Histories – Wilson."

124 Gale, "Oral Histories – Young."
125 Gale, "Oral Histories – Davis."
126 Ibid.
127 Bryder, *Below the Magic Mountain*, 203.
128 Esslemont, "Sanatoriums from Within," 1639.
129 "Bury Dr W.J. Dobbie, Long Hospital Chief."
130 *Toronto Sunday World*, 9 May 1915, 37.
131 "Noted Fighter against T.B. Dr W.J. Dobbie Stricken."
132 Dobbie, *History of the Toronto Hospital for Consumptives*, 2.
133 Gale, *Changing Years*, 118.
134 "On Dit," *Daily Mail and Empire*, 25 September 1900.
135 "Hospital and Training-School Items," *American Journal of Nursing* 6, no. 3 (1905): 199–200.
136 Jardine, "Urban Middle-Class Calling," 188.
137 Ibid.
138 Randal, "Editorial," *Canadian Nurse and Hospital Review* 26, no. 8 (1920): 478.
139 "Edith MacPherson Dickson, c. 1876–1966," Canadian Nurses Association Memorial: www.cna-aiic.ca/~/media/cna/page-content/pdf-en/cna-memorial-book-2017.pdf?la=en; Dickson, "Report of the Thirteenth Annual Convention"; "The Graduate Nurses' Association of Ontario Incorporated 1908," *Canadian Nurse and Hospital Review* 16, no. 6 (1920): 375; Canadian Nurses' Association, "Dominion Registration of Nurses."
140 International Council of Nurses, "Tentative Programme."
141 Gale, *Changing Years*, 38.
142 During her training at the Toronto General Hospital School for Nurses, Dickson studied under Mary Agnes Snively, the superintendent of nurses from 1884 to 1910; see Jardine, "Urban Middle-Class Calling."
143 "Edith MacPherson Dickson, c. 1876–1966."
144 Gale, *Changing Years*.
145 Dobbie, *History of the Toronto Hospital for Consumptives*, 2.
146 Bryder, *Below the Magic Mountain*.
147 Kirby and Madsen, "Institutionalised Isolation."
148 Esslemont, "Sanatoriums from Within," 1640.
149 Jardine, "Urban Middle-Class Calling," 185.

150 Gale, *Changing Years,* 37.
151 Jardine, "Urban Middle-Class Calling," 180.
152 Gale, *Changing Years,* 38.
153 Ibid.
154 Gale, *Changing Years*; Jardine, "Urban Middle-Class Calling."
155 Gale, "Oral Histories – Davis."
156 Gale, "Oral Histories – Grant."
157 Jardine, "Urban Middle-Class Calling," 179.
158 Gale, "Oral Histories – Grant."
159 Jardine, "Urban Middle-Class Calling," 183.
160 Gale, "Oral Histories – Davis."
161 Ibid.
162 Ibid.
163 Ibid.
164 Gale, *Changing Years,* 118. With the departure of Wilkinson in 1943, Miss A. Bell served as lady superintendent from 1943 to 1950, followed by Miss Edith Eldridge from 1950 to 1971.
165 Wilkinson, "Four Score and Ten," 20.
166 Ibid., 22.
167 Introduced by Dr Gallie, professor of surgery and surgeon-in-chief at the Toronto General Hospital, in 1931. See surgery.utoronto.ca/history.
168 Gale, "Oral Histories – Garrett."
169 "Information for Resident Physicians," ca. 1940, West Park Health Centre Archives (hereafter WPHCA).
170 "Resident Physicians," June 1929, WPHCA.
171 Ibid.
172 "Information for Resident Physicians," ca. 1940, WPHCA.
173 Ibid.
174 Ibid.
175 Ibid.
176 "Resident Physicians," June 1929, WPHCA.
177 "Information for Resident Physicians," ca. 1940, WPHCA.
178 Gale, "Oral Histories – Garrett."
179 Ibid.
180 Ibid.
181 Brink, "Division of Tuberculosis Prevention."

182 "News Items," *Canadian Medical Association Journal* 41, no. 1 (1939): 100.
183 Gale, *Changing Years*, 76.
184 "Routine of Physician," June 1929, WPHCA.
185 Gale, *Changing Years*, 80.
186 Ibid., 76.
187 Gale, "Oral Histories – Clark"; Gale, "Oral Histories – Davis."
188 Gale, "Oral Histories – King."
189 Gale, "Oral Histories – Davis."
190 Gale, *Changing Years*, 53-54.
191 Connor, "Adoption and Effects of X-rays in Ontario," 101.
192 Holbrook, "Tuberculosis in General Practice," 123.
193 Gale, "Oral Histories – Garrett."
194 Gale, "Oral Histories – Davis."
195 Ibid.
196 Gale, *Changing Years*, 54.
197 Grzybowski and Allen, "Tuberculosis: 2. History of the Disease in Canada," 1027.
198 Ibid.
199 Hobbs, "After the Sanatorium."
200 Gale, "Oral Histories – Garrett."
201 Gale, *Changing Years*, 66.
202 Kirby and Madsen, "Institutionalised Isolation," 127.
203 Gale, "Oral Histories – Grant."
204 Marcellus, "Tiny Cripples and the Sunshine of Life," 418.
205 Anderson, "Nursing the Patient with Bone and Joint Tuberculosis," 216.
206 Gale, "Oral Histories – Grant."
207 Gale, "Oral Histories – Young."
208 Gale, *Changing Years*, 36.
209 Rothman, *Living in the Shadow of Death*.
210 For physicians, the wearing of laboratory coats in practice can be traced back to the late nineteenth century when "the medical profession turned to science" to build its credibility. Physicians seeking to represent themselves as scientists donned lab coats, the symbolism of which came to be associated with modern, scientific medicine, or biomedicine. While nineteenth-century lab coats were originally beige, physicians chose

white to convey "purity," "cleanliness," and "seriousness of purpose" in medical professionalism and compassion. See Jones, "White Coat."

211 "Hospital Rules for Physicians, Nurses, Employees, and Others," June 1929, WPHCA.

212 Shaw and Reeves, *The Children of Craig-y-nos*, 69.

213 Barratt, Shaban, and Moyle, "Patient Experience of Source Isolation"; Hansel et al., "Quality of Life in Tuberculosis"; Madeo, "Understanding the MRSA Experience"; Mayho, "Barrier Grief."

214 Gale, "Oral Histories – Young."

215 Ibid.

216 "Hospital Rules for Physicians, Nurses, Employees, and Others," June 1929, WPHCA.

217 A focus on hand-washing to prevent disease transmission in hospitals caring for patients with infectious diseases was also noted in a 1913 publication by Toronto's Riverdale Isolation Hospital's medical superintendent. See Whyte, "How Can Cross-Infection Be Prevented in a Hospital for Communicable Disease."

218 Gale, "Oral Histories – Young."

219 Gale, "Oral Histories – Davis."

220 Sepkowitz, "Tuberculosis and the Health Care Worker."

221 Wells, "On Airbone Infection, Study II."

222 Brown, "Proper Dosage of Air, Food and Rest in Pulmonary Tuberculosis," 530.

223 Riley, "Aerial Dissemination of Pulmonary Tuberculosis"; Riley, Mills, and Nyka, "Aerial Dissemination of Tuberculosis"; Riley et al., "Infectiousness of Air from a Tuberculosis Ward."

224 Daniel, Bates, and Downes, "History of Tuberculosis"; Escombe et al., "Upper-Room Ultraviolet Light and Negative Air Ionization."

225 Sepkowitz, "Tuberculosis and the Health Care Worker," 76.

226 Escombe et al., "Upper-Room Ultraviolet Light and Negative Air Ionization"; Memarzadeh, Olmsted, and Bartley, "Applications of Ultraviolet Germicidal Irradiation Disinfection."

227 For insights on the design of the National Sanitarium Association buildings in Muskoka and Toronto, see Adams and Burke, "Not a Shack in the Woods."

228 Hobday, "Sunlight Therapy and Solar Architecture," 456.

229 See Maitland, "Design of Tuberculosis Sanatoria"; Adams and Burke, "Not a Shack in the Woods."

230 "Rules for Employees' Quarters," 1915, WPHCA.

231 Perhaps challenged by this rule, Dobbie wrote to the Liquor Control Board of Ontario some years later, in 1934, enquiring whether employees living at the hospital could keep liquor in their bedrooms. The solicitor responding on behalf of the Liquor Control Board affirmed that employees could have liquor since they were occupying a "residence" under the terms of the Act (although the solicitor noted, somewhat confusingly, that the hospital could enforce its own rules independent of the Act).

232 "Rules for Employees' Dining Room," 1915, WPHCA.

233 Shaw and Reeves, *Children of Craig-y-nos*, 66.

CHAPTER THREE

1 Stobie, "Prognosis in Pulmonary Tuberculosis," 507.

2 Tomes, "Making of a Germ Panic."

3 Sakula, "Robert Koch: The Story," S7.

4 A sterile solution of specially cultured, boiled, filtered, and concentrated *Mycobacterium tuberculosis*.

5 Myers et al., *Tuberculosis among Children and Young Adults*, 62–3.

6 Ibid., 310.

7 Parsons, "Tuberculosis Contacts," 502.

8 Canadian Tuberculosis Association, *Handbook for Tuberculosis Patients*, 22.

9 Ibid.

10 Myers et al., *Tuberculosis among Children and Young Adults*, 343.

11 Ibid.

12 Elliott, "Treatment of Pulmonary Tuberculosis," 380.

13 Dobbie, "What Should Be Taught To-day about the Prevention of Tuberculosis," 229.

14 Bayne, "I'm Afraid It's Bad News," 258.

15 Jeanes, "Tuberculosis," 34.

16 Gagneux, "Host-Pathogen Coevolution in Human Tuberculosis," 856.

17 Armstrong, "Patient's View," 740–1.

18 Esslemont, "Sanatoriums from Within," 1639.

19 Shorter, *Bedside Manners*, 118–19.
20 Ibid., 57.
21 Chronic cough is still "one of the most common complaints for which patients seek medical attention"; see Irwin, "Introduction to the Diagnosis and Management of Cough," S25; Irwin and Madison, "Symptom Research on Chronic Cough"; Dalal and Geraci, "Office Management of the Patient with Chronic Cough."
22 Shorter, *Bedside Manners*, 119.
23 Thanks to Ann Herring (Anthropology, McMaster University) for suggesting the importance of the 1918–19 influenza pandemic.
24 Starr, "Politics of Therapeutic Nihilism," 26.
25 Shorter, *Bedside Manners*, 107.
26 Wood, "Phthisis in Adolescence and Early Adult Life," 509.
27 Shorter, *Bedside Manners*, 93.
28 Shorter, *Bedside Manners*.
29 Ibid., 92.
30 Stobie, "Prognosis in Pulmonary Tuberculosis," 509.
31 Rosenberg, "Therapeutic Revolution"; Shorter, *Bedside Manners*.
32 Paine and Hershfield, "Tuberculosis," 55.
33 Pope, "Role of the Sanatorium," 327.
34 Rothman, *Living in the Shadow of Death*.
35 Hurt, "Tuberculosis Sanatorium Regimen," 350.
36 Seabrook, *Working-Class Childhood*, 61.
37 Ibid., 62.
38 Ibid., 63.
39 Deming, *Home Care of Tuberculosis*, 20.
40 McCuaig, *The Weariness, the Fever, and the Fret*, 171–2.
41 Deming, *Home Care of Tuberculosis*, 20.
42 Shaw and Reeves, *Children of Craig-y-nos*.
43 Ibid., 52, 43, 84.
44 Ibid., 83.
45 Ibid., 84.
46 Ibid., 52.
47 Ripley, *Thine Own Keeper*, 175–6.
48 Bashford, "Cultures of Confinement," 131.
49 Ibid., 134.

50 Jeanes, "Tuberculosis," 35.
51 Though whether or not Estelle actually had TB remained contentious. The home-town physician attending to Estelle did not think she was tuberculous, much to the disgust of Estelle's daughter, who, when her mother was admitted, wrote to the sanatorium stating that the local doctor "went around town telling everyone that Mother had no more tuberculosis than he has … All this Doctor is good for is maternity cases and extracting children's teeth."
52 A Moro test was similar to the tuberculin skin test used for detecting histories of tuberculosis infection. While the tuberculin skin test consists of an injection of tuberculin, the Moro test procedure involved rubbing an ointment containing tuberculin on the skin. Results could be read from the skin within one to two days; when positive for infection, reddish papules appeared on the skin.
53 Myers et al., *Tuberculosis among Children and Young Adults.*
54 Ibid., 282.
55 Ibid.
56 Ibid.
57 Ibid., 283.
58 Holbrook, "Tuberculosis in General Practice," 129.
59 Myers, *Tuberculosis among Children and Young Adults*, 161.
60 Holbrook, "Tuberculosis in General Practice," 129.
61 Minns, "Practical Management of Pulmonary Tuberculosis."
62 Ibid., 160.
63 Ibid.
64 Ibid., 167.
65 Myers, *Tuberculosis among Children and Young Adults*, 271–2.
66 Minns, "Practical Management of Pulmonary Tuberculosis," 163.
67 Gale, "Oral Histories – Wilson."
68 Ibid.
69 Shaw and Reeves, *Children of Craig-y-nos*, 44.
70 Gale, "Oral Histories – Wilson."
71 Hobbs, "Before the Sanatorium."
72 See Crockett *et al.,* "Nosocomial Transmission of Congenital Tuberculosis"; Smith, "Congenital Tuberculosis"; Winters et al., "Congenital Tuberculosis and Management of Exposure."

73 Gale, "Oral Histories – Garrett."
74 See Murray, "Governing 'Unwed Mothers' in Toronto."
75 Neff, "Government Approaches to Child Neglect and Mistreatment," 202.
76 Ibid.
77 In recognition that children interact with their environments in ways different from adults, such as mouthing and sharing toys in communal settings, more focused guidelines for the prevention of microbial transmission have been developed. See, for example, Avila-Aguero et al., "Toys in a Pediatric Hospital"; Canadian Partnership for Children's Health and Environment, *Advancing Environmental Health in Child Care Settings.*
78 "News." *Canadian Medical Association Journal* 3, no. 3 (1913): 240.
79 Struthers, "In the Interests of the Children," 66.
80 Neff, "Role of the Toronto Girls' Home."
81 Kendig Jr and Inselman, "Tuberculosis in Children," 241.
82 *ARNSA*, 1936, 26.
83 *ARNSA*, 1913–14, 38.
84 *ARNSA*, 1936, 25.
85 Strange, "'She Cried a Very Little,'" 146.
86 Dubos and Dubos, *White Plague*, 67; Myers, *Tuberculosis among Children and Young Adults*, 312. This phenomenon has also been described as the "favored age," for its lower active case rate; see Agrons, Markowitz, and Kramer, "Pulmonary Tuberculosis in Children," 158.
87 Myers, *Tuberculosis among Children and Young Adults*, 316.
88 According to Poutanen et al., at Montreal's Mount Sinai Sanatorium, morbidly ill patients could be discharged "since the sanatorium, from the physician's perspective, was an institution for cure." Poutanen et al., "Tuberculosis in Town," 101.
89 See the City of Toronto Archives' Web Exhibit "An Infectious Idea: Hospitals and Ambulance Services."
90 Miliary tuberculosis has been described as an "acute generalized tuberculosis, marked by the presence of numerous minute tubercles in the affected organs or tissues." *Stedman's Medical Dictionary* 1949, 739.
91 Also known as the Sacrament of the Anointing of the Sick, for Catholics, last rites are intended to replace fear with hope in death, and to secure forgiveness for sins if Confession is not possible.

92 Jones, "Politicizing the Laboring Body," 58.
93 Ibid., 58.
94 Strange, "'She Cried a Very Little,'" 144.
95 The hospitalization charges of residents of unorganized territories and Indigenous patients living on reserves were paid by the provincial and federal governments, respectively.
96 Strange, "'She Cried a Very Little,'" 149.
97 Rales are varied adventitious sounds that are heard on auscultation; moist rales are "of a bubbling character caused by the pressure of a fluid secretion in the bronchial tubes or a cavity." *Stedman's Medical Dictionary* 1949, 1013.
98 Gale, "Oral Histories – Wilson."
99 Shaw and Reeves, *Children of Craig-y-nos*, 48.
100 Ibid., 42.
101 Duffin, *History of Medicine*, 330.
102 Canadian Tuberculosis Association, *Handbook for Tuberculosis Patients*, 27–8.
103 Shorter, *Bedside Manners*, 107.

CHAPTER FOUR

1 Myers et al., *Tuberculosis among Children and Young Adults*, 318.
2 Horsburgh Jr, "Priorities for the Treatment of Latent Tuberculosis Infection."
3 Farmer, "Anthropology of Structural Violence."
4 Cassidy, "Address to the Association of Executive Health Officers of Ontario," 147–8.
5 Kline and Lorin, "Childhood Tuberculosis," 138.
6 Ibid.
7 Jackson and McLeod, "Tuberculosis in Infants, Children, and Adolescents," 414.
8 Versus T_h2, or T helper 2, type immunity, also known as humoral or antibody-mediated immunity, an immune response effective against extracellular pathogens present in body fluids such as the bloodstream.
9 Jackson and McLeod, "Tuberculosis in Infants, Children, and Adolescents," 414.
10 Armstrong and Hart, "Response of Cultured Macrophages to *Mycobacterium tuberculosis*."

11 Jacobs and Eisenach, "Childhood Tuberculosis," 24; Jackson and McLeod, "Tuberculosis in Infants, Children, and Adolescents," 414.
12 Marais et al., "Natural History of Childhood Intra-Thoracic Tuberculosis."
13 Kendig Jr and Inselman, "Tuberculosis in Children," 235.
14 Pezzella and Fang, "Surgical Aspects of Thoracic Tuberculosis," 793.
15 Ibid.
16 Myers et al., *Tuberculosis among Children and Young Adults*, 198.
17 Grzybowski and Allen, "History and Importance of Scrofula."
18 Jadvar et al., "Still the Great Mimicker."
19 Price, "Mediastinal Gland Tuberculosis in Young Children," 200.
20 Zychowicz, "Osteoarticular Manifestations of *Mycobacterium tuberculosis* Infection."
21 Kline and Lorin, "Childhood Tuberculosis," 139-40.
22 Erb, "Pathology of Mediastinal Tuberculosis," 506.
23 Kline and Lorin, "Childhood Tuberculosis," 139–40.
24 *Stedman's Medical Dictionary* 1949, 544.
25 In a 1924 publication, Griffith called for the abandonment of the use of the term *scrofula* altogether since he felt it was used too liberally: "It is a mistake to call the delicate, flabby children with enlarged glands and sore eyes 'scrofulous.' Some of them are tuberculous, some syphilitic, and some owe their ailments to other causes. The term, if used at all, should be applied only to tuberculous inflammation of the glands of the neck." Griffith, *Care of the Baby*, 353.
26 Jacobs and Eisenach, "Childhood Tuberculosis," 28.
27 Gale, "Oral Histories – Wilson."
28 Myers et al., *Tuberculosis among Children and Young Adults*, 202.
29 Ibid., 203.
30 Starr, "Treatment of Tuberculous Affections of Bones and Joints"; Wilson, "Treatment of Tuberculous Hip Disease."
31 Marais et al., "The Natural History of Childhood Intra-Thoracic Tuberculosis," 393.
32 Ibid., 394.
33 Kline and Lorin, "Childhood Tuberculosis," 139–40.
34 Belcher, "Surgical Collapse Therapy in Pulmonary Tuberculosis," 300.
35 *Stedman's Medical Dictionary* 1949, 940.

36 Marais et al., "Natural History of Childhood Intra-Thoracic Tuberculosis," 393.

37 Murray, "Bill Dock and the Location of Pulmonary Tuberculosis."

38 Another laboratory test popular in the sanatorium era evaluated the relative proportions of young, mature, and old lymphocytes in blood samples. Lymphocytes generally increase in number as the body attempts to heal tissues damaged by TB bacteria (or other pathogens). In a typical blood sample, a ratio of 4 per cent young, 48 per cent mature, and 48 per cent old lymphocytes was expected. In active tuberculosis, when "large numbers of lymphocytes are in demand" and "when there is rapid destruction of lymphocytes," fewer lymphocytes survive to the old stage. As a result, an old lymphocyte proportion of 30 per cent or less was considered a strong indication of active disease. See Myers et al., *Tuberculosis among Children and Young Adults*, 266, 274.

39 "Erythrocyte Sedimentation Rate."

40 Myers, *Tuberculosis among Children and Young Adults*, 270.

41 See Hesseling et al., "Mycobacterial Genotype is Associated with Disease Phenotype."

42 Shaw and Reeves, *Children of Craig-y-nos*, 51.

43 It was generally recommended that patients not swallow any sputum that was coughed up, since "the bacilli may be carried to a new growing ground other than the lungs." Minns, "Practical Management of Pulmonary Tuberculosis," 168. It was believed that women were more likely to swallow their sputum than men. Neal, "Early Diagnosis of Pulmonary Tuberculosis."

44 Starke, "Childhood Tuberculosis in the 1990s," 558–9.

45 See Ferrer, "Pleural Tuberculosis."

46 The pleural cavity occupies the space between a two-layer membrane composed of the outer pleura, a membrane lining the chest wall, and the inner pleura, a membrane that covers the lungs and bronchi.

47 Fanning, "Tuberculosis: 6. Extra-Pulmonary Disease," 1600.

48 Kline and Lorin, "Childhood Tuberculosis," 147; Jacobs and Eisenach, "Childhood Tuberculosis," 28.

49 Elliott, "Treatment of Pulmonary Tuberculosis," 379–80; Agrons, Markowitz, and Kramer, "Pulmonary Tuberculosis in Children," 159; McCuaig, *The Weariness, the Fever, and the Fret*.

50 Girdlestone, "Pott's Disease and Pott's Paraplegia."

51 Hesseling *et al.*, "Mycobacterial Genotype Is Associated with Disease Phenotype in Children," 1252.

52 Ibid.

53 Ibid., 1256.

54 After the 1779 disease description by British surgeon Percivall Pott (1714–1788) in *Remarks on That Kind of Palsy of the Lower Limbs Which Is Frequently Found to Accompany a Curvature of the Spine and Is Supposed to Be Caused by It. Together with Its Method of Cure*, 1779. See Johnson, Hillman, and Southwick, "Importance of Direct Surgical Attack."

55 Aufderheide and Rodriguez-Martin, with Langsjoen, *Cambridge Encyclopedia of Human Paleopathology.*

56 Moon, "Tuberculosis of the Spine," 1791.

57 Aufderheide and Rodriguez-Martin, with Langsjoen, *Cambridge Encyclopedia of Human Paleopathology.*

58 Morse, "Prehistoric Tuberculosis in America."

59 Pezzella and Fang, "Surgical Aspects of Thoracic Tuberculosis," 795.

60 Ibid.

61 Ibid.

62 Marais et al., "Spectrum of Disease in Children Treated for Tuberculosis,"

63 Starke, "Tuberculosis: An Old Disease but a New Threat."

64 Kendall, "Of What Value are Sanitoria as a Public Health Measure," 206.

65 Canadian Tuberculosis Association, *Handbook for Tuberculosis Patients*, 22.

66 Holbrook, "Present Need of the Tuberculosis Campaign," 462.

67 Gillis, "History of the Patient History," 506.

68 Parsons, "Tuberculosis Contacts," 503.

69 Dow and Lloyd, "Incidence of Tuberculous Infection"; Lloyd and Macpherson, "Pulmonary Tuberculosis in Young Adults."

70 Neff, "Government Approaches to Child Neglect and Mistreatment," 181–3.

71 Parsons, "Tuberculosis Contacts," 503.

72 Canadian Public Health Association, "Minutes of the Section of Infant and Child Welfare."

73 Sakula, "Robert Koch: Centenary."

74 Ontario Provincial Department of Health, "Development of Public Health in Ontario," 112.
75 Elliott, *Present Status of Antituberculosis Work in Canada – 1908*, 6.
76 Hodgetts, "National and Provincial Responsibility in the Tuberculosis Crusade," 220.
77 Holbrook, "Present Need of the Tuberculosis Campaign," 469.
78 Collins, "Tuberculosis in Animals," S19; similar concerns over the transmission of pathogens between species has also been explored by Blue and Rock, "Trans-Biopolitics: Complexity in Interspecies Relations," in the case of BSE.
79 McCuaig, *The Weariness, the Fever, and the Fret*, 169.
80 Ibid., 170.
81 Ibid.
82 Ibid., 171.
83 Ibid., 168.
84 Myers et al., *Tuberculosis among Children and Young Adults*, 208.
85 Ontario Provincial Board of Health, *Report of the International Commission on the Control of Bovine Tuberculosis*, 54.
86 Singer, "Doorways in Nature," 997.
87 Marais et al., "Spectrum of Disease in Children Treated for Tuberculosis"; Schaaf et al., "Adult-to-Child Transmission of Tuberculosis."
88 Schaaf et al., "Adult-to-Child Transmission of Tuberculosis."
89 Gale, "Oral Histories – Garrett."
90 Fanning, "Tuberculosis: 6. Extra-Pulmonary Disease," 1601.
91 Myers, *Tuberculosis among Children and Young Adults*, 162.
92 Ibid.
93 Ibid., 162–5.
94 Ibid., 166.
95 Ibid., 274.
96 Jessel et al., "Modern Developments in the Tuberculosis Scheme," 253.
97 Myers, *Tuberculosis among Children and Young Adults*, 274.
98 Shaw and Reeves, *Children of Craig-y-nos*, 15.
99 Ibid., 16.
100 Gale, "Oral Histories – Wilson."
101 Ripley, *Thine Own Keeper*, 175.
102 von Pirquet, "Das Verhalten der Kutanen Tuberkulinreaktion Während der Masern."

103 Brody, Overfield, and Hammes, "Depression of the Tuberculin Reaction by Viral Vaccines"; Bentzon, "Effect of Certain Infectious Diseases on Tuberculin Allergy."

104 Reed, Olds, and Kisch, "Decreased Skin-Test Reactivity Associated with Influenza."

105 Noymer and Garenne, "1918 Influenza Epidemic's Effects on Sex Differentials in Mortality"; Herring and Sattenspiel, "Social Contexts, Syndemics, and Infectious Disease"; Sawchuk, "Rethinking the Impact of the 1918 Influenza Pandemic."

106 Alexander, "Rôles of Medicine and Surgery in the Management of Bronchiectasis," 569.

107 Ibid.

108 Connolly and Gibson, "'White Plague' and Color," 235.

109 Alexander, "Rôles of Medicine and Surgery in the Management of Bronchiectasis," 577–8.

110 Milk pasteurization became mandatory in Canada in 1938.

111 Even today, the average interval between the initial appearance of suspected symptoms and a final diagnosis of spinal tuberculosis has been found to range between three to six months. Ivo et al., "Tuberculous Spondylitis and Paravertebral Abscess Formation."

112 See Giessler, "Tuberculosis of the Bones and Joints," 216.

113 Ibid.

114 As TB burdens lessened in industrialized countries, psoas abscess diagnoses became rare and more often associated with other infections. In recent years, lack of familiarity has led to delayed diagnoses of TB due to confusion with conditions such as arthritis and abdominal disorders. See, for example, Franco-Paredes and Blumberg, "Psoas Muscle Abscess Caused by *Mycobacterium tuberculosis* and *Staphylococcus aureus*"; Garner et al., "Psoas Abscess: Not as Rare as We Think?"; Gruenwald, Abrahamson, and Cohen, "Psoas Abscess: Case Report and Review of the Literature"; Harrigan, Kauffman, and Love, "Tuberculous Psoas Abscess"; Muckley et al., "Psoas Abscess."

115 Steinbock, *Paleopathological Diagnosis and Interpretation.*

116 Aufderheide and Rodriguez-Martin, with Langsjoen, *Cambridge Encyclopedia of Human Paleopathology.*

117 Robert Inkerman Harris (1889–1966), who specialized in orthopedic

surgery, held weekly clinics at the Toronto sanatorium for thirty-five years. Harris was known to have suffered tuberculosis as a child. See "Robert Inkerman Harris" in Mostofi, *Who's Who in Orthopedics*, 126–7.

118 Though less common in comparison to pulmonary infection, tuberculosis could be transmitted via cutaneous contact with open draining wounds. See Kendig Jr and Inselman, "Tuberculosis in Children," 241.

119 See Smith, "Tuberculosis in Children and Adolescents."

120 Kline and Lorin, "Childhood Tuberculosis"; Long, Njoo, and Hershfield, "Tuberculosis: 3. Epidemiology of the Disease in Canada," 1186.

121 Escombe et al., "Natural Ventilation for the Prevention of Airborne Contagion."

122 See Nardell, "Environmental Control of Tuberculosis."

123 Long, Njoo, and Hershfield, "Tuberculosis: 3. Epidemiology of the Disease in Canada," 1186.

124 Starke, "Childhood Tuberculosis in the 1990s."

125 Dobbie, "What Should Be Taught To-Day about the Prevention of Tuberculosis."

126 Ibid., 230–1.

127 Altet-Gómez et al., "Clinical and Epidemiological Aspects of Smoking and Tuberculosis."

128 Arcavi and Benowitz, "Cigarette Smoking and Infection."

129 Cook, "'Liberation Sticks' or 'Coffin Nails'?," 395.

130 Warsh and Tinkler, "In Vogue: North American and British Representations of Women Smokers."

131 Holbrook, "'Present Need of the Tuberculosis Campaign," 462–3.

132 Editorial, "Anti-Spitting By-Law in Toronto," 953.

133 Ibid.

134 Kluger, *Ashes to Ashes*.

135 Chandra, "Nutrition, Immunity and Infection."

136 See reviews in Cegielski and McMurray, "The Relationship between Malnutrition and Tuberculosis"; Chandra, "Nutrition, Immunity and Infection"; Vijayakumar, Bhaskaram, and Hemalatha, "Malnutrition and Childhood Tuberculosis."

137 Stapleford, "Neighbourhood Workers' Association," 327.

138 Cegielski and McMurray, "Relationship between Malnutrition and

Tuberculosis"; Chan et al., "Effects of Protein Calorie Malnutrition on Tuberculosis in Mice"; Schaible and Kaufmann, "Malnutrition and Infection."

139 Barnes et al., "γδ T Lymphocytes in Human Tuberculosis."

140 Schaible and Kaufmann, "Malnutrition and Infection," 0808–9.

141 Cegielski and McMurray, "Relationship between Malnutrition and Tuberculosis," 294. See also Vijayakumar, Bhaskaram, and Hemalatha, "Malnutrition and Childhood Tuberculosis," 297.

142 Cegielski and McMurray, "Relationship between Malnutrition and Tuberculosis," 294.

143 Boyd, "Streptomycin in Childhood Tuberculosis," 479.

144 Schaible and Kaufmann, "Malnutrition and Infection."

145 Katona and Katona-Apte, "Interaction between Nutrition and Infection."

146 Ibid.; Ramachandran *et al.*, "Vitamin A Levels in Sputum-Positive Pulmonary Tuberculosis Patients."

147 Chandra, "Increased Bacterial Binding to Respiratory Epithelial Cells in Vitamin A Deficiency."

148 Kosek and Oberhelman, "Unraveling the Contradictions of Vitamin A and Infectious Diseases in Children," 965.

149 Varughese, "Measles in Canada."

150 King et al., "Measles Elimination in Canada."

151 Ibid.; Varughese, "Measles in Canada."

152 For a textbook introduction to this subject, see Molnar, *Human Variation.*

153 Stone et al., "Tuberculosis and Leprosy in Perspective."

154 Larcombe et al., "Differential Cytokine Genotype Frequencies."

155 Ibid.

156 Reviewed by Donoghue et al., "Tuberculosis: From Prehistory to Robert Koch."

157 Brosch et al., "New Evolutionary Scenario."

158 Waldram, Herring, and Young, "Aboriginal Health in Canada."

159 The federal government was responsible for funding sanatorium care for Indigenous patients admitted from reserves or residential schools.

160 According to the Truth and Reconciliation Commission of Canada, see www.trc.ca.

161 Elliott and de Leeuw, "Our Aboriginal Relations"; Macaulay, "Improving Aboriginal Health."

162 Waldram, Herring, and Young, "Aboriginal Health in Canada"; Grzybowski and Allen, "Tuberculosis: 2. History of the Disease in Canada"; Grygier, *Long Way from Home*; see also Roberts and Buikstra, *Bioarchaeology of Tuberculosis.*
163 Scambler and Hopkins, "Being Epileptic."
164 Gale, "Oral Histories – Wilson."
165 Bashford, "Cultures of Confinement," 126.
166 Ibid., 127.
167 Ibid., 131.
168 Rothman, *Living in the Shadow of Death.*
169 Hobbs, "Before the Sanatorium."
170 Ibid.
171 Ripley, *Thine Own Keeper*, 176-177.
172 Ludwig, "Emotional Factors in Tuberculosis," 884.
173 McCuaig, *The Weariness, the Fever, and the Fret.* See chapter 2, "Tuberculosis and the Great War."
174 Park, "Causes of Rejection from the Army," 412.
175 Park, "Causes of Rejection from the Army."
176 For a brief review, see Burke and Sawchuk, "Tuberculosis Mortality and Recent Childbirth."
177 Smith, *Retreat of Tuberculosis, 1850-1950.*
178 Snider, "Pregnancy and Tuberculosis."
179 Mathad and Gupta, "Tuberculosis in Pregnant and Postpartum Women," 1534.
180 See Blaser and Kirschner, "The Equilibria That Allow Bacterial Persistence in Human Hosts"; Gagneux, "Host-Pathogen Coevolution in Human Tuberculosis."
181 Lerner, "Constructing Medical Indications."
182 Myers, *Tuberculosis among Children and Young Adults*, 201.
183 Ibid.

CHAPTER FIVE

1 Canadian Tuberculosis Association, *Handbook for Tuberculosis Patients*, 17–18.
2 Warner, "From Specificity to Universalism in Medical Therapeutics," 87–8.
3 Ibid., 91–2.

4 Rosenberg, "Therapeutic Revolution," 13.
5 Ibid., 9; Warner, "From Specificity to Universalism in Medical Therapeutics."
6 Rosenberg, "Therapeutic Revolution," 5.
7 Warner, "From Specificity to Universalism in Medical Therapeutics," 91.
8 Osborne and Fogarty, "Medical Climatology in France," 544.
9 Warner, "From Specificity to Universalism in Medical Therapeutics," 92.
10 Rosenberg, "Therapeutic Revolution."
11 Starr, "Politics of Therapeutic Nihilism," 24.
12 Rosenberg, "Therapeutic Revolution," 11.
13 Ibid.
14 Starr, "Politics of Therapeutic Nihilism," 24.
15 Lawrence, "Still Incommunicable," 102.
16 Currow and Abernethy, "Therapeutic Nihilism," 69.
17 Rosenberg, "Therapeutic Revolution," 15.
18 The idea of "conservative treatment," which I read as related to therapeutic nihilism, is mentioned in Winnett, "Bier's Hyperemic Treatment," 330.
19 Rosenberg, "Therapeutic Revolution," 8.
20 Ibid., 8.
21 Ibid.
22 Ibid., 18.
23 Warner, "From Specificity to Universalism in Medical Therapeutics," 87–8.
24 Proctor, "Pulmonary Tuberculosis: Its Treatment and Prevention," 155 (italics in original).
25 Starr, "Treatment of Tuberculous Affections of Bones and Joints," 160.
26 Bethune, "Plea for Early Compression in Pulmonary Tuberculosis," 37.
27 For a detailed review, see Inhorn and Whittle, "Feminism Meets the 'New' Epidemiologies."
28 The black-and-white silent film, with a playtime of just over eighteen minutes, has been uploaded to YouTube by Library and Archives Canada; see http://www.youtube.com/watch?v=HfLirbpOD-w.
29 For a discussion on the problems inherent in the individualizing of risk, see Inhorn and Whittle, "Feminism Meets the 'New' Epidemiologies."
30 See, for example, Uhlin et al., "Adjunct Immunotherapies for Tuberculosis."

31 Rosenberg, "Therapeutic Revolution," 17.
32 Ibid.
33 Elliott, "Sanatorium," 33.
34 Brown, "Proper Dosage of Air, Food and Rest in Pulmonary Tuberculosis," 534.
35 Cassidy, "Prevention of Tuberculosis," 114.
36 Brown, "Proper Dosage of Air, Food and Rest in Pulmonary Tuberculosis," 533.
37 Elliott, "Sanatorium," 117–18.
38 Ibid.
39 Marshall, "My Personal Experience of Tuberculosis," 495.
40 Ibid.
41 Norton, "*Whole Little City by Itself*," 59.
42 Recent research suggests that a cholesterol-rich diet (and eggs and milk are cholesterol-rich) may shorten the duration of active disease among patients treated with antibiotics; biologically, a cholesterol-rich diet is believed to influence the fluidity of macrophage membranes, and more fluid membranes may enhance the ability of macrophages to ingest tuberculosis bacteria and, therefore, result in more effective control of infection. See Pérez-Guzmán et al., "Cholesterol-Rich Diet Accelerates Bacteriologic Sterilization in Pulmonary Tuberculosis."
43 Minns, "Practical Management of Pulmonary Tuberculosis."
44 Dobbie, "Hygienic, Dietetic and Medicinal Treatment of Tuberculosis," 156.
45 Kendall, "Observations Relating to Diet in Tuberculosis," 673.
46 Esslemont, "Sanatoriums from Within," 1640.
47 Minns, "Practical Management of Pulmonary Tuberculosis," 166.
48 Myers, *Tuberculosis among Children and Young Adults*, 283.
49 Dobbie, "Hygienic, Dietetic and Medicinal Treatment of Tuberculosis," 157.
50 Cassidy, "Prevention of Tuberculosis," 114.
51 Kendall, "Observations Relating to Diet in Tuberculosis," 674.
52 Jarman, "Awaiting Sanatorium Treatment," 261.
53 Knox-Macaulay, "Tuberculosis and the Haemopoietic System"; Weiss and Goodnough, "Anemia of Chronic Disease."
54 Kent, Weinberg, and Stuart-Macadam, "The Etiology of the Anemia of Chronic Disease and Infection."

55 Zhang and Rovin, "Beyond Anemia: Hepcidin, Monocytes and Inflammation," 234.
56 Knox-Macaulay, "Tuberculosis and the Haemopoietic System"; Weiss and Goodnough, "Anemia of Chronic Disease."
57 Kent, Weinberg, and Stuart-Macadam, "Etiology of the Anemia of Chronic Disease and Infection"; Stuart-Macadam, "Integrative Anthropology: A Focus on Iron-Deficiency Anemia."
58 Patricia Stuart-Macadam notes the influence that American microbiologist Eugene Weinberg's concept of "iron-withholding" had on her reinterpretations of porotic hyperostosis in paleopathological studies of past populations. See Stuart-Macadam, "Integrative Anthropology: A Focus on Iron-Deficiency Anemia"; Stuart-Macadam, "Porotic Hyperostosis: A New Perspective"; Weinberg, "Iron and Susceptibility to Infectious Disease."
59 Weiss and Goodnough, "Anemia of Chronic Disease."
60 Kent, Weinberg, and Stuart-Macadam, "Etiology of the Anemia of Chronic Disease and Infection," 26.
61 Ibid.
62 See Wagner-Jauregg, "Nobel Lecture."
63 Myers, *Tuberculosis among Children and Young Adults*, 285.
64 Cassidy, "Formula for Giving Alcohol in Fevers," 273.
65 Rosenberg, "Therapeutic Revolution," 17.
66 Cassidy, "Formula for Giving Alcohol in Fevers," 271.
67 Ellman, "Co-relation of Calcium Metabolism, Parathyroid Function and Pulmonary Tuberculosis," 163.
68 Ibid., 163–4.
69 Ibid.
70 Symons, "Treatment of Tuberculosis with Colloid Calcium."
71 Moe, "Disorders Involving Calcium, Phosphorus, and Magnesium."
72 Prest, "Treatment of Tuberculosis with Colloid of Calcium."
73 Myers, *Tuberculosis among Children and Young Adults*, 284.
74 Arnup, "Raising the Dionne Quintuplets."
75 Gillis, "Taking the Medical History in Childhood Illness," 398.
76 Arnup, "Raising the Dionne Quintuplets."
77 Gale, "Oral Histories – Wilson."
78 The idea of an evolving "fashion" in tuberculosis treatments is from Spriggs, "Rest and Exercise in Pulmonary Tuberculosis."

79 Ibid.
80 Fowler, "Therapeutic Value of Sanatorium Treatment in Pulmonary Tuberculosis."
81 Ibid., 5.
82 Wilson, "Treatment of Tuberculous Hip Disease by Weight-Bearing and Fixation," 440.
83 Spriggs, "Rest and Exercise in Pulmonary Tuberculosis."
84 Ibid., 460.
85 For a more detailed analysis, see Adams and Burke, "Not a Shack in the Woods."
86 Rogers, "Rise and Decline of the Altitude Therapy of Tuberculosis," 14.
87 Spriggs, "Rest and Exercise in Pulmonary Tuberculosis," 460.
88 Paine and Hershfield, "Tuberculosis: Past, Present and Future," 56.
89 Spriggs, "Rest and Exercise in Pulmonary Tuberculosis," 461.
90 Fowler, "Therapeutic Value of Sanatorium Treatment in Pulmonary Tuberculosis," 5.
91 Cassidy's biography is detailed in MacDougall, "Cassidy, John Joseph."
92 Cassidy, "Prevention of Tuberculosis."
93 Fowler, "Therapeutic Value of Sanatorium Treatment in Pulmonary Tuberculosis," 5.
94 Ibid., 6.
95 Ibid.
96 Esslemont, "Sanatoriums from Within," 1640.
97 Trudeau, "Adirondack Cottage Sanitarium for the Treatment of Incipient Pulmonary Tuberculosis," 377.
98 Ibid.
99 Ibid.
100 Minns, "Practical Management of Pulmonary Tuberculosis," 162.
101 Canadian Tuberculosis Association, *Handbook for Tuberculosis Patients*, 15.
102 Cassidy, "Address to the Association of Executive Health Officers of Ontario," 150.
103 Allbutt et al., "Value of Sanatorium Treatment," 180.
104 Ibid.
105 Ibid., 181.
106 Ibid.
107 Murray, "Bill Dock and the Location of Pulmonary Tuberculosis," 1029.

108 Colbeck and Pritchard, "Explanation of the Vulnerability of the Apices in Tuberculosis of the Lungs."
109 As reviewed by Murray, "Bill Dock and the Location of Pulmonary Tuberculosis," 1029.
110 Bryan, "Distribution of Ventilation and Perfusion in the Normal Lung," 3.
111 See Blessing, *Pathways of Homeopathic Medicine*, chap. 3.
112 Winnett, "Bier's Hyperemic Treatment, with Demonstration of Technique," 330.
113 Ibid.
114 Ibid.
115 Ibid.
116 Bennett, "Induced Hyperaemia as a Means of Treatment," 1533.
117 Waterhouse, "Address on Professor Bier's Treatment by Means of Induced Hyperaemia," 125.
118 Ibid.
119 Ibid.
120 Ibid., 126.
121 Walsh, "Pulmonary Activity Greatest at the Apex and Least at the Base."
122 Bennett, "Induced Hyperaemia as a Means of Treatment," 1533.
123 Waterhouse, "Address on Professor Bier's Treatment by Means of Induced Hyperaemia," 125.
124 Phelps, "Light Therapy," 876.
125 Ibid.
126 Stoney, "Bier's Method of Treatment by Hyperaemia," 146.
127 Ibid.
128 Tileston, "Passive Hyperemia of the Lungs and Tuberculosis."
129 Ibid., 1181.
130 Ibid.
131 Ibid., 1182.
132 Howarth, "Tuberculosis of the Larynx," 164.
133 Ewart, "Treatment of Bronchiectasis."
134 Wise, "Treatment of Pulmonary Tuberculosis by a Postural Method," 1546.
135 Peter Warren notes that Hermann Brehmer, who founded in the sanatorium movement in 1854, was also concerned with blood circulation to

the lungs, but for different reasons. Brehmer believed that TB was a hereditary disease caused by a weak heart that could not deliver sufficient blood flow or nutrients to the lungs. As a result, Brehmer advised medically supervised exercise to "strengthen the heart, improve the circulation and so heal the lungs." Warren, "Evolution of the Sanatorium," 462.

136 Wise, "Treatment of Pulmonary Tuberculosis by a Postural Method," 1547.

137 Ibid.

138 Ewart, "Treatment of Pulmonary Tuberculosis by a Postural Method," 1654.

139 Prisk et al., "Pulmonary Perfusion in the Prone and Supine Postures."

140 Shaw and Reeves, *Children of Craig-y-nos*, 123.

141 Pottenger, "Physiologic Nature of Protective and Healing Principles in Tuberculosis," 225.

142 Odell, "History of Surgery for Pulmonary Tuberculosis," 260.

143 Ibid., 261.

144 An interview with Dr Dock, conducted in 1981, is included in Washington University School of Medicine's Oral History Project. Both a written transcript and an MP3 recording of the interview are available through the Bernard Becker Medical Library at http://beckerexhibits.wustl.edu/oral/transcripts/dock.html. For a brief but candid biography on Dock, see Zoneraich, "Legacy of William Dock." William Dock was born in Ann Arbor, Michigan, in 1898 and died at ninety-one years of age in Guadeloupe in 1990. Dock's publications reviewed here include Dock, "Apical Localization of Phthisis"; and Dock, "Effect of Posture on Alveolar Gas Tension in Tuberculosis."

145 Dock, "Apical Localization of Phthisis," 301.

146 Ibid., 298.

147 Ibid., 300.

148 Ibid., 302.

149 "More Health Talk over the Teacups – Dr W.J. Dobbie Says Great Need in Fighting Tuberculosis Was Publicity – Urges Rest, Nutrition," *Globe*, 14 February 1928, scrapbook article from "Dr William James Dobbie," University of Toronto Archives, file A73-0026/85 (38).

150 Bryan, *Distribution of Ventilation and Perfusion in the Normal Lung*, 3.

151 Rhoades, "Pulmonary Circulation and Ventilation-Perfusion."

152 Bryan, *Distribution of Ventilation and Perfusion in the Normal Lung*, 3.
153 Glenny, "Determinants of Regional Ventilation and Blood Flow in the Lung."
154 Ibid., 1839.
155 Rhoades, "Pulmonary Circulation and Ventilation-Perfusion," 370.
156 Murray, "Bill Dock and the Location of Pulmonary Tuberculosis"; Rhoades, "Pulmonary Circulation and Ventilation-Perfusion."
157 Bryan, *Distribution of Ventilation and Perfusion in the Normal Lung*, 4.
158 Corper, "Organic Tuberculosis in Man," 1757.
159 Ibid., 1760.
160 Walsh, "Pulmonary Activity Greatest at the Apex and Least at the Base."
161 Gordon, "Mechanism and Effects of Abdominal Compression," 197.
162 Ibid., 198.
163 Dock, "Effect of Posture on Alveolar Gas Tension in Tuberculosis."
164 Ibid., 701.
165 Ibid., 706.
166 Ibid., 705.
167 Ibid., 706.
168 Mure et al., "Regional Ventilation-Perfusion Distribution."
169 Glenny et al., "Gravity Is an Important but Secondary Determinant of Regional Pulmonary Blood Flow."
170 Dock, "Effect of Posture on Alveolar Gas Tension in Tuberculosis," 706.
171 Ibid., 707.
172 Abebe and Bjune, "Protective Role of Antibody Responses," 235.
173 Ibid., 236; see also Begg et al., "Does a Th1 over Th2 Dominancy Really Exist"; Glatman-Freedman, "Role of Antibody-Mediated Immunity"; Glatman-Freedman and Casadevall, "Serum Therapy for Tuberculosis Revisited."
174 Glatman-Freedman, "Role of Antibody-Mediated Immunity," 192.
175 Abebe and Bjune, "Protective Role of Antibody Responses," 241.
176 Glatman-Freedman and Casadevall, "Serum Therapy for Tuberculosis Revisited."
177 Abebe and Bjune, "Protective Role of Antibody Responses," 241.
178 Murray, "Bill Dock and the Location of Pulmonary Tuberculosis," 1029–30; Long, "Canadian Lung Association/Canadian Thoracic Society," 428.

179 Glatman-Freedman and Casadevall, "Serum Therapy for Tuberculosis Revisited," 520.

180 Sever and Youmans, "The Relation of Oxygen Tension to Virulence of Tubercle Bacilli," 201, 202.

181 Ibid., 201.

182 Riboldi et al., "Hypoxia-Mediated Regulation of Macrophage Functions," 70.

183 Rustad et al., "Hypoxia," 1152.

184 Nickel et al., "Hypoxia Triggers the Expression of Human β Defensin 2 and Antimicrobial Activity," 4005.

185 Ibid., 4006.

CHAPTER SIX

1 Bethune, "Plea for Early Compression in Pulmonary Tuberculosis," 40.

2 Rosenberg, "Therapeutic Revolution," 9.

3 Ibid.

4 Shorter, *Bedside Manners*.

5 Bethune, "Plea for Early Compression in Pulmonary Tuberculosis," 38.

6 See Adams and Burke, "Not a Shack in the Woods."

7 Daniel, "History of Tuberculosis," 1866.

8 In 1912, Gerardo Balboni, a Boston physician, also credited the early work of James Carson, though he positions Carson's experiments in 1842. Balboni, "Treatment of Pulmonary Tuberculosis by Artificial Pneumothorax," 756.

9 Sakula, "Carlo Forlanini," 327.

10 Thomas Daniel also notes that London's F.H. Ramadge induced a successful pneumothorax in 1834 and reported that his tuberculous patient had been cured. Daniel, "History of Tuberculosis," 1866.

11 Sakula, "Carlo Forlanini," 327.

12 Ibid.

13 Ibid., 331.

14 Long, "Artificial Pneumothorax in Tuberculosis," 265.

15 Balboni, "Treatment of Pulmonary Tuberculosis by Artificial Pneumothorax," 755–6.

16 Robinson and Floyd, "Artificial Pneumothorax as a Treatment of Pulmonary Tuberculosis," 304.

17 Ibid.

18 Winslow, "Initiation," 20.

19 Balboni, "Treatment of Pulmonary Tuberculosis by Artificial Pneumothorax," 757–8.

20 Esmond Long, an American physician, received his PhD in 1918 and his MD in 1926. He was a second-year medical student in 1913 when active tuberculosis was diagnosed. According to his biographers, "He coughed up several mouthfuls of blood while playing tennis, and that evening he went back to the laboratory, stained his sputum, and found it full of tubercle bacilli." As a track athlete specializing in the mile run in his pre–medical school days, tuberculosis had never been suspected. During his TB convalescence, Long eventually ended up as a laboratory assistant at Saranac Lake in 1918 and some years later resumed and completed his medical degree. Nowell and Delpino, "Esmond R. Long," 286.

21 Long, "Artificial Pneumothorax in Tuberculosis," 265.

22 Ibid.

23 Canadian Tuberculosis Association, *Handbook for Tuberculosis Patients*, 18.

24 Camblos, "Artificial Pneumothorax Therapy as Observed by a Nurse," 571.

25 Robinson and Floyd, "Artificial Pneumothorax as a Treatment of Pulmonary Tuberculosis," 289.

26 Ibid., 290.

27 Ibid., 452.

28 Ibid., 289.

29 Balboni, "Treatment of Pulmonary Tuberculosis by Artificial Pneumothorax," 757–8.

30 Colgan, Whang, and Gillies, "Atelectasis and Pneumothorax"; see also Liu et al., "Sequential Changes of Hemodynamics and Blood Gases."

31 Glenny, "Determinants of Regional Ventilation and Blood Flow in the Lung," 1833.

32 Christophe et al., "Hemodynamics in the Pulmonary Artery of a Patient," 725.

33 Grainger, "Pulmonary Circulation," 103.

34 Christophe et al., "Hemodynamics in the Pulmonary Artery of a Patient," 731.

35 Liu et al., "Sequential Changes of Hemodynamics and Blood Gases."
36 Murray, "Bill Dock and the Location of Pulmonary Tuberculosis," 1032.
37 Long, "Canadian Lung Association."
38 In this respect, there are some similarities with the earlier use of Koch's tuberculin to render the lung "unfavourable soil" for tuberculosis bacteria.
39 Nickel et al., "Hypoxia Triggers the Expression of Human β Defensin 2 and Antimicrobial Activity."
40 Shneerson, "Respiratory Failure in Tuberculosis," 73.
41 Balboni, "Treatment of Pulmonary Tuberculosis by Artificial Pneumothorax," 761.
42 Long, "Artificial Pneumothorax in Tuberculosis," 267.
43 Dobbie, "Provincial Program for the Control of Tuberculosis," 501.
44 Robinson and Floyd, "Artificial Pneumothorax as a Treatment of Pulmonary Tuberculosis," 299.
45 Long, "Artificial Pneumothorax in Tuberculosis," 266.
46 Camblos, "Artificial Pneumothorax Therapy as Observed by a Nurse," 571–2.
47 Ibid., 572.
48 Long, "Artificial Pneumothorax in Tuberculosis," 266.
49 Camblos, "Artificial Pneumothorax Therapy as Observed by a Nurse," 572.
50 Birath, "Prophylaxis against Air Embolism."
51 Long, "Artificial Pneumothorax in Tuberculosis," 267.
52 Gale, "Oral Histories – Garrett."
53 Long, "Artificial Pneumothorax in Tuberculosis," 268.
54 Breitling, "Compressing Consumption," 195.
55 Critical of the authoritarian and paternalistic undertone associated with "non-compliance" terminology, the language has now been softened to "non-adherence." The terminology is still problematic, however. See Lerner, "From Careless Consumptives to Recalcitrant Patients."
56 See Breitling, "Compressing Consumption," 195.
57 Subotic et al., "Uncertainties in the Current Understanding of Gas Exchange," 1147.
58 Long, "Artificial Pneumothorax in Tuberculosis," 266.
59 Ibid., 267.

60 Myers, *Tuberculosis among Children and Young Adults*, 288.
61 Long, "Artificial Pneumothorax in Tuberculosis," 266.
62 Myers, *Tuberculosis among Children and Young Adults*, 282.
63 Ibid.
64 Ibid., 279.
65 Ibid., 280.
66 Dobbie, *History of the Toronto Hospital for Consumptives*.
67 A rod with a sharp three-cornered tip that is inserted with the cannula, with the sharpened tip pushing into a cavity; the trocar is then pulled out after piercing the cavity and the cannula remains in place (*Stedman's Medical Dictionary* 1949).
68 A tube inserted into a cavity that works as a channel for draining fluid, administering medicine, or acting as a conduit for surgical instruments (*Stedman's Medical Dictionary* 1949).
69 At this time, the thoracoscope would have been a tube that the surgeon could look through to see inside the patient's body; see Adams and Schwartzman, "Pneumothorax Then and Now."
70 Paine and Hershfield, "Tuberculosis: Past, Present and Future," 56.
71 In 1936, it was noted that refills ran about $2.00 per treatment, and municipalities "sometimes" paid for the treatments.
72 Ringer, "Management of Pulmonary Tuberculosis in Relation to Hemorrhage," 136.
73 Trimble and Wood, "Pulmonary Hemorrhage."
74 Polverino et al., "Anatomy and Neuro-Pathophysiology of the Cough Reflex Arc."
75 Gale, "Oral Histories – Davis."
76 Ringer, "Management of Pulmonary Tuberculosis in Relation to Hemorrhage," 136.
77 Shorter, *Bedside Manners*.
78 Ringer, "Management of Pulmonary Tuberculosis in Relation to Hemorrhage," 136.
79 Ibid.; Hawes, "Hemorrhage in Pulmonary Tuberculosis."
80 Ringer, "Management of Pulmonary Tuberculosis in Relation to Hemorrhage," 137.
81 Ibid.; Bennett, "How Not to Treat Tuberculosis"; Moorman, "Hemoptysis in Tuberculosis," 453.

82 Thearle, "Radical Phrenicotomy for Pulmonary Tuberculosis."
83 Adams, Schwartzman, and Theodore, "Collapse and Expand," 924.
84 Gale, "Oral Histories – Garrett."
85 Davies, "Provocative Talk on Pulmonary Tuberculosis," 194.
86 Gordon, "Mechanism and Effects of Abdominal Compression," 198.
87 Shepherd, "Plombage in the 1980s," 328. British surgeon Hugh Morriston Davies also switched a number of his patients from artificial pneumothorax to oleothorax at the beginning of the Second World War in the event that his patients would encounter difficulties getting air refills; see Davies, "Provocative Talk on Pulmonary Tuberculosis," 193.
88 For an X-ray perspective on the in vivo appearance of a Lucite sphere plombage (in addition to a photograph of Lucite spheres obtained from another patient upon autopsy), under the "Images in Medicine" feature, see Mond and Khan, "Lucite Ball Plombage."
89 Shepherd, "Plombage in the 1980s," 328.
90 Gale, "Oral Histories – Garrett."
91 See, for example, Horowitz et al., "Late Complications of Plombage"; Vigneswaran and Ramasastry, "Paraffin Plombage of the Chest Revisited."
92 Alarcón, "Extrapleural Pneumothorax: Prejudices and Facts," 137.
93 Bethune, "Plea for Early Compression in Pulmonary Tuberculosis," 42.
94 Grzybowski and Allen, "Tuberculosis: 2. History of the Disease in Canada."
95 Bayne, "I'm Afraid It's Bad News."
96 Gough et al., "Results of Thoracoplasty," 251.
97 Alarcón, "Extrapleural Pneumothorax: Prejudices and Facts," 138–9.
98 Ibid.
99 Ibid.
100 Gale, "Oral Histories – Young."
101 Bayne, "I'm Afraid It's Bad News."
102 Breitling, "Compressing Consumption," 196.
103 Loynes, "Scoliosis after Thoracoplasty."
104 Ibid.
105 Ibid. For arguments against the increased risk of scoliosis with the removal of transverse processes, see Davies, "Provocative Talk on Pulmonary Tuberculosis," 196.

106 Gale, "Oral Histories – Garrett."
107 Peppas et al., "Thoracoplasty in the Context of Current Surgical Practice."
108 Bredin, "Pulmonary Function in Long-term Survivors of Thoracoplasty"; Jackson et al., "Long Term Non-Invasive Domiciliary Assisted Ventilation"; O'Connor et al., "Airways Obstruction in Survivors of Thoracoplasty"; Tsuboi et al., "Ventilatory Support during Exercise."
109 Paine and Hershfield, "Tuberculosis: Past, Present and Future," 56–7.
110 Carter, "Technic of Thoracoplasty for Pulmonary Tuberculosis."
111 Ibid., 712.
112 Belcher, "Surgical Collapse Therapy in Pulmonary Tuberculosis."
113 Law, "Some Surgical Problems Attending the Operation of Extrapleural Thoracoplasty"; Carter, "Technic of Thoracoplasty for Pulmonary Tuberculosis."
114 Carter, "The Technic of Thoracoplasty for Pulmonary Tuberculosis"; Davies, "Provocative Talk on Pulmonary Tuberculosis," 211.
115 Carter, "Technic of Thoracoplasty for Pulmonary Tuberculosis," 722.
116 Ibid.
117 Semb, "Thoracoplasty with Extrafascial Apicolysis," 651.
118 Gale, "Oral Histories – Young."
119 Cosnett and Linton, "Thoracoplasty for Large Tuberculous Cavities."
120 Semb, "Thoracoplasty with Extrafascial Apicolysis."
121 Brock, "Present Position of Thoracic Surgery."
122 Semb, "Thoracoplasty with Extrafascial Apicolysis."
123 Alexander, "Some Advances in the Technic of Thoracoplasty."
124 Odell, "History of Surgery for Pulmonary Tuberculosis," 264.
125 Hobbs, "Before the Sanatorium."
126 Ibid.
127 Dobbie, "Hygienic, Dietetic and Medicinal Treatment of Tuberculosis."
128 Clark, "Probable Amount of Ultra-Violet Radiation Obtained Indoors."
129 Gale, "Oral Histories – Garrett."
130 Hobday, "Sunlight Therapy and Solar Architecture."
131 Rollier et al., *Heliotherapy*, vi.
132 Roelandts, "History of Phototherapy."
133 Woloshyn, "Our Friend, the Sun."
134 Reyn, "Discussion on the Artificial Light Treatment of Lupus."

135 Roelandts, "New Light on Niels Finsen," 116.
136 Ibid.
137 Hobday, "Sunlight Therapy and Solar Architecture"; Reyn, "Discussion on the Artificial Light Treatment of Lupus."
138 Myers, *Tuberculosis among Children and Young Adults*, 285.
139 Hobday, "Sunlight Therapy and Solar Architecture."
140 Billings Jr, "Memorial: August Rollier, M.D.," lii.
141 Ibid.
142 Hobday, "Sunlight Therapy and Solar Architecture," 460.
143 Reyn, "Discussion on the Artificial Light Treatment of Lupus," 502.
144 Rollier, *Heliotherapy*.
145 Ibid., 41.
146 Ibid.
147 Rollier, *Heliotherapy*.
148 Ibid., 42.
149 Billings Jr, " Memorial: August Rollier, M.D.," lii.
150 Ibid.
151 Hobday, "Sunlight Therapy and Solar Architecture," 464.
152 Reyn, "Discussion on the Artificial Light Treatment of Lupus."
153 Rosselet, "Scientific Basis of Heliotherapy."
154 Phelps, "Light Therapy," 877.
155 Myers, *Tuberculosis among Children and Young Adults*, 286.
156 Reyn, "Discussion on the Artificial Light Treatment of Lupus," 502.
157 Rollier, *Heliotherapy*, 10.
158 Anderson, "Nursing the Patient with Bone and Joint Tuberculosis," 217.
159 Myers, *Tuberculosis among Children and Young Adults*, 286.
160 Rollier, *Heliotherapy*, 4–5.
161 Phelps, "Light Therapy," 877.
162 Gale, "Oral Histories – Garrett."
163 Rollier, *Heliotherapy*, 109–10.
164 Woloshyn, "Our Friend, the Sun."
165 Martin et al., "Changes in Skin Tanning Attitudes."
166 Ibid.
167 Wejse, "Tuberculosis and Vitamin D."
168 Luong and Nguyen, "Impact of Vitamin D in the Treatment of Tuberculosis."

169 Ibid., 494–6.
170 Liu et al., "Toll-Like Receptor Triggering of a Vitamin D–Mediated Human Antimicrobial Response"; for a review on this research and other associated work, see Mandavilli, "Sunshine Cure."
171 This novel vitamin D/cathelicidin pathway is shared by humans, apes, Old World monkeys, and New World monkeys, all anthropoid primates, but is not shared with prosimian primates; this suggests that the pathway is a derived trait, emerging in anthropoid primates following their evolutionary split from prosimians. See Gombart, Saito, and Koeffler, "Exaptation of an Ancient Alu Short Interspersed Element."
172 Liu et al., "Toll-Like Receptor Triggering of a Vitamin D–Mediated Human Antimicrobial Response"; Gombart, Saito, and Koeffler, "Exaptation of an Ancient Alu Short Interspersed Element."
173 Giessler, "Tuberculosis of the Bones and Joints," 218.
174 Ibid., 221.
175 Wilson, "Treatment of Tuberculous Hip Disease," 441.
176 Ibid.
177 Ibid.
178 Ibid., 443.
179 Starr, "Treatment of Tuberculous Affections of Bones and Joints."
180 Moon, "Tuberculosis of the Spine," 1791.
181 Designed by Hugh Owen Thomas, a general practitioner who had apprenticed with his father, "an established bone setter." Thomas's "waiting rooms were packed with patients, mostly drawn from dock yards and work rooms ... Whether the affection be spinal caries or fractured thigh, [the patient] is able to return home in an hour, fitted with a simple and appropriate splint." Whitman, "Development of Orthopaedic Surgery," 408.
182 Jones, "Notes on the Uses and Application of Thomas's Hip Splint," 715.
183 Nissen, "Editorial," 227.
184 The differences between Bradford and Whitman frames as detailed by Greff, "Care of the Child on a Bradford Frame or a Whitman Frame."
185 Anderson, "Nursing the Patient with Bone and Joint Tuberculosis," 218.
186 Ibid.
187 Ibid.
188 Ibid., 219.

189 See https://archive.org/details/Filletandspicaplaster-wellcome (the Wellcome Library has also uploaded the documentary to Youtube).
190 Anderson, "Nursing the Patient with Bone and Joint Tuberculosis," 217.
191 Ibid., 218.
192 Bradford, "Treatment of Pott's Disease," 459.
193 Anderson, "Nursing the Patient with Bone and Joint Tuberculosis," 218.
194 Ibid.
195 Whitman, "Development of Orthopaedic Surgery"; Zampini and Sherk, "Lewis A. Sayre."
196 Sayre, *Spinal Disease and Spinal Curvature.*
197 Rutkow, "Lewis Albert Sayre and the Suspension Treatment of Spinal Disease." In the particular photo that accompanies this article, of Sayre with a twenty-year-old woman in a tripod, unclothed from the waist up and her back to the camera, Rutkow notes a "subtle degree of eroticism" suggested in this case.
198 Bernard, "Experience of Sayre's Plaster Jacket," 558.
199 See Holding, "Improved Methods of Applying Plaster Spicas and Jackets"; for another horizontal extension apparatus, see also Hawley, "Fracture and Orthopedic Table."
200 Davy, "Clinical Lecture on the Treatment of Spinal Curvature."
201 Ridlon, "Forcible Straightening of Spinal Curvature," 120.
202 Ibid., 125.
203 Grattan, "Treatment of Spinal Curvature by Means of the Cuirass," 693.
204 Ibid.
205 Bradford, "Treatment of Pott's Disease by the Plaster-of-Paris Jacket," 459.
206 Grattan, "Treatment of Spinal Curvature by Means of the Cuirass," 693.
207 Howell, "Use and Abuse of Plaster of Paris."
208 Charlie "Chuck" Conacher (1909–1967), Toronto Maple Leaf #9, right wing. Conacher played for the Leafs from 1929 to 1938, and was team captain in the 1937/8 season. As a Maple Leaf, he played 326 games, scored 200 goals, and earned 124 assists. Conacher was inducted into the Hockey Hall of Fame in 1961. See the "Legends Spotlight" tab at www.legendsofhockey.net.
209 Charles Joseph Sylvanus "Syl" Apps (1915–1998), Toronto Maple Leaf

#10, centre. Apps played for the Leafs from 1936 to 1948,and was team captain from 1940 to1943 and 1945 to 1948 (he left the NHL to join the Canadian Army from 1943 to 1945). As a Maple Leaf, he played 423 games, scored 201 goals, and earned 231 assists. Apps was inducted into the Hockey Hall of Fame in 1961. See the "Legends Spotlight" tab at www.legendsofhockey.net.

210 Moon, "Tuberculosis of the Spine," 1794.

211 Hurwitz, "Form and Representation in Clinical Case Reports," 230.

212 Brittain, "Ischiofemoral Arthrodesis."

213 Nissen, "Editorial," 227.

214 Ibid.

215 Ibid., 228.

216 Myers, *Tuberculosis among Children and Young Adults*, 284.

217 Ibid.

218 Boyd, "Streptomycin in Childhood Tuberculosis."

219 Ronald, "Some Aspects of Tuberculosis in Ontario," 793.

220 Ibid.

221 Johnson, Hillman, and Southwick, "Importance of Direct Surgical Attack."

222 Ibid., 18.

223 Gale, *Changing Years*, 80.

224 Ryan, *Forgotten Plague*.

225 Ibid., 88.

226 Ibid., 88–9.

227 Ryan, *Forgotten Plague*.

228 Ibid., 122–3.

229 Ibid., 218.

230 Taylor, *Conquest of Bacteria*.

231 McClelland, "Anuria: A Report of Three Types of Cases."

232 Mellon, "Chemotherapy of Tuberculosis," 166.

233 Ibid., 171.

234 Birkhaug, "Treatment of Experimental Tuberculosis," 54.

235 Hoggarth, Martin, and Young, "Studies in the Chemotherapy of Tuberculosis," 154.

236 Waksman, "Award Ceremony Speech."

237 Gale, *Changing Years*, 80.

238 Solotorovsky, Bugie, and Frost, "Effect of Penicillin."

239 Gale, *Changing Years*, 80.
240 Ibid., 88.
241 Dr Mulligan's obituary appeared in the *Canadian Medical Association Journal* 54, no. 3 (1946): 319.
242 Boyd, "Streptomycin in Childhood Tuberculosis," 476, 479.
243 Aronovitch and Lewin, "Streptomycin in Tuberculosis," 578.
244 Ronald, "Some Aspects of Tuberculosis in Ontario," 792.
245 Jeanes, "Tuberculosis," 35.
246 Aronovitch and Lewin, "Streptomycin in Tuberculosis," 578.
247 Ibid.
248 Lee, "Streptomycin in Pulmonary Tuberculosis," 242.
249 Kincade et al., "Streptomycin in the Treatment of Tuberculosis," 105.
250 Lee, "Streptomycin in Pulmonary Tuberculosis," 243.
251 Ronald, "Some Aspects of Tuberculosis in Ontario," 792.
252 Aronovitch and Lewin, "Streptomycin in Tuberculosis," 577.
253 Committee on Chemotherapy and Antibiotics of the American College of Chest Physicians, "Information: The Use of Streptomycin in Tuberculosis."
254 Aronovitch and Lewin, "Streptomycin in Tuberculosis," 577.
255 Ibid.
256 See, for example, Boyd, "Streptomycin in Childhood Tuberculosis"; Editorial, "Effects of Streptomycin in Tuberculosis"; Kincade et al., "Streptomycin in the Treatment of Tuberculosis"; Lee, "Streptomycin in Pulmonary Tuberculosis"; MacGregor, "Case of Tuberculous Meningitis"; Wood and Scott, "Case of Pulmonary and Meningeal Tuberculosis."
257 Aronovitch and Lewin, "Streptomycin in Tuberculosis," 578.
258 Ibid.
259 Ibid.
260 Ibid., 579.
261 Ibid., 580.
262 Ibid., 582.
263 Hinshaw, Feldman, and Pfuetze, "Present Status of Chemotherapy in Tuberculosis."
264 The planogram (or tomogram) is the image produced by a planograph (or tomograph). According to Bryder, tomography "enabled the lungs to be viewed without any of the details being obscured by the normal bone

markings of the ribs. In this way the position and size of the cavity could be determined in terms of length, breadth, and depth in a precise way which had previously been impossible." Bryder, *Below the Magic Mountain*, 181.

265 Gale, *Changing Years*, 88.

266 Ibid.

267 According to patient LHW, in Gale, *Changing Years*, 100.

268 Ibid., 73, 88.

269 Ronald, "Some Aspects of Tuberculosis in Ontario," 792.

270 Boyd, "Streptomycin in Childhood Tuberculosis."

271 Ibid., 478.

272 Ronald, "Some Aspects of Tuberculosis in Ontario," 793.

273 Kincade et al., "Streptomycin in the Treatment of Tuberculosis," 111.

274 According to Dr Garrett, a drug of "last resort," because it typically caused irreversible deafness. Gale, "Oral Histories – Garrett."

CHAPTER SEVEN

1 Scheper-Hughes and Lock, "Mindful Body," 30.

2 Bashford, "Cultures of Confinement," 133.

3 Ibid.

4 Paine and Hershfield, "Tuberculosis: Past, Present and Future," 57.

5 For a discussion on childhood agency, see Minnett and Poutanen, "Swatting Flies for Health."

6 Dobbie, "Toronto Hospital for Consumptives, Weston, Ontario: 'The Future.'"

7 Bryder, *Below the Magic Mountain*, 205.

8 Rothman, *Living in the Shadow of Death*.

9 Haugh, "Hill of Health," 6–7.

10 Marcellus, "Tiny Cripples and the Sunshine of Life," 416.

11 The Webster's dictionary description is "a custardlike dessert of flavored milk curded with rennet."

12 Gale, "Oral Histories – Wilson."

13 Fleitas, "To Tell You the Truth," 197.

14 Ibid.

15 Gale, "Oral Histories – Wilson."

16 Ibid.

17 Gale, *Changing Years*, 23–4.
18 Gale, "Oral Histories – Wilson."
19 Shaw and Reeves, *Children of Craig-y-nos*, 136.
20 This is a condition characterized by an abnormal persistent widening of the bronchial tubes. The walls of the bronchial tubes become damaged by the distension, in turn damaging the cilia (tiny hairs) that line the bronchial tubes and sweep them free of dust, germs, and excess mucus. The destruction of the cilia causes dust, mucus, and bacteria to accumulate, and infection may result. Certain genetic/congenital and mechanical factors may result in this rare condition; pneumonias associated with measles or whooping cough infections may also be implicated by weakening the walls of the bronchial tubes.
21 Rothman, *Living in the Shadow of Death*, 236–8.
22 Bayne, "I'm Afraid It's Bad News," 258.
23 Rothman, *Living in the Shadow of Death*, 235.
24 Shaw and Reeves, *Children of Craig-y-nos*.
25 There was actually a far worse incident, involving a six-year-old boy named Bernard. Apparently Bernard had urinated directly into another little boy's mouth. Dr McHugh "gave him a severe caution and let him know very forcibly that this was detestable." McHugh did not think that Bernard would do it again, and while he may have preferred to simply discharge the boy, he was not physically ready to leave the sanatorium.
26 On 23 May 1952, a fire did eventually destroy these pavilions. According to Gale, despite the efforts of the York Township Fire Department and the Weston Fire Brigade, "the fire spread rapidly, and destroyed not only the patients' quarters and personal possessions (including one man's false teeth which he dropped as he rushed out), but also the adjacent Assembly Hall, the Walker Cottage for employees, the physiotherapy exercise room, the occupational therapy workshop, and the last remaining [Toronto Transit Commission] horse-drawn street car" (a handful of old streetcars had been donated to the original Toronto Free Hospital for Consumptives for use as patient accommodation when the TTC went electric). There were no fatalities and alternate accommodations were found for all twenty-four patients. See Gale, *Changing Years*, 89.
27 Bryder, *Below the Magic Mountain*, 207.
28 Cassidy, "Physical Exercise in the Treatment of Tuberculosis," 114.

29 Connolly and Gibson, "The "White Plague' and Color," 235.
30 Wood, "Bowlby's Children," 127.
31 Shaw and Reeves, *Children of Craig-y-nos*, 15.
32 Ibid., 44.
33 Ibid., 29.
34 Ibid., 93.
35 Ibid., 61.

CHAPTER EIGHT

1 "Report of the Samaritan Club," *ARNSA*, 1921–22, 48.
2 Wherrett, *Miracle of the Empty Beds*; McCuaig, *The Weariness, the Fever, and the Fret*.
3 *ARNSA*, 1913–14, 52.
4 Or, in the case of Indigenous patients, the federal government.
5 McCuaig, *The Weariness, the Fever, and the Fret*.
6 Draus, *Consumed in the City*, 53.
7 Ibid., 53; Farmer, *Infections and Inequalities*.
8 Dusel, "Fashioning the Schooled Self through Uniforms," 93.
9 Shaw and Reeves, *Children of Craig-y-nos*, 45.
10 Ibid., 56.
11 Ibid.
12 Elliott, *Present Status of Antituberculosis Work in Canada – 1908*, 8.
13 Chappell, *Social Welfare in Canadian Society*.
14 Holbrook, "'Present Need of the Tuberculosis Campaign in Canada," 464.
15 "Report of the Physician-in-Chief, W.J. Dobbie," *ARNSA*, 1919–20, 21.
16 McCuaig, *The Weariness, the Fever, and the Fret*, 142–5.
17 Hodgetts, "National and Provincial Responsibility in the Tuberculosis Crusade," 217.
18 Ibid.
19 *ARNSA*, 1938.
20 McCuaig, *The Weariness, the Fever, and the Fret*, 146.
21 Ibid., 142–5.
22 *ARNSA*, 1938.
23 McCuaig, *The Weariness, the Fever, and the Fret*, 144–5.
24 Dodd, "Advice to Parents"; Little, "'Manhunts and Bingo Blabs'"; Struthers, "'In the Interests of the Children'"; Young, "'Little Sufferers.'"

25 Young, "Divine Mission," 71.
26 Jones, *Influenza 1918*.
27 Bates, *Bargaining for Life*, 231.
28 "Report of the Samaritan Club," *ARNSA*, 1914–15, 47.
29 Stewart, "Samaritan Club of Toronto, 1912–1933."
30 "Report of the Samaritan Club," *ARNSA*, 1928–29, 44. Julia Stewart died in 1934 ("Report of the Samaritan Club," *ARNSA*, 1935, 35).
31 "Report of the Visiting Nurse, Julia Stewart," *ARNSA*, 1913–14, 45.
32 See McCuaig, *The Weariness, the Fever, and the Fret*, 160.
33 "Report of the Visiting Nurse, Julia Stewart," *ARNSA*, 1913–14, 44.
34 "Report of the Samaritan Club," *ARNSA*, 1914–15, 47.
35 "Report of the Samaritan Club," *ARNSA*, 1917–18, 29.
36 "Report of the Samaritan Club," *ARNSA*, 1921–22, 46.
37 "Report of the Visiting Nurse, Julia Stewart," *ARNSA*, 1914–15, 43.
38 See McCullagh, *Legacy of Caring*; "Report of the Samaritan Club," *ARNSA*, 1919–20, 29.
39 Stewart, "Samaritan Club of Toronto, 1912–1933," 6–7.
40 "Report of the Samaritan Club," *ARNSA*, 1921–22, 46.
41 "Report of the Samaritan Club," *ARNSA*, 1914–15, 48.
42 Ibid.
43 "Report of the Samaritan Club," *ARNSA*, 1915–16, 27.
44 "Report of the Samaritan Club," *ARNSA*, 1921–22, 47.
45 The Orde Street Public School is located at 18 Orde Street, Toronto. The school opened in September 1915, with an enrolment of 372 students. According to researchers with the Toronto Branch of the Ontario Genealogical Society, the school had "third-floor and rooftop space for children who had tuberculosis. [The] Board believed sick children could attend school if taken outside on gurneys for some time in the fresh air. The weight increase of the children was graphed to show the benefits of fresh air, food, and rest." See http://torontofamilyhistory.org/kingandcountry/tdsb/elementary-n-q.
46 Poutanen et al., "Tuberculosis in Town," 85.
47 "Report of the Samaritan Club," *ARNSA*, 1914–15, 49.
48 Ibid.
49 Ibid.
50 "Report of the Samaritan Club," *ARNSA*, 1916–17, 30.
51 Mrs Walter Massey, among others, is also credited with support of the

Rest Home at Glen Sibbald, Jackson's Point, Lake Simcoe. See Stewart, *Samaritan Club of Toronto, 1912–1933*, 8.

52 "Report of the Samaritan Club," ARNSA, 1917–18, 29.
53 "Report of the Samaritan Club," ARNSA, 1925–26, 46.
54 Ibid.
55 Ibid.
56 "Report of the Samaritan Club," ARNSA, 1939. The newspaper began its own Fresh Air Fund in 1901, which continues to operate today, sending children to accredited camps in Ontario. More recently, organizations such as the Tim Horton Children's Foundation continue to expand the summer camp experience.
57 Perretz, "Study of the Samaritan Club of Toronto"; McKergow, "Outline of History of the Samaritan Club of Toronto."
58 "Report of the Samaritan Club," ARNSA, 1922–23, 45.
59 Ibid.
60 Samaritan Club, *History 1912–1971*.
61 In a later annual report, the name change was chalked up to "some confusion … owing to the similarity in name of the Western Hospital." "Report of the Weston Sanitarium Club," ARNSA, 1937, 24.
62 "Report of the Weston Sanitarium Club," ARNSA, 1937, 23.
63 "Report of the Weston Hospital Sewing Club," ARNSA, 1913–14, 47.
64 "Report of the Weston Sanitarium Club," ARNSA, 1915–16, 28.
65 "Report of the Weston Hospital Sewing Club," ARNSA, 1914–15, 50.
66 "Report of the Weston Sanitarium Club," ARNSA, 1925–26, 45.
67 In reference the New Testament, Gospel of Matthew 25:40.
68 "Report of the Samaritan Club," ARNSA, 1925–26, 47.
69 "Report of the Weston Hospital Sewing Club," ARNSA, 1914–15, 47.
70 Florence Gooderham Huestis served as president of the Local Council of Women in Toronto for eight years. She "worked tirelessly for the welfare of children and single mothers" in projects such as Mother's Pension, Big Sisters, and milk pasteurization. See Southee, "Florence Gooderham Huestis."
71 "Report of the Weston Hospital Sewing Club," ARNSA, 1914–15, 51.
72 "Report of the Weston Sanitarium Club," ARNSA, 1915–16, 28.
73 "Report of the Weston Sanitarium Club," ARNSA, 1924–25, 47.
74 "Report of the Weston Sanitarium Club," ARNSA, 1916–17, 32.

75 "Report of the Weston Sanitarium Club," *ARNSA*, 1919–20, 30.
76 "Report of the Weston Sanitarium Club," *ARNSA*, 1924–25, 47.
77 "Report of the Weston Sanitarium Club," *ARNSA*, 1927–28, 47.

CHAPTER NINE

1 Bates, *Bargaining for Life*, 340.
2 Lienhardt et al., "Global Tuberculosis Control."
3 Kochi, "Global Tuberculosis Situation."
4 Grange et al., "Biosocial Dynamics of Tuberculosis," 128.
5 Fukuda, "Foreword," ix.
6 See World Health Organization, "End TB Strategy."
7 On this latter point, see the great discussion by Tomes, "Making of Germ Panic."
8 Farmer, "Anthropology of Structural Violence," 315.
9 Draus, *Consumed in the City*.
10 Larcombe et al., "Differential Cytokine Genotype Frequencies"; Waldram, Herring, and Young, *Aboriginal Health in Canada*.
11 McCuaig, *The Weariness, the Fever, and the Fret*; McKeown, *Role of Medicine*; McKeown, *Origins of Human Disease*.
12 McCuaig, *The Weariness, the Fever, and the Fret*, 8.
13 Draus, *Consumed in the City*, 71.
14 Roberts and Buikstra, *Bioarchaeology of Tuberculosis*, 43.
15 Paluzzi, "A Social Disease/A Social Response."
16 Porter and Ogden, "Commentary on 'The Resurgence of Disease'"; Gandy and Zumla, "Theorizing Tuberculosis."

Bibliography

Abebe, F., and G. Bjune. "The Protective Role of Antibody Responses during *Mycobacterium tuberculosis* Infection." *Clinical & Experimental Immunology* 157, no. 2 (2009): 235–43.

Adams, Annmarie. *Medicine by Design: The Architect and the Modern Hospital, 1893–1943*. Minneapolis: University of Minnesota Press, 2008.

Adams, Annmarie, and Stacie Burke. "A Doctor in the House: The Architecture of Home-Offices for Physicians in Toronto, 1885–1930." *Medical History* 52, no. 2 (2008): 163–94.

– "'Not a Shack in the Woods': Architecture for Tuberculosis in Muskoka and Toronto." *Canadian Bulletin of Medical History* 23, no. 2 (2006): 429–55.

Adams, Annmarie, and Kevin Schwartzman. "Pneumothorax Then and Now." *Space and Culture* 8, no. 4 (2005): 435–48.

Adams, Annmarie, Kevin Schwartzman, and David Theodore. "Collapse and Expand: Architecture and Tuberculosis Therapy in Montreal, 1909, 1933, 1954." *Technology and Culture* 49, no. 4 (2008): 908–42.

Adams, William. "Remarks on the Subcutaneous Division of the Neck of the Thigh-Bone, as Compared with Other Operations for Rectifying Extreme Distortion at the Hip–Joint, with Bony Anchylosis." *British Medical Journal* 2, no. 521 (24 December 1870): 673–6.

Agrons, Geoffrey A., Richard I. Markowitz, and Sandra S. Kramer. "Pulmonary Tuberculosis in Children." *Seminars in Roentgenology* 28, no. 2 (1993): 158–72.

Alarcón, Donato A. "Extrapleural Pneumothorax: Prejudices and Facts." *Chest* 9, no. 2 (1943): 137–50.

Alexander, John. "Rôles of Medicine and Surgery in the Management of Bronchiectasis." *Annals of Internal Medicine* 21, no. 4 (1944): 565–79.

– "Some Advances in the Technic of Thoracoplasty." *Annals of Surgery* 104, no. 4 (1936): 545–51.

Allbutt, Clifford, Lauder Brunton, Arthur Latham, and William Osler. "The Value of Sanatorium Treatment." *Lancet* 178, no. 4585 (1911): 180–2.

Altet-Gómez, M.N., J. Alcaide, P. Godoy, M.A. Romero, and I. Hernández del Rey. "Clinical and Epidemiological Aspects of Smoking and Tuberculosis: A Study of 13308 Cases." *International Journal of Tuberculosis and Lung Disease* 9, no. 4 (2005): 430–6.

Anderson, Helen C. "Nursing the Patient with Bone and Joint Tuberculosis." *American Journal of Nursing* 48, no. 4 (1948): 215–20.

Arcavi, Lidia, and Neal L. Benowitz. "Cigarette Smoking and Infection." *Archives of Internal Medicine* 164, no. 8 (2004): 2206–16.

Armstrong, David. "The Patient's View." *Social Science and Medicine* 18, no. 9 (1984): 737–44.

Armstrong, J.A., and D'Arcy Hart. "Response of Cultured Macrophages to *Mycobacterium tuberculosis*, with Observations on Fusion of Lysosomes with Phagosomes." Part 1. *Journal of Experimental Medicine* 134, no. 3 (1971): 713–40.

Arnup, Katharine. "Raising the Dionne Quintuplets: Lessons for Modern Mothers." *Journal of Canadian Studies* 29, no. 4 (1994): 65–85.

Aronovitch, M., and N. Lewin. "Streptomycin in Tuberculosis." *Canadian Medical Association Journal* 61, no. 6 (1949): 577–83.

Aufderheide, Arthur C., and Conrado Rodriguez-Martin, with Odin Langsjoen. *The Cambridge Encyclopedia of Human Paleopathology*. Cambridge: Cambridge University Press, 1998.

Avila-Aguero, Maria L., Gabriela German, Maria M. Paris, and José F. Herrera. "Toys in a Pediatric Hospital: Are They a Bacterial Source?" *American Journal of Infection Control* 32, no. 5 (2004): 287–90.

Balboni, Gerardo M. "The Treatment of Pulmonary Tuberculosis by Artificial Pneumothorax, According to the Method of Forlanini." *Boston Medical and Surgical Journal* 167, no. 22 (1912): 755–61.

Barnes, Peter F., Cara L. Grisso, John S. Abrams, Hamid Band, Thomas H. Rea, and Robert L. Modlin. "γδ T Lymphocytes in Human Tuberculosis." *Journal of Infectious Diseases* 165, no. 3 (1992): 506–12.

Baron, Richard J. "An Introduction to Medical Phenomenology: I Can't Hear You While I'm Listening." *Annals of Internal Medicine* 103, no. 4 (1985): 606–11.

Barratt, Ruth Linda, Ramon Shaban, and Wendy Moyle. "Patient Experience of Source Isolation: Lessons for Clinical Practice." *Contemporary Nurse* 39, no. 2 (2011): 180–93.

Barton, Ellen. *Driven by a Dream: The Story of Ongwanada, 1948–1998*. Kingston: Ontario Quarry, 1998.

Bashford, Alison. "Cultures of Confinement: Tuberculosis, Isolation and the Sanatorium." In *Isolation: Places and Practices of Exclusion*, edited by Alison Bashford and Carolyn Strange, 125–40. New York: Routledge, 2005.

Baston, Andrea. *Curing Tuberculosis in Muskoka: Canada's First Sanatoria*. Toronto: Old Stone Books, 2013.

Bates, Barbara. *Bargaining for Life: A Social History of Tuberculosis, 1876–1938*. Philadelphia: University of Pennsylvania Press, 1992.

Bayne, Ronald. "I'm Afraid It's Bad News." *Canadian Medical Association Journal* 159, no. 3 (1998): 258.

Begg, D.J., K. de Silva, N. Carter, K.M. Plain, A. Purdie, and R.J. Whittington. "Does a T_h1 over T_h2 Dominancy Really Exist in the Early Stages of *Mycobacterium avium* subspecies *paratuberculosis* Infections?" *Immunobiology* 216, no. 7 (2011): 840–6.

Belcher, J.R. "Surgical Collapse Therapy in Pulmonary Tuberculosis." *Postgraduate Medical Journal* 30, no. 344 (1954): 300–4.

Bennett, Edwin S. "How Not to Treat Tuberculosis." *Chest* 1, no. 4 (1935): 9–21.

Bennett, William. "Induced Hyperaemia as a Means of Treatment, with Special Reference to Tuberculous Joint Disease and Stiffened Joints." *British Medical Journal* 2 (21 November 1908): 1533–5.

Bentzon, Johanne W. "The Effect of Certain Infectious Diseases on Tuberculin Allergy." *Tubercle* 34, no. 2 (1953): 34–41.

Bernard, Walter. "Experience of Sayre's Plaster Jacket." *British Medical Journal* 2, no. 1238 (1884): 558.

Bethune, Norman. "A Plea for Early Compression in Pulmonary Tuberculosis." *Canadian Medical Association Journal* 27, no. 1 (1932): 36–42.

Billings Jr, F.T. "Memorial: Auguste Rollier, M.D." *Transactions of the American Clinical and Climatological Association* 68 (1957): lii–liii.

Birath, Gösta. "Prophylaxis against Air Embolism from Puncture of the Lungs and Pleurae; With Special Reference to Refills of Artificial Pneumothorax." *Chest* 27, no. 6 (1955): 649–53.

Birkhaug, Konrad. "Treatment of Experimental Tuberculosis with Sulphonamide." *British Medical Journal* 2, no. 4096 (1939): 54–7.

Blaser, Martin J., and Denise Kirschner. "The Equilibria That Allow Bacterial Persistence in Human Hosts." *Nature* 449, no. 7164 (2007): 843–9.

Blessing, Bettina. *Pathways of Homeopathic Medicine*. Heidelberg: Springer Medizin Verlag, 2011.

Bliss, Michael. "Davies, William." Dictionary of Canadian Biography Online, http://www.biographi.ca/en/bio/davies_william_15E.html.

Bloom, B.R., and C.J. Murray. "Tuberculosis: Commentary on a Reemergent Killer." *Science* 257, no. 5073 (1992): 1055–64.

Blue, Gwendolyn, and Melanie Rock. "Trans-Biopolitics: Complexity in Interspecies Relations." *Health* 15, no. 4 (2010): 353–68.

Boyd, Gladys L. "Streptomycin in Childhood Tuberculosis." *Canadian Medical Association Journal* 60, no. 5 (1949): 476–80.

Boye, Seika. "Finding Amy Sternberg." *Dance Collection Danse: The Magazine* 59 (2005): 24–7.

Bradford, Edward H. "The Treatment of Pott's Disease by the Plaster-of-Paris Jacket." *Boston Medical and Surgical Journal* 102 (13 May 1880): 459–63.

Bredin, Charles P. "Pulmonary Function in Long-term Survivors of Thoracoplasty." *Chest* 95, no. 1 (1989): 18–20.

Breitling, Magnus. "Compressing Consumption: The Surgery of Pulmonary Tuberculosis." In *Proceedings of the 13th Annual History of Medicine Days*, edited by W.A. Whitelaw, 193–7. Calgary: Health Sciences Centre, 2004.

Brink, G.B. "Division of Tuberculosis Prevention." Sessional Papers, Volume LXX, Part IV, Second Session of the Twentieth Legislature of the Province of Ontario. Session 1938. Toronto: T.E. Bowman, 1938.

Brittain, H.A. "Ischiofemoral Arthrodesis." *British Journal of Surgery* 29, no. 113 (1941): 93–104.

Brock, R.C. "The Present Position of Thoracic Surgery." *British Medical Bulletin* 2, no. 2 (1944): 33–6.

Brody, Jacob A., Theresa Overfield, and Laurel M. Hammes. "Depression of the Tuberculin Reaction by Viral Vaccines." *New England Journal of Medicine* 271, no. 25 (1964): 1294–6.

Brosch, R., S.V. Gordon, M. Marmiesse, P. Brodin, C. Buchrieser, K. Eiglmeier, T. Garnier, C. Gutierrez, G. Hewinson, K. Kremer et al. "A New Evolutionary Scenario for the *Mycobacterium tuberculosis* Complex." *Proceedings of the National Academy of Sciences* 99, no. 6 (2002): 3684–9.

Brown, Alan. "Infant and Child Welfare Work." *Public Health Journal* 9, no. 4 (1918): 145–56.

Brown, Lawrason. "The Proper Dosage of Air, Food and Rest in Pulmonary Tuberculosis." *Canadian Practitioner* 37, no. 9 (1912): 529–37.

Bryan, A.C. "The Distribution of Ventilation and Perfusion in the Normal Lung, Studied with Xenon." PhD diss., McGill University, 1964.

Bryder, Linda. *Below the Magic Mountain: A Social History of Tuberculosis in Twentieth-Century Britain.* Oxford: Clarendon, 1988.

Bergey, Lorna L. "Martin, Jesse Bauman (1897–1974)." Global Anabaptist Mennonite Encyclopedia. gameo.org/index.php?title=Martin,_Jesse_Bauman_(1897-1974)

Burke, Donald S. "Of Postulates and Peccadilloes: Robert Koch and Vaccine (Tuberculin) Therapy for Tuberculosis." *Vaccine* 11, no. 8 (1993): 795–804.

Burke, Stacie, and Lawrence Sawchuk. "Tuberculosis Mortality and Recent Childbirth: A Retrospective Case-Control Study of Gibraltarian Women, 1874–1884." *Social Science and Medicine* 56, no. 3 (2003): 477–90.

Camblos, Cynthia. "Artificial Pneumothorax Therapy as Observed by a Nurse." *American Journal of Nursing* 28, no. 6 (1928): 571–3.

Canadian Nurses' Association. "Dominion Registration of Nurses for Canada." *British Journal of Nursing* 84 (1936): 126.

Canadian Partnership for Children's Health and Environment. *Advancing Environmental Health in Child Care Settings: A Checklist for Child Care Practitioners and Public Health Inspectors.* Toronto: CPCHE, 2010.

Canadian Public Health Association. "Minutes of the Section of Infant and Child Welfare of the Canadian Public Health Association Held at the Royal Connaught Hotel, Hamilton (1918)." *Public Health Journal* 9, no. 4 (1918): 319–22.

Canadian Tuberculosis Association. *A Handbook for Tuberculosis Patients: What You Should Know about Tuberculosis.* Ottawa: CTA, ca. 1935.

Canadian Tuberculosis Committee. "Housing Conditions That Serve as Risk Factors for Tuberculosis Infection and Disease: An Advisory Committee Statement." *Canada Communicable Disease Report* 33, ACS-9 (2007): 1–13.

Carter, B. Noland. "The Technic of Thoracoplasty for Pulmonary Tuberculosis." *Annals of Surgery* 103, no. 5 (1936): 711–24.

Cassidy, J.J. "Address to the Association of Executive Health Officers of Ontario." *Canadian Journal of Medicine and Surgery* 7, no. 3 (1900): 145–57.

– "The Bacteriological Diagnosis of Diphtheria." *Canadian Journal of Medicine and Surgery* 5, no. 2 (1899): 129–30.

– "A Formula for Giving Alcohol in Fevers." *Canadian Journal of Medicine and Surgery* 13, no. 4 (1903): 271–4.

– "Physical Exercise in the Treatment of Tuberculosis." *Canadian Journal of Medicine and Surgery* 28, no. 2 (1910): 114–15.

– "The Prevention of Tuberculosis." *Canadian Journal of Medicine and Surgery* 8, no. 2 (1900): 113–16.

– "Unhealthy Dwellings Cause Tuberculosis." *Canadian Journal of Medicine and Surgery* 25, no. 6 (1909): 371–3.

Cegielski, J.P., and D.N. McMurray. "The Relationship between Malnutrition and Tuberculosis: Evidence from Studies in Humans and Experimental Animals." *International Journal of Tuberculosis and Lung Disease* 8, no. 3 (2004): 286–98.

Chan, John, Yu Tian, Kathryn E. Tanaka, Ming S. Tsang, Keming Yu, Padmini Salgame, Dinah Carroll, Yvonne Kress, Rachel Teitelbaum, and Barry R. Bloom. "Effects of Protein Calorie Malnutrition on Tuberculosis in Mice." *Proceedings of the National Academy of Science* USA 93, no. 25 (1996): 14857–61.

Chandra, R.K. "Increased Bacterial Binding to Respiratory Epithelial Cells in Vitamin A Deficiency." *British Medical Journal* 297, no. 6652 (1988): 834–5.

– "Nutrition, Immunity and Infection: From Basic Knowledge of Dietary Manipulation of Immune Responses to Practical Application of Ameliorating Suffering and Improving Survival." *Proceedings of the National Academy of Science,* USA 93, no. 25 (1996): 14304–7.

Chappell, Rosalie. *Social Welfare in Canadian Society*. Toronto: International Thomson Publishing, 1997.

Christophe, J.-J., T. Ishikawa, Y. Imai, K. Takase, M. Thiriet, and T. Yamaguchi. "Hemodynamics in the Pulmonary Artery of a Patient with Pneumothorax." *Medical Engineering and Physics* 34, no. 6 (2012): 725–32.

Clark, Janet H. "The Probable Amount of Ultra-Violet Radiation Obtained Indoors through Ultra-Violet Transmitting Glass." *Science* 68, no. 1755 (1928): 165–6.

Colbeck, E.H., and Eric Pritchard. "An Explanation of the Vulnerability of the Apices in Tuberculosis of the Lungs." *Lancet* 157, no. 4058 (1901): 1595–7.

Colgan, Frank J., Tae B. Whang, and Alastair J. Gillies. "Atelectasis and Pneumothorax: Effect on Lung Function and Shunting." *Anesthesiology* 29, no. 5 (1968): 923–30.

Collins, J.D. "Tuberculosis in Animals." *Irish Journal of Medical Science* 154, S1 (1985): S15–S23.

Committee for Survey of Hospital Needs in Metropolitan Toronto. *Tuberculosis Care, Part Ten of a Study*. December 1963.

Committee on Chemotherapy and Antibiotics of the American College of Chest Physicians. "Information: The Use of Streptomycin in Tuberculosis." *California Medicine* 70, no. 1 (1949): 81–2.

Condrau, Flurin. "The Patient's View Meets the Clinical Gaze." *Social History of Medicine* 20, no. 3 (2007): 525–40.

Connolly, Cynthia A., and Mary E. Gibson. "The 'White Plague' and Color: Children, Race, and Tuberculosis in Virginia 1900–1935." *Journal of Pediatric Nursing* 26, no. 3 (2011): 230–8.

Connor, J.T.H. "The Adoption and Effects of X-rays in Ontario." *Ontario History* 79, no. 1 (1987): 92–107.

Cook, Sharon Anne. "'Liberation Sticks' or 'Coffin Nails'? Representations of the Working Woman and Cigarette Smoking in Canada, 1919–1939." *Canadian Bulletin of Medical History* 24, no. 2 (2007): 367–401.

Corish, J.L. *Health Knowledge: A Thorough and Concise Knowledge of the Prevention, Causes, and Treatments of Disease, Simplified for Home Use*. Vol. 1. New York: Medical Book Distributors, 1928.

Corper, H.J. "Organic Tuberculosis in Man Analyzed from Postmortem and Experimental Data." *Journal of the American Medical Association* 89, no. 21 (1927): 1756–60.

Cosnett, J.E., and W.S. Linton. "Thoracoplasty for Large Tuberculous Cavities." *South African Medical Journal* 25, no. 12 (1951): 207–9.

Creswell, John W. *Qualitative Inquiry and Research Design: Choosing among Five Approaches*. 3rd ed. Thousand Oaks, CA: Sage Publications, 2013.

Crichton-Browne, James. "An Address on the Treatment of Tuberculosis in Sanatoria." *Lancet* 158, no. 4069 (1901): 505–8.

Crockett, Maryanne, Susan M. King, Ian Kitai, Frances Jamieson, S. Richardson, P. Malloy, B. Yaffe, D. Reynolds, J. Hellmann, E. Cutz et al. "Nosocomial Transmission of Congenital Tuberculosis in a Neonatal Intensive Care Unit." *Clinical Infectious Diseases* 39, no. 11 (2004): 1719–23.

Currow, David C., and Amy P. Abernethy. "Therapeutic Nihilism: The Next Hurdle in Improving the Treatment of Breathlessness." *Current Opinion in Supportive and Palliative Care* 5, no. 2 (2011): 69–70.

Dalal, Bhavin, and Stephen A. Geraci. "Office Management of the Patient with Chronic Cough." *American Journal of Medicine* 124, no. 3 (2011): 206–9.

Daniel, Thomas M. "The History of Tuberculosis." *Respiratory Medicine* 100, no. 11 (2006): 1862–70.

Daniel, Thomas M., Joseph H. Bates, and Katharine A. Downes. "History of Tuberculosis." In *Tuberculosis: Pathogenesis, Protection and Control*, edited by Barry R. Bloom, 13–24. Washington, DC: American Society for Microbiology, 1994.

DasGupta, Sayantani. "Between Stillness and Story: Lessons of Children's Illness Narratives." *Pediatrics* 119, no. 6 (2007): 1384–91.

Davies, Hugh Morriston. "A Provocative Talk on Pulmonary Tuberculosis." *Thorax* 3, no. 4 (1948): 189–213.

Davies, Megan J. "Night Soil, Cesspools, and Smelly Hogs on the Streets: Sanitation, Race, and Governance in Early British Columbia." *Histoire sociale – Social History* 38, no. 75 (2005): 1–35.

Davy, Richard. "Clinical Lecture on the Treatment of Spinal Curvature by Hammock Suspension, and the Application of the Plaster, Felt, or Glue Jacket." *British Medical Journal* 1, no. 1017 (1880): 959–60.

Deming, Dorothy. *Home Care of Tuberculosis: A Guide for the Family*. New York: National Tuberculosis Association, 1949.

Dickson, Edith MacPherson. "Report of the Thirteenth Annual Convention of the Canadian Association of Nursing Education." *Canadian Nurse and Hospital Review* 26, no. 8 (1920): 454–7.

Dobbie, William James. "The History of the Toronto Hospital for Consumptives." West Park Healthcare Centre Archives, ca. 1937.

– "The Hygienic, Dietetic and Medicinal Treatment of Tuberculosis." *Canadian Practitioner* 36, no. 3 (1911): 152–64.

– "A Provincial Program for the Control of Tuberculosis." *Canadian Public Health Journal* 26, no. 10 (1935): 494–505.
– "The Toronto Hospital for Consumptives, Weston, Ontario: The Future, 1935–1955." West Park Healthcare Centre Archives, 1936.
– "What Should Be Taught To-day about the Prevention of Tuberculosis." *Canadian Practitioner* 45, no. 7 (1920): 229–34.
Dock, William. "Apical Localization of Phthisis: Its Significance in Treatment by Prolonged Rest in Bed." *American Review of Tuberculosis* 53 (April 1946): 297–305.
– "Effect of Posture on Alveolar Gas Tension in Tuberculosis: Explanation for Favored Sites of Chronic Pulmonary Lesions." *Archives of Internal Medicine* 94, no. 5 (1954): 700–8.
Dodd, Dianne. "Advice to Parents: The Blue Books, Helen MacMurchy, MD, and the Federal Department of Health, 1920–34." *Canadian Bulletin of Medical History* 8, no. 2 (1991): 203–30.
Donoghue, Helen D., Mark Spigelman, Charles L. Greenblatt, G. Lev-Meor, G.K. Bar-Gal, C. Matheson, K. Vernon, A.G. Nerlich, and A.R. Zink. "Tuberculosis: From Prehistory to Robert Koch, as Revealed by Ancient DNA." *Lancet Infectious Diseases* 4, no. 9 (2004): 584–92.
Dow, Dorothy J., and W. Ernest Lloyd. "The Incidence of Tuberculous Infection and Its Relation to Contagion in Children under 15." *British Medical Journal* 2, no. 3862 (1931): 183–6.
Draus, Paul. *Consumed in the City: Observing Tuberculosis at Century's End.* Philadelphia: Temple University Press, 2004.
Drees, Laurie Meijer. *Healing Histories: Stories from Canada's Indian Hospitals*. Edmonton: University of Alberta Press, 2013.
Dubos, René Jules, and Jean Dubos. *The White Plague: Tuberculosis, Man, and Society*. New Brunswick: Rutgers University Press, 1987.
Duffin, Jacalyn. *History of Medicine: A Scandalously Short Introduction.* Toronto: University of Toronto Press, 1999.
Dusel, Inés. "Fashioning the Schooled Self through Uniforms: A Foucauldian Approach to Contemporary School Policies." In *Dangerous Coagulations?: The Uses of Foucault in the Study of Education*, edited by Bernadette M. Baker and Katharine E. Heyning, 85–199. New York: Peter Lang Publishing, 2004.
Editorial. "Anti-Spitting By-law in Toronto." *Canada Lancet* 37, no. 10 (1904): 953–4.

– "Effects of Streptomycin in Tuberculosis." *Canadian Medical Association Journal* 58, no. 1 (1948): 83–4.

– "Promizole in Tuberculosis." *Canadian Medical Association Journal* 58, no. 2 (1948): 195.

Editorial Comment. "Trends in Tuberculosis." *Canadian Medical Association Journal* 61, no. 6 (1949): 626–7.

Editorial Comments. "The Sulfa Derivatives in the Treatment of Tuberculosis." *Canadian Medical Association Journal* 51, no. 5 (1944): 467.

Elliott, Catherine T., and Sarah N. de Leeuw. "Our Aboriginal Relations: When Family Doctors and Aboriginal Patients Meet." *Canadian Family Physician* 55, no. 4 (2009): 443–4.

Elliott, J.H. *The Present Status of Antituberculosis Work in Canada – 1908*. Prepared for the Canadian Committee of the International Congress on Tuberculosis for presentation at the Washington Meeting, September 1908. Ottawa: Printed by James Hope & Sons, 1909.

– "The Sanatorium: Its Importance in the Crusade against Tuberculosis." *St Paul Medical Journal* 5 (February 1903): 112–25.

– "The Treatment of Pulmonary Tuberculosis." *Canadian Practitioner* 49 (1924): 379–85.

Ellman, Philip. "Co-relation of Calcium Metabolism, Parathyroid Function and Pulmonary Tuberculosis." *Tubercle* 9, no. 4 (1928): 162–7.

Erb, I.H. "The Pathology of Mediastinal Tuberculosis. *Canadian Practitioner* 48 (1923): 505–6.

"Erythrocyte Sedimentation Rate." Lab Tests Online. https://labtestsonline.org/understanding/analytes/esr/tab/test/.

Escombe, A. Roderick, David A.J. Moorse, Robert H. Gilman, Marcos Navincopa, Eduardo Ticona, Bailey Mitchell, Catherine Noakes, Carlos Martínez, Patricia Sheen, Rocio Ramirez et al. "Upper-Room Ultraviolet Light and Negative Air Ionization to Prevent Tuberculosis Transmission." *PLoS Medicine* 6, no. 3 (2009). doi:10.1371/journal.pmed.1000043.

Escombe, A. Roderick, Clarissa C. Oeser, Robert H. Gilman, Marcos Navincopa, Eduardo Ticona, William Pan, Carlos Martínez, Jesus Chacaltana, Richard Rodriguez, David A. Moore et al. "Natural Ventilation for the Prevention of Airborne Contagion." *PLoS Medicine* 4, no. 2 (2007). doi: 10.1371/journal.pmed.0040068.

Esslemont, J.E. "Sanatoriums from Within." *Lancet* 177, no. 4581 (1911): 1639–41.

Ewart, William. "The Treatment of Bronchiectasis and of Chronic Bronchial Affectations by Posture and by Respiratory Exercises." *Lancet* 158, no. 4063 (1901): 70–2.

– "The Treatment of Pulmonary Tuberculosis by a Postural Method." *Lancet* 171, no. 4423 (1908): 1654.

Fanning, Anne. "Tuberculosis: 6. Extra-Pulmonary Disease." *Canadian Medical Association Journal* 160, no. 11 (1999): 1597–1603.

Farmer, Paul. "An Anthropology of Structural Violence." *Current Anthropology* 45, no. 3 (2004): 305–25.

– *Infections and Inequalities: The Modern Plagues*. Berkeley: University of California Press, 1999.

Ferrer, J. "Pleural Tuberculosis." *European Respiratory Journal* 10, no. 4 (1997): 942–7.

Filey, Mike. *Mount Pleasant Cemetery: An Illustrated Guide*. 2nd ed., rev., expanded. Toronto: Dundurn, 1999.

Firestone, William A. "Meaning in Method: The Rhetoric of Quantitative and Qualitative Research." *Educational Researcher* 16, no. 7 (1987): 16–21.

Flanagan, Clara Raina, and Anne Raina. *Clara's Rib: A True Story of a Young Girl Growing Up in a Tuberculosis Hospital*. Self-published by Anne Raina, 2010.

Fleitas, Joan D. "To Tell You the Truth: Children Reflect on Hospital Care." *Issues in Comprehensive Pediatric Nursing* 20, no. 4 (1997): 195–206.

Fleming, A. Grant. "Responsibilities and Opportunities of the Private Practitioner in Preventive Medicine." *Canadian Medical Association Journal* 20, no. 1 (1929): 11–13.

Flyvbjerg, Bent. "Five Misunderstandings about Case-Study Research." *Qualitative Inquiry* 12, no. 2 (2006): 219–45.

Foster-Carter, A.F. "Sanatoria." *Lancet* 265, no. 6862 (1955): 508–9.

Fowler, J. Kingston. "The Therapeutic Value of Sanatorium Treatment in Pulmonary Tuberculosis." *Lancet* 167, no. 4297 (1906): 4–7.

Franco-Paredes, Carlos, and Henry Blumberg. "Psoas Muscle Abscess Caused by *Mycobacterium tuberculosis* and *Staphylococcus aureus*: Case Report and Review." *American Journal of the Medical Sciences* 321, no. 6 (2001): 415–17.

Fukuda, Keiji. "Foreword." In *Antimicrobial Resistance: Global Report on Surveillance*, ix. Geneva: World Health Organization, 2014.

Gagneux, Sebastien. "Host-Pathogen Coevolution in Human Tuberculosis."

Philosophical Transactions of the Royal Society of London B Biological Sciences 367, no. 1590 (2012): 850–9.

Gaikwad, A.N., and Sudhir Sinha. "Determinants of Natural Immunity against Tuberculosis in an Endemic Setting: Factors Operating at the Level of Macrophage–*Mycobacterium tuberculosis* Interaction." *Clinical and Experimental Immunology* 151, no. 3 (2008): 414–22.

Gale, Godfrey L. *The Changing Years: The Story of Toronto Hospital and the Fight against Tuberculosis*. Toronto: West Park Hospital, 1979.

Gale, Godfrey L. Research Notes, 12 pages, West Park Healthcare Centre Archives, n.d.

– "Toronto Hospital – Oral Histories. Autobiography by Dr Roy Garrett, May 1981." West Park Healthcare Centre Archives, 1981.

– "Toronto Hospital – Oral Histories. Interview with Della Robinson (pseudonym), 29 June 1983." West Park Healthcare Centre Archives, 1983.

– "Toronto Hospital – Oral Histories. Interview with Jane Clark (pseudonym), 9 January 1981." West Park Healthcare Centre Archives, 1981.

– "Toronto Hospital – Oral Histories. Interview with Jean Grant (pseudonym), 5 June 1981." West Park Healthcare Centre Archives, 1981.

– "Toronto Hospital – Oral Histories. Interview with Lillian Wilson (pseudonym), 8 November 1983." West Park Healthcare Centre Archives, 1983.

– "Toronto Hospital – Oral Histories. Interview with Lorene Young (pseudonym). 9 June 1981." West Park Healthcare Centre Archives, 1981.

– "Toronto Hospital – Oral Histories. Interview with Marilyn King (pseudonym), 11 January 1983." West Park Healthcare Centre Archives, 1983.

– "Toronto Hospital – Oral Histories. Interview with Sara Davis (pseudonym), 28 April 1982." West Park Healthcare Centre Archives, 1982.

Gandy, Matthew, and Alimuddin Zumla. "Theorizing Tuberculosis: A Reply to Porter and Ogden." *Social Science and Medicine* 55, no. 3 (2002): 399–401.

Garner, J.P., P.D. Meiring, K. Ravi, and R. Gupta. "Psoas Abscess: Not as Rare as We Think?" *Colorectal Disease* 9, no. 3 (2007): 269–74.

Giessler, Paul W. "Tuberculosis of the Bones and Joints." In *Tuberculosis among Children and Young Adults*, J. Arthur Myers, 215–31. Springfield, IL: Charles C. Thomas, 1946.

Gillis, Jonathan. "The History of the Patient History since 1850." *Bulletin of the History of Medicine* 80, no. 3 (2006): 490–512.

– "Taking the Medical History in Childhood Illness: Representations of Parents in Pediatric Texts since 1850." *Bulletin of the History of Medicine* 79, no. 3 (2005): 393–429.

Girdlestone, G.R. "Pott's Disease and Pott's Paraplegia." *Annals of the Royal College of Surgeons of England* 4, no. 4 (1949): 214–31.

Glatman-Freedman, Aharona. "The Role of Antibody-Mediated Immunity in Defense against *Mycobacterium tuberculosis*: Advances toward a Novel Vaccine Strategy." *Tuberculosis* 86, nos 3–4 (2006): 191–7.

Glatman-Freedman, Aharona, and Arturo Casadevall. "Serum Therapy for Tuberculosis Revisited: Reappraisal of the Role of Antibody-Mediated Immunity against *Mycobacterium tuberculosis*." *Clinical Microbiology Reviews* 11, no. 3 (1998): 514–32.

Glenny, Robb W. "Determinants of Regional Ventilation and Blood Flow in the Lung." *Intensive Care Medicine* 35, no. 11 (2009): 1833–42.

Glenny, Robb W., Susan Bernard, H. Thomas Robertson, and Michael Hlastala. "Gravity Is an Important but Secondary Determinant of Regional Pulmonary Blood Flow in Upright Primates." *Journal of Applied Physiology* 86, no. 2 (1999): 623–32.

Goffman, Erving. *Asylums: Essays on the Social Situation of Mental Patients and Other Inmates*. New York: Anchor Books, 1961.

Gombart, Adrian F., Tsuyako Saito, and H. Philip Koeffler. "Exaptation of an Ancient Alu Short Interspersed Element Provides a Highly Conserved Vitamin D-Mediated Innate Immune Response in Humans and Primates." *BMC Genomics* 10 (July 2009): 321.

Gooderham, Mrs. Albert E. "What the Daughters of the Empire Are Doing toward the Prevention of Tuberculosis." *Public Health Journal* 4, no. 4 (1913): 190–4.

Gordon, Burgess. "The Mechanism and Effects of Abdominal Compression in the Treatment of Pulmonary Tuberculosis." *New England Journal of Medicine* 214, no. 5 (1936): 195–8.

Gough, J.H., D. Barlow, T. Holmes Sellors, and V.C. Thompson. "The Results of Thoracoplasty in the Treatment of Pulmonary Tuberculosis." *Thorax* 12, no. 3 (1957): 241–52.

Grainger, Ronald G. "The Pulmonary Circulation: The Radiology of Adaptation." *Clinical Radiology* 36, no. 2 (1985): 103–16.

Grange, John M., Nathan Kapata, Duncan Chanda, Peter Mwaba, and

Alimuddin Zumla. "The Biosocial Dynamics of Tuberculosis." *Tropical Medicine and International Health* 14, no. 2 (2009): 124–30.

Grattan, Nicholas. "The Treatment of Spinal Curvature by Means of the Cuirass." *British Medical Journal* 1, no. 1115 (1882): 693–4.

Greff, Hazel. "The Care of the Child on a Bradford Frame or a Whitman Frame." *American Journal of Nursing* 29, no. 8 (1929): 922–4.

Griffith, J.P. Crozer. *The Care of the Baby: A Manual for Mothers and Nurses*. Philadelphia: W.B. Saunders, 1924.

Gruenwald, I., J. Abrahamson, and O. Cohen. "Psoas Abscess: Case Report and Review of the Literature." *Journal of Urology* 147, no. 6 (1992): 1624–6.

Grygier, Pat Sandiford. *A Long Way from Home: The Tuberculosis Epidemic among the Inuit*. Montreal and Kingston: McGill-Queen's University Press, 1994.

Grzybowski, Stefan, and Edward A. Allen. "History and Importance of Scrofula." *Lancet* 346, no. 8988 (1995): 1472–4.

– "Tuberculosis: 2. History of the Disease in Canada." *Canadian Medical Association Journal* 160, no. 7 (1999): 1025–8.

Hansel, Nadia N., Albert W. Wu, Betty Chang, and Gregory B. Diette. "Quality of Life in Tuberculosis: Patient and Provider Perspectives." *Quality of Life Research* 13, no. 3 (2004): 639–52.

Harper, John E. "Guaiacol Carbonate in Phthisis" (abstract from the *Medical Standard*), *Western Medical Reporter* 15, no. 4 (April 1893): 86.

Harrigan, Richard A., Frederic H. Kauffman, and Michael B. Love. "Tuberculous Psoas Abscess." *Journal of Emergency Medicine* 13, no. 4 (1995): 493–8.

Haugh, Susan. "The Hill of Health: Aspects of Community at the Waipiata Tuberculosis Sanatorium, 1923–1961." *Health and History* 11, no. 2 (2009): 1–20.

Hawes, John B. "Hemorrhage in Pulmonary Tuberculosis." *New England Journal of Medicine* 204 (21 May 1931): 1088–91.

Hawley, George W. "Fracture and Orthopedic Table." *Journal of the American Medical Association* 60, no. 24 (1913): 1850–1.

Heron, Craig. "Baillie, Sir Frank Wilton." Dictionary of Canadian Biography Online. http://www.biographi.ca/en/bio/baillie_frank_wilton_15E.html.

Herring, D. Ann, and Lisa Sattenspiel. "Social Contexts, Syndemics, and Infectious Disease in Northern Aboriginal Populations." *American Journal of Human Biology* 19, no. 2 (2007): 190–202.

Hesseling, A.C., B.J. Marais, H.L. Kirchner, A.M. Mandalakas, W. Brittle, T.C. Victor, R.M. Warren, and H.S. Schaaf. "Mycobacterial Genotype Is Associated with Disease Phenotype in Children." *International Journal of Tuberculosis and Lung Disease* 14, no. 10 (2010): 1252–8.

Hinshaw, H. Corwin, William H. Feldman, and Karl. H. Pfuetze. "Present Status of Chemotherapy in Tuberculosis." *Annals of Internal Medicine* 22, no. 5 (1945): 696–703.

Hobbs, Sidney [pseud]. "After the Sanatorium: An Autobiography by Sidney Hobbs." West Park Healthcare Centre Archives, 1991.

– "Before the Sanatorium: An Autobiography by Sidney Hobbs." West Park Healthcare Centre Archives. 1991.

Hobday, Richard A. "Sunlight Therapy and Solar Architecture." *Medical History* 41, no. 4 (1997): 455–72.

Hodgetts, Charles A. "National and Provincial Responsibility in the Tuberculosis Crusade." *Canadian Practitioner* 37, no. 4 (1912): 214–22.

Hoggarth, E., A.R. Martin, and E.H.P. Young. "Studies in the Chemotherapy of Tuberculosis: Part II. Sulphonamides." *British Journal of Pharmacology* 3, no. 2 (1948): 153–5.

Holbrook, John Howard. "Present Need of the Tuberculosis Campaign in Canada." *Public Health Journal* 11, no. 10 (1920): 461–73.

– "Tuberculosis in General Practice." *Ontario Medical Review* 12 (1945): 122–34.

Holding, Arthur. "Improved Methods of Applying Plaster Spicas and Jackets." *Journal of the American Medical Association* 52, no. 6 (1909): 466–7.

Hopkins, J. Castell. *The Canadian Annual Review of Public Affairs*. Vol. 13. Toronto: Annual Review Publishing, 1913.

Horowitz, M.D., M. Otero, R.J. Thurer, and H. Bolooki. "Late Complications of Plombage." *Annals of Thoracic Surgery* 53, no. 5 (1992): 803–6.

Horsburgh Jr., C. Robert. "Priorities for the Treatment of Latent Tuberculosis Infection in the United States." *New England Journal of Medicine* 350, no. 20 (2004): 2060–7.

Howarth, Walter. "Tuberculosis of the Larynx, with Considerable Dysphagia, Treated and Relieved by Congestion Hyperaemia." *Proceedings of the Royal Society of Medicine* 3 (Laryngol Sect) (1910): 164–5.

Howell, B. Whitchurch. "The Use and Abuse of Plaster of Paris." *Postgraduate Medical Journal* 8, no. 76 (1932): 17–21.

Hurt, Raymond. "Tuberculosis Sanatorium Regimen in the 1940s: A Patient's Personal Diary." *Journal of the Royal Society of Medicine* 97, no. 7 (2004): 350–3.

Hurwitz, Brian. "Form and Representation in Clinical Case Reports." *Literature and Medicine* 25, no. 2 (2006): 216–40.

Iles, Elizabeth A. *Ask the Grey Sisters: Sault Ste Marie and the General Hospital, 1898–1998*. Sault Ste Marie: Sault Area Hospitals, 1998.

Inhorn, Marcia C., and K. Lisa Whittle. "Feminism Meets the 'New' Epidemiologies: Toward an Appraisal of Antifeminist Biases in Epidemiological Research on Women's Health." *Social Science and Medicine* 53, no. 5 (2001): 553–67.

International Council of Nurses. "Tentative Programme for the Congress at Helsingfors, July 20 to 25, 1925." *British Journal of Nursing* 73 (1925): 100.

Irwin, Richard S. "Introduction to the Diagnosis and Management of Cough: ACCP Evidence-Based Clinical Practice Guidelines." *Chest* 129, no. S1 (2006): S25–S27.

Irwin, Richard S., and J. Mark Madison. "Symptom Research on Chronic Cough: A Historical Perspective." *Annals of Internal Medicine* 134, no. 9 (part 2) (2001): 809–14.

Ivo, Roland, Rolf Sobottke, Harald Seifert, M. Ortmann, and P. Eysel. "Tuberculous Spondylitis and Paravertebral Abscess Formation after Kyphoplasty: A Case Report." *Spine* 35, no. 12 (2010): 559–63.

Jackson, Marguerite McMillan, and Renee P. McLeod. "Tuberculosis in Infants, Children, and Adolescents: An Update with Case Studies." *Pediatric Nursing* 23, no. 5 (1998): 411–20.

Jackson, Mark, Ian Smith, Martin King, and John Shneerson. "Long Term Non-Invasive Domiciliary Assisted Ventilation for Respiratory Failure following Thoracoplasty." *Thorax* 49, no. 9 (1994): 915–19.

Jacobs, Richard F., and Kathleen D. Eisenach. "Childhood Tuberculosis." *Advances in Pediatric Infectious Diseases* 8 (1993): 23–51.

Jadvar, Hossein, Robert E. Mindelzun, Eric W. Olcott, and Diana B. Levitt. "Still the Great Mimicker: Abdominal Tuberculosis." *American Journal of Roentgenology* 168, no. 6 (1997): 1455–60.

Jardine, Pauline O. "An Urban Middle-Class Calling: Women and the Emer-

gence of Modern Nursing Education at the Toronto General Hospital, 1881–1914." *Urban History Review* 17, no. 3 (1989): 177–90.
Jarman, T. Francis. "Awaiting Sanatorium Treatment." *Lancet* 244, no. 6312 (1944): 261.
Jeanes, C.W.L. "Tuberculosis." *Canadian Family Physician* 15, no. 1 (1969): 34–40.
Jessel, George, G.T. Hebert, Peter Edwards, R.C. Wingfield, and F.T.H. Wood. "Modern Developments in the Tuberculosis Scheme." *Public Health* 47 (May 1934): 252–61.
Johnson, Robert W., John W. Hillman, and Wayne O. Southwick. "The Importance of Direct Surgical Attack upon Lesions of the Vertebral Bodies, Particularly in Pott's Disease." *Journal of Bone and Joint Surgery* 35–A, no. 1 (1953): 17–24.
Jones, Esyllt W. *Influenza 1918: Disease, Death, and Struggle in Winnipeg.* Toronto: University of Toronto Press, 2007.
– "Politicizing the Laboring Body: Working Families, Death, and Burial in Winnipeg's Influenza Epidemic, 1918–1919." *Labor* 3, no. 3 (2006): 57–75.
Jones, Greta. *"Captain of All These Men of Death": The History of Tuberculosis in Nineteenth and Twentieth Century Ireland.* Amsterdam: Rodopi, 2001.
Jones, Robert. "Notes on the Uses and Application of Thomas's Hip Splint." *British Medical Journal* 2, no. 1396 (1887): 715–16.
Jones, Valerie A. "The White Coat: Why Not Follow Suit?" *Journal of the American Medical Association* 281, no. 5 (1999): 478.
Katona, Peter, and Judit Katona-Apte. "The Interaction between Nutrition and Infection." *Clinical Infectious Diseases* 46, no. 10 (2008): 1582–8.
Kaufmann, Stefan H.E., and Ulrich E. Schaible. "100th Anniversary of Robert Koch's Nobel Prize for the Discovery of the Tubercle Bacillus." *Trends in Microbiology* 13, no. 10 (2005): 469–75.
Kelm, Mary-Ellen. *Colonizing Bodies: Aboriginal Health and Healing in British Columbia, 1900–50.* Vancouver: UBC Press, 1999.
Kendall, W.B. "Observations Relating to Diet in Tuberculosis." *Canadian Medical Association Journal* 2, no. 8 (1912): 670–9.
– "Of What Value Are Sanitoria as a Public Health Measure?" *Canadian Journal of Public Health* 4, no. 4 (1913): 205–8.
Kendig Jr., Edwin L., and Laura S. Inselman. "Tuberculosis in Children." *Advances in Pediatrics* 38 (1991): 233–55.

Kent, S., E.D. Weinberg, and P. Stuart-Macadam. "The Etiology of the Anemia of Chronic Disease and Infection." *Journal of Clinical Epidemiology* 47, no. 1 (1994): 23–33.

Kincade, G.F., G.D. Saxton, P.W. Morse, and A.K. Mathisen. "Streptomycin in the Treatment of Tuberculosis: A Report of Its Use in a Series of 100 Cases." *Canadian Medical Association Journal* 59, no. 2 (1948): 105–12.

King, Arlene, Paul Varughese, Gaston De Serres, Graham A. Tipples, John Waters, and Members of the Working Group on Measles Elimination. "Measles Elimination in Canada." *Journal of Infectious Diseases* 189, S1 (2004): S236–S42.

Kirby, Stephanie, and Wendy Madsen. "Institutionalised Isolation: Tuberculosis Nursing at Westwood Sanatorium, Queensland, Australia 1919–1955." *Nursing Inquiry* 16, no. 2 (2009): 122–32.

Klaver, Elizabeth. "The Illness Memoir." *Contemporary Literature* 49, no. 2 (2008): 307–10.

Kline, Mark W., and Martin I. Lorin. "Childhood Tuberculosis." *Advances in Pediatric Infectious Disease* 2 (1987): 135–60.

Kluger, Richard. *Ashes to Ashes: America's Hundred-Year Cigarette War, the Public Health, and the Unabashed Triumph of Philip Morris*. New York: Alfred A. Knopf, 1996.

Knox-Macaulay, Huxley H.M. "Tuberculosis and the Haemopoietic System." *Baillière's Clinical Haematology* 5, no. 1 (1992): 101–29.

Koch, Robert. "Die Aetiologie der Tuberculose." *Berliner Klinische Wochenschrift* 19 (April 1882): 221–30.

Kochi, Arata. "The Global Tuberculosis Situation and the New Control Strategy of the World Health Organization." *Tubercle* 72, no. 1 (1991): 1–6.

Kosek, Margaret, and Richard A. Oberhelman. "Unraveling the Contradictions of Vitamin A and Infectious Diseases in Children." *Journal of Infectious Diseases* 196, no. 7 (2007): 965–6.

Larcombe, Linda, Julia D. Rempel, Iga Dembinski, K. Tinckam, C. Rigatto, and P. Nickerson. "Differential Cytokine Genotype Frequencies among Canadian Aboriginal and Caucasian Populations." *Genes and Immunity* 6, no. 2 (2005): 140–4.

Law, Arthur A. "Some Surgical Problems Attending the Operation of Extrapleural Thoracoplasty." *Annals of Surgery* 86, no. 2 (1927): 227–8.

Lawrence, Christopher. "Still Incommunicable: Clinical Holists and Medical

Knowledge in Interwar Britain." In *Greater Than the Parts: Holism in Biomedicine 1920–1950*, edited by Christopher Lawrence and George Weisz, 94–111. Oxford: Oxford University Press, 1998.

Lee, Jos. H. "Streptomycin in Pulmonary Tuberculosis." *Canadian Medical Association Journal* 60, no. 3 (1949): 241–3.

Lerner, Barron H. "Constructing Medical Indications: The Sterilization of Women with Heart Disease or Tuberculosis, 1905–1935." *Journal of the History of Medicine and Allied Sciences* 49, no. 3 (1994): 362–79.

– "From Careless Consumptives to Recalcitrant Patients: The Historical Construction of Noncompliance." *Social Science and Medicine* 45, no. 9 (1997): 1423–31.

Levine, Carol. "The Good Doctor: The Carer's Perspective." *Clinical Medicine* 4, no. 3 (2004): 244–5.

Levy, Jack S. "Case Studies: Types, Designs, and Logics of Inference." *Conflict Management and Peace Science* 25, no. 1 (2008): 1–18.

Lienhardt, Christian, Philippe Glaziou, Mukund Uplekar, Knut Lönnroth, Haileyesus Getahun, and Mario Raviglione. "Global Tuberculosis Control: Lessons Learnt and Future Prospects." *Nature Reviews Microbiology* 10, no. 6 (2012): 407–16.

Lindsay, Mary. "Comments on the Article 'Changing Attitudes towards the Care of Children in Hospital: A New Assessment of the Influence of the Work of Bowlby and Robertson in the UK, 1940–1970.'" *Attachment & Human Development* 11, no. 6 (2009): 563–7.

Little, Margaret Hillyard. "'Manhunts and Bingo Blabs': The Moral Regulation of Ontario Single Mothers." In *Moral Regulation and Governance in Canada: History, Context, and Critical Issues*, edited by Amanda Glasbeek, 217–32. Toronto: Canadian Scholars', 2006.

Liu, Jiangqin, Chloe Joynt, Corinne Tymafichuk, and Po-Yin Cheung. "Sequential Changes of Hemodynamics and Blood Gases in Newborn Piglets with Developing Pneumothorax." *Pediatric Pulmonology* 44, no. 1 (2009): 70–5.

Liu, Philip T., Steffen Stenger, Huiying Li, L. Wenzel, B.H. Tan, S.R. Krutzik, M.T. Ochoa, J. Schauber, K. Wu, C. Meinken et al. "Toll-Like Receptor Triggering of a Vitamin D–Mediated Human Antimicrobial Response." *Science* 311, no. 5768 (2006): 1770–3.

Lloyd, W. Ernest, and A. Margaret C. Macpherson. "Pulmonary Tuberculosis in Young Adults." *British Medical Journal* 2, no. 3961 (1936): 1130–3.

Long, Esmond R. "Artificial Pneumothorax in Tuberculosis." *American Journal of Nursing* 19, no. 4 (1919): 265–8.

Long, Richard. "The Canadian Lung Association/Canadian Thoracic Society and Tuberculosis Prevention and Control." *Canadian Respiratory Journal* 14, no. 7 (2007): 427–31.

Long, Richard, Howard Njoo, and Earl Hershfield. "Tuberculosis: 3. Epidemiology of the Disease in Canada." *Canadian Medical Association Journal* 160, no. 8 (1999): 1185–90.

Loynes, R.D. "Scoliosis after Thoracoplasty." *Journal of Bone and Joint Surgery* 54 B, no. 3 (1972): 484–98.

Ludwig, Alfred O. "Emotional Factors in Tuberculosis." *Public Health Reports* 63, no. 27 (1948): 883–8.

Luong, Khanh vinh quoc, and Lan Thi Hoang Nguyen. "Impact of Vitamin D in the Treatment of Tuberculosis." *American Journal of the Medical Sciences* 341, no. 6 (2011): 493–8.

Lux, Maureen. *Medicine That Walks: Medicine, Disease and Canadian Plains Native People, 1880–1940*. Toronto: University of Toronto Press, 2001.

– *Separate Beds: A History of Indian Hospitals in Canada, 1920s–1980s*. Toronto: University of Toronto Press, 2016.

Lyman, Henry M., Christian Fenger, H. Webster Jones, and W.T. Belfield. *The Practical Home Physician: A Popular Guide for the Household Management of Disease, Giving the History, Cause, Means of Prevention and Symptoms of All Diseases of Men, Women and Children and the Most Approved Methods of Treatment, with Plain Instructions for the Care of the Sick*. Albany, NY: Selleck, Ross, 1886.

Macaulay, Ann C. "Improving Aboriginal Health: How Can Health Care Professionals Contribute?" *Canadian Family Physician* 55, no. 4 (2009): 334–6.

MacDougall, Heather. "Cassidy, John Joseph." *Dictionary of Canadian Biography Online*. http://www.biographi.ca/en/bio/cassidy_john_joseph_14E.html.

MacGregor, R.R. "A Case of Tuberculous Meningitis Treated with Streptomycin and Promin." *Canadian Medical Association Journal* 59, no. 1 (1948): 69–70.

Madeo, M. "Understanding the MRSA Experience." *Nursing Times* 97, no. 30 (2001): 36–7.

Maitland, Leslie. "The Design of Tuberculosis Sanatoria in Late Nineteenth-Century Canada." *Bulletin of the Society for the Study of Architecture in Canada* 14, no. 1 (1989): 5–13.

Mandavilli, Apoorva. "The Sunshine Cure." *Nature Medicine* 13, no. 4 (2007): 396–7.

Marais, B.J., R.P. Gie, H.S. Schaaf, A.C. Hesseling, D.A. Enarson, and N. Beyers. "The Spectrum of Disease in Children Treated for Tuberculosis in a Highly Endemic Area." *International Journal of Tuberculosis and Lung Disease* 10, no. 7 (2006): 732–8.

Marais, B.J., R.P. Gie, H.S. Schaaf, A.C. Hesseling, C.C. Obihara, J.J. Starke, D.A. Enarson, P.R. Donald, and N. Beyers. "The Natural History of Childhood Intra-Thoracic Tuberculosis: A Critical Review of Literature from the Pre-Chemotherapy Era." *International Journal of Tuberculosis and Lung Disease* 8, no. 4 (2004): 392–402.

Marcellus, Lenora. "Tiny Cripples and the Sunshine of Life: 15 Years of Children's Nursing at Vancouver Island's Queen Alexandra Solarium, 1927–1942." *Journal of Pediatric Nursing* 19, no. 6 (2004): 411–20.

Marshall, Marion. "My Personal Experience of Tuberculosis." *Canadian Journal of Public Health* 4, no. 9 (1913): 491–8.

Martin, Jo M., Jessica M. Ghaferi, Deborah L. Cummins, Adam J. Mamelak, Chrys D. Schmults, Mona Parikh, Lark-Aeryn Speyer, Alice Chuang, Hazel V. Richardson, David Stein et al. "Changes in Skin Tanning Attitudes: Fashion Articles and Advertisements in the Early 20th Century." *American Journal of Public Health* 99, no. 12 (2009): 2140–6.

Mathad, Jyoti S., and Amita Gupta. "Tuberculosis in Pregnant and Postpartum Women: Epidemiology, Management, and Research Gaps." *Clinical Infectious Diseases* 55, no. 11 (2012): 1532–49.

Mayho, P. "Barrier Grief." *Nursing Times* 95, no. 31 (1999): 24–5.

McClelland, J.C. "Anuria: A Report of Three Types of Cases." *Canadian Medical Association Journal* 45, no. 4 (1941): 332–5.

McConnachie, Kathleen. "Methodology in the Study of Women in History: A Case Study of Helen MacMurchy, MD." *Ontario History* 75, no. 1 (1983): 61–70.

McCuaig, Katherine. *The Weariness, the Fever, and the Fret: The Campaign against Tuberculosis in Canada, 1900–1950*. Montreal and Kingston: McGill-Queen's University Press, 1999.

McCullagh, John. *A Legacy of Caring: A History of the Children's Aid Society of Toronto*. Toronto: Dundurn Group, 2002.

McKeown, Thomas. *The Origins of Human Disease*. Oxford: Basil Blackwell, 1988.

– *The Role of Medicine: Dream, Mirage, or Nemesis?* Princeton: Princeton University Press, 1979.

McKergow, Mrs F.C. "Outline of History of the Samaritan Club of Toronto." West Park Healthcare Centre Archives, ca. 1950.

Mellon, Ralph R. "Chemotherapy of Tuberculosis and the Mode of Action of the Sulfonamide Compounds." *Chest* 8, no. 6 (1942): 166–72.

Memarzadeh, Farhad, Russell N. Olmsted, and Judene M. Bartley. "Applications of Ultraviolet Germicidal Irradiation Disinfection in Health Care Facilities: Effective Adjunct, but Not Stand-Alone Technology." *American Journal of Infection Control* 38, no. 5, S1 (2010): S13–S24.

Merriam, Sharan B. *Qualitative Research and Case Study Applications in Education*. San Francisco: Jossey-Bass Publishers, 1998.

Mierau, Maurice. *Memoir of a Living Disease: The Story of Earl Hershfield and Tuberculosis in Manitoba and Beyond*. Winnipeg: Great Plains Publications, 2005.

Minnett, Valerie, and Mary-Anne Poutanen. "Swatting Flies for Health: Children and Tuberculosis in Early Twentieth-Century Montréal." *Urban History Review* 36, no. 1 (2007): 32–44.

Minns, F.S. "The Practical Management of Pulmonary Tuberculosis." *Canadian Practitioner and Review* 37, no. 3 (1912): 159–70.

Moe, Sharon M. "Disorders Involving Calcium, Phosphorus, and Magnesium." *Primary Care: Clinics in Office Practice* 35, no. 2 (2008): 215–37.

Moffatt, Jessica, Maria Mayan, and Richard Long. "Sanitoriums and the Canadian Colonial Legacy: The Untold Experiences of Tuberculosis Treatment." *Qualitative Health Research* 23, no. 12 (2013): 1591–9.

Molnar, Stephen. *Human Variation: Races, Types, and Ethnic Groups*. 6th ed. Upper Saddle River, NJ: Pearson / Prentice Hall, 2005.

Mond, David J., and Arfa Khan. "Lucite Ball Plombage." *New England Journal of Medicine* 330, no. 24 (1994): 1723.

Moon, Myung-Sang. "Tuberculosis of the Spine: Controversies and New Challenge." *Spine* 22, no. 15 (1997): 1791–7.

Moorman, Lewis J. "Hemoptysis in Tuberculosis, with a Differential Discussion of Other Causes." *Annals of Internal Medicine* 121, no. 3 (1944): 447–54.

Morland, Egbert. "Contact with the Tubercle Bacillus." *Lancet* 244, no. 6312 (1944): 249–51.

– "Essay and Plans for the Erection of a Sanatorium for Tuberculosis." *Lancet* 161, no. 4140 (1903): 59–68.

Morse, D. "Prehistoric Tuberculosis in America." *American Review of Respiratory Diseases* 83 (1961): 489–504.

Mostofi, Seyed Behrooz. *Who's Who in Orthopedics*. London: Springer-Verlag, 2005.

Muckley, Thomas, Tanja Schutz, Martin Kirschner, Michael Potulski, Gunther Hofmann, and Volker Buhren. "Psoas Abscess: The Spine as a Primary Source of Infection." *Spine* 28, no. 6 (2003): 106–13.

Mure, Margareta, Karen B. Domino, Sten G.E. Lindahl, M.P. Hlastala, W.A. Altemeier, and R.W. Glenny. "Regional Ventilation-Perfusion Distribution Is More Uniform in the Prone Position." *Journal of Applied Physiology* 88, no. 3 (2000): 1076–83.

Murray, John F. "Bill Dock and the Location of Pulmonary Tuberculosis: How Bed Rest Might Have Helped Consumption." *American Journal of Respiratory and Critical Care Medicine* 168, no. 9 (2003): 1029–33.

Murray, Karen Bridget. "Governing 'Unwed Mothers' in Toronto at the Turn of the Twentieth Century." *Canadian Historical Review* 85, no. 2 (2004): 1–13.

Myers, J. Arthur, with C.A. Stewart, Paul W. Giessler, and Allen K. Krause. *Tuberculosis among Children and Young Adults*. 2nd ed. Springfield, IL: Charles C. Thomas, 1946.

Nardell, Edward A. "Environmental Control of Tuberculosis." *Medical Clinics of North America* 77, no. 6 (1993): 1315–34.

National Sanitarium Association (NSA). *Annual Report* (various years).

Neal, F.C. "The Early Diagnosis of Pulmonary Tuberculosis." *Canadian Practitioner and Review* 36, no. 9 (1911): 531–9.

Neff, Charlotte. "The Education of Destitute Homeless Children in Nineteenth-Century Ontario." *Journal of Family History* 29, no. 1 (2004): 3–46.

– "Government Approaches to Child Neglect and Mistreatment in Nineteenth-Century Ontario." *Histoire sociale/Social History* 41, no. 81 (2008): 165–214.

– "The Role of Protestant Children's Homes in Nineteenth-Century Ontario: Child Rescue or Family Support?" *Journal of Family History* 34, no. 1 (2009): 48–88.

– "The Role of the Toronto Girls' Home, 1863–1910. *Journal of Family History* 36, no. 3 (2011): 286–315.

Nickel, Daniel, Martin Busch, Daniel Mayer, Benjamin Hagemann, Valeska Knoll, and Steffen Stenger. "Hypoxia Triggers the Expression of Human β Defensin 2 and Antimicrobial Activity against *Mycobacterium tuberculosis* in Human Macrophages." *Journal of Immunology* 188, no. 8 (2012): 4001–7.

Nissen, K.I. "Editorial." *Postgraduate Medical Journal* 24, no. 271 (1948): 227–8.

Noll, Steven. "Patient Records as Historical Stories: The Case of Caswell Training School." *Bulletin of the History of Medicine* 68, no. 3 (1994): 411–28.

Norton, Wayne. *"A Whole Little City by Itself": Tranquille and Tuberculosis.* Kamloops, BC: Plateau, 1999.

Nowell, Peter C., and Louis B. Delpino. "Esmond R. Long." In *Biographical Memoirs: National Academy of Sciences of the United States of America*, 56:284–311. Washington, DC: National Academy, 1987.

Noymer, Andrew, and Michel Garenne. "The 1918 Influenza Epidemic's Effects on Sex Differentials in Mortality in the United States." *Population and Development Review* 26, no. 3 (2000): 565–81.

O'Connor, Terence M., Deirdre M. O'Riordan, Maria Stack, and Charles P. Bredin. "Airways Obstruction in Survivors of Thoracoplasty: Reversibility Is Greater in Non-smokers." *Respirology* 9, no. 1 (2004): 130–3.

Odell, John A. "The History of Surgery for Pulmonary Tuberculosis." *Thoracic Surgery Clinics* 22, no. 3 (2012): 257–69.

Ontario Provincial Board of Health. *Twenty-Ninth Annual Report of the Provincial Board of Health of Ontario, for the Year 1910*. Toronto: Printed by L.K. Cameron, 1911.

Ontario Provincial Department of Health. "The Development of Public Health in Ontario." *Canadian Public Health Journal* 26, no. 3 (1935): 110–23.

Osborne, Michael A., and Richard S. Fogarty. "Medical Climatology in France: The Persistence of Neo-Hippocratic Ideas in the First Half of the Twentieth Century." *Bulletin of the History of Medicine* 86, no. 4 (2012): 543–63.

Paine, A.L., and Earl S. Hershfield. "Tuberculosis: Past, Present and Future." *Canadian Family Physician* 25 (1979): 55–8.

Paluzzi, Joan E. "A Social Disease/A Social Response: Lessons in Tuberculosis from Early 20th Century Chile." *Social Science and Medicine* 59, no. 4 (2004): 763–73.

Park, F.S. "Causes of Rejection from the Army and Incidence of Defects in Recruits." *Canadian Medical Association Journal* 51, no. 5 (1944): 412–16.

Parker, George. "Distributors, Agents, and Publishers: Creating a Separate Market for Books in Canada, 1900–1920." *Papers of the Bibliographical Society of Canada* 43, no. 2 (2005): 7–66.

Parsons, Harold C. "Tuberculosis Contacts." *Canadian Practitioner* 48 (1923): 501–4.

Peppas, George, Thomas F. Molnar, Kumarasingham Jeyasingham, and Alan B. Kirk. "Thoracoplasty in the Context of Current Surgical Practice." *Annals of Thoracic Surgery* 56, no. 4 (1993): 903–9.

Pérez-Guzmán, Carlos, Mario H. Vargas, Francisco Quiñonez, Norma Bazavilvazo, and Adriana Aguilar. "A Cholesterol-Rich Diet Accelerates Bacteriologic Sterilization in Pulmonary Tuberculosis." *Chest* 127, no. 2 (2005): 643–51.

Perretz, Edgar A., "A Study of the Samaritan Club of Toronto, Conducted for the Social Planning Council of Metropolitan Toronto." West Park Healthcare Centre Archives, n.d.

Pezzella, A.T., and W. Fang. "Surgical Aspects of Thoracic Tuberculosis: A Contemporary Review – Part 2." *Current Problems in Surgery* 45, no. 10 (2008): 771–829.

Phelps, Winthrop M. "Light Therapy." *American Journal of Nursing* 28, no. 9 (1928): 875–80.

Polverino, Mario, Francesca Polverino, Marco Fasolino, Filippo Andò, Antonio Alfieri, and Francesco de Blasio. "Anatomy and Neuro-Pathophysiology of the Cough Reflex Arc." *Multidisciplinary Respiratory Medicine* 7 (2012).

Pope, Alton S. "The Role of the Sanatorium in Tuberculosis Control." *Milbank Memorial Fund Quarterly* 16, no. 4 (1938): 327–37.

Porter, George D. "On the Choice of a Climate." *Canadian Journal of Medicine and Surgery* 24, no. 6 (1908): 341–8.

– "Tuberculosis Association." *Canadian Practitioner* 41 (1916): 511–13.

Porter, John D.H., and Jessica A. Ogden. "Commentary on 'The Resurgence of Disease': Social and Historical Perspectives on the 'New' Tuberculosis." *Social Science and Medicine* 55, no. 3 (2002): 397–8.

Pottenger, F.M. "The Physiologic Nature of Protective and Healing Principles in Tuberculosis." *British Journal of Tuberculosis* 30, no. 4 (1936): 219–27.

Poutanen, Mary Anne, Sherry Olson, Raphael Fischler, and Kevin Schwartzman. "Tuberculosis in Town: Mobility of Patients in Montreal, 1925–1950." *Histoire Sociale/Social History* 42, no. 83 (2009): 69–106.

Prest, Edward E. "The Treatment of Tuberculosis with Colloid of Calcium." *British Medical Journal* 1, no. 3185 (January 1922): 53–4.

Price, Dorothy. "Mediastinal Gland Tuberculosis in Young Children." *Irish Journal of Medical Science* 11, no. 5 (1936): 200–8.

Price-Brown, J. "Treatment of Laryngeal Tuberculosis." *Canadian Journal of Medicine and Surgery* 11, no. 2 (1902): 75–83.

Prisk, G. Kim, Kei Yamada, A. Cortney Henderson, Tatsuya J. Arai, David L. Levin, Richard B. Buxton, and Susan R. Hopkins. "Pulmonary Perfusion in the Prone and Supine Postures in the Normal Human Lung." *Journal of Applied Physiology* 103, no. 3 (2007): 883–94.

Proctor, A.P. "Pulmonary Tuberculosis: Its Treatment and Prevention." *Canadian Journal of Medicine and Surgery* 11, no. 3 (1902): 153–9.

Pulver Ungar, Molly, and Vicky Bach. "Gage, Sir William James." Dictionary of Canadian Biography Online. http://www.biographi.ca/en/bio/gage_william_james_15E.html.

Rajakumar, Kumaravel. "Vitamin D, Cod-Liver Oil, Sunlight, and Rickets: A Historical Perspective." *Pediatrics* 112, no. 2 (2003): 132–5.

Ramachandran, G., T. Santha, R. Garg, D. Baskaran, S.A. Iliayas, P. Venkatesan, R. Fathima, and P.R. Narayanan. "Vitamin A Levels in Sputum-Positive Pulmonary Tuberculosis Patients in Comparison with Household Contacts and Healthy 'Normals.'" *International Journal of Tuberculosis and Lung Disease* 8, no. 9 (2004): 1130–3.

Randal, Helen. "Editorial." *Canadian Nurse and Hospital Review* 16, no. 8 (1920): 478.

Reed, William P., John W. Olds, and Alexander L. Kisch. "Decreased Skin-Test Reactivity Associated with Influenza." *Journal of Infectious Diseases* 125, no. 4 (1972): 398–402.

Reyn, Axel. "Discussion on the Artificial Light Treatment of Lupus and Other Forms of Tuberculosis." *British Medical Journal* 2, no. 3273 (1923): 499–503.

Rhoades, Rodney A. "Pulmonary Circulation and Ventilation-Perfusion." In *Medical Physiology: Principles for Clinical Medicine*, 3rd ed., edited by Rodney A. Rhoades and David R. Bell, 361–73. Baltimore, MD: Lippincott Williams & Wilkins, 2009.

Riboldi, Elena, Chiara Porta, Sara Morlacchi, A. Viola, A. Mantovani, and A. Sica. "Hypoxia-Mediated Regulation of Macrophage Functions in Pathophysiology." *International Immunology* 25, no. 2 (2012): 67–75.

Ridlon, John. "Forcible Straightening of Spinal Curvature." *Transactions of the American Orthopedic Association* 1 (May 1898): 120–31.

Riley, Richard L. "Aerial Dissemination of Pulmonary Tuberculosis." *American Review of Tuberculosis* 76, no. 6 (1957): 931–41.

Riley, Richard L., C. Mills, and W. Nyka. "Aerial Dissemination of Tuberculosis: A Two-Year Study of Contagion on a Tuberculosis Ward." *American Journal of Hygiene* 70, no. 2 (1959): 185–96.

Riley, Richard L., C.C. Mills, F. O'Grady, L.U. Sultan, F. Wittstadt, and D.N. Shivpuri. "Infectiousness of Air from a Tuberculosis Ward. Ultraviolet Irradiation of Infected Air: Comparative Infectiousness of Different Patients." *American Review of Respiratory Disease* 85 (April 1962): 511–25.

Ringer, Paul H. "Management of Pulmonary Tuberculosis in Relation to Hemorrhage." *Chest* 6, no. 5 (1940): 136–8.

Ripley, Donald F. *Thine Own Keeper: Life at the Nova Scotia Sanatorium, 1904–1977*. Hantsport, NS: Lancelot, 1992.

Risse, Guenter B. *Mending Bodies, Saving Souls: A History of Hospitals*. Cary, NC: Oxford University Press, 1999.

Risse, Guenter B., and John Harley Warner. "Reconstructing Clinical Activities: Patient Records in Medical History." *Social History of Medicine* 5, no. 2 (1992): 183–205.

Roberts, Charlotte A., and Jane E. Buikstra. *The Bioarchaeology of Tuberculosis: A Global View on a Reemerging Disease*. Gainesville: University Press of Florida, 2003.

Roberts, David. "Massey, Hart Almerrin." Dictionary of Canadian Biography Online. http://www.biographi.ca/en/bio/massey_hart_almerrin_12E.html.

Robertson, Joyce, and Katharine McGilly. "Comments on 'Changing Attitudes towards the Care of Children in Hospital: A New Assessment of the Influence of the Work of Bowlby and Robertson in the UK, 1940–1970.'" *Attachment & Human Development* 11, no. 6 (2009): 557–61.

Robinson, Samuel, and Cleaveland Floyd. "Artificial Pneumothorax as a Treatment of Pulmonary Tuberculosis." *Archives of Internal Medicine* 9, no. 4 (1912): 452–83.

– "Artificial Pneumothorax as a Treatment of Pulmonary Tuberculosis."

Transactions of the American Climatological Association 27 (1911): 289–383.

Roelandts, Rik. "The History of Phototherapy: Something New under the Sun?" *Journal of the American Academy of Dermatology* 46, no. 6 (2002): 926–30.

– "A New Light on Niels Finsen, a Century after His Nobel Prize." *Photodermatology, Photoimmunology and Photomedicine* 21, no. 3 (2005): 115–17.

Rogers, Frank B. "The Rise and Decline of the Altitude Therapy of Tuberculosis." *Bulletin of the History of Medicine* 43, no. 1 (1969): 1–16.

Rollier, Auguste, with A. Rosselet, H.J. Schmid, and E. Amstad. *Heliotherapy*. London: Oxford Medical Publications, 1923.

Ronald, Alfred C. "Some Aspects of Tuberculosis in Ontario, Canada." *South African Medical Journal* 29, no. 34 (1955): 791–4.

Rooke, Patricia T., and R.L. Schnell. "Child Welfare in English Canada, 1920–1948." *Social Service Review* 55, no. 3 (1981): 484–506.

Rosenberg, Charles E. "The Therapeutic Revolution: Medicine, Meaning, and Social Change in Nineteenth-Century America." In *The Therapeutic Revolution: Essays in the Social History of American Medicine*, edited by Morris J. Vogel and Charles E. Rosenberg, 3–25. Philadelphia: University of Pennsylvania Press, 1979.

Rosselet, A. "The Scientific Basis of Heliotherapy," In *Heliotherapy*, A. Rollier, with the collaboration of A. Rosselet, H.J. Schmid, and E. Amstad, 158–214. London: Oxford Medical Publications, 1923.

Rothman, Sheila M. *Living in the Shadow of Death: Tuberculosis and the Social Experience of Illness in American History*. New York: Basic Books, 1994.

Rubaie, Talal Al. "The Rehabilitation of the Case-Study Method." *European Journal of Psychotherapy* 5, no. 1 (2002): 31–47.

Ruddin, Lee Peter. "You Can Generalize Stupid! Social Scientists, Bent Flyvbjerg, and Case Study Methodology." *Qualitative Inquiry* 12, no. 4 (2006): 797–812.

Rustad, Tige R., Ashley M. Sherrid, Kyle J. Minch, and David R. Sherman. "Hypoxia: A Window into *Mycobacterium tuberculosis* Latency." *Cellular Microbiology* 11, no. 8 (2009): 1151–9.

Rutkow, Ira M. "Lewis Albert Sayre and the Suspension Treatment of Spinal Disease." *Archives of Surgery* 136, no. 1 (2001): 119.

Ryan, Frank. *The Forgotten Plague: How the Battle against Tuberculosis was Won – and Lost*. Boston: Back Bay Books – Little, Brown, 1992.

Sakula, Alex. "Carlo Forlanini, Inventor of Artificial Pneumothorax for Treatment of Pulmonary Tuberculosis." *Thorax* 38, no. 5 (1983): 326–32.
– "Robert Koch: Centenary of the Discovery of the Tubercle Bacillus, 1882." *Thorax* 37, no. 4 (1982): 246–51.
– "Robert Koch: The Story of His Discoveries in Tuberculosis." *Irish Journal of Medical Science* 154, no. 5, S1 (1985): S3–S9.
Samaritan Club. "History 1912–1971." West Park Healthcare Centre Archives, n.d.
Sawchuk, Lawrence A. "Rethinking the Impact of the 1918 Influenza Pandemic on Sex Differentials in Mortality." *American Journal of Physical Anthropology* 139, no. 4 (2009): 584–90.
Sayre, Lewis Albert. *A New Operation for Artificial Hip-Joint in Bony Anchylosis: Illustrated by Two Cases*. New York: D. Appleton, 1869.
– *Spinal Disease and Spinal Curvature: Their Treatment by Suspension, and by the Use of the Plaster of Paris Bandage*. London: Smith Elder, 1877.
Scambler, Graham, and Anthony Hopkins. "Being Epileptic: Coming to Terms with Stigma." *Sociology of Health and Illness* 8, no. 1 (1986): 26–43.
Schaaf, H.S., I.A. Michaelis, M. Richardson, C.N. Booysen, R.P. Gie, R. Warren, P.D. van Helden, and N. Beyers. "Adult-to-Child Transmission of Tuberculosis: Household or Community Contact?" *International Journal of Tuberculosis and Lung Disease* 7, no. 5 (2003): 426–31.
Schaible, Ulrich E., and Stefan H.E. Kaufmann. "Malnutrition and Infection: Complex Mechanisms and Global Impacts." *PLoS Medicine* 4, no. 5 (2007). doi: 10.1371/journal.pmed.0040115.
Scheper-Hughes, Nancy, and Margaret M. Lock. "The Mindful Body: A Prolegomenon to Future Work in Medical Anthropology." *Medical Anthropology Quarterly* 1, no. 1 (1987): 6–41.
Seabrook, Jeremy. *Working-Class Childhood: An Oral History*. London: Victor Gollancz, 1982.
Semb, Carl. "Thoracoplasty with Extrafascial Apicolysis." *British Medical Journal* 2, no. 4014 (1937): 650–6.
Sepkowitz, Kent A. "Tuberculosis and the Health Care Worker: A Historical Perspective." *Annals of Internal Medicine* 120, no. 1 (1994): 71–9.
Sever, John L., and Guy P. Youmans. "The Relation of Oxygen Tension to Virulence of Tubercle Bacilli and to Acquired Resistance in Tuberculosis." *Journal of Infectious Diseases* 101, no. 2 (1957): 193–202.
Shaw, Ann, and Carole Reeves. *The Children of Craig-y-nos: Life in a Welsh*

Tuberculosis Sanatorium, 1922–1959. London: Wellcome Trust Centre for the History of Medicine at UCL, 2009.

Shepherd, Mary P. "Plombage in the 1980s." *Thorax* 40, no. 5 (1985): 328–40.

Shneerson, John M. "Respiratory Failure in Tuberculosis: A Modern Perspective." *Clinical Medicine* 4, no. 1 (2004): 72–6.

Shorter, Edward. *Bedside Manners: The Troubled History of Doctors and Patients*. New York: Simon and Schuster, 1985.

Shortt, S.E.D. "The Canadian Hospital in the Nineteenth Century: An Historiographic Lament." *Journal of Canadian Studies* 18, no. 4 (1983–84): 3–14.

Shumsky, Neil Larry, James Bohland, and Paul Knox. "Separating Doctors' Homes and Doctors' Offices: San Francisco, 1881–1941." *Social Science and Medicine* 23, no. 10 (1986): 1051–7.

Sims, Diane. *A Life Consumed: Lilly Samson's Dispatches from the TB Front*. Sudbury: Scrivener, 2008.

Singer, Merrill C. "Doorways in Nature: Syndemics, Zoonotics, and Public Health. A Commentary on Rock, Buntain, Hatfield and Hallgrímsson." *Social Science and Medicine* 68, no. 6 (2009): 996–9.

Singer, Merrill, and Scott Clair. "Syndemics and Public Health: Reconceptualizing Disease in Bio-Social Context." *Medical Anthropology Quarterly* 17, no. 4 (2003): 423–41.

Smith, Francis B. *The Retreat of Tuberculosis, 1850–1950*. London: Croom Helm, 1988.

Smith, Kim Connelly. "Congenital Tuberculosis: A Rare Manifestation of a Common Infection." *Current Opinion in Infectious Diseases* 15, no. 3 (2002): 269–74.

Smith, Margaret H.D. "Tuberculosis in Children and Adolescents." *Clinics in Chest Medicine* 10 (1989): 381–95.

Smith, Susan L., and Dawn D. Nickel. "From Home to Hospital: Parallels in Birthing and Dying in Twentieth-Century Canada." *Canadian Bulletin of Medical History* 16, no. 1 (1999): 49–64.

Snider, Dixie E. "Pregnancy and Tuberculosis." *Chest* 86, S3 (1984): S10–S13.

Solotorovsky, Morris, Elizabeth J. Bugie, and Bettina M. Frost. "The Effect of Penicillin on the Growth of *Mycobacterium tuberculosis* in Dubos' Medium." *Journal of Bacteriology* 55, no. 4 (1948): 555–9.

Southam, W.J. "Secretary's Report." *Hamilton Health Association, Second Annual Report of the Mountain Sanatorium*, 1907.

Southee, Kathy Weekes. "Florence Gooderham Huestis." Ban Righ Foundation, 2015. banrighcentre.queensu.ca/tributes/florence-gooderham-huestis/.

Spriggs, Edmund Anthony. "Rest and Exercise in Pulmonary Tuberculosis: A Study of Fashion in Treatment." *Tubercle* 41, no. 6 (1960): 455–62.

Stake, Robert E. *The Art of Case Study Research*. Thousand Oaks, CA: Sage Publications, 1995.

Stanton, Judith Anne. "Aesculapius: A Modern Tale." *Journal of the American Medical Association* 281, no 5 (1999): 476–7.

Stapleford, F.N. "Neighbourhood Workers' Association, Toronto: Summary of Operation for the Year." *Public Health Journal* 11, no. 7 (1920): 326–31.

Starke, Jeffrey R. "Childhood Tuberculosis in the 1990s." *Pediatric Annals* 22, no. 9 (1993): 550–60.

– "Tuberculosis: An Old Disease but a New Threat to the Mothers, Fetus, and Neonate." *Clinics in Perinatology* 24, no. 1 (1997): 107–27.

Starks, Helen, and Susan Brown Trinidad. "Choose Your Method: A Comparison of Phenomenology, Discourse Analysis, and Grounded Theory." *Qualitative Health Research* 17, no. 10 (2007): 1372–80.

Starr, Clarence L. "Treatment of Tuberculous Affections of Bones and Joints." *Canadian Journal of Medicine and Surgery* 11, no. 3 (1902): 160–2.

Starr, Paul. "The Politics of Therapeutic Nihilism." *Hastings Center Report* 6, no. 5 (1976): 24–30.

– *The Social Transformation of American Medicine*. New York: Basic Books, 1982.

Steinbock, R. Ted. *Paleopathological Diagnosis and Interpretation*. Springfield, IL: C.C. Thomas, 1976.

Stewart, Julia. "The Samaritan Club of Toronto, 1912–1933." Toronto: Gage Institute. West Park Healthcare Centre Archives, n.d.

Stobie, W. "Prognosis in Pulmonary Tuberculosis." *British Medical Journal* 1, no. 3768 (1933): 507–9.

Stone, Anne C., Alicia K. Wilbur, Jane E. Buikstra, and Charlotte A. Roberts. "Tuberculosis and Leprosy in Perspective." *American Journal of Physical Anthropology* 140, S49 (2009): S66–S94.

Stoney, R. Atkinson. "Bier's Method of Treatment by Hyperaemia." *Transactions of the Royal Academy of Medicine in Ireland* 27, no. 1 (1909): 145–57.

Strange, Julie-Marie. "'She Cried a Very Little': Death, Grief and Mourning in Working-Class Culture, c. 1880–1914." *Social History* 27, no. 2 (2002): 143–61.

Street, Alice. "Affective Infrastructure: Hospital Landscapes of Hope and Failure." *Space and Culture* 15, no. 1 (2012): 44–56.

Struthers, James. "'In the Interests of the Children': Mothers' Allowances and the Origins of Income Security in Ontario, 1917–1930." In *Social Fabric or Patchwork Quilt: The Development of Social Policy in Canada*, edited by Raymond B. Blake and Jeffrey A. Keshen, 59–87. Peterborough, ON: Broadview, 2006.

Stuart, Meryn. "Ideology and Experience: Public Health Nursing and the Ontario Rural Child Welfare Project, 1920–25." *Canadian Bulletin of Medical History* 6, no. 2 (1989): 111–31.

Stuart-Macadam, Patricia. "Integrative Anthropology: A Focus on Iron-Deficiency Anemia." *Archaeological Papers of the American Anthropological Association* 16, no. 1 (2006): 129–37.

– "Porotic Hyperostosis: A New Perspective." *American Journal of Physical Anthropology* 87, no. 1 (1992): 39–47.

Subotic, D., D. Mandaric, M. Gajic, and M. Vukcevic. "Uncertainties in the Current Understanding of Gas Exchange in Spontaneous Pneumothorax: Effective Lung Ventilation May Persist in a Smaller-Sized Pneumothorax." *Medical Hypotheses* 64, no. 6 (2005): 1144–9.

Symons, A.D. "Treatment of Tuberculosis with Colloid Calcium." *British Medical Journal* 1, no. 3186 (January 1922): 123–4.

Taylor, Frank Sherwood. *The Conquest of Bacteria: From Salvarsan to Sulphapyridine*. Freeport, NY: Books for Libraries Press, 1971. First published in 1940.

Taylor, James Frater. "In the Limelight: A Series of Short Sketches of Prominent Canadians." *Journal of Commerce*, 5 September 1914.

Thearle, William H. "Radical Phrenicotomy for Pulmonary Tuberculosis." *Journal of the American Medical Association* 86, no. 12 (1926): 811–13.

Tileston, Wilder. "Passive Hyperemia of the Lungs and Tuberculosis." *Journal of the American Medical Association* 50, no. 15 (1908): 1179–82.

Tomes, Nancy. "The Making of Germ Panic, Then and Now." *American Journal of Public Health* 90, no. 2 (2000): 191–8.

Tremblay, G.A. "Historical Statistics Support a Hypothesis Linking Tuberculosis and Air Pollution Caused by Coal." *International Journal of Tuberculosis and Lung Disease* 11, no. 7 (2007): 722–32.

Trimble, Harold Guyon, and James Robert Wood. "Pulmonary Hemorrhage:

Its Control by the Use of Intravenous Pituitrin." *Chest* 18, no. 4 (1950): 345–51.

Trudeau, Edward L. "The Adirondack Cottage Sanitarium for the Treatment of Incipient Pulmonary Tuberculosis." *Canadian Journal of Medicine and Surgery* 5, no. 6 (1899): 370–80.

Tsuboi, Tomomasa, Motoharu Ohi, Kazuo Chin, H. Hirata, N. Otsuka, H. Kita, and K. Kuno. "Ventilatory Support during Exercise in Patients with Pulmonary Tuberculosis Sequelae." *Chest* 112, no. 4 (1997): 1000–7.

Uhlin, Michael, Jan Andersson, Alimuddin Zumla, and Markus Maeurer. "Adjunct Immunotherapies for Tuberculosis." *Journal of Infectious Diseases* 205, S2 (2012): S1–S10.

van der Geest, Sjaak, and Kaja Finkler. "Hospital Ethnography: Introduction." *Social Science and Medicine* 59, no. 10 (2004): 1995–2001.

van der Horst, Frank C.P., and Rene van der Veer. "Changing Attitudes towards the Care of Children in Hospital: A New Assessment of the Influence of the Work of Bowlby and Robertson in the UK, 1940–1970." *Attachment & Human Development* 11, no. 2 (2009): 119–42.

Varughese, Paul. "Measles in Canada: 1986 Update." *Canadian Medical Association Journal* 135, no. 5 (1986): 499–501.

Vassar, Matt, and Matthew Holzmann. "The Retrospective Chart Review: Important Methodological Considerations." *Journal of Educational Evaluation for Health Professions* 10 (2013). doi: 10.3352/jeehp.2013.10.12.

Velayati, Ali Akbar, Parissa Farnia, and Mohammad Reza Masjedi. "The Totally Drug-Resistant Tuberculosis (TDR–TB)." *International Journal of Clinical and Experimental Medicine* 6, no. 4 (2013): 307–9.

Vigneswaran, Wickii T., and Sai S. Ramasastry. "Paraffin Plombage of the Chest Revisited." *Annals of Thoracic Surgery* 62, no. 6 (1996): 1837–9.

Vijayakumar, M., P. Bhaskaram, and P. Hemalatha. "Malnutrition and Childhood Tuberculosis." *Journal of Tropical Pediatrics* 36, no. 6 (1990): 294–8.

von Pirquet, Clemens. "Das Verhalten der Kutanen Tuberkulinreaktion Während der Masern." *Deutsche Medizinische Wochenschrift* 34, no. 30 (1908): 1297–1300.

Wagner-Jauregg, Julius. "Nobel Lecture: The Treatment of Dementia Paralytica by Malaria Inoculation." Nobelprize.org, 1927. www.nobelprize.org nobel_prizes/medicine/laureates/1927/wagner-jauregg-lecture.html.

Waksman, Selman A. "Award Ceremony Speech: Nobel Prize in Physiology or Medicine." Nobelprize.org, 1952. http://nobelprize.org/nobel_prizes/medicine/laureates/1952/press.html.

Waldram, James B., D. Ann Herring, and T. Kue Young. *Aboriginal Health in Canada: Historical, Cultural, and Epidemiological Perspectives.* 2nd ed. Toronto: University of Toronto Press, 2006.

Walsh, Joseph. "Pulmonary Activity Greatest at the Apex and Least at the Base." *American Review of Tuberculosis* 14, no. 2 (1926): 142–63.

Warner, John Harley. "From Specificity to Universalism in Medical Therapeutics: Transformation in the 19th-Century United States." In *Sickness and Health in America: Readings in the History of Medicine and Public Health.* 3rd ed., rev., edited by Judith Walzer Leavitt and Ronald L. Numbers, 87–101. Madison: University of Wisconsin Press, 1997.

– "The Uses of Patient Records by Historians: Patterns, Possibilities, and Perplexities." *Health and History* 1, nos 2/3 (1999): 101–11.

Warren, Peter. "The Evolution of the Sanatorium: The First Half-Century, 1854–1904." *Canadian Bulletin of Medical History* 23, no. 2 (2006): 457–76.

Warsh, Cheryl Krasnick, and Penny Tinkler. "In Vogue: North American and British Representations of Women Smokers in *Vogue*, 1920s–1960s." *Canadian Bulletin of Medical History* 24, no. 1 (2007): 9–47.

Waterhouse, Herbert F. "An Address on Professor Bier's Treatment by Means of Induced Hyperaemia." *British Medical Journal* 2, no. 2481 (1908): 125–9.

Weinberg, Eugene. "Iron and Susceptibility to Infectious Disease." *Science* 184, no. 4140 (1974): 952–6.

Weiss, Guenter, and Lawrence T. Goodnough. "Anemia of Chronic Disease." *New England Journal of Medicine* 352, no. 10 (2005): 1011–23.

Wejse, Christian. "Tuberculosis and Vitamin D: What Is the Evidence for Interaction?" *European Infectious Disease* 2, no. 1 (2008): 107–10.

Wells, William Firth. "On Airborne Infection, Study II. Droplets and Droplet Nuclei." *American Journal of Hygiene* 20 (1934): 611–18.

Wherrett, George Jasper. *The Miracle of the Empty Beds: A History of Tuberculosis in Canada.* Toronto: University of Toronto Press, 1977.

Whitman, Royal. "The Development of Orthopaedic Surgery: A Critical Estimate of the Influence of Three Pioneers – Lewis A. Sayre, Hugh Owen Thomas, and James Knight." *Journal of Bone and Joint Surgery* 26, no. 2 (1944): 408–10.

Whyte, M.B. "How Can Cross-Infection Be Prevented in a Hospital for Communicable Disease." *Canadian Journal of Public Health* 4 (August 1913): 452–4.

Wilkinson, Maude. "Four Score and Ten." *Canadian Nurse* 73, no. 12 (1977): 16–23.

Williams, C. Theodore. "Oration on the Sanatorium Treatment of Pulmonary Tuberculosis." *Lancet* 1 (30 January) (1904): 278–81.

Williams, J. Ivan, Eileen N. Healey, and Christina Gow. "The Death Throes of Tradition: Change in a Tuberculosis Sanatorium." *Social Science and Medicine* 5, no. 6 (1971): 545–59.

Wilson, H. Augustus. "Treatment of Tuberculous Hip Disease by Weight-Bearing and Fixation by the Lorenz Short Hip Spica." *Southern Medical Journal* 2, no. 1 (1909): 440–44.

Winnett, Frederick. "Bier's Hyperemic Treatment, with Demonstration of Technique." *Canadian Journal of Medicine and Surgery* 23, no. 6 (1908): 330–4.

Winslow, E.J. "Initiation." *Sanitarium Sun* 3, no. 12 (1932): 20.

Winters, A., T.B. Agerton, C.R. Driver, L. Teu, T. O'Flaherty, and S.S. Munsiff. "Congenital Tuberculosis and Management of Exposure in Three Neonatal Intensive Care Units." *International Journal of Tuberculosis and Lung Disease* 14, no. 12 (2010): 1641–3.

Wise, A.T. Tucker. "The Treatment of Pulmonary Tuberculosis by a Postural Method, Encouraging Drainage of the Lung and Inducing Artificial Hyperaemia of the Apex." *Lancet* 171, no. 4422 (1908): 1546–47.

Wolf, George. "The Discovery of Vitamin D: The Contribution of Adolf Windaus." *Journal of Nutrition* 134, no. 6 (2004): 1299–1302.

Woloshyn, Tania Anne. "Our Friend, the Sun: Images of Light Therapeutics from the Osler Library Collection, c. 1901–1944." Osler Library of the History of Medicine, McGill University Exhibition, 2011. www.mcgill.ca/files/_nea/170546_ourfriendsun.pdf.

Wood, G.W., and J.A. Scott. "A Case of Pulmonary and Meningeal Tuberculosis." *Canadian Medical Association Journal* 59, no. 1 (1948): 67–70.

Wood, Jeanette. "Bowlby's Children: The Forgotten Revolution in Australian Children's Nursing." *Contemporary Nurse* 30, no. 2 (2008): 119–32.

Wood, W. Burton. "Phthisis in Adolescence and Early Adult Life." *British Medical Journal* 1, no. 3768 (1933): 509–12.

World Health Organization. "The End TB Strategy." www.who.int/tb/strategy/en.

Yin, Robert K. *Case Study Research: Design and Methods*. 5th ed. Los Angeles: Sage Publications, 2014.

Young, Judith. "A Divine Mission: Elizabeth McMaster and the Hospital for Sick Children, Toronto, 1875–92." *Canadian Bulletin of Medical History* 11, no.1 (1994): 71–90.

– "'Little Sufferers.' Sick Children in Late-Nineteenth-Century Toronto." *Nursing History Review* 3 (1995): 129–42.

Zampini, Jay M., and Henry H. Sherk. "Lewis A. Sayre: The First Professor of Orthopaedic Surgery in America." *Clinical Orthopedics and Related Research* 466, no. 9 (2008): 2263–7.

Zhang, Xiaolan, and Brad H. Rovin. "Beyond Anemia: Hepcidin, Monocytes and Inflammation." *Biological Chemistry* 394, no. 2 (2013): 231–8.

Zoneraich, Samuel. "The Legacy of William Dock: A Giant of American Cardiology." *Clinical Cardiology* 17, no. 2 (1994): 95–7.

Zychowicz, Michael E. "Osteoarticular Manifestations of *Mycobacterium tuberculosis* Infection." *Orthopaedic Nursing* 29, no. 6 (2010): 400–6.

Index